MALIGNANT LYMPHOPROLIFERATIVE DISEASES

BOERHAAVE SERIES
FOR POSTGRADUATE
MEDICAL EDUCATION
Vol. 17

PROCEEDINGS OF A BOERHAAVE COURSE
organized by
THE FACULTY OF MEDICINE,
UNIVERSITY OF LEIDEN
and co-sponsored by
UNIVERSITY OF SOUTHERN CALIFORNIA
SCHOOL OF MEDICINE,
LOS ANGELES

MALIGNANT LYMPHOPROLIFERATIVE DISEASES

edited by

J.G. VAN DEN TWEEL

Department of Pathology, De Wever Hospital, Heerlen

in collaboration with

C.R. TAYLOR

Department of Pathology, University of Southern California, Los Angeles

F.T. BOSMAN

Department of Pathology, Leiden University, Leiden

1980
LEIDEN UNIVERSITY PRESS
THE HAGUE/BOSTON/LONDON

Distributors:

for the United States and Canada

Kluwer Boston, Inc.
190 Old Derby Street
Hingham, MA 02043
USA

for all other countries

Kluwer Academic Publishers Group
Distribution Center
P.O. Box 322
3300 AH Dordrecht
The Netherlands

ISBN 90-6021-451-X (this volume)
ISBN 90-6021-455-2 (series)

Cover design: Paul Burg

PRINTED IN THE NETHERLANDS

CONTENTS

Contributors   ix

Introduction   xiii

I. BASIC CONCEPTS AND METHODOLOGY IN LYMPHOMA CLASSIFICATION

1. Histophysiology of normal lymphoid tissue and immune
   reactions   3
   P. NIEUWENHUIS and K. LENNERT

2. Development and differentiation of the T-cell and B-cell
   systems: a perspective   13
   H. STEIN and G. TOLKSDORF

3. B-cell differentiation and characterization   31
   P. BIBERFELD and K. NILSSON

4. T-cell differentiation and characterization   49
   E.J. HENSEN

5. Different reticulum cells of the lymph node: microecological.
   concept of lymphoid tissue organization   57
   H.K. MÜLLER-HERMELINK and E. KAISERLING

6. HLA studies in malignant lymphomas   71
   J.G. VAN DEN TWEEL

7. Regulatory properties of T lymphocytes: implications for
   studies on malignant lymphoid cells   77
   R.E. BALLIEUX

8. Immunological approach to lymphoid neoplasms   85
   J.W. PARKER

9. Immunoperoxidase techniques in lymphoma research 111
    C.R. TAYLOR

10. Immunofluorescence methods 133
    W. HIJMANS

11. Cytochemical methods 137
    E.-W. SCHWARZE

12. Electron microscopy in the study of human lymphomas 149
    J.W. PARKER

13. Changing concepts in the classification of lymphoma 175
    C.R. TAYLOR

                          II. B-CELL LYMPHOMAS

14. The functional approach to the pathology of malignant
    lymphomas 187
    R.J. LUKES

15. Germinal center cell lymphomas and the Kiel classification . . . 213
    K. LENNERT

16. Malignant lymphomas of germinal center cell origin: preval-
    ence, type of presentation, stages and survival (preliminary
    data) 221
    F. RILKE, R. CANETTA, and M.R. CASTELLANI

17. Immunoglobulin expression in B-cell leukemias and B-cell
    lymphomas 229
    B. CHRISTENSSON, G. BIBERFELD, and P. BIBERFELD

18. Lymphoplasmacytic/lymphoplasmacytoid lymphoma (LP
    immunocytoma) (modified abstract) 245
    K. LENNERT and M. BURKERT

19. Lymphoproliferative diseases and monoclonal gammopathy . . 249
    D.Y. MASON

20. Immunoblastic lymphoma arising in angioimmunoblastic
    lymphadenopathy 273

B.N. Nathwani, H. Rappaport, G. Pangalis, E.M. Moran,
and H. Kim

21. Interrelations of B-cell neoplasms 281
C.R. Taylor

22. Clinical manifestations, staging, and management of the
non-Hodgkin's lymphomas: an overview 295
S.A. Rosenberg

III. T-CELL LYMPHOMAS

23. T-cell derived neoplasms: an overview 305
J.C. van den Tweel

24. T-cell neoplasia in the perspective of normal T-cell differentiation 315
H. Stein, G. Tolksdorf, and K. Lennert

25. Clinical manifestations of T-cell lymphomas 331
A.M. Levine

26. Cutaneous T-cell lymphoma: morphological and immuno-
logical aspects 341
C.J.L.M. Meijer, E.M. van der Loo, W.A. van Vloten,
C.J. Cornelisse, and E. Scheffer

27. Cutaneous T-cell lymphomas: clinical aspects 355
W.A. van Vloten and L. Hamminga

28. Systemic manifestations of mycosis fungoides 369
H. Rappaport

29. Early involvement of lymph nodes in mycosis fungoides 373
E. Scheffer and C.J.L.M. Meijer

IV. HODGKIN'S DISEASE

30. Natural history of Hodgkin's disease in relation to non-
Hodgkin's lymphoma 389
H. Kim

31. Immunopathology of Hodgkin's disease 399
   C.R. TAYLOR

32. The results of the treatment of Hodgkin's disease:
   an overview of current approaches and future directions . . . 417
   S.A. ROSENBERG

V. SPECIAL TOPICS

33. Epithelioid cellular lymphogranulomatosis (lymphoepithelioid cell lymphoma): histologic and clinical observa-
   tions 433
   H. NOEL, D. HELBRON, and K. LENNERT

34. The pathology of childhood lymphomas 447
   H. KIM

35. Extranodal lymphomas 459
   H. KIM

36. Hairy-cell leukemia 469
   J. JANSEN, H.R.E. SCHUIT, C.J.L.M. MEIJER, and W. HIJMANS

37. The prognostic relevance of leukemic cell typing in acute
   lymphoblastic leukemia 481
   R. WILLEMZE

38. The significance of fine-needle aspiration cytology for the
   diagnosis and treatment of malignant lymphomas 489
   P. LOPES CARDOZO

Index 503

CONTRIBUTORS

Ballieux, R.E., Department of (Clinical) Immunology, Utrecht University Hospital, Catharijnesingel 101, 3511 GV Utrecht, The Netherlands (and Wilhelmina Kinderziekenh).

Biberfeld, Gunner, The National Bacteriological, Laboratory, Stockholm, Sweden.

Biberfeld, P., Department of Pathology, Karolinska Institute, Stockholm, Sweden.

Burkert, M., Institute of Pathology, Hospitalstrasse 42, 2300 Kiel, Bundesrepublik Deutschland.

Canetta, Renzo, Istituto Nazionale per lo Studio, e la Cura dei Tumori, Milan, Italy.

Castellani, Maria Rita, Istituto Nazionale per lo Studio, e la Cura dei Tumori, Milan, Italy.

Christensson, B., Department of Pathology, Karolinska Institute, Stockholm, Sweden.

Cornelisse, C.J., Department of Pathology, Leiden University, Medical Center, Wassenaarseweg 62, 2333 AL Leiden, The Netherlands.

Hamminga, L., Leiden University Hospital, Department of Dermatology, Rijnsburgerweg 10, 2333 AA Leiden, The Netherlands.

Helbron, Dagmar, Institute of Pathology, Hospitalstrasse 42, 2300 Kiel Bundesrepublik Deutschland.

Hensen, E.J., Department of Immunohematology, Leiden University Hospital, Rijnsburgerweg 10, 233 AA Leiden, The Netherlands.

Hijmans, W., Department of Pathology, Leiden University Medical Center, Wassenaarseweg 62, 2333 AL Leiden, The Netherlands.

Jansen, J., Department of Hematology, Leiden University Medical Center, Rijnsburgerweg 10, 2333 AA Leiden, The Netherlands.

Kaiserling, E., Institute for Pathology, Hospitalstrasse 42, 2330 Kiel, Bundesrepublik Deutschland.

Kim, Hun, Department of Anatomic Pathology, City of Hope National Medical Center, Duarte, CA 91010, U.S.A.

Lennert, K., Institute for Pathology, Hospitalstrasse 42, 2300 Kiel, Bundesrepublik Deutschland

Levine, Alexandra, M., Department of Hematology, Los Angeles County Hospital, Los Angeles, CA 90033, U.S.A.

Loo, E.M. van der, Department of Pathology, Leiden University Medical Center, Wassenaarseweg 62, 2333 AL Leiden, The Netherlands.

Lopes Cardozo, P., Department of Hematomorphology and Clinical Cytology, Leiden University Hospital, Rijnsburgerweg 10, 2333 AA Leiden, The Netherlands.

Lukes, Robert J., Department of Pathology, University of Southern California, School of Medicine, Los Angeles, CA, U.S.A.

Mason, D.Y., Department of Pathology, University of Oxford, John Radcliffe Infirmary, Oxford, United Kingdom.

Meijer, C.J.L.M., Department of Pathology, Leiden University Medical Center, Wassenaarseweg 62, 2333 AL Leiden, The Netherlands.

Müller-Hermelink, E.K., Institute for Pathology, Hospitalstrasse 42, 2300 Kiel, Bundesrepublik Deutschland.

Nathwani, Bharat N., Department of Anatomic Pathology, City of Hope National Medical Center, Duarte, CA 91010, U.S.A.

Nieuwenhuis, P., Department of Histology, Groningen University, Oostersingel 69/1, 9713 EZ Groningen, The Netherlands.

Nilsson, K., The Wallenberg Laboratory, University of Uppsala, Uppsala, Sweden.

Noel, H., Service d'Anatomie Pathologique, Clinique Universitaire Saint-Luc, Avenue Hippocrate 10, Bruxelles, Belgique.

Pangalis, Gerassimos, University of Athens School of Medicine, 1st Department of Internal Medicine, Hospital "Vassilevs Pavlos", Athens 609, Greece.

Parker, John W., Department of Pathology, University of Southern California, School of Medicine, Los Angeles, CA, U.S.A.

Rappaport, Henry, Department of Anatomic Pathology, City of Hope National Medical Center, Duarte, CA 91010, U.S.A.

Rilke, Franko, Istituto Nazionale per lo Studio e la Cura dei Tumori, Milan, Italy.

Rosenberg, Saul A., Divisions of Oncology and Radiotherapy, Departments of Medicine and Radiology Stanford University School of Medicine, Stanford, CA 94305, U.S.A.

Scheffer, E., Leiden University Medical Center, Department of Pathology, Wassenaarseweg 62, 2333 AL Leiden, The Netherlands.

Schuit, H.R.E., Leiden University Medical Center, Department of Pathology, Wassenaarseweg 62, 2333 AL Leiden, The Netherlands.

Schwarze, E.-W., Institute for Pathology, Hospitalstrasse 42, 2300 Kiel, Bundesrepublik Deutschland.

Stein, H., Institute for Pathology, Hospitalstrasse 42, 2300 Kiel, Bundesrepublik Deutschland.

Taylor, Clive R., Department of Pathology, University of Southern California, School of Medicine, Los Angeles, CA, U.S.A.

Tolksdorf, G., Institute for Pathology, Hospitalstrasse 42, 2300 Kiel, Bundesrepublik Deutschland.

Tweel, J.G. van den, Department of Pathology, De Wever Hospital, Henri Dunantstraat, 6419 PB Heerlen, The Netherlands.

Vloten, W.A. van, Department of Dermatology, Leiden University Hospital, Rijnsburgerweg 10, 2333 AA Leiden, The Netherlands.

Willemze, R., Department of Hematology, Leiden University Medical Center, Rijnsburgerweg 10, 2333 AA Leiden, The Netherlands.

INTRODUCTION

During the last five years the histological classification of the non-Hodgkin lymphomas has become a complex subject. Even experienced pathologists and clinicians find it increasingly difficult to make their way through the extensive and often confusing literature. The confusion is mainly due to the fact that different "schools" use different starting points for their classification. Moreover, since many immunological problems related to classification have not been completely resolved yet, even researchers who use the same approach do not always arrive at the same classification scheme.

This book represents an attempt to find common elements in three most important classifications for non-Hodgkin lymphomas (the Rappaport classification, the Lukes-Collins classification and the Kiel classification) and to provide a scientific basis for the classification of this disease group. It therefore defines the two main groups of lymphocytes and their specific distribution pattern in the lymphoid organs and discusses the methods by which these cells and related tumors can be recognized. The various malignant B- and T-cell lymphomas are described in detail by expert authors, who deal not only with the morphological details, but also with the relevant clinical aspects. Finally, some related special topics are dealt with to complete the contents of this book.

SECTION I

BASIC CONCEPTS AND METHODOLOGY IN LYMPHOMA CLASSIFICATION

1. HISTOPHYSIOLOGY OF NORMAL LYMPHOID TISSUE AND IMMUNE REACTIONS

P. NIEUWENHUIS AND K. LENNERT

INTRODUCTION

Not so long ago (1) the lymphocyte was defined as:" . . . a somewhat incon-spicuous cell, with no particularly striking functional or morphological characteristics . . . . Comparing it with other cells, one thinks of the lym-phocyte in negative terms, defining it rather by the absence of characteristics which other white cells possess than by positive attributes of its own. Yet it has been for many years, and still is the cell around which a violent haema-tological controversy has been waged" (1). And, quoting Lewis (1933), they remark: "its fate . . . is the subject of religious beliefs."

Better knowledge about the normal cells of the lymphoid system would seem to be a prerequisite for a better understanding of malignant lympho-mas. The past two decades have certainly added to this knowledge, which has had great impact on both the diagnosis and the treatment of lymphoid tumours.

T and B lymphocytes

The first major achievement was the characterization of T and B cell sub-populations among lymphoid cells and their association with separate and distinct "central" lymphoid organs like the thymus (for T cells) and the Bursa of Fabricius (for B cells) (2, 3). After a period of hectic research to identify the Bursa equivalent in mammals, it became evident (4, 5) that in this species B cells are bone marrow derived. Chromosome marker studies (6) showed that T cells are likewise bone marrow derived but while passing through the thymus undergo an extra maturation step. Both types of cell are believed to derive originally from a common universal haemopoietic stem cell (see Figure 1). Differentiation pathways for T and B cells are described in more detail in the papers by Stein and Biberfelt (this volume).

In routine haematoxylin-eosin-stained sections T and B cells usually cannot be distinguished morphologically. It is, however, clear that, for instance, in the spleen and lymph nodes T and B cell areas can be recognized

J.G. van den Tweel et al. (eds.), Malignant Lymphoproliferative Diseases, 3–12
All rights reserved.
Copyright © 1980 by Martinus Nijhoff Publishers bv, The Hague/Boston/London.

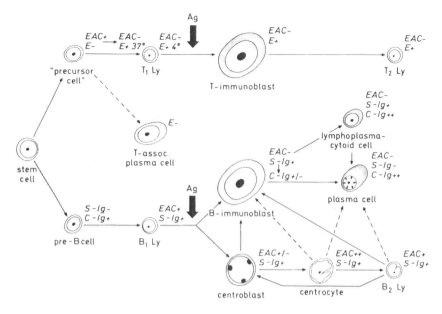

Figure 1. Simplified scheme of the T- and B-lymphocyte systems (from (7)).

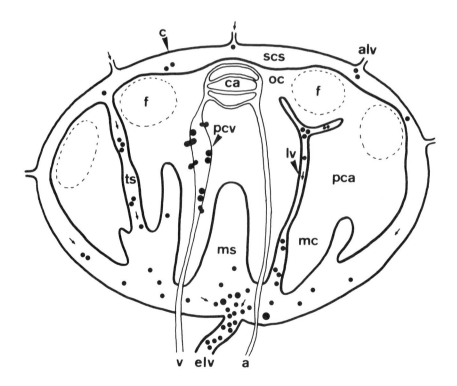

Figure 2. Schematic presentation of the lymph node. (Courtesy Dr. W. van Ewijk.)
c = capsule; alv = afferent lymph vessel; scs = subcapsular sinus; oc = outer cortex;
f = follicle; pca = paracortical area; mc = medullary cord; ts = trabecular sinus; ms =
medullary sinus; lv = lymph vessel; a = arteriole; ca = capillary plexus; pcv = postcapillary
venule; v = vene; elv = efferent lymph vessel. The arrows indicate the direction of lymph
flow. The black dots represent lymphoid cells.

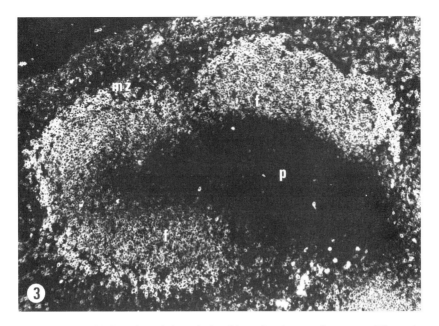

Figure 3. Frozen dried section of the splenic white pulp of a germfree mouse. The section was incubated with rabbit anti mouse —Ig and stained with fluorescent goat anti rabbit—Ig. Primary follicles (f) and marginal zone (mz) are positive, whereas the PALS (p) is negative (10 × oc., 10 × obj.). (Courtesy Dr. W. van Ewijk.)

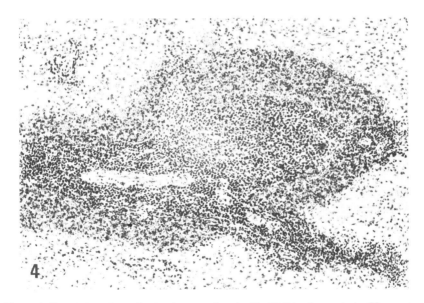

Figure 4. Cryostat section of rat spleen overlayed with EAC to demonstrate C3 receptor bearing B lymphocytes. Note EAC binding to cells in the lymphocyte corona and the marginal zone but not in the periarteriolar lymphocyte sheath (10 × oc., 10 × obj.).

(see Figures 2–5): in the spleen the periarteriolar lymphocyte sheath (T area) and the follicular structures (B area), and in lymph nodes the paracortical area (T area) and again follicular structures (B area).

When special staining techniques such as immunofluorescence and/or (immuno)-histiochemical procedures are used, individual T and B cells (and subsets) can be visualized. For instance, T suppressor cells show azurophil granules (visible in imprints only), whereas the other T lymphocytes (the helper cells definitely, and the cytotoxic cells possibly) show spotlike acid phosphatase and acid nonspecific esterase activity. B cells display the membrane enzymes 5-nucleotidase and adenosine triphosphatase, whereas T cells are negative for these enzymes (for illustrations see (7)). Figure 3 gives an example of the immunofluorescent staining results obtained when the fluorescent antiserum reacts with the surface immunoglobulin (sIg) of B-cells occurring in a follicular structure in the spleen. With the same method (using an anti-T-cell serum), individual T cells have been demonstrated, inside germinal centres (8).

For comparison, Figure 4 shows the results obtained when another membrane marker is used to identify B cells, viz., the C_3 receptor. When SRBC coated with IgM anti-SRBC and complement (EAC, erythrocyte-antibody-complement) are applied to cryostat sections, the EAC specifically react with and bind to the C_3 receptor present on B cells.

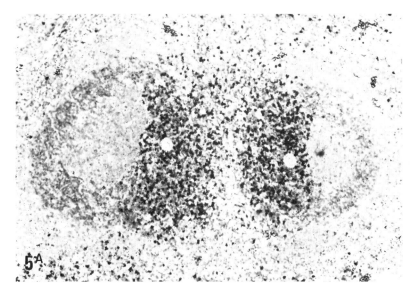

Figure 5a. Autoradiograph of rat spleen, 4 hours after the i.v. injection of ^{3}H-uridine labeled thoracic duct lymphocytes showing heavily labeled T-cells in the periarteriolar lymphocyte sheaths. Weakly labeled B cells are not distinguishable at this time and magnification (10× oc., 10× obj.).

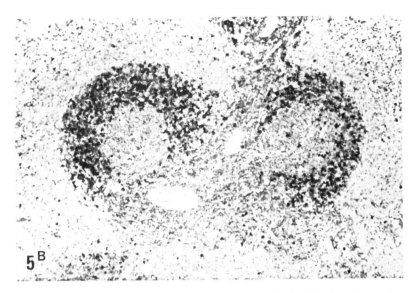

Figure 5b. Autoradiograph of rat spleen, 24 hours after the i.v. injection of complement receptor bearing thoracic duct (B-) lymphocytes, showing heavily labeled B cells in lymphocyte coronas of follicular structures (10× oc., 10× obj.).

T and B immunoblasts

T and B cells can also occur in another form, i.e., as immunoblasts (see Figure 1). T and B immunoblasts too cannot be distinguished with simple light microscopy. Both appear as large pyroninophilic cells when staining with menthylgreen-pyronin. However, in the electron microscope T immunoblasts show numerous polyribosomes in their cytoplasm, whereas B immunoblasts have ribosomes attached to the endoplasmic reticulum (rough endoplasmic reticulum), which indicates the protein (= antibody) synthesizing and secreting nature of these cells (9). Nevertheless, even with the light microscope a calculated speculation can be made as to the nature of an immunoblast when the actual location (e.g., at the border of a follicular structure or in the periarteriolar lymphocyte sheath or paracortex for B and T immunoblasts, respectively) is taken into consideration. This consideration is based on studies concerning the various types of immune responses that can occur after antigenic stimulation (9).

Nonlymphoid cells in lymphoid tissues

Lymphoid tissues contain not only lymphocytes but various other cell types constituting the basic framework as well. Essentially, the infrastructure is provided by (fiber-associated) reticulum cells. Among these cells other nonlymphoid cells have been identified, viz., the dendritic reticulum cells present in the follicles and the interdigitating cells in the T-dependent areas (periarteriolar lymphocyte sheath, paracortex) (10); (see also the chapter by Müller-Hermelink in this volume). Of these two cell types the dendritic reticulum cell (DRC) is considered to be a special manifestation form of the reticulum cell having numerous cytoplasmic dendrites extending between neighboring lymphoid cells. The DRC is thought to be nonphagocytic and presumably has a function in antigen presentation to B cells. The inter-digitating cell (IDC) has been postulated to be part of the mononuclear-phagocyte system and perhaps instrumental in antigen presentation to T cells (see also (11)).

Recirculating lymphocytes

From the above description one might gain a rather static picture of lymphoid tissues. That the oppositie is the case has been shown by the work of Gowans, Ford et al. (for a review, see (12)), who found that lymphocytes recirculate continuously, leaving lymphoid tissues via efferent lymphatics and, after a short time in the circulation, leaving the blood again by way of specialized vascular structures (high endothelial venules, HEVs) in, e.g., lymph nodes and Peijer's patches or in the marginal sinus bordering follicular structures in the spleen. The transit time through a lymph node has been roughly calculated to be of the order of 5–6 hr for T cells and > 24 hr for B cells (12). Once inside a node or in the spleen, T and B cells follow different routes to "home" in their respective T and B areas. Figure 5 gives examples of the respective localization patterns for T and B cells in the spleen as observed 4 or 24 hr, respectively after i.v. injection. Apparently the sorting out of T and B lymphocytes occurs after they have entered the lymphoid organ.

It has been suggested that the common pathway followed initially by both T and B cells upon entry might be functional in T–B collaboration in the initiation of an immune response. Obviously, this continuous re-circulation of lymphocytes from blood to lymph via lymphoid tissues and reentry into the bloodstream would contribute greatly to the postulated "immune surveillance" function of lymphocytes, the recirculation leading to continuous redistribution of available lymphoid cells of all specificities all over the organism.

Immune reactions

That lymphocytes are not end cells but can transform into what has be-come known as immunoblasts was first shown unequivocally by Gowans (13) in 1962. After the i.v. injection of parental thoracic-dust lymphocytes into an F_1 recipient, some of the inoculated cells transformed into large pyroninophilic cells in the recipient's spleen. Transformation of lympho- cytes into large pyroninophilic cells has since been recognized to be the first step in the various types of immune reactions to all kinds of antigenic stimuli.

The type of blast cell originating from a B cell may be morphologically indistinguishable (at least with the light microscope) from its T cell coun- terpart, but its functional commitment is quite different, because eventually these B immunoblasts (plasmablasts) will differentiate into plasma cells, unlike T immunoblasts, which will eventually end up as small but specifi- cally sensitized lymphocytes (effector cells, memory cells) (see Figure 1). For a more detailed description of the above-mentioned immune reactions, see the paper by Stein in this volume.

Germinal center reaction

Besides the above-described two types of immune reactions (the plasma cell reaction and the specific lymphocyte reaction, leading to humoral and cellular immunity, respectively) a third type of immune reaction occurs inside the central part of follicular structures after antigenic stimulation, i.e., the accumulation of large pyroninophilic cells from which a germinal center develops. These large pyroninophilic cells were formerly called lymphoblasts, because it was assumed on the basis of the numerous mitotic figures among these cells, that germinal centers were sites of lymphocyte production (Flemming's *Keimzentren*). Later experiments (14, 15) have shown this to be the case. Recent nomenclature no longer uses the word lymphoblast but, in referring to its site of origin, gives preference to the term germinoblast or centroblast (see Figure 1).

In due course centroblasts will give rise—by cell division—to centrocytes which eventually, as small- or medium-sized lymphoid cells, will emigrate from the germinal center. The sequence small to large-cleaved to small- and large-noncleaved cells, proposed by Lukes (this volume) seems unlikely to us, because experimental evidence obtained in animal models does not support this view (15). Moreover, the small- and large-cleaved cells cannot be identified in germinal centers in various rodents.

Lymphocyte production by germinal centers is essentially an antigen- dependent process, in contrast to lymphocyte production in the thymus and bone marrow. Germ-free animals lack germinal centers, but both T and B cell populations are present in presumably normal quantities and qualities. After the appearance, some 3–4 days after antigenic stimulation, of large pyroninophilic cells centrally inside a follicular structure (see Figure 6), mitotic figures appear, and are soon followed (by day 5) by "tingible bodies" macrophages which give rise to the characteristic "starry-sky" appearance

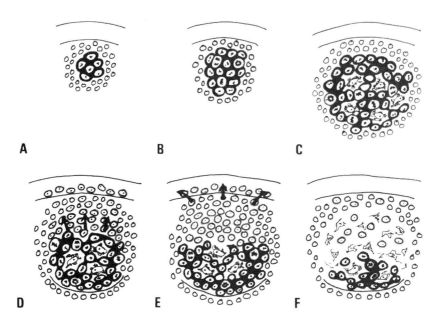

Figure 6. Schematic representation of a germinal center reaction as seen in a rabbit popliteal lymph node following subcutaneous injection of Salm. Java paratyphoid vaccine (times indicated are approximate).
A. 3 days after injection. Appearance of large pyroninophilic cells in the central part of a primary follicle.
B. 4 days. First appearance of mitotic figures.
C. 5 days. First appearance of "tingible bodies" macrophages.
D. 7 days. Beginning differentiation (arrows): centroblasts giving rise to centrocytes which subsequently will traverse the lymphocyte corona towards the marginal sinus.
E. 14–21 days. Steady state production: newly formed centrocytes are exported from the follicle (arrows) to leave the node by way of the efferent lymphatics.
F. 28 days. Residual germinal center activity in a secondary nodule.

of this stage of germinal center development. Possible clues to the significance of these tingible-body macrophages are still lacking. By the 7th day, newly centroblast-derived medium-sized lymphoid cells, or centrocytes, appear above the area containing centroblasts. From there, germinal center-derived lymphoid cells traverse the lymphocyte corona to reach the marginal zone. Via the efferent lymph—or in the spleen, directly—these cells may enter the circulation to become distributed over other peripheral lymphoid tissues where they home to the lymphocyte corona of the follicular structures (15). Depending upon the strength of the antigenic stimulus, this stage of lymphocyte production takes about 2–4 weeks, after which mitotic activity subsides and only some residual activity is seen at the base of the follicle (densely populated area) separated by a now almost empty lighter (or thinly populated) area from the lymphocyte corona, thus leaving a typical secondary nodule.

Continuous antigenic stimulation leads to a continuing germinal center reaction, as indicated by the proliferative activity in germinal centers in Peijer's patches and the appendix.

Germinal centers and B-cell differentiation

Some of the germinal center-generated lymphocytes are specifically sensitized to the inducing antigen and serve as memory B-cells for that particular antigen (14). However, experiments on the functional capacities of lymphocytes produced by appendix germinal centers in the rabbit have provided evidence pointing to a nonspecific proliferation of B lymphocytes unrelated to the specificity of the germinal center inducing antigen (16). Thus, besides the production of specific memory B-cells, germinal centers were found to be a source of virginal primary antibody-forming cell precursors (AFCP). These germinal center-derived B lymphocytes were then called B_2 cells. It is an open question how the cell from which a germinal center originates (i.e., the germinal center precursor cell, GCPC), is related to the known stages of B-cell differentiation. Originally, it was assumed that GCPC were directly bone marrow derived and, to distinguish these cells from the germinal center-derived lymphocytes (B_2 cells), they were called B_1 cells. From bone marrow reconstitution experiments (17) it is clear that like other B cells, GCPC indeed originally arise in the bone marrow. However, the characteristics of the immediate germinal center precursor cell are not known.

The question now arises as to what determines the sequence of events happening when a B cell meets antigen. Two possible types of reaction have been described, viz., the plasma cell reaction and the germinal-center reaction, each with its own location, kinetics, and outcome and a choice between them seems difficult. Theoretically, there are at least two possibilities:

1) the GCPC is identical to a primary (or secondary) AFCP, in which case the direction of the reaction must be regulated by extraneous (non-B-cell) factors such as (i) different T cell regulatory influence (help vs. suppression?), (ii) the way in which antigen is presented to either T or B cell, or (iii) unknown micro-environmental factors; or
2) GCPC differ from primary AFCP, in a way resulting in a different reaction pattern.

Perhaps GCPC are relatively immature B-cells and thereby prohibited from terminal differentiation into plasma cells upon antigenic contact. GCPC thus might constitute a hitherto unknown subpopulation of B cells. When the functional capacities of the B_1 cell, as shown in Figure 1, are considered, the above observations should be taken into account.

REFERENCES

1. Yoffey, F.M., and Courtice, F.C.: Lymphatics, lymph and lymphoid tissue. Edward Arnold, London, 1956.
2. Warner, N.L., and Szenberg, A.: Effect of neonatal thymectomy in the chicken. Nature, 196:784 1962.
3. Cooper, M.D., Peterson, R.D.A., and Good, R.A.: Delineation of the thymic and bursal lymphoid systems in the chicken. Nature, 205:143, 1965.
4. Mitchell, G.F., and Miller, J.F.A.P.: Cell to cell interaction in the immune response. II. The source of hemolysin forming cells in irradiated mice given bone-marrow and thymus or thoracic duct lymphocytes. J. Exp. Med., 128:821, 1968.
5. Osmond, D.G.: Potentials of bone marrow lymphocytes. In: Stem cells of renewing cell populations, Cairnie, A.B., Lala, P.K., and Osmond, D.G., (eds.), p. 195, 1976.
6. Ford, C.E.: Traffic of lymphoid cells in the body. In: The thymus. Experimental and Clinical Studies Ciba Foundation Symp., p. 131, 1966.
7. Lennert, K., Stein, H., Mohri, U., Kaiserling, E., and Müller-Hermelink, H.K.: In: Malignant lymphomas other than Hodgkin's Disease. Springer Verlag, New York, Heidelberg, Berlin, 1978.
8. Gutman, G.A., and Weisman, I.L.: Lymphoid tissue architecture. Experimental analysis of the origin and distribution of T and B cells. Immunology, 23:465, 1972.
9. Veldman, J.E., Keuning, F.J., and Molenaar, I.: Site of initiation of the plasma cell reaction in the rabbit lymph node. Virchows Arch. B Cell Path., 28:187, 1978.
10. Veldman, J.E., Molenaar, I., and Keuning, F.J., Electron microscopy of cellular immunity in B-cell deprived rabbits. Virchows Arch. B Cell Path., 28:217, 1978.
11. Hoefsmit, E.C.M., Kamperdijk, E.W.A., and Balfour, B.M.: Reticulum cells and macrophages in the immune response. In: Mononuclear phagocytes: functional aspects. Furth, R.v., (ed.), Martinus Nijhoff, The Hague, in press.
12. Ford, W.L.: Lymphocyte migration and immune responses. Progr. Allergy, 19:1, 1975.
13. Gowans, J.L.: The fate of parental strain lymphocytes in F_1 hybrid rats. Ann. N.Y. Acad. Sci., 99:335, 1962.
14. Thorbecke, G.J., Romano, T.J., and Lerman, S.P.: Regulatory mechanisms in proliferation and differentiation of lymphoid tissue, with particular reference to germinal centre development. In: Progress in immunology II, vol. 3, p. 25, Brent, L., and Holborow, J., (eds.), North Holland, Amsterdam, 1974.
15. Nieuwenhuis, P., and Keuning, F.J.: Germinal Centres and the origin of the B-cell system. II: Germinal centres in the rabbit spleen and lymph nodes. Immunology, 26:509, 1974.
16. Nieuwenhuis, P., van Nouhuys, C.E., Eggens, J.H., and Keuning, F.J.: Germinal centres and the origin of the B-cell system I: Germinal centres in the rabbit appendix. Immunology, 26:497, 1974.
17. Rozing, J., Brons, N.H.C., van Ewijk, W., and Benner, R.: B lymphocyte differentiation in lethally irradiated and reconstituted mice. IV. A histological study using immunofluorescent detection of B lymphocytes. Cell. Tiss. Res., 189:19, 1978.

2. DEVELOPMENT AND DIFFERENTIATION OF THE T-CELL AND B-CELL SYSTEMS: A PERSPECTIVE

H. STEIN AND G. TOLKSDORF

INTRODUCTION

The past decade has brought substantial progress in the understanding, the development and differentiation of the T- and B-cell systems. The present paper attempts to give a survey of this topic, with special reference to the various maturation and differentiation forms of the T-cell and B-cell axes and their immunologic, enzyme-cytochemical, and cytologic features.

THE PLURIPOTENT STEM CELL

There is ample evidence supporting the concept that the lymphoid B-cell and T-cell lineages outlined in Figure 1 and the myelopoietic lineage are derived from a common progenitor, called the pluripotent stem cell. This concept is mainly based on data obtained from functional studies and from the investigation of neoplasms of lymphoid and myeloid cells.

The neoplastic equivalent of the pluripotent stem cell is thought by some authors (25, 26) to be the so-called common acute lymphoblastic leukemia (ALL) cell, which lacks all of the specific properties of lymphoid or myeloid cells. Instead, the common ALL cell displays not only the common ALL antigen (CALLA) (20) which a glycoprotein with a molecular weight of 100,000 to 125,000 daltons (27, 28, 50) but also an intracytoplasmic human thymus/leukemia-associated antigen (HTHY-L) (11) Ia-like antigens (15, 56) receptors for polyarcrylic acid beads (PAAB) (24) and terminal deoxynucleotidyl transferase (TdT) (33). A link between the common ALL cell and myeloid cells is documented by the presence of Ia-like antigen (15, 56) and receptors for PAAB on myeloid cells (24), and the presence of CALLA and TdT on lymphoid blast crisis cells of chronic myeloid leukemia (CML) (26). A connection between the common ALL cell and the B-cell system is indicated by the presence of Ia-like antigens and receptors for PAAB on B cells and by the observation that pre-B cells and pre-B-ALL cells and by the observation that pre-B cells and pre-B-ALL cells both contain cyto-

J.G. van den Tweel et al. (eds.), Malignant Lymphoproliferative Diseases, 13–29

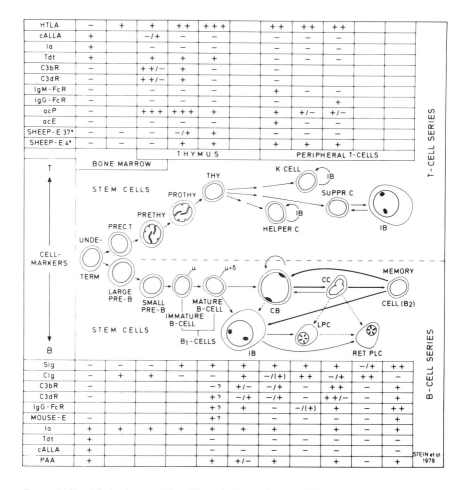

Figure 1. Simplified scheme of the differentiation pathways of the T-cell and B-cell systems, and their immunologic and cytochemical markers. HTLA = human T-lymphocyte antigen; cALLA = common ALL antigen (Greaves' antigen); Ia = Ia-like antigen; Tdt = terminal deoxynucleotidyl transferase; C3bR = receptor for C3b. C3dR = receptor for C3d; IgM-FcR = receptor for the Fc pieces of IgM; IgG-FcR = receptor for the Fc pieces of IgG; acP = acid phosphatase; acE = acid nonspecific esterase; SHEEP-E 37° = rosette formation with sheep erythrocytes at 37°C; SHEEP-E 4° = rosette formation with sheep erythrocytes at 37°C followed by incubation at 4°C for 1 hour; SIg = surface immunoglobulin; CIg = cytoplasmic immunoglobulin; MOUSE-E = rosette formation with mouse erythrocytes; PAA = binding of polyacrylic acid beads; UNDETERM. = undetermined stem cell; PREC.T = precursor T-cell; PRETHY. = prethymocyte; PROTHY. = prothymocyte; THY. = postnatal or mature thymocyte; K. Cell = killer T cell; IB = immunoblast; SUPPR.C. = suppressor T-cell; HELPER C. = helper T-cell; CB = centroblast; CC = centrocyte; LPC = lymphatic plasma cell; RET.PLC = reticular (Marschalkó type) plasma cell.

plasmic IgM and express CALLA (13, 19, 55). A link between the common ALL cell and the T-cell system is suggested by the presence of TdT and HTHY-L in thymocytes and the cells of the mature thymocytic type of ALL (11) and also by the presence of CALLA on the cells in 10% of the cases of the immature thymocytic type of ALL (44). The detection of a few CALLA⁺ cells in normal bone marrow (44), the demonstration of Ia-like antigen on colony-forming units of bone marrow cells (12), and the presence of TdT in normal thymocyte precursors (45) offer additional argument in favor of the concept that lymphoid and myeloid-determined stem cells are generated by the physiologic equivalent of the common ALL cell.

DEVELOPMENT OF T CELLS

Precursor T cells

In response to appropriate stimuli, lymphoid stem cells develop into precursor T cells. This has been experimentally confirmed by the finding that murine bone marrow "null" cells (lymphoid cells devoid of B and T markers) give rise to cells expressing specific T-cell surface antigen in the course of a response to phytohemagglutinin (PHA) (40). In vivo, the production of precursor T cells probably occurs first in the fetal liver and later in the bone marrow. Asma et al. (3) found cells that stained for human T-lymphocyte antigen (HTLA), but did not rosette with sheep erythrocytes (E), in fetal liver as early as 5½ weeks after the beginning of gestation. No information is available concerning the expression of other surface markers, including complement (C3) receptors, on precursor T cells.

Maturation of thymocytes

Precursor T cells enter the thymus anlage during the ninth or tenth week of gestation, apparently under the influence of epithelial cells of the thymus anlage, which might be capable of recognizing precursor T cells (57). On the basis of studies by Gatien et al. (18) and our own investigations (46), we conclude that the first thymocytes recognizable in the thymus bear C3 receptors, lack sheep E receptors, and show strong focal acid phosphatase activity. We called these cells prethymocytes (48).

Double labeling experiments have revealed that prethmocytes mature into cells that express sheep E receptors in addition to C3 receptors. We called these cells prothymocytes. Recent studies have shown that the C3 receptors present on pre- and prothymocytes have an affinity for both sub-types (C3b and C3d) (48).

Before birth, all prothymocytes develop into mature thymocytes, which are characterized by the absence of C3 receptors, the presence of sheep E receptors that are capable of binding 37°C, and large amounts of HTLA (48).

Prethymocytes display strong focal acid phosphatase activity and com-pletely negative staining with acid nonspecific esterase. This reaction pattern is typical of all maturation forms of thymocytes, with the exception of a small proportion made up of medium-sized mature thymocytes, which show a dotlike acid nonspecific esterase reaction product.

Peripheral T cells

As mentioned above, all maturation forms of the thymocyte contain large amounts of TdT. After emigration from the thymus, the cells of the T axis are called T cells. T cells differ from thymocytes by their lack of TdT (10, 33), the instability of their sheep E receptors at 37°C (34), and their smaller amount of HTLA (51). At present, we still do not know when and where the differentiation of specialized T cells, such a cytotoxic T cells, suppressor T cells, helper T cells and activator cells takes place. It has become clear, however, that specialized T cells, such as helper T cells and suppressor T cells, are not cells that acquire their special functional capacity directly in response to appropriate signals. It has now been proven that help and suppression are performed by two distinct subpopulations of T cells, each genetically programmed to carry out only one of these functions (6, 7, 36).

Recently, it became possible to identify the T-cell fractions that show helper or suppressor activity at the single-cell level. Helper T cells usually express receptors for IgM and contain dotlike acid nonspecific esterase activity. Suppressor T cells exhibit IgG-Fc receptors, are acid nonspecific esterase negative, and may contain azurophil granules (21, 36).

T immunoblasts

On the basis of studies on blast transformation curves and on acid non-specific esterase (31, 52) and glycoprotein patterns induced by different means (2), we conclude that each T-cell subset can regenerate itself via a blast-cell stage, the cell in this stage generally being called an immuno-blast. In other words, each lymphoid cell subset appears to have its own immunoblast. Accordingly, we define immunoblasts as lymphoid cells that are transformed for division and, in some instances, for differentiation. Thus, immunoblasts exhibit a uniform "blastic" morphology, but differ in origin and fate.

DEVELOPMENT OF B CELLS

Early events in B-cell differentiation

The development of the B-cell system is outlined in the lower part of Figure 1. Information about the early events in the differentiation pathway of the B-cell lineage is increasing. The first B cells that are recognizable in fetal life contain small amounts of μ chains in their cytoplasm ($C\mu$), but are devoid of μ chains at the cell surface and of light chains both in the cytoplasm and at the cell surface (13, 17, 42). The $C\mu^+$ and surface immunoglobulin (Ig)$^-$ negative cells are called pre-B cells.

Pre-B cells appear in the liver during the seventh week of gestation and later in the bone marrow. There are two types of pre-B cells, one large and the other small. Pulse-labeling experiments with ^{3}H-thymidine have shown that large pre-B cells from human fetal liver and also from adult bone marrow divide rapidly and give rise to small pre-B cells (17). Thus, large pre-B cells might be identical to the postulated B-determined stem cells. In mice and rabbits, large and small pre-B cells are found only in the liver and bone marrow; the fetal spleen, blood, and lymph nodes of these animals contain only small pre-B-cells. In humans after birth, the bone marrow appears to be the primary repository of pre-B cells (17).

Pre-B cells develop into surface IgM$^+$ and $C\mu^-$ immature B cells, which are detectable in the human fetus two weeks later than pre-B cells. The B cells that express exclusively surface IgM may be called immature B cells. These might give rise to different B-cell subsets, each devoted to the synthesis of a different Ig class. This path of development is not included in Figure 1.

Pre-B-cells and the surface IgM$^+$ immature B cells are highly susceptible to tolerance induction (35, 43). It appears that B-cell tolerance to self antigens is aquired at this level of B-cell development. The immature B cells apparently develop into mature B cells by the acquisition of surface IgD. With the appearance of surface IgD on the surface-IgM-bearing lymphocytes, the high susceptibility of the cells to induction of tolerance by antigen is lost (9, 54).

The antigenically unstimulated, surface Ig$^+$B cells have been called B_1 cells by some authors. Except for the certainty that B_1 cells bear surface Ig, there are merely assumptions as to the markers of this type of cell. It has been speculated that B_1 cells have the same surface markers as the cells of common chronic lymphocytic leukemia of the B type (B-CLL), namely, receptors for C3d but not for C3b, receptors for IgG, and receptors for mouse E.

Antigen-dependent differentiation of B cells

The B_1 cell can enter either of two distinct, antigen-dependent B-cell reactions, viz.: the germinal center reaction (GCR) or the plasma cell reaction (PCR), which are outlined in Figure 1. The GCR chiefly serves the proliferation of B cells, whereas the main function of the PCR is the production of antibody-secreting cells, i.e., plasma cells.

Germinal center reaction

We call the B cells generated by the GCR "B_2 cells". In a primary immune response B_1 cells, and in a secondary immune response B_2 cells are probably the starter cells of the GCR (30, 37, 39). Since adults have memory cells for most antigenix stimuli their GCR probably usually begins with B_2 cells.

It seems likely that when B_1 and B_2 cells are activated by antigenic stimulation, they migrate to the lymph-node cortex, where they accumulate in the form of primary follicles. Four days after antigenic stimulation (8, 53) and under the obligatory influence of immunoregulatory T cells (16, 23) the GCR starts with the appearance of centroblasts, often, although not always,

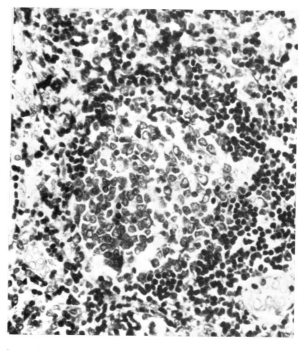

Figure 2. Fresh germinal center consisting of centroblasts and surrounded by a narrow rim of follicular mantle cells. Giemsa. × 350.

in the primary follicles. Figure 2 shows a fresh germinal center consisting of centroblasts, surrounded by a narrow rim of follicular mantle lymphocytes (FML). Centroblasts are morphologically well characterized cells (32). They are medium-sized or large and have a round or oval, pale nucleus containing two or three nucleoli usually located at the nuclear membrane. Cytoplasm is very sparse and intensely basophilic. Centroblasts divide actively.

After one week, large pale macrophages appear among the centroblasts, producing the so-called starry-sky pattern. After one to three more weeks, the centroblasts transform into centrocytes. This transformation begins in the lighter zone of the germinal center facing the marginal sinuses. It is easy to identify centrocytes by their morphology: they are small or medium-sized cells with a cleaved or irregularly shaped nucleus. Cytoplasm is usually sparse, weakly basophilic, and difficult to recognize in sections (Figure 3).

The usual fate of centrocytes appears to depend on the intensity and duration of the antigenic stimulation and its immunoregulation. The first possibility, which has not yet been proven, is that centrocytes retransform into centroblasts, which divide and thus multiply further. The usual fate of centrocytes, however, appears to be to leave the germinal center. In that

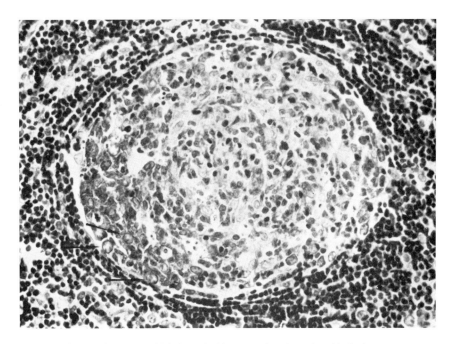

Figure 3. Germinal center, which is probably more than 3 weeks old. It shows two zones, namely, a darker and a lighter one. The darker zone abounds with centroblasts (arrows), whereas the lighter zone is made up of centrocytes. Giemsa. × 350.

case, their nuclei become small and round. These cells may circulate in the blood as B$_2$ memory cells, rejoin the GCR (39), or migrate to the submarginal areas of the same or other lymph nodes, where they give rise to cells of the PCR (37).

In sum, the cells of the GCR usually include three main types of lymphoid cell, namely, FML, centroblasts, and centrocytes.

Immunologic properties of the cells of the germinal center reaction

FML have a dense layer of surface Ig (Figure 4). Most of the cells in the germinal center show a much weaker surface staining, and some of them do not stain at all with the immunoperoxidase technique. It is, however difficult, to evaluate the surface Ig staining of germinal center cells (GCC) in sections because of the intercellular Ig network pattern (Figure 4). Staining of suspended cells prepared from hyperplastic tonsils established that a varying number of GCC are surface Ig$^+$.

Besides surface Ig, GCC may also have Ig in the cytoplasm. In non-neoplastic germinal centers, cytoplasmic Ig is mainly demonstrable in cells with the features of centrocytes, with some exceptions. This is evident in

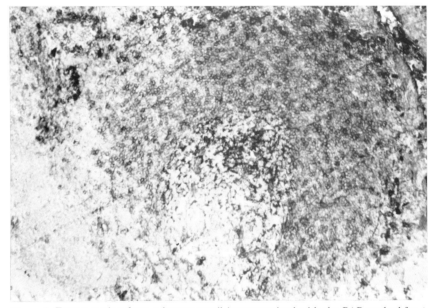

Figure 4. Frozen section from a human tonsil immunostained with the PAP method for λ chains. On the right, a germinal center is seen with a characteristic immunoglobulin network pattern. Only some of the germinal center cells are surface Ig$^+$. Follicular mantle cells are strongly positive for surface Ig. Intensely stained plasma cells are evident around the follicular mantle. The unstained area at the lower left is part of a T-dependent region. × 90.

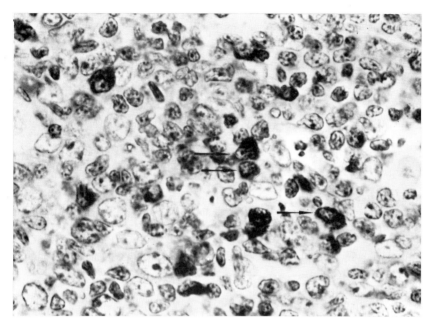

Figure 5. Part of a germinal center immunostained for cytoplasmic IgM. Note that some centrocytes (arrows), identifiable by their cleaved nuclei, are positively stained. × 800.

Figure 5, which shows a paraffin section stained for IgM. According to experimental findings in animals, the number of cytoplasmic Ig$^+$ GCC increases with the intensity and duration of the antigenic stimulation. In hyperimmune conditions, germinal centers may show a predominance of cytoplasmic Ig$^+$ cells. Such cells have some features of plasma cells and often some features of centrocytes as well (Figure 6a and b). These observations suggest that, under special conditions, GCC can directly transform into antibody-producing cells.

Studies on the occurrence and distribution of C3b and C3d receptors in frozen sections from tonsils have indicated that a major proportion of FML and GCC express receptors for both complement receptor subtypes (47). Investigations on suspended cells prepared from lymphoid tissue containing many germinal centers have revealed that the EAC rosette-forming cell population includes a large number of centrocytes but only a few centroblasts. This might explain why neoplasms whose morphology indicates that they are derived from centroblasts are often complement receptor negative.

The most relevant of the known characteristics of the cells of the GCR are summarized in Figure 7. As mentioned above, FML consistently express large amounts of surface Ig but lack cytoplasmic Ig. A varying number of centroblasts and centrocytes are also surface Ig$^+$, but the staining is only mo-

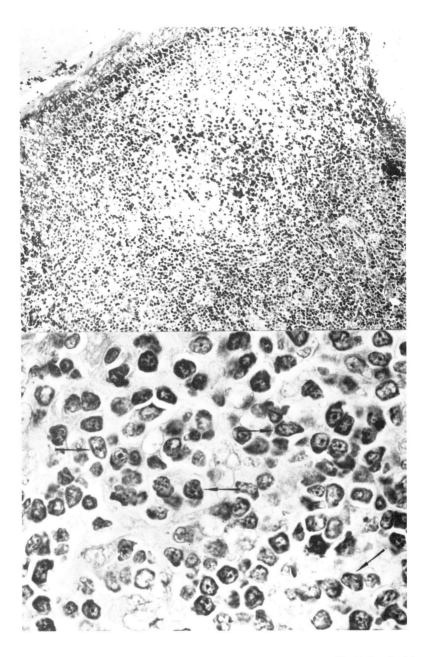

Figure 6. (a) Germinal center with many basophilic cells. Giemsa. × 120. (b) Detail of the germinal center in (a) at a higher magnification. This shows that the basophilic cells resemble plasma cells in cytoplasmic features and centrocytes in nuclear features (arrows). Giemsa. × 800.

Cytology	Immunology			
		FML	CB	CC
	S - Ig	+ + +	+ - + +	+ - + +
	C - Ig	−	−	− / +
	C3b receptor	+ + +	− / +	+ + / −
	C3d receptor	+ +	− / +	+ + / −
	IgG - Fc receptor	− /(+)	− /(+)	− /(+)
	Mouse - E rosettes	− / +	−	−
	Ia - like antigen	+	+	+

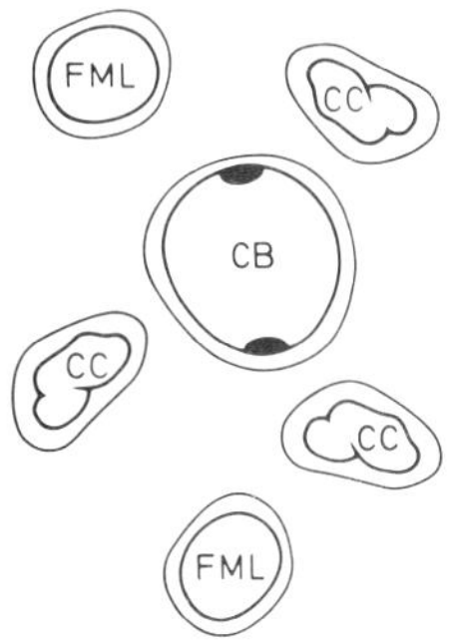

Figure 7. Cytologic and immunologic features of the cells of the germinal center reaction. FML = follicular mantle lymphocyte; CB = centroblast; CC = centrocyte; S-Ig = surface immunoglobulin; C-Ig = cytoplasmic immunoglobulin; E = erythrocyte.

derately intense. FML are constantly C3b and C3d receptor positive, with the exception of those in the outer rim, which are not always C3d receptor positive. The vast majority of centrocytes express both C3 receptor subtypes in a high density. A large but not yet exactly determined proportion of centroblasts are devoid of C3 receptors. All three types of cell of the GCR lack IgG-Fc receptors detectable with IgG-EA. About 20% of the cells found in tissue with follicular hyperplasia form rosettes with mouse E. The mouse E-rosette-forming cells display the morphologic features of FML. In non-neoplastic tissue we have not observed any cells resembling centroblasts or centrocytes among the mouse E-rosetting cells.

Plasma cell reaction

The other antigen-induced reaction of the B-cell system is the PCR. The PCR is not directly dependent on the GCR, and becomes manifest one or two days after exposure to antigen (53), i.e., two or three days before the GCR starts.

The PCR has been studied in detail by Veldman (53). According to his findings the PCR is started by cells located in the outer lymph node cortex. These starter cells are probably derived from B_1 cells or, with increasing age from B_2 (memory?) cells. It is difficult to investigate the PCR in normally reacting lymphoid tissue because of the simultaneous occurrence of the T-cell reaction and the GCR, both of which usually overlap with the PCR; Veldman succeeded in studying an isolated PCR by means of lethal irradiation and application of various antigens. Under the conditions chosen by Veldman, some of the antigens induced an isolated PCR.

In man, there are apparently a few virus infections that are associated with an almost isolated PCR. Rubella is one example. A rubella-induced hyperplastic PRC with marked suppression of both the T-cell reaction and the GCR is illustrated in Figure 8a. Between "atrophic" germinal centers, there is a broad corridor which extends from the outer cortex to the medulla of the lymph node and contains a large number of immunoblasts. These cells are large and have a pale nucleus that usually shows a prominent central nucleolus; the cytoplasm is relatively abundant and intensely basophilic (Figure 8b). The immunoblasts, most of which are generated in the lymph-node cortex, move towards the medulla and transform into plasmablasts and plasma cells (53)(Figure 8b).

At the stage of immunoblastic differentiation, the cells of the PCR switch from the synthesis of surface Ig to the synthesis of secretory Ig (4). Secretory Ig, which is Ig destined for secretion, is readily detectable in the cytoplasm of many B immunoblasts, all plasmablasts, and all plasma cells. With the switch to secretory Ig synthesis, the cells of the PCR lose their surface Ig (first IgD and later the other Ig classes) and their IgG-Fc receptors (41); they also lose their C3 receptors. In vitro experiments have indicated that 24 hours after antigenic stimulations, σ chains are no longer necessary for the differentiation of B cells into plasma cells (9).

With respect to blast transformation occurring in the PCR, it has often been asked whether B cells can transform directly into plasma cells without going through an immunoblast stage. Recently, Fu et al. (14) showed that this question can be answered in the affirmative. In a pokeweed mitogen cocultivation study on surface Ig$^+$ and cytoplasmic Ig$^-$ leukemic B cells and T cells from normal individuals, these authors found that up to 50% of the leukemic B cells matured into (cytoplasmic Ig$^+$) plasma cells without dividing.

The PCR varies greatly, depending on the kind of antigen (T-independent or T-dependent) and the incidence of exposure to antigen (5, 22). The extremes among the various types of PCR might be the following: one type of PCR occurring mainly in response to a primary, T-independent antigenic stimulus and another in response to a secondary, T-dependent antigenic stimulus (5). Apparently, the cells generated after primary, T-independent antigenic stimulation are almost exclusively IgM-secreting plasma cells, and these cells usually exhibit the features of what are called lymphatic plasma cells (see Figure 1). Secondary, T-dependent antigenic induction of the PCR apparently favors the generation of IgG-secreting plasma cells, which usually correspond in morphology to the Marschalkó type of plasma cells (see Figure 1).

There is accumulating evidence supporting the view that, in vivo, the secondary type of PCR starts with memory B_2 cells generated by a prior GCR, whereas the primary type of PCR begins with B_1 cells (22). The ex-

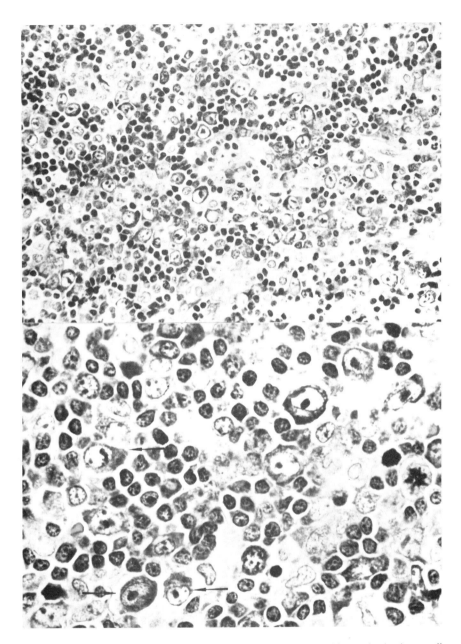

Figure 8. (a) Cortical area of a lymph node with a rubella-induced hyperplastic plasma cell reaction (PCR). Note the large number of immunoblasts. Giemsa. × 350. (b) Higher magnification of the medulla of the same lymph node as in (a). It contains numerous immuno-blasts that are destined to transform into plasma cells via plasmablasts (arrows). Giemsa. × 800.

periments of many investigators have indicated that a large proportion, although certainly not all, of the IgG-secreting plasma cells develop from surface IgM$^+$ B cells via a switch from the synthesis of IgM to that of IgG (1, 29, 38, 49). The number of cells that switch depends on the regulatory influence, probably of T cells (1). At present, it is not clear whether the IgG-secreting Marschalkó type of plasma cells usually arise from IgM-secreting lymphatic plasma cells, or whether the development of the IgG-secreting Marschalkó type of plasma cell takes place directly, i.e., without passing through a morphologic transition form similar or identical to the lymphatic type of the plasma cell.

REFERENCES

1. Andersson, J., Coutinho, A., and Melchers, F.: The switch from IgM to IgG secretion in single mitogen-stimulated B-cell clones. J. Exp. Med., 148:1744–1754, 1978.
2. Andersson, L.C., and Gahmberg, C.G.: Membrane glycoprotein patterns of normal and malignant human leukocytes. In: Function and structure of the immune system. Advances in experimental medicine and biology, vol. 114, pp. 623–628, Müller-Ruchholtz, W., and Müller-Hermelink, H.K. (eds), Plenum Press, New York and London, 1979.
3. Asma, G.E.M., Pichler, W., Schuit, H.R.E., Knapp, W., and Hijmans, W.: The development of lymphocytes with T- or B-membrane determinants in the human foetus. Clin. exp. Immunol., 29:278–285, 1977.
4. Avrameas, S., and Leduc, E.H.: Detection of simultaneous antibody synthesis in plasma cells and specialized lymphocytes in rabbit lymph nodes. J. Exp. Med., 131:1137–1168, 1970.
5. Black, S.J., van der Loo, W., Loken, M.R., and Herzenberg, L.A.: Expression of IgD by murine lymphocytes. Loss of surface IgD indicates maturation of memory B cells. J. Exp. Med., 147:984–996, 1978.
6. Broder, S., Edelson, R.L., Lutzner, M.A., Nelson, D.L., MacDermott, R.P., Durm, M.E., Goldman, C.K., Meade, B.D., and Waldmann, T.A.: The Sézary syndrome. A malignant proliferation of helper T cells. J. clin. Invest., 58:1297–1306, 1976.
7. Broder, S., Poplack, D., Whang-Peng, J., Durm, M., Goldman, C., Muul, L., and Waldmann, T.A.: Characterization of a suppressor-cell leukemia. Evidence for the requirement of an interaction of two T cells in the development of human suppressor effector cells. New Engl. J. Med., 198:66–72, 1978.
8. van Buchem, F.L.: Histologisch onderzoek van de plasmacellulaire reactie en zijn plaats in de histophysiologie van de lymphklier. Doctoral thesis, University of Groningen, 1962.
9. Cambier, J.C., Vitetta, E.S., Kettman, J.R., Wetzel, G.M., and Uhr, J.W.: B-cell tolerance. III. Effect of papain-mediated cleavage of cell surface IgD on tolerance susceptibility of murine B cells. J. Exp. Med. 146:107–117, 1977.
10. Chang, L.M.S.: Development of terminal deoxynucleotidyl transferase activity in embryonic calf thymus gland. Biochem. biophys. Res. Commun., 44:124–131, 1971.
11. Chechik, B.E., Pyke, K.W., and Gelfand, E.W.: Human thymus/leukemia-

associated antigen in normal and leukemic cells. Int. J. Cancer 18 :551–556, 1976.

12. Cline, M.J., and Billing, R.: Antigens expressed by human B lymphocytes and myeloid stem cells. J. Exp. Med. 146:1143–1145, 1977.

13. Cooper, M.D.: Early events in B-cell differentiation/maturation. Paper read at: Norsk Hydro's Institute for Cancer Research, The Norwegian Cancer Society Symposium, "B-cell neoplasia in the perspective of normal B-cell differentiation", Oslo, 14–15 June, 1979.

14. Fu, S.M., Chiorazzi, N., Kunkel, H.G., Halper, J.P., and Harris, S.R.: Induction of in vitro differentiation and immunoglobulin synthesis of human leukemic B lymphocytes. J. Exp. Med., 148:1570–1578, 1978.

15. Fu, S.M. Winchester, R.J., and Kunkel, H.G.: The occurrence of the HL-B allo-antigens on the cells of unclassified acute lymphoblastic leukemias. J. Exp. Med., 142:1334–1338, 1975.

16. Gastkemper, N.A., Wubbena, A.S., and Nieuwenhuis, P.: Germinal centres and the B-cell system: A search for the germinal centre precursor cell in the rat. In: Function and structure of the immune system. Advances in experimental medicine and biology, vol. 114, pp. 43–49, Müller-Ruchholtz, W., and Müller-Hermelink, H.K., (eds.), Plenum Press, New York and London, 1979.

17. Gathings, W.E., Lawton, A.R., and Cooper, M.D.: Immunofluorescent studies of the development of pre-B cells, B lymphocytes and immunoglobulin isotype diversity in humans. Eur. J. Immunol., 7:804–810, 1977.

18. Gatien, J.G., Schneeberger, E.E., and Merler, E.: Analysis of human thymocyte subpopulations using discontinuous gradients of albumin: Precursor lymphocytes in human thymus. Eur. J. Immunol., 5:312–317, 1975.

19. Greaves, M.F.: Neoplasia in early B cells. Paper read at: Norsk Hydro's Institute for Cancer Research, The Norwegian Cancer Society Symposium "B-cell neoplasia in the perspective of normal B-cell differentiation", Oslo, 14–15 June, 1979.

20. Greaves, M.F., Brown, G., Rapson, N.T., and Lister, T.A.: Antisera to acute lymphoblastic leukemia cells. Clin. Immunol. Immunopath., 4:67–84, 1975.

21. Grossi, C.E., Webb, S.R., Zicca, A., Lydyard, P.M., Moretta, L., Mingari, M.C., and Cooper, M.D.: Morphological and histochemical analyses of two human T-cell subpopulations bearing receptors for IgM or IgG. J. Exp. Med., 147:1405–1417, 1978.

22. Howard, M.C., Baker, J.A., and Shortman, K.: Antigen-initiated B lymphocyte differentiation. XV. Existence of "pre-progenitor" and "direct progenitor" subsets among secondary B cells. J. Immunol., 121:2066–2069, 1978.

23. Jacobsen, E.B., Caporale, L.H., and Thorbecke, G.J.: Effect of thymus cell injections on germinal center formation in lymphoid tissues of nude (thymus-less) mice. Cell. Immunol., 13:416, 1974.

24. Jäger, G., Pachmann, C., Rodt, H., and Huhn, D.: Polyacrylsäure-Kügelchen als Nachweis von B-Lymphocyten (abstract). Blut 35:335, 1977.

25. Janossy, G., Greaves, M.F., Revesz, T., Lister, T.A., Roberts, M., Durrant, J., Kirk, B., Catovsky, D., and Beard, M.E.J.: Blast crisis of chronic myeloid leukemia (CML). II. Cell surface marker analysis of "lymphoid" and myeloid cases. Brit. J. Haemat., 34:179–192, 1976.

26. Janossy, G., Roberts, M., and Greaves, M.F.: Target cell in chronic myeloid leukemia and its relationship to acute lymphoid leukemia. Lancet, II: 1058–1061, 1976.

27. Kabisch, H., Arndt, R., Becker, W.M., Thiele, H.-G., and Landbeck, G.:

Serological detection and partial characterization of the common-ALL-cell associated antigen in the serum of ALL-patients. Leuk. Res., 3:83–91, 1979.

28. Kabisch, H., Arndt, R., Thiele, H.-G., Winkler, K., and Landbeck, G.: Partial molecular characterization of an antigenic structure associated to cells of common acute lymphocytic leukaemia (ALL). Clin. Exp. Immunol., 32:399–404, 1978.

29. Kearney, J.F.M., Cooper, M.D., and Lawton, A.R.: B-lymphocyte differentiation induced by lipopolysaccharide. III. Suppression of B-cell maturation by anti-mouse immunoglobulin antibodies. J. Immunol., 116:1664, 1976.

30. Keuning, F.J.: Dynamics of immunoglobulin forming cells and their precursors. In: Immunoglobulins, pp. 1–14, North-Holland, Amsterdam, 1972.

31. Knowles, D.M., II, Hoffman, T., Ferrarini, M., and Kunkel, H.G.: The demonstration of acid α-naphthyl acetate esterase activity in human lymphocytes: Usefulness as a T-cell marker. Cell.Immunol., 35:112–123, 1978.

32. Lennert, K.: Über die Erkennkung von Keimzentrumszellen im Lymphknotenausstrich. Klin. Wschr., 35:1130–1132, 1957.

33. McCaffrey, R., Harrison, T.A., Kung, P.C., Parkman, R., Silverstone, A.E., and Baltimore, D.: Terminal deoxynucleotidyl transferase in normal and neoplastic hematopoietic cells. In: Modern trends in human leukemia II. Hämatologie und Blut-transfusion, vol. 19, pp. 503–513, Neth, R., Gallo, R.C., Mannweiler, K., and Moloney, W.C., (eds.), Lehmanns, München, 1976.

34. Mendes, N.F., Tolnai, M.E.A., Silveira, N.P.A., Gilbertsen, R.B., and Metzgar, R.S.: Technical aspects of the rosette tests used to detect human complement receptor (B) and sheep erythrocyte-binding (T) lymphocytes. J. Immunol., 111: 860–867, 1973.

35. Metcalf, E.S., and Klinman, N.R.: In vitro tolerance induction of neonatal murine B cells. J. Exp. Med., 143:1327–1340, 1976.

36. Moretta, L., Webb, S.R., Grossi, C.E., Lydyard, P.M., and Cooper, M.D.: Functional analysis of two human T-cell subpopulations: Help and suppression of B-cell responses by T cells bearing receptors for IgM or IgG. J. Exp. Med., 146:184–200, 1977.

37. Nieuwenhuis, P., Van Nouhuijs, C.E., Eggens, J.H., and Keuning, F.J.: Germinal centers and the origin of the B-cell system. I. Germinal centers in the rabbit appendix. Immunology, 26: 497–567, 1974.

38. Nossal, G.J.V., Szenberg, A., Ada, G.L., and Austin, C.M.: Single cell studies on 19 S antibody production. J. Exp. Med. 119: 485, 1964.

39. Opstelten, D., van der Heijden, D., Stikker, R., and Nieuwenhuis, P.: Germinal centers and the B-cell system: B-cell differentiation in rabbit appendix germinal centers. In: Function and structure of the immune system. Advances in experimental medicine and biology, vol. 114, pp. 125–131, Müller-Ruchholtz, W., and Müller-Hermelink, H.K., (eds.), Plenum Press, New York and London, 1979.

40. Press, O.W., Rosse, C., and Clagett, J.: Phytohemagglutinin-induced differentiation and blastogenesis of precursor T cells from mouse bone marrow. J. Exp. Med., 146:735–746, 1977.

41. Preud'Homme, J.L.: Loss of surface IgD by human B lymphocytes during polyclonal activation. Eur. J. Immunol., 7:191–193, 1977.

42. Raff, M.C., Megson, M., Owen, J.J.T., and Cooper, M.D.: Early production of intracellular IgM by B-lymphocyte precursors in mouse. Nature, 259:224–226, 1976.

43. Raff, M.C., Owen, J.J.T., Cooper, M.D., Lawton, A.R., III, Megson, M., and

Gathings, W.E.: Differences in susceptibility of mature and immature mouse B lymphocytes to anti-immunoglobulin-induced immunoglobulin suppression in vitro. Possible implications for B-cell tolerance to self. J. Exp. Med., 142: 1052–1064, 1975.

44. Roberts, M., Greaves, M., Janossy, G., Sutherland, R., and Pain, C.: Acute lymphoblastic leukaemia (ALL) associated antigen—I. Expression in different haematopoietic malignancies. Leuk. Res., 2:105–114, 1978.

45. Silverstone, A.E., Cantor, H., Goldstein, G., and Baltimore, D.: Terminal deoxynucleotidyl transferase is found in prothymocytes. J. Exp. Med., 144:543–548, 1976.

46. Stein, H., and Müller-Hermelink, H.K.: Simultaneous presence of receptors for complement and sheep red blood cells on human fetal thymocytes. Brit. J. Haemat., 36:227–233, 1977.

47. Stein, H. Siemssen, U., and Lennert, K.: Complement receptor subtypes C3b and C3d in lymphatic tissue and follicular lymphoma. Brit. J. Cancer, 37:520–529., 1978.

48. Stein, H., Tolksdorf, G., and Lennert, K.: T-cell lymphomas. A cell origin-related classification on the basis of cytologic, immunologic, and enzyme cytochemical criteria. Path. Res. Pract., in press.

49. Sterzl, J., and Nordin, A.: The common cell precursor for cells producing different immunoglobulins. In: Cell interactions and receptor antibodies in immune responses. Mäkelä, O., Cross, A., and Kosunen, T.U., (eds.). p. 213, Academic Press, New York, (1971).

50. Sutherland, R., Smart, J., Niaudet, P., and Greaves, M.: Acute lymphoblastic leukaemia associated antigen—II. Isolation and partial characterization. Leuk. Res., 2:115–126, 1978.

51. Thiel, E., Rodt, H., Huhn, D., and Thierfelder, S.: Decrease and altered distribution of human T antigen on chronic lymphatic leukemia cells of T type, suggesting a clonal origin. Blood, 47:723–736, 1976.

52. Tötterman, T.H., Ranki, A., and Häyry, P.: Expression of the acid α-naphtyl acetate esterase marker by activated and secondary T lymphocytes in man. Scand. J. Immunol., 6:305–310, 1977.

53. Veldman, J.E.: Histophysiology and electron microscopy of the immune response. Thesis, University of Groningen, 1970.

54. Vitetta, E.S., Melcher, U., McWilliams, M., Lamm, M.E., Phillips-Quagliata, J.M., and Uhr, J.W.: Cell surface immunoglobulin. XI. The appearance of an IgD-like molecule on murine lymphoid cells during ontogeny. J. Exp. Med., 141:206–215, 1975.

55. Vogler, L.B., Crist, W.M., Bockman, D.E., Pearl, E.R., Lawton, A.R., and Cooper, M.D.: Pre-B-cell leukemia. A new phenotype of childhood lymphoblastic leukemia. New Engl. J. Med., 298:872–878, 1978.

56. Wernet, P., Schunter, F., Wilms, K., and Waller, H.D.: New aspects in the classification of leukemic cell types by Ia alloantigens and complement receptors. In: Immunological diagnosis of leukemias and lymphomas. Haematology and blood transfusion, vol. 20, pp. 333–338, Thierfelder, S., Rodt, H., and Thiel, E., (eds.), Springer, Berlin, Heidelberg and New York, 1977.

57. Zinkernagel, R.M., Callahan, G.N., Althage, A., Cooper, S., Klein, P.A., and Klein, J.: On the thymus in the differentiation of "H-2 self-recognition" by T cells: Evidence for dual recognition? J. Exp. Med., 147:882–896, 1978.

3. B-CELL DIFFERENTIATION AND CHARACTERIZATION*

P. BIBERFELD AND K. NILSSON

B-CELL DIFFERENTIATION

Compared with T-cell differentiation, the differentiation of lymphoid cells of the B-cell lineage is poorly understood (for reviews, see (1, 2)). The following presentation will therefore by necessity be subjective and incomplete, but an attempt is made to collect facts from the numerous reports on animal and human B-cell differentiation into a coherent picture, which will be useful as background for the understanding of the diverse B-cell systems from which most human lymphomas originate.

Ontogeny of the human immune B-cell system   (Figure 1)

The first immunological function in the fetus can be demonstrated at about the fifth week of gestation, when MLC-reactive cells are found in the liver (3). By the seventh week of gestation, cells with cytoplasmic IgM are detectable in the liver, and about two weeks later, surface (s) IgM-positive lymphocytes are found in the liver and subsequently in the bone marrow, spleen, blood, and lymph nodes. By the twelfth week of gestation, cells bearing sIG can be detected before those bearing sIgD or sIgA (4). Antigen-binding cells (ABC) have been demonstrated in the liver and spleen of mice at about the same time as the appearance of sIg$^+$ cells (5).

The structural differentiation of the lymphoid tissues, for instance germinal centers, is not completed until after birth. Experimental evidence indicates that the adult histology of the lymphoid apparatus is largely dependent on stimulation by exogenous, specific and possibly nonspecific factors (6, 7, 8).

Differentiation of the adult immune B-cell system

From experimental evidence obtained in murine and human systems,

*Supported by grants from the Swedish Cancer Society.

J.G. van den Tweel et al. (eds.), Malignant Lymphoproliferative Diseases, 31–48

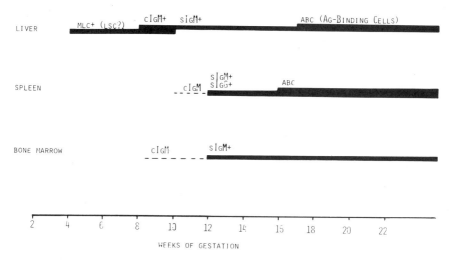

Figure 1. Ontogeny of the human B-immune system (from (3)). MLC = mixed lymphocyte culture; cIg, sIg = cytoplasmic and surface localized Ig.

five major cell categories or compartments within the B-cell differentiation lineage can be recognized (1, 8, 9, 10, 11) (Figure 2).

Physically not yet very well defined *lymphoid stem cells* (LSC) develop in the bone marrow and become seeded into the circulation and peripheral lymphoid organs. The further differentiation into functionally mature B cells seems to be a highly ordered sequential process leading at the same time to diversity with respect to antigen specificity within the mature B-cell population (12). This step-wise differentiation occurs within proliferative cell compartments (LSC, pre-B cells, and undefined in-between B-cell types) and seems to be influenced mainly by as yet undefined micro-environmental factors (8, 13, 14) (Figure 2).

The environment for specific differentiation of prethymic LSC to T cells is recognized both in birds and mammals to be the thymus and thymus-dependent areas in peripheral lymphoid tissue. In birds, the Bursa of Fabricius serves as the corresponding B-cell specific maturation environment, but in mammals no bursa or any corresponding tissue with capacity for selective induction of LSC to B-cell differentiation has been identified, although the so-called gut-associated lymphoid tissue (GALT) has been implicated in that respect. The in vitro studies by Owen et al. (15) rather strengthen the notion that the B-cell differentiation in mammals may take place multifocally in various lymphoid tissues.

It should be emphasized, however, that any compartmentalization of the differentiation of the B-cell lineage is at present schematic and probably artificial and that a substantial heterogeneity with regard to cell phenotypes is present within each of the cell compartments discussed below.

The extent of recruitment of LSC from the multipotent stem cell population is unknown. Also, the inductive signals required for the sequential steps involved in the generation of antigen-sensitive B cells from the stem cells have not been indentified. Most observations seem to indicate the existence of an intermediate step (steps) morphologically represented by relatively large, rapidly dividing cells producing cytoplasmic IgM but lacking B-cell surface markers and apparently committed to the generation of B cells (4).

These so-called *pre-B cells*, which constitute the second compartment, multiply in the bone marrow but probably also circulate through extramedullary sites (4, 16, 17). Transfer experiments and in vitro studies seem to indicate that pre-B cells indeed can generate mature antigen-receptor carrying B cells outside the bone marrow environment.

Little is known about the extent of heterogeneity within the pre-B-cell population and Ig surface receptor bearing B cells generated from pre-B cells.

The post-mitotic maturation of the pre-B to the primary (virgin Ig receptor positive) B cell is morphologically reflected by the transition of the relatively large undifferentiated cells to medium-to-small lymphocytes in the bone marrow, and in extramedullary sites.

The third compartment is made up of the *virgin B cells (B1 cells)*. These cells develop mainly in extramedullary lymphoid tissues but to some extent also in the bone marrow (8). In the lymphoid tissues they are progenitors of the cells of the germinal center reaction.

Up to this stage, differentiation is probably independent of specific (antigen) induction. However, by virtue of its Ig receptors, and usually by T-cell and macrophage help, the virgin B cell can now be specifically induced by antigen to differentiate through a lymphoblast intermediate form to a clone of antibody-forming cells by division and step-wise functional maturation (18) or to develop into a *secondary B memory cell (MB)*. Nonspecific stimulation by polyclonal B-cell activators and microbial factors other than antigens, may also stimulate the expansion of primary B cells (8, 19, 20, 21).

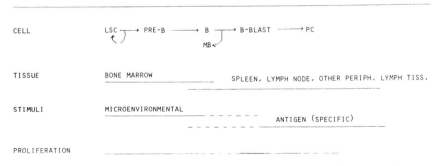

Figure 2. B-cell differentiation and compartmentalization. For abreviations see the text.

It has also been suggested that B cells at this stage of development might be susceptible to tolerogenic events and that expansion and maturation might require the combined or additive effects of nonspecific and specific stimuli (8, 22).

Development of immunological memory coincides with the germinal-center proliferation (6).

The fourth cell compartment consists of the *secondary B cells (B2, B-blasts)*, which, by definition, are generated by specific stimulation of primary B cells (18, 23). As in the B1-cell compartment, there is probably heterogeneity within the B2-cell population with several sequential stages of maturation which require specific and "helper" or nonspecific stimulation leading eventually to the development of the fifth cell compartment, the *plasma cells (PC)* (23).

The PC are end cells which secrete Ig at a high rate and undergo no further differentiation. Like other end cells, they have a finite life-span, as has been demonstrated by transfer experiments in the mouse (23). Some degree of heterogeneity exists within the PC compartment, too. Although all cells are characterized functionally by their capacity for Ig secretion, some ultrastructural heterogeneity has been demonstrated, and it has been suggested that this is correlated with the type and the rate of Ig secretion (24).

Several major functional aspects of B-cell differentiation are poorly understood. For instance, to what extent are B cells within the different schematic compartments thymus-dependent or independent, what kind of stimuli determine the immunoglobulin isotype diversification during the differentiation within the pre-B and primary B-cell compartments, and at what stage of B-cell differentiation does tolerance induction or clonal abortion occur?

To elucidate these and other questions concerning the nature of the B-cell differentiation lineage, cell markers allowing physical separation and characterization of various cellular subsets have to be used. In the following, the most important markers currently available for the identification and subdivision of the B-cell system will be reviewed.

CHARACTERIZATION OF DIFFERENTIATING B CELLS

Morphology

According to several observations, B cells can be distinguished from T cells on the basis of their villous surface topography seen by electron microscopy (Figure 3, 4) (25). However, other observations suggest these differences to be technical artifacts (26).

(3)

(4)

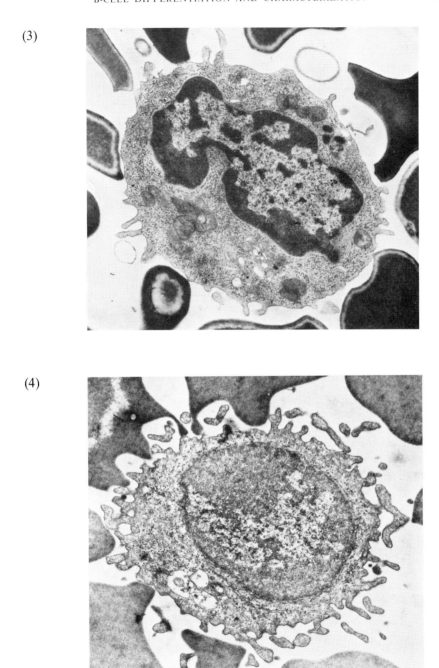

Figures 3, 4. Electron micrographs of an E$^+$ (3) and a CR$^+$ (4) cell from human blood.

(5)

(6)

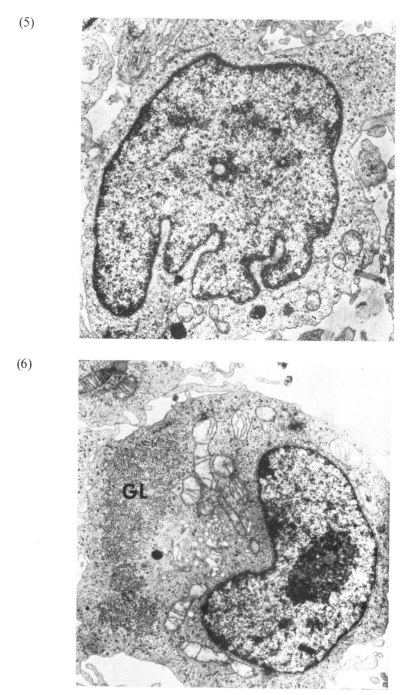

Figures 5–8. Electron micrographs of lymphoblasts (5 and 6) and immature plasma cells (7 and 8) in cultures of human blood lymphocytes stimulated by pokeweed mitogen (PWM).

(7)

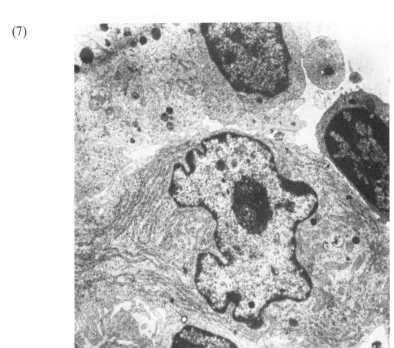

(8)

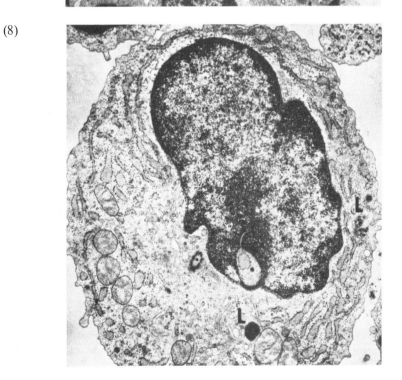

Other fine-structural features have been described as distinctive for either
T or B lymphocytes (27), e.g., size, amount of ER, number of lysosomes
and mitochondria, and size of the Golgi zone, but in general these features
do not allow distinction between individual B and T cells, at least not at
the light-microscopical level.

Attempts to define the LSC morphologically have resulted in disparate
and controversial statements (24). They have been defined, alternatively,
as lymphocyte-like, monocytoid, or so-called transitional cells. Larger and
smaller subsets of B lymphocytes have been separated by gradient sedimentation techniques, but on the whole no detailed morphological analyses
have been reported (9).

Primary and secondary lymphocytes are heterogeneous in size but are
morphologically indistinguishable.

After stimulation either specifically by antigen or nonspecifically by
appropriate mitogens (PBA), B cells transform to blast cells. Depending
on the kind and degree of stimulation, B-blasts may or may not mature
subsequently and step-wise to plasma cells. In the early stages of blast
transformation individual B-blast cannot be distinguished morphologically
from T-blasts (7, 28, 29).

There is of course no difficulty in the cytological distinction between
lymphocytes and the mature plasma cell. Furthermore incompletely differentiated plasma cells, so-called plasma blasts, and lymphoplasmacytoid
cells can be distinguished by EM and also with a certain confidence at the
light-microscopical level (Figure 5–8).

Cytochemistry

Cytochemical stains are not discriminatory for the various stages of B-cell
differentiation. Generally, B-lymphoid cells, in contrast to T-lymphoid
cells, are PAS positive, but no clear differences between the different subsets of B cells have been demonstrated. β-glucuronidase (B-glu) staining can
be used to some extent to discriminate between B cells and plasmacytoid
cells. The B-glu is diffuse and weak in B cells but strong and granular in
plasmacytoid cells (30).

In B-blasts the B-glu activity is somewhat stronger than in B cells but
less intense than in plasmacytoid cells (30).

Immunoglobulin expression

By definition, B-lymphoid cells synthesize Ig. The Ig produced may
be destined for cell surface expression and/or for secretion. The surface
and secreted Ig is probably synthesized along separate pathways (7).

The relative amounts of surface and secretory Ig in B-lymphoid cells
vary depending on the stage of B-cell differentiation (Figure 9).

EXPRESSION	LSC	PRE-B	B	B-BLAST	PC
mIg	-	-	+-+++ M,MD	+ MD,MG,MA M,D	(+) G,M,A D,E
cIg	-	++ M	-	+-++ M,G,A D,E	+++ G,M,A D,E

Figure 9. Ig expression during B-cell differentiation. M,D,G,A,E = heavy-chain isotypes.

Several basic questions concerning Ig production during B-cell differentiation have not yet been unequivocally answered, e.g., at what stage of differentiation is immunoglobulin first expressed, at what stage is Ig-isotype diversity determined, and what is the functional importance of the different isotypes for stimulation and tolerance induction in maturing B cells?

By current methodology LSC are Ig−. Most studies in both human and mouse systems indicate that large and small pre-B cells (maturing stem cells?) first found in the fetal liver and later in the fetal and adult bone marrow, spleen, blood, and lymph nodes contain intracytoplasmic IgM (16). sIg is not detectable by conventional immunofluorescence techniques. However, on the basis of a sensitive rosetting assay, a low density of sIg has been claimed to be present on pre-B cells (31).

The primary B cell expresses sIgM but not intracellular Ig and is committed with respect to antibody specificity and allotype. During maturation of the B1 cell compartment these cells acquire and express increasing amounts of IgD (4, 22). The B-blasts (secondary B lymphocytes) are usually μ^+ and diversity during their proliferation into lymphocytes expressing either μ^+ and γ, μ and α, and transitionally also δ (4, 32, 33). Certain subsets also have cytoplasmic Ig.

The small amount of sIg that can be demonstrated on the maturing plasma cells by conventional techniques, represents surface-bound Ig and not Ig in the process of secretion.

Complement receptors (CR)   (Figure 10)

A receptor for complement, distinct from sIg and Fc receptors, is present on the surface of most Ig$^+$ B lymphocytes (34). A similar receptor is also found on monocytic and myeloid cells but not on T lymphocytes. The presence of CR during ontogeny of the B-cell lineage has been studied by several groups (1). Their results essentially indicate that CR expression is well correlated with the appearance of Ig^+ cells in various fetal tissues. Some studies have indicated that circulating pre-B cells are CR^- but pre-T cells are possibly CR^+. During maturation to plasma cells, CR are no longer demonstrable.

Studies on the distribution of CR^+ cells in various tissues have shown their presence on mononuclear bone marrow cells (5–8%), thoracic duct cells (< 20%), spleen cells (30–40%), and lymphnode cells (10–25%) but CR^+ cells are characteristically absent in the thymus (1).

The histological distribution of CR can be demonstrated in cryo-sections (35). Such investigations have shown that CR is predominantly confined to so-called thymus-independent areas of lymph nodes, spleen, and Peyer's patches.

More recent studies have shown that CR actually consists of two receptor sites, one for C3b and the other for C3d, located on either the same or different molecular structures. It has also been shown that polymorphonuclear cells preferentially react with C3b, whereas B lymphocytes usually have both receptors.

In frozen sections of lymphoid tissues C3b and C3d are predominantly found over the follicular areas, whereas interfollicular cells react predominantly with C3b (36).

Studies on malignant lymphomas have shown that CR is a convenient marker for most B lymphomas, particularly B-CLL and those derived from follicle center cells (37). However, CR alone should probably not be unequivocally considered a B-cell marker in view of its presence on myeloid, monocytic, and possibly also some stem cells.

The function (s) of CR are not very well understood, but they have been suggested to be of importance in antigen localization during antigen-mediated B-cell differentiation and also for the release of cell-bound soluble complexes (1).

Fc receptors (FCR)   (Figure 10)

A receptor for the Fc part of IgG can be demonstrated on B lymphocytes by their binding of aggregated immunoglobulin or antibodies on erythrocytes (38). Initially, the FCR was thought to be a specific B-cell marker, but it is now clear that certain T-subsets and so-called null cells with effector functions in ADCC (antibody-dependent cell cytotoxicity) (K-cells), also have FCR. In addition, FCR are present on moncytes, macrophages, and to some extent on myeloid cells (1).

It has been shown that during ontogeny there is an increased overlapping of FCR + and Ig + cells. FCR are present on immature and mature B cells but not on plasma cells and not on stem cells and pre-B cells (1).

Redistribution and capping experiments have shown a nonreciprocal association of FCR and Ig, i.e., co-capping of FCR with Ig but not the reverse. The hypothesis is that there is a allosteric or conformational change in sIg complexed with anti-Ig, thereby exposing the Fc portion of sIg to the FCR. A possible association of FCR with Ia antigens has been suggested, but the issue is controversial.

In cryo-sections of lymphoid tissues FCR are usually present over both follicular and interfollicular areas in accordance with their presence on both B cells and cells of mononuclear phagocytic systems (36).

The function of FCR of B cells is by no means clear. FCR of K cells have been shown to mediate the necessary contact between the effector and target cells (39).

Within the B-cell system FCR can be used for identification of the B1 and B2 stages in B-cell maturation but is of little use for differentiation between B, T, and other leukocyes.

Ia-like antigen(s)   (Figure 10)

The I region-associated antigens (Ia) of the mouse have been extensively studied as to tissue distribution (1). Ia antigens are expressed not only on B lymphocytes but also on macrophages, epidermal cells, sperm cells, and some subsets of T cells.

Recently, human allo-antigens preferentially expressed on B lymphocytes have been identified by rabbit antisera (40–44). These antisera detect a bimolecular surface-membrane complex with chemical similarities to the Ia antigens of the mouse.

The human Ia-like antigen(s) are strongly expressed on B cells but also on other cell types such as monocytes, some epithelial cells, and the Langerhan's cells of the epidermis (44). Studies on leukemic and malignant lymphoid cell lines have also demonstrated the expression of Ia-like antigen in immature myeloid cells (42, 45, 45).

Figure 10 summarizes present knowledge about the expression of Ia-like antigen in the differentiating B-cell compartments. The Ia-like antigens seem to be expressed by the LSC and on pre-B cells, as judged from studies on human leukemias (45, 46). Studies on normal resting and mitogen-stimulated B cells have shown that these cells also express Ia antigen strongly (40, 43). Whether lymphoplasmacytoid cells and plasma cells express Ia-like antigen is less clear. However, Halpern et al. (43) and Nilsson (10) have

SURFACE MARKER	LSC	PRE-B	B	B-BLAST	PC
SIG	-	-	+	+	(+)
C3R	?	?	+	+	-
FCR	-	-	+	+	-
IA[1]	+	+[3]	+	+	+;-
ALL[2]	+	+	-	-	-
EBVR	-[4]	-[3]	+	+	-

[1]. IA-LIKE ANTIGENS

[2]. "COMMON ALL ANTIGEN" AS DEFINED BY ANTISERUM PREPARED BY M. GREAVES.

[3]. INDIRECT EVIDENCE FROM STUDIES ON HUMAN ACUTE LEUKEMIAS.

[4]. A SMALL FRACTION OF NON-T, NON-B CELLS IN HUMAN PERIPHERAL BLOOD BINDS EBV.

Figure 10. Expression of surface markers during B-cell differentiation.

shown that some, but not all cases of Waldenström's disease and multiple myeloma tumors express Ia-like antigen.

Ia-like antigen is easily demonstrable by conventional immunofluorescence. The diagnostic usefulness of Ia-like antigen in human malignant lymphoma seems to be restricted, because the expression of the antigen is not limited to any particular stage of B-lymphoid differentiation.

"Common ALL antigen" (CALL antigen)   (Figure 10)

Using a rabbit antiserum against the common form of acute lymphocytic leukemia (ALL), Greaves et al. (47) identified a surface antigen on ALL cells. This antigen has since been isolated and partially characterized as a glycoprotein of an apparent molecular weight of 100,000 daltons (48). The antigen, although first detected on leukemic cells, seems to be a normal gene product of immature haemopoietic cells, since it is also expressed on a small population of normal bone marrow cells.

Similar antisera were recently produced by Rodt et al. (49) and by Koshiba et al. (46).

Taken together the results of studies on normal bone marrow, fresh leukemic cells, and on leukemia and lymphoma cell lines suggest that the "common ALL antigen" is present on immature B cells (LSC, pre-B) but absent on B cells, B-blasts, and plasma cells. However, two B-lymphoma lines carrying sIg have been found to express the CALL antigen (46), which perhaps suggests that a minority of cells within the heterogeneous B-cell population continue to express the gene coding for CALL antigen.

EBV receptor   (Figure 10)

A receptor for Epstein-Barr virus (EBV) has been demonstrated on B lymphocytes by Jondal & Klein (50) and by Greaves et al. (51). The EBV receptor is expressed on all B cells and B-blasts but does not occur on LSC, pre-B cells, or plasma cells. To date, besides B cells, only a small fraction of so-called O-cells from human peripheral blood have been found to express EBV receptors (52). The EBV receptor, although difficult to assay, is therefore apparently a quite specific B-cell marker.

The EBV receptor is associated with, but not identical to, the CR of the B lymphocyte (53) as shown by co-expression of the two receptors on a large number of cell lines, by co-capping experiments, and by blocking experiments demonstrating that addition of complement blocks the EBV receptor and that addition of EBV inhibits the binding of complement.

Surface glycoprotein pattern of B lymphocytes

Recently, lactoperoxidase catalyzed iodination and the galactoseoxidase tritiated sodium borohydrine surface labelling techniques have been used to identify specific surface glycoproteins on mouse and human T and B B cells (54, 55).

Such studies have later been extended to mitogen-stimulated B cells and a panel of B lymphomas and B leukemias which, according to surface marker studies, represent various stages of B-lymphoid differentiation (56). Taken together, these findings suggest that it is possible to differentiate B cells, B-blasts, and plasma cells, and in addition consistent differences were found between normal B cells and B lymphomas. If such distinguishing surface glycoproteins could be purified, it is possible that hetero-antisera to B-cell differentiation associated surface antigen could be prepared.

DISCUSSION

In this brief review we have mainly discussed features of B-cell differentiation and characterization which may be useful in diagnostic efforts to characterize B cell-derived lymphoproliferative diseases.

It should be emphasized that with the exception of Ig, the functional importance of most of the above-mentioned markers is poorly understood.

At present, they are only indirectly correlated with functional properties of cells that express these markers. The demonstration of these functional properties usually involves elaborate in vitro and in vivo experiments and are therefore less applicable in clinical practice.

Most malignant lymphomas and lymphocytic leukemias are B-cell derived (24, 33, 57). Evidence is accumulating that in adults, non-B lymphomas and leukemias in general have a worse prognosis than B-derived tumors (58). If so, an immunological classification of lymphoproliferative diseases seems justified as a complement to conventional histology. However, the immunological classification of B-derived lymphomas and leukemias is at present restricted by our incomplete knowledge of B-cell differentiation. Furthermore such classifications rest on the assumption that each individual tumor is a phenotypically stable clone of cells arrested in a particular stage of differentiation. Results from work on tumor-derived cell lines have in several instances supported this hypothesis (10). Thus, several established lymphoid cell lines could be related to corresponding properties of differentiating B cells (Figure 11). On the basis of such morphological, immunological, and functional correlates a relationship between various lymphomas/leukemias and different cell compartments of the B-cell lineage has been suggested by Nilsson (10, 11) (Figure 11).

For the further elucidation of B-lymphoid cell differentiation, malignant lymphomas and leukemias have already been and will undoubtedly be important models. Conversely, further elucidation of B-cell differentiation will probably allow a better immunological classification of lymphoid tumors according to their origin in the B-cell differentiation lineage.

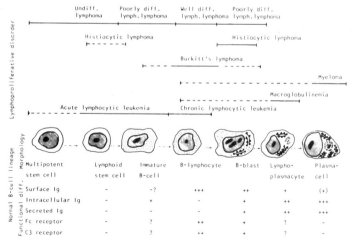

Figure 11. Lymphoproliferative disorders. Tentative morphological and functional differentiation and relationship to the normal B-cell lineage (from (10)).

REFERENCES

1. Katz, D.H.: Lymphocyte differentiation, recognition and regulation, Academic Press, New York, 1977.
2. INSERM Symposium No. 8: Serron, B., and Rosenfeld, C., (eds.), Elsevier/ North Holland Biochemical Press, 1978.
3. Parkman, R.: Treatment of immunodeficiency diseases by organ transplantation. In: Progress in clinical immunology, Schwartz, R.S., (eds.), p. 85, 1977.
4. Cathings, W.E., Lawton, A.R., and Cooper, M.D.: Immunofluorescent studies of the development of pre-B cells. By lymphocytes and immunoglobulin isotype diversity in humans. Eur. J. Immunol., 7:804, 1977.
5. D'Eustachio, P., and Edelman, G.M.: Frequency and avidity of specific antigen-binding cells in developing mice. J. Exp. Med., 142:1978, 1975.
6. Thorbecke, G.J., Romano, T.J., and Lerman, S.P.: Regulatory mechanisms in proliferation and differentiation of lymphoid tissue, with particular reference to germinal center development. In: Progress in immunology II, Brent, L., and Holborow, J., (eds.), vol. 3, p. 25, 1974.
7. Janossy, G., and Greaves, M.: Functional analysis of murine and human B lymphocyte subsets. Transplant. Rev., 24:177, 1975.
8. Nossal, G.Y.V., Shortman, K., Howard, M., and Pike, B.L.: Current problem areas in the study of B-lymphocyte differentiation. Immunological Rev., 37:187, 1977.
9. Strober, S.: Immune function, cell surface characteristics and maturation of B cell subpopulations. Transpl. Rev. 24:84, 1975.
10. Nilsson, K.: Established human lymphoid cell lines as models fœr B-lymphocyte differentiation (abstract). INSERM Symposium No. 8, 307, 1978.
11. Seligmann, M., Preud'homme, J-L., and Brouet, J-C.: Human lymphocyte differentiation, its application to cancer, INSERM Symposium No. 8:133, 1978.
12. Lydyard, P.M., Crossi, C.E., and Coopes, M.D.: Ontogeny of B cells in the chicken. I. Segmental development of clonal diversity in the bursa. J. Exp. Med., 144:79, 1976.
13. Metcalf, E.S., Sigal, N.H., and Klinman, N.R.: In vitro tolerance induction of neonatal murine B cells. as a probe for the study of B cell diversification. J. Exp. Med., 145:1382–1386, 1977.
14. Sherr, D., Szewczuh, M.R., and Suskind, G.W.: Ontogeny of B lymphocyte function. IV. Kinetics of maturation of B lyphocytes from fetal and neonatal mice when transferred into adult irradiated hosts. J. Immunol., 119:1674–1679, 1977.
15. Owen, J.J.T., Cooper, M.D., and Raff, M.C.: In vitro generation of B lymphocytes in mouse foetal liver. A mammalian "bursa equivalent". Nature 249:361, 1974.
16. Raff, M.C., Megson, M., Owen, J.J.T., and Cooper, M.D.: Early production of intracellular IgM by B lymphocyte precursors in the mouse. Nature 259:224, 1976.
17. Melchers, F., von Boehmer, H., and Phillips, R.A.: B lymphocyte sub-populations in the mouse. Transplant. Rev., 25:26–57, 1975.
18. Anofsky, R., Ikari, N.S., and Hylton, M.B.: The relationship of specific antigenic stimulation of serum Ig or levels in germfree mice. In: Advances in germfree research and gnotobiology, Miyakawa, M., and Lucker, T.D., (eds.), Chemical Rubber Co. p. 219, 1968.

19. Melchers, F., von Bohmer, H. and Phillips, R.A. B lymphocyte subpopulations in the mouse. Transpl. Rev., 25:26, 1975.
20. Smith, C.I.E., and Hammarström, L.: Sodium polyanethole sulfonate: a new macrophage dependent polymyxin-inhibitable, polyclonal B cell activation. Immunol., 121:823, 1978.
21. Gronowicz, E., and Coutinho, A.: Functional analysis of B cell heterogenity. Transpl. Rev., 24:3, 1975.
22. Vitetta, Ellen S., and Uhr, G.W., IgD and B cell differentiation. Transpl. Rev., 37:50, 1977.
23. Askonas, B.A., Williamson, A.R., and Wright, B.E.G.: Selection of single antibody forming cell alone and its propagation in syngeneic mice. PNAS, 67:1398, 1970.
24. Lennert, K., Mohri, N., Stein, H., Kaiserlung, E., Muller-Hermelink, H.K:In: Malignant lymphomas, Springer-Verlag 1978.
25. Polliak, A., Lampen, N., Clarkson, B.D., de Harven, E., Bentwich, Z., Siegel, F.P., Kunkel, H.G., Identification of human B and T lymphocyte by scanning election microscopy. J. Exp. Med., 138:607, 1973.
26. Alexander, E., Sanders, S., and Braylan, R.: Purported difference between human T- and B-cell surface morphology in an artifact. Nature, 261:239, 1976.
27. Matter, A., Lisowska-Bernstein, B., Ryser, Y.E., Lamelin, J.P., Vassalli, P.: Mouse thymus independent and thymus-derived lymphoid cells: Ultrastructural studies. J. Exp. Med., 136:1008, 1972.
28. Biberfeld, P.: Morphogenesis in blood lymphocytes stimulated with phytohaemagglutinin (PHA). A light and election microscopic study. Acta Path. Microbiol. Scand. A suppl., 223, 1971.
29. Biberfeld, P. and Mellstedt, H.: Selective activation of human B-lymphocytes by suboptimal doses of pokeweed mitogen. (PWM). Exp. Cell Res., 89:377, 1974.
30. Sundström, C., and Nilsson, K.: Cytochemical profile of human hematopietic biopsy cells and derived cell lines. Br. J. Haematol., 37:489–501, 1977.
31. Rosenberg, Y.J., and Parish, C.R.: Ontogeny of antibody forming cell line in mice. IV: Appearance of cells bearing Fc receptors, complement receptors, and surface immunoglobulin. Immunol., 18:612, 1977.
32. Parkhouse, R.M.E., and Cooper, M.D.: A model for the differentiation of B lymphocytes with implications for the biological role of IgD. Immunological Rev., 37:105, 1977.
33. Preud'homme, J.L., Brouet, J-C., Seligmann, M.: Membrane-bound IgD on human lymphoid cells with special reference to immunodeficiency and immunoproliferative diseases. Immunological Rev., 37:127, 1977.
34. Lay, W.H., and Nussenzweig, V.: Receptions for complement on leukocytes. J. Exp. Med., 128:991, 1968.
35. Dukor, P., Bianco, C., Nussenzweig, V.: Tissue localization of lymphocytes bearing a membrane receptor for antigen-antibody-complement complexes. Proc. Nat. Acad. Sci. (Wash.), 67:991, 1970.
36. Christensson, B. and Biberfeld, P.: Distribution of the Fc and complement receptors in spleen sections. I. Comparison of various erythrocyte indicator systems. Immunol. Method, 19:13, 1978.
37. Stein, H.: The immunologic and immunochemical basis for the Kiel classification. In: Malignant lymphomas, Lennert, K., (ed.), Springer-Verlag, 1978.
38. Dickler, H.B., and Kunkel, H.G.: Interaction of aggregated γ-globulin with B-lymphocytes. J. Exp. Med., 136:191, 1972.

39. Biberfeld, P., Perlmann, P.: Morphological observations on the cytotoxicity of human blood lymphocytes for antibody-coated chicken erythrocytes. Exp. Cell. Res., 62:433, 1970.
40. Billing, R., Rafizadeh, B., Drew, I., Hartman, G., Gale, R., and Terasaki, P.: Human B-lymphocyte antigens expressed by lymphocytic and myelocytic leukemia cells. I. Detection by rabbit antisera. J. Exp. Med., 144:167, 1976.
41. Schlossman, S.F., Chess, L., Humphreys, R.E., and Strominger, J.L.: Distribution of Ia-like molecules on the surface of normal and leukemic human cells. Proc. Nat. Acad. Sci., 73:1288–1292, 1976.
42. Hoffman, T., Yi Wang, Ch., Winchester, R.J., Ferrarini, M., and Kunkel, H.G.: Human lymphocytes bearing "Ia-like" antigens; absence in patients with infantile agammaglobilinemia. J. Immunol., 119:1977.
43. Halper, J., Fu, S.M., Wang, C.Y., Winchester, R., and Kunkel, H.G.: Patterns of expression of human "Ia-like" antigens during the terminal stages of B cell development. J. Immunol., 120:1480, 1978.
44. Klareskog, L.: On the structure, function and tissue distribution of HLA-DR and IA antigens. Thesis, Uppsala, 1978.
45. Janossy, G., Goldstone, A.H., Capellaro, D., Greaves, M.F., Kulenkampff, J., Pippard, M., and Welsh, K.: Differentiation linked expression of p. 28, 33 (Ia-like) structures on human leukaemic cells. Br. J. Haematol., 37, 391, 1977.
46. Koshiba, H., Minowada, J. and Pressman, D.: Rabbit antiserum against a non-T, non-B leukemia cell line that carries the Ph Chromosome (NALM-1): Antibody specific to a non-T, non-B acute lymphoblastic leukemia antigen. J. Natl. Cancer Inst., 61:987, 1978.
47. Greaves, M.F., Brown, G., Rapson, N., and Lister, T.A., Antisera to acute lymphoblastic leukaemia cells. Clin. Immun. Immunopath., 4:67, 1975.
48. Sutherland, R., Smart, J., Niaudet, P., and Greaves, M.: Acute lymphoblastic leukaemia associated antigen-II. Isolation and partial characterisation. Leukemia Research, 2:115–126, 1978.
49. Rodt, H., Netzel, B., Thiel, E., Jäger, G., Huhn, D., Haas, R., Götze, D., and Thierfelder, S.: Classification of leukemic cells with T- and O-ALL-specific antisera. In: Immunological diagnosis of leukemias and lymphomas, Thierfelder et al. (eds), Springer Verlag, 1977.
50. Jondal, M., and Klein, G.: surface markers on human B and T lymphocytes. II. Presence of Epstein-Barr virus receptors on B lymphocytes. J. Exp. Med., 138:1365–1378, 1973.
51. Greaves, M.F., Brown, G., and Rickinson, A.B.: Epstein-Barr virus binding sites on lymphocyte subpopulations and the origin of lymphoblasts in cultured lymphoid cell lines and in the blood of patients with infectious mononucleosis. Clin. Immunol. Immunopathol. 3, 514–524, 1975.
52. Einhorn, L., Steinitz, M., Yefenof, E., Ernberg, I., Bakacs, T. and Klein, G.: Epstein-Barr virus (EBV) receptors, complement receptors, and EBV infectibility of different lymphocyte fractions of human peripheral blood. II. Epstein-Barr Virus Studies. Cellular Immunol. 35:43–58, 1978.
53. Yefenof, E.: Plasma membrane functions and dynamics of normal and trans-human lymphoid cells. Thesis, 1978. Karolinska Institute, Stockholm.
54. Trowbridge, I.S., Hyman, R. and Masauskas, C. Surface molecules of cultured human lymphoid cells. Europ. J. Immunol., 6:77, 1976.
55. Andersson, L.C., Wasastjerna, C. and Gahmberg, C.G.: Different surface glycoprotein patterns on human T-, and B and leukemic lymphocytes. Int. J. Cancer 17:40–46, 1976.

56. Nilsson, K., Andersson, L.C., Gahmberg, C.G., and Wigzell, H.: Surface glyco-protein patterns of normal and malignant human lymphoid cells. II. B cells, B blasts and Epstein-Barr virus (EBV)-positive and negative B lymphoid cell lines. Int. J. Cancer 20:708–716, 1977.

4. T-CELL DIFFERENTIATION AND CHARACTERIZATION

E.J. HENSEN

Since the finding in the early 1970s that lymphocytes could be classified into B and T lymphocytes on the basis of cell-surface determinants, it has become clear that the heterogeneity within the T-lymphocyte population is considerably greater than was expected at that time.

The main defined function of T lymphocytes is the expression of cellular immunity. It is now clear that this cellular immunity includes a diversity of functions. Distinct subpopulations of T lymphocytes have been shown to be involved in those functions that can be *effector* functions, such as delayed-type hypersensitivity, cellular cytotoxicity, and graft rejection, as well as *regulator* functions controlling the magnitude, specificity, and type of both humoral and cellular immune responses (1, 2).

The thymus plays a major role in the maturation sequence of T lymphocytes. Precursors of T lymphocytes originate from pluripotent hematopoietic stem cells and migrate to the thymus. It is assumed that all mature peripheral T lymphocytes (or their progenitors) have been processed within the micro-environment of the thymus. The mechanism by which the thymus influences the maturation and differentiation of T lymphocytes is poorly understood (3).

The way in which T lymphocytes can be recognized will be discussed (in the first and second sections), as well as the sites where differentiation into specialized subpopulations might occur during maturation (in the third and fourth sections). Most of our knowledge of T-lymphocyte characterization and maturation derives from findings in the mouse. The mouse data will be used a guideline, and human equivalents mentioned where possible (2, 4). There is good correlation between the maturation sequences of these two species, but the information about the human system is much more fragmentary.

J.G. van den Tweel et al. (eds.), Malignant Lymphoproliferative Diseases, 49–56
All rights reserved.
Copyright © 1980 by Martinus Nijhoff Publishers bv, The Hague/Boston/London.

PROPERTIES AND CHARACTERISTICS FOR RECOGNITION

Cell-membrane determinants

These can be all structures on the cell surface that can be recognized by:

1) Antibodies directed against those structures. Binding of the antibodies can be demonstrated by several methods, such as cytotoxicity by complement lysis or immunofluorescent staining techniques.
2) Molecules (or cells) which interact specifically with membrane determinants on the cell surface. The best-known example is the spontaneous rosette formation of human T lymphocytes with sheep red blood cells, which is still the main method to recognize human T lymphocytes. The sheep red blood cells bind to a structure only present on those T lymphocytes, and by definition cells not forming E-rosettes are not T lymphocytes. The binding of sheep red blood cells to T lymphocytes is strictly limited to the human situation. The phenomenon was originally observed by chance.

Functional properties

The interest of immunologists in the differentiation of T lymphocytes is a consequence of the divergent functional characteristics of these cells. These functional differences can be demonstrated in a number of in vitro and in vivo essays. Only a few in vitro assays will be mentioned here, i.e., those based on the ability of T lymphocytes to proliferate in vitro on polyclonal stimulation by mitogens such as phytohaemagglutinin (PHA) or concanavalin A (Con A), or to proliferate on specific stimulation by soluble antigens or allogeneic cells in lymphocyte cultures.

Another widely used type of in vitro assay is the cell-mediated lympholysis assay used to test the ability of T lymphocytes to function as cytotoxic effector cells.

Physical properties

The use of differences in physical properties made it possible to obtain enriched populations of lymphocytes with distinct functions and helped to characterize several subpopulations. The methods used were based on special features: The differences in buoyant density of the cells permitted density gradient centrifugation. Differences in size allowed separation by means of velocity sedimentation. Specific differences in electrophoretic mobility could select the cells by cell electrophoresis.

Susceptibility to physical or chemical agents

Susceptibility to various agents can be strikingly different among different subpopulations and can be important, especially for those studying the lymphocytes of patients treated with various drugs. Differences can be found in the susceptibility of subpopulations to X-irradiation, corticosteroids, and anti-lymphocyte sera. Most immunocompetent lymphocytes, for example, are relatively radioresistant and corticosteroid resistant. Immature thymocytes are highly sensitive to radiation or corticosteroid treatment.

Homing properties

Various techniques can be used to demonstrate that migrant cells from the thymus differ in their preference to migrate to lymph node or spleen (lymph-node-seeking or spleen-seeking). There is evidence that this preference might be due to differences in carbohydrate structures on the T lymphocytes.

Enzyme content

Chemical and histochemical techniques can be used to show differences in the enzyme content of cells. Two enzymes will be mentioned here. Terminal deoxynucleotidyl transferase is an intriguing enzyme only present in "T-precommitted" bone marrow stem cells, in immature thymocytes, and some leukemic cells (5). The second enzyme is α-naphtyl acid esterase. Differences in the activity of this enzyme, shown by histochemical techniques, discriminate between subpopulations of human T lymphocytes (6).

DIFFERENTIATION ANTIGENS

Differentation antigens are cell-membrane determinants with differences in expression on the cell during different stages of maturation or specialization of the lymphocytes. Commonly, they are recognized by antibodies. These structures might be of great value for the study and treatment of leukemic patients. In addition, differentiation antigens can contribute to the better classification and characterization of lymphocyte disorders.

The mouse is the species which has been studied most intensively because of the availability of unique congenic strains which make it easy to raise antisera to allogeneic variations of a variety of membrane molecules. In man, some antisera have been described which can recognize a few comparable determinants on human cells, but the sera are still extremely rare.

Table 1. Relative amounts of differentiation antigens detectable on the cell surface of (sub) populations of T lymphocytes during the stages of the maturation sequence.

		Thy 1	H-2	TL	Lyt
Pre-thymic	Thymocyte precursor	$-/+$	$+$	$-$	
Intra-thymic	Cortical thymocytes (85%)	$+++$	$+$	$+++$	1, 2, 3
	Medullary thymocytes (15%)	$+$	$+++$	$+/-$	{ 1, 2, 3 1 or 2, 3
Post-thymic	Early post-thymic T cells (60%)	$++$ $+$	$++$ $+++$	$-$ $-$	1, 2, 3 1, 2, 3
	T helper cells (30%)	$+$	$+++$	$-$	1
	T cytotoxic and suppressor cells (10%)	$+$	$+++$	$-$	2, 3

Note: The density of the differentiation antigens are indicated as low $(+)$, medium $(++)$, high $(+++)$, or absent $(-)$. For Lyt antigens, only those that can be recognized are indicated. The estimated percentages of lymphocytes that can be assigned to a subpopulation are indicated between parentheses.

Mouse differentiation antigens for T lymphocytes (see Table 1) and the presumed human equivalents will be discussed below.

Thy 1 (or θ)

Thy 1 is present on all T lymphocytes, but in different concentrations on distinct populations. Two allelic forms can be detected in the mouse (by alloantisera). Heterologous antisera (raised in other species) do not recognize allospecific determinants on the molecules. Such heterologous antisera can be raised to recognize human T lymphocytes (for example, rabbit-anti-human-T-lymphocyte serum). Such sera have to be extensively absorbed with human cells lacking the relevant antigen (4).

H-2 antigens

These are determinants expressed on the cell surface and coded for by the MHC (major histocompatibility complex) of the mouse. The human homologue of H-2 is HLA (7). Differences in the amount of H-2D and K determinants (human homologues HLA-A and HLA-B, respectively) are found on the cell surface during differentiation. Ia (Immune response associated) determinants are allogeneic determinants on different molecules coded for by the I region of the MHC. They are of particular importance for cell interaction during the immune response. Only some of the mature T lymphocytes express detectable amounts on their surface. The human equivalent of the Ia determinants are very probably the HLA-DR determinants (8).

TL antigens

These determinants were originally found on leukemic cells in certain mouse strains. Their expression is under genetic control by a locus close to the H-2 complex. Healthy mice of several strains express the TL antigens on their immature thymocytes. Chess and Schlossman reported an antiserum which, after extensive absorptions, may recognize a human homologue of the TL antigens present on both thymocytes and leukemic lymphocytes of some patients with T-cell variety of acute lymphoblastic leukemia (4).

Ly(t) antigens

Lyt (or Ly) alloantigens in mice were originally described by Boyse. Each locus (1, 2, and 3) codes for allelic variants. Different combinations of Ly antigens have been described in functionally distinct T lymphocyte subpopulations (2). Recently, Evans et al. reported on a possible human homologue for the Lyt 2 or 3 antigens (9). The results obtained with rosette formation of human T lymphocytes with IgM *versus* IgG coated erythrocytes also suggest the existence of different subpopulations of human T lymphocytes (6).

MATURATION SEQUENCE OF T LYMPHOCYTES

Three separate maturation stages (see Table 1) can be recognized, but it is not known which cells make the transition from one stage to the next.

Pre-thymic

In the bone marrow (or in the liver in early life) some of the "pluripotent" stem cells differentiate to a prethymic precursor cell, committed to a T-cell program. The stimulus for this step is unknown. In the mouse, these cells are at least in part Thy 1 negative (the commitment to "T" may be determined by the presence of the enzyme terminal deoxynucleotidyl transferase). These Thy 1-negative cells can be induced to express Thy 1 antigen by soluble thymic factors (10).

By the induction of Thy 1 expression on the cell or some other (unknown) trigger, thymic factors might cause the precommitted cells to migrate to the thymus via the blood circulation.

Many cells enter the thymus, but only the priviliged precursor cells with the right key determinants on their surface will be allowed to pass through the epithelial barrier around the vessels and enter the parenchyme of the thymus.

Intrathymic

The precursor cells migrate in the thymus, presumably to the outer cortex, and proliferate under the selective control of the micro-environment of epithelial cells. The cortical thymocyte population is, at least in part, the result of the proliferation of these immigrant cells.

Two major populations of lymphocytes can be recognized inside the thymus, each in a separate compartment. The cortex contains the cortical thymocytes (approximately 85% of the total), which are small and have a relatively high buoyant density, low expression of H-2 antigens, and high expression of Thy 1 and all three Lyt antigens. The medulla contains a functionally relatively mature population of medullary thymocytes (about 15% of the total). They are medium-sized or large, have a low density, and express a high amount of H-2 antigens and low amounts of Thy 1. Some of these cells express either Lyt 1 or the combination Lyt 2 and 3 and have the functional characteristics of the mature T lymphocytes, which also carry either Lyt 1 or Lyt 2 and 3. Recently, evidence has been accumulating that the thymus is not only a site of random proliferation but also a site for the selection of cells.

Experimental results suggest that either only selected precursor cells can develop in the thymus or only selected "mature" thymocytes are allowed to leave the thymus. Zinkernagel et al. (11) and Waldmann (12) have pointed out that the abilities of T lymphocytes to interact in the immune response are imposed by the thymic environment.

Post-thymic

It is still not clear which cells of the thymus migrate to the periphery, and under what conditions they do so. Homing properties of the cells like spleen-seeking or lymph-node-seeking have been described, but they cannot be explained in relation to the later mature function. A residual population might remain under the influence of a thymic humoral factor.

MATURE SUBPOPULATIONS

A classification of mature T lymphocytes into subpopulations cannot be reached as a logical consequence of the maturation sequence. A few years ago, Cantor presented considerable evidence for the existence of at least two subpopulations of mature T lymphocytes in the mouse on the basis of Lyt phenotypes and functional properties (2):

a) helper T lymphocytes, which increase the magnitude of an immune response, are characterized by the expression of only Lyt 1 (no Lyt 2 or 3), and b) suppressor cells and cytotoxic cells, which can inhibit an immune response or have specific cytolytic activity, respectively. These cells are characterized by the expression of both Lyt 2 and 3 exclusively (no Lyt 1). Differentiation into subpopulations must occur before antigen-specific immunocompetence is realized, but the exact moment is unknown.

In man the results obtained on the basis of rosette formation with IgM *versus* IgG coupled to erythrocytes as well as by histochemical techniques can be used to discriminate between subpopulations expressing either helper or suppressor functions in immune response assays (6).

New data obtained from functional-assay studies in both humans and mice have shown that there may be several more specialized subpopulations of T lymphocytes for controlling the immune response (Figure 1), but the characterization of these subpopulations is still incomplete (13). More data on the mature subpopulations of the human system are discussed elsewhere in this book (chapters 2 and 7).

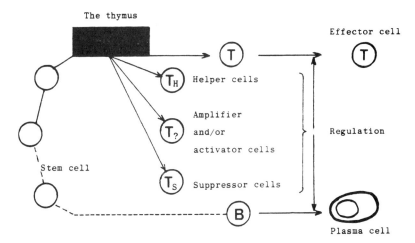

Figure 1. Simplified schematic representation of T-cell maturation and differentiation. A presumed stem cell differentiates into either a T- or B-committed precursor cell. The T-committed precursor cells migrate to the thymus where they proliferate and develop under the selective control of the thymic environment. Cells leaving the thymus give rise to the peripheral T lymphocytes, which in turn become the potential effector cells for cellular immunity or members of a family of regulator lymphocytes controlling both humoral and cellular immune responses.

ACKNOWLEGEMENT
I wish to acknowledge the valuable critical comments I received from Dr. J. D'Amaro during the preparation of this paper.

REFERENCES

1. Cantor, H., and Weissman, I.: Development and function of subpopulations of thymocytes and T lymphocytes. Progr. Allergy, 20:1–64, 1976.
2. Cantor, H., and Boyse, E.: Regulation of the immune response by T-cell subclasses. In: T cells. Contemporary topics in immunobiology, Vol. 7, pp. 47–65, Stutman, O., (ed.), Plenum Press, New York, 1977.
3. Stutman, O.: Intrathymic and extrathymic T-cell maturation. Immunol. Rev., 42:139–184, 1978.
4. Chess, L., and Schlossman, S.F.: Human lymphocyte subpopulations. Adv. Immunol., 25:213–241, 1977.
5. McCaffrey, R., Harrison, T.A., Parkman, R., and Baltimore, D.: Terminal deoxynucleotidyl transferase activity in human leukemic cells and in normal human thymocytes. N. Engl. J. Med., 292:775–780, 1975.
6. Grossi, C.E., Webb, S.R., Zicca, A., Lydyard, P.M., Moretta, L., Mingari, M.C., and Cooper, M.C.: Morphological and histochemical analyses of two human subpopulations bearing receptors for IgM or IgG. J. Exp. Med., 147:1405–1417, 1978.
7. Bach, F.H., and van Rood, J.J.: The major histocompatibility complex— Genetics and biology. N. Engl. J. Med., 295:806–813, 872–878, 927–936, 1976.
8. van Rood, J.J., and van Leeuwen, A.: The serology of HLA-DR. In: Clinical immunobiology, chapter IV, Good, R.A., and Bach, F.H., (eds.), Academic Press, New York, in press.
9. Evans, R.L., Lazarus, H., Penta, A.C., and Schlossman, S.F.: Two functionally distinct subpopulations of human T cells, that collaborate in the generation of cytotoxic cells, responsible for cell mediated lympholysis. J. Immunol., 120:1423–1428, 1978.
10. Bach, J.F., and Carnaud, C.: Thymic factors. Progr. Allergy., 21:342–408, 1978.
11. Zinkernagel, R.M.: Thymus and lymphopoietic cells: their role in T-cell maturation. Immunol. Rev., 42:224–270, 1978.
12. Waldmann, H.: The influence of the MHC on the function of T helper cells in antibody formation. Immunol. Rev., 42:202–223, 1978.
13. Broder, S., and Waldmann, T.A.: The suppressor-cell network in cancer. N. Engl. J. Med., 299:1281–1284, 1335–1341, 1978.

5. DIFFERENT RETICULUM CELLS OF THE LYMPH NODE: MICROECOLOGICAL CONCEPT OF LYMPHOID TISSUE ORGANIZATION

H.K. MÜLLER-HERMELINK AND E. KAISERLING

INTRODUCTION

Both immunological reactivity to antigens and polyclonal lymphocyte activation by mitogens can only be induced in vitro by the cooperative action of different types of cell (39, 50). The magnitude of the resulting immune phenomena is determined not only by the number of active partners but also by the absence or presence of inhibiting factors or cells, or by the "quality" of the cooperation. There are indications that the number of macrophages present determines whether immunostimulation or immunotolerance will occur in antigen-induced B-cell activation at a given dose of antigen and a given number of B and T cells.

In vivo, the complicated process of cooperation among various types of cells in immune reactions has to be optimal for biologically meaningful immune reactions to occur. That means that the cooperation must be structurally organized at places where immune reactions are induced, namely, in lymphoid tissue.

These considerations and speculations led to a detailed study of the structural cells in human lymphoid tissue.

NOMENCLATURE OF RETICULUM CELLS

According to the original definition, reticulum cells make up the stationary part of "lymphoreticular" tissue. With their cellular processes, they form a loose network within which lymphocytes and other free cells can circulate. In histology textbooks reticulum cells are described as stellate cells with slender processes, a pale, oval or polymorphic, leptochromatic nucleus, a distinct nuclear membrane, a small nucleolus, and nonbasophilic cytoplasm (21). This description is inaccurate, however, because several types of cell with a pale nucleus have been included under the term reticulum cell.

As early as the time of Aschoff, reticulum cells were considered to have

J.G. van den Tweel et al. (eds.), Malignant Lymphoproliferative Diseases, 57–70
All rights reserved.
Copyright © 1980 by Martinus Nijhoff Publishers bv, The Hague/Boston/London.

two functions: (a) fiber formation and (b) phagocytosis. At present, it is recognized that these functions are fulfilled by different types of cells, one of them being a true primary stationary cell and the other probably a mono-cyte-derived cell that secondarily migrates to the lymphoid tissue. The whole concept of the reticuloendothelial system (RES) has been challenged and has been replaced by the mononuclear phagocyte system (MPS) (11, 12).

Numerous hypotheses and speculations presented in the past twenty years have led to a chaotic situation around the term reticulum cell. Some new proposals that a distinction be made between reticul*um* and reticul*ar* cells (5) have added even more confusion. Nevertheless, what still holds since the original definition and is well known to all students of histology, is the concept of cells forming a stationary framework in which freely cir-culating cells can home, or pass through, or transform to fulfill special func-tions.

FOUR TYPES OF RETICULUM CELLS

During the last ten years, experimental work on the histophysiology of lymphoid tissue in rabbits (15, 48, 49) and rats (9, 47) and morphologic studies on human lymphoid tissue (18, 19, 29, 32, 33) have led to a more precise understanding of the nonlymphoid cells in lymphoid tissue. Using electron microscopy, enzyme histochemistry, and cytochemistry, we can now differentiate four types of reticulum cell (29, 32, 33). These cells are distributed unevenly in the cortical tissue of lymph nodes, one type is speci-fically located in B areas and another in T areas; the other two types of reticulum cell are not specifically confined to either of these areas. The four types comprise

1) Fibroblastic reticulum cells, which are seen in various regions of the lymph node and are associated with, and probably also produce, argyrophil fibers.

2) Dendritic reticulum cells, which are found only in the lymph follicles and in adjacent B regions. They are most prominent in germinal centers.

3) Histiocytic reticulum cells, which correspond to tissue macrophages and probably belong to the MPS. They are seen as so-called starry-sky mac-rophages containing cellular debris in germinal centers. In paracortical regions, histiocytic reticulum cells show other substances within their phagolysosomes, e.g., melanin, ceroid, and other lipoid substances.

4) Interdigitating reticulum cells, which are seen exclusively in T regions.

These different types of cell can be differentiated by enzyme histochemical methods and electron microscopy. We should point out, however, that with routine light microscopy they are only recognizable with great difficulty, if at all. Thus, the reason we use the conventional term reticulum cell to cover all these cell types is more pragmatic than cytogenetically justified. Each type appears to have a different function, origin, and turnover. Our understanding of these parameters is incomplete. For this reason, and to facilitate general understanding, we at present qualify the term reticulum cell with an adjective indicating a certain functional or morphologic attribute of the cells traditionally defined as nonlymphoid structural cells. Until more information is available, we prefer this terminology to more sophisticated names.

FUNCTIONAL, ULTRASTRUCTURAL, AND HISTOCHEMICAL FEATURES OF
RETICULUM CELLS IN HUMAN LYMPH NODES

Fibroblastic reticulum cells (synonym: fiber-associated reticulum cells)

Fibroblastic reticulum cells of lymph nodes are localized mainly in the neighborhood of intermediary sinuses and small blood vessels, especially at the borderline of T regions. This type of reticulum cell is identifiable by a positive alkaline phosphatase reaction; neutral nonspecific esterase and acid phosphatase activities are weak or moderate. Fibroblastic reticulum cells form a continuum with adventitial cells of blood vessels. These two types of cell cannot be clearly distinguished by ultrastructural features or cytochemistry unless their relation to other structures (blood vessels, lymphoid cells) is taken into consideration.

Ultrastructurally, fibroblastic reticulum cells show an oblong nucleus with a finely indented margin. Nuclear chromatin is coarse. The nucleolus is small; nucleospheroids are seen occasionally. The cytoplasm contains a moderate amount of ergastoplasm. In addition, there are varying amounts of fine filaments, which are probably actin fibrils. Immunocytochemical demonstration of the actin content of reticulum cells in lymph nodes revealed a relatively high actin content in cells that could be assumed to be fibroblastic reticulum cells (7).

A special characteristic of fibroblastic reticulum cells is their relationship to reticulin fibers. Hemidesmosomal junctions are seen at the cytomembrane adjacent to associated reticulin fibers. On the cytoplasmic side of the membrane, filaments converge toward the membrane, condense there, and appear to break through the membrane and penetrate into the adjacent fibers. This peculiar relationship between cells and adjacent fibers is not found for the other types of reticulum cell or for fibroblasts or fibrocytes in connective tissue. In the latter, the fibers are of another collagen type and there is only sparse interfibrillar basement membranelike material.

Fibroblastic reticulum cells are often extremely electron-dense. They might correspond to the so-called dark reticulum cells described in animals and man (17, 27). This type of staining might also be a consequence of intra- or supravital damage to the cells (30). There is still no definite answer, however, to the question as to whether "dark" reticulum cells are special functional differentiation forms or merely artifacts. An investigation of fibroblastic reticulum cells and their relationship to myofibroblasts in scarring lymph node lesions would thus be of interest.

Dendritic reticulum cells

Dendritic reticulum cells are found exclusively in B-cell regions of lymphoid tissue. Their ultrastructure has been known for a long time. Swartzen-druber (44, 49) and Milanesi (26) described nonphagocytosing cells connected by desmoses in cortical lymphoid tissue of lymph nodes of rats and dogs, respectively. The capacity of dendritic reticulum cells to retain antigen at their cytoplasmic processes, and the importance of this capacity for antibody formation was demonstrated by Nossal et al. (34). Recently, the nondegradation and persistence of antigen at the cellular processes of dendritic reticulum cells in immune lymph nodes was related to the regulation of serum antibody formation (46). The fixation of antigen is probably mediated via an antibody connected by its Fc fragments to Fc receptors on the cytomembrane of the cells. In contrast to antigen that comes into contact with macrophages, this antigen does not become internalized and degraded in phagolysosomes (46).

Cytochemically, dendritic reticulum cells are recognizable by high activity of 5'-nucleotidase and neutral nonspecific esterase. The acid phosphatase reaction is usually negative, as are the alkaline phosphatase and ATPase reactions. Double-staining and specific inactivation studies clearly established the distinction between fibroblastic reticulum cells and dendritic reticulum cells at the margins of B-cell regions of lymphoid tissue (28).

Ultrastructurally, dendritic reticulum cells have an oval or angular nucleus with relatively coarse chromatin. They are frequently binucleate. The nucleolus is composed of interwoven nucleolonemata; nucleospheroids are frequent. In germinal centers the fine, elongated projections of dendritic reticulum cells form a myceliumlike web with other dendritic reticulum cells and adjacent centroblasts. The cellular processes of dendritic reticulum cells are often connected by desmosomes. At the margins of germinal centers, the dendritic reticulum cells are elongated and show a bipolar orientation. A similar pattern of dendritic reticulum cells is found in primary follicles of lymphoid tissue. Membrane activation and cellular proliferation of dendritic reticulum cells apparently occur during the formation of germinal centers.

Histiocytic reticulum cells

Histiocytic reticulum cells are found in various areas of lymphoid tissue and fulfill various duties. In lymph-node sinuses this type of reticulum cell takes the form of a round cell. In the lymph-node parenchyme, they show a sub-sinusoidal localization in the paracortical pulp, and in germinal centers they occur as so-called starry-sky cells.

It is not yet clear to what extent blood-borne moncytes and/or macrophages in the afferent lymph contribute to the population of histiocytic reticulum cells and their turnover in lymph nodes. Nevertheless, a majority of histiocytic reticulum cells are apparently part of the MPS. Once settled in the lymph node, they are relatively long-lived and occasionally show mitotic division as a sign of local regeneration.

The distribution of histiocytic reticulum cells in lymphoid tissue has a characteristic pattern and does not appear to be related to inflammatory or phagocytotic stimuli. This pattern is already recognizable during ontogeny. On the basis of differences in ultrahistochemical features Daems and co-workers (6) discuss the possibility that noninflammatory, fixed ("tissue-type") macrophages, which correspond to histiocytic reticulum cells, constitute a separate type of cell differing from the wandering moncyte-derived macrophages of the MPS.

Histo- and cytochemically, histiocytic reticulum cells are characterized by high activity of acid phosphatase and neutral nonspecific esterase. The ATPase reaction is weak or negative. The alkaline phosphatase and 5'-nucleotidase reactions are negative.

Ultrastructurally, histiocytic reticulum cells have an oval nucleus with finely dispersed chormatin and a medium-sized nucleolus. The cytoplasm often has relatively large Golgi areas and well-developed smooth and rough endoplasmic reticulum. The rough endoplasmic reticulum is usually made up of short strands. There are numerous phagolysosomes with varying contents. On the basis of the contents of the phagolysosomes, two different functions can be distinguished: (a) intrinsic clearance of cellular debris at sites of high cellular turnover (such phagolysosomes are found in starry-sky cells in germinal centers and malignant tumors such as Burkitt's lymphoma), and (b) extrinsic clearance of bacteria, antigens, and any type of foreign substance transported mainly via afferent lymph. The second of these functions is chiefly fulfilled by intrasinusoidal, subsinusoidal, and paracortical histiocytic reticulum cells, whose phagolysosomes contain residual bodies with various structures, lipoid substances, ceroid, melanin, etc.

Interdigitating reticulum cells

Interdigitating reticulum cells are found exclusively in T-cell areas of peripheral lymphoid tissue and in the thymic medulla. It is not yet known whether these cells have a proliferative potential. Experimental investigations (47, 48, 49), ontogenetic analyses of thymuses and lymph nodes (25, 32), and studies on human diseases (18, 22, 38) have indicated that the formation of interdigitating reticulum cells is related to cells that enter the lymphoid tissue and become secondarily fixed in T-cell areas, where they come into special contact with T lymphocytes (49). Two cell types have been discussed as possible progenitors of interdigitating reticulum cells: (a) monocytes, as suggested by studies done in the spleen (47) and thymus (14) and on the ontogeny of lymph node (25), and (b) Langerhans cells of the skin, as suggested by experimental investigations of rat lymph nodes (20) and studies on human dermatopathic lymphadenitis (38). These two possibilities need not be exclusive, since Langerhans cells, or their precursors, might be closely related to monocytes.

The function of interdigitating reticulum cells is unknown. Some very indirect evidence suggests that precursors of interdigitating reticulum cells (e.g., Langerhans cells of the skin) migrate to lymph nodes via the afferent lymph and are then involved in antigen presentation to T cells (20). Fc receptors for IgG have been found both on Langerhans cells of the skin (43) and on some interdigitating reticulum cells (40). These might be receptors related to antigen presentation. The very intimate contact between interdigitating reticulum cells and adjacent T cells in T-cell areas and in the thymic medulla also suggests that interdigitating reticulum cells have some function in T-cell differentiation and proliferation (18, 48).

Histo- and cytochemically, interdigitating reticulum cells can be identified by the high ATPase reactivity of their cytomembrane. Furthermore, neutral nonspecific esterase activity is very weak, and acid phosphatase is found only in the paranuclear Golgi region. The alkaline phosphatase and 5'-nucleotidase reactions are negative (33).

The ultrastructure of interdigitating reticulum cells was first described by Veldman (48) who found that it characterized a separate type of cell in the paracortical region of rabbit lymph nodes. The nucleus is very irregular in shape and often deeply indented. Chromatin is finely dispersed. There is usually a marginal nucleolus. Cytoplasm tends to be abundant and electron-transparent. Very near the nucleus there is a relatively large Golgi area with numerous vesicles, some of which contain electron-dense material and thus suggest a secretory function. Phagolysosomes are usually absent (even when histiocytic reticulum cells in the direct vicinity have engulfed large amounts of various substances). There are numerous short profiles and vesicles of rough and smooth endoplasmic reticulum forming the so-called tubulovesicular system, which is sometimes arranged in concentric layers. This system stains positively with silver methenamine. The cell surface shows broad cytoplasmic projections, which interdigitate with those of other "interdigitating" reticulum cells and establish intimate contact with adjacent T cells by fingerlike cytoplasmic indentations. Sometimes, lymphocytes appear to be engulfed in the cytoplasm of interdigitating reticulum cells. Degradation of cells or formation of phagosomes is never seen, however. This suggests emperipolesis, which may be interpreted as a distinct expression of cellular contacts.

ONTOGENY OF HUMAN LYMPH NODES, WITH EMPHASIS ON RETICULUM CELLS

Lymph-node development starts during the sixth week of gestation with the formation of primitive vascular and mesenchymal buds in the close vicinity of dilatations of lymph channels (1, 4, 8, 15). The cellularity of these mesenchymal buds increases until the 12th week of gestation. Hematopoietic cells (mostly granulocytopoietic cells and monocytes) and some lymphoid cells are evenly distributed in the lumen of the lymph vessel and in early lymphnode tissue. Histiocytic reticulum cells first appear between the 10th and 12th weeks; they are interspersed among sinus endothelial cells. During the 12th week, some cells that are morphologically reminiscent of interdigitating reticulum cells or promonocytes (which are also seen in the hematopoietic foci) are found in the close vicinity of lymph sinuses; some of these cells must pass through the sinus walls. By the 13th week, nodular areas are evident; these contain a characteristic mixture of interdigitating reticulum cells and lymphoid cells. Fibroblastic cells derived from the perivascular mesenchyme are found at the margins of such areas. The T-cell areas reach maturity by the end of the 16th week.

Dendritic reticulum cells are first seen at subsinusoidal and perivascular localizations in the outer cotex of developing lymph nodes during the 13th and 16th weeks of gestation. The formation of primary follicles and the maturation of B areas in the lymph node do not occur, however, until the 22nd week.

From these ontogenetic findings, one may conclude that the various types of reticulum cell differ in origin. Fibroblastic and dendritic reticulum cells are probably derived from the perivascular mesenchyme, whereas histiocytic and interdigitating recticulum cells appear to be related to the cells in the hematopoietic foci, particularly monocytes.

THE MICROECOLOGICAL CONCEPT OF LYMPHOID TISSUE ORGANISATION

The demonstration of different types of reticulum cell in lymphoid tissue provides a formal explanation of the phenomenon of ecotaxis (42), the mechanism by which T and B lymphocytes "home" to different places in lymphoid tissue. The T- and B-cell areas are constant tissue compartments organized by different sets of reticulum cells. During ontogeny, the "lymphoid" structure of the early T- and B-cell areas is not formed until characteristic reticulum cells have appeared. In view of the different origins of reticulum cells, primarily fixed reticulum cells (fibroblastic and dendritic) may be distinguished from secondarily fixed reticulum cells (interdigitating and histiocytic). Although pre-B cells, surface immunoglobulinbearing mature B lymphocytes, and functionally active T lymphocytes are found somewhat earlier than histologically mature T- and B-cell compartments in fetal liver, blood, and lymphoid tissue (13, 35), the maturation of these compartments and the differentiation of their specific reticulum cells coincide with the functional maturation of the immune response.

Thus, the microecological concept not only takes into account the topographical association between fixed and circulating cells, but also describes the structural basis of normal immune reactivity and immune regulation.

THE MICROECOLOGICAL CONCEPT IN RELATION TO PATHOLOGICAL CHANGES IN LYMPHOID TISSUE

For obvious reasons, only a few examples can be given here. They have been selected to elucidate some special aspects of the relationship between interdigitating reticulum cells and other types of cell (Langerhans cells, monocytes) and of the relationship between the different types of reticulum cell and neoplastic lymphoid cells.

Dermatopathic lymphadenitis

Dermatopathic lymphadenitis (18, 38) is a good human model in which to investigate interdigitating reticulum cells. On light microscopy, the paracortical region of the lymph node is enlarged, owing to an increase in the number of reticulum cells. These cells have been identified by electron microscopy as interdigitating reticulum cells (18, 38). Their ultrastructural appearance and enzyme-cytochemical reaction pattern are identical to those of interdigitating reticulum cells seen in normal lymphoid tissue. Dermatopathic lymphadenitis is found only in skin-associated lymph nodes.

A remarkable finding was the presence of Langerhans cells with typical Birbeck granules among the interdigitating reticulum cells in all of the cases of dermatopathic lymphadenitis we have studied so far. The Langerhans cells were connected to the interdigitating reticulum cells in a fashion corresponding to the typical structural relationship between cells of the latter type. Furthermore, there were no ultrastructural or histochemical (ATPase, acid phosphatase, neutral nonspecific esterase) differences between the two cell types except for the presence of Birbeck granules in the Langerhans cells.

Langerhans cells were found not only in the paracortical region, but also in the marginal sinuses of lymph nodes. This finding indicates that Langerhans cells enter the lymph node by migration from the skin to the node via the afferent lymph. Experiments in rabbits have shown that Langerhans cells containing antigen are present in dermal afferent lymphatics (41).

The cytogenetic and functional relationships between Langerhans cells and interdigitating reticulum cells are still unclear. Since dermatopathic lymphadenitis is a special reaction of skin-associated lymph nodes, findings in this lesion do not apply to other lymphoid tissues, such as deep lymph nodes, the spleen, or the thymic medulla.

Sarcoidosis

In lymph nodes subtotally involved by sarcoidosis, it is obvious that the epithelioid cell granulomas are initially formed in T-cell regions. Even when the lymph node is almost completely infiltrated by epithelioid cells, the 5'-nucleotidase reactions and the demonstration of complement receptors (the latter are markers of B-cell regions) reveal that the intergranulomatous lymphoid tissue belongs to B-cell regions; T-cell regions are not seen.

In view of the close relationship of interdigitating reticulum cells and monocytes, the question arose whether interdigitating reticulum cells are altered by the granulomatous process. Electron microscopy has revealed "untouched" interdigitating reticulum cells even within epithelioid cell granulomas in sarcoidosis. The interdigitating reticulum cells were easily distinguishable from epithelioid cells, because the former showed no structural alterations. One may conclude that monocytes and interdigitating reticulum cells behave in different ways in the formation of epithelioid cell granulomas: monocytes transform into epithelioid cells and form granulomas, whereas interdigitating reticulum cells in the altered T regions of the lymph node do not appear to change to any significant degree.

These observations indicate that even if interdigitating reticulum cells are derived from monocytes (47), they may behave differently from monocytes under functional or pathological conditions.

Malignant lymphomas

The microecological concept has also been evaluated in malignant lymphomas (22). The distribution of reticulum cells in non-Hodgkin's lymphomas of low-grade malignancy, which are monoclonal proliferations of various types of lymphoid cell, reveals that most tumors of B-lymphocytic origin contain dendritic reticulum cells, whereas tumors of T-lymphocytic origin contain interdigitating reticulum cells.

The microecological pattern of normal lymphoid tissue has been found to be preserved in low-grade malignant lymphomas. This is shown best by comparing centroblastic/centrocytic lymphoma (formerly known as giant follicular lymphoma) with T-zone lymphoma. Centroblastic/centrocytic lymphoma regularly shows the specific reticulum cells of normal primary follicles and germinal centers, namely, dendritic reticulum cells. These are connected by desmosomes (23) and exhibit the typical enzyme histochemical reaction pattern of normal dendritic reticulum cells. Interfollicular areas can be identified as nonneoplastic T zones by the presence of opithelioid venules and interdigitating reticulum cells, whereas in T-zone lymphoma the neoplastic polymorphic T lymphocytes are found in close contact with interdigitating reticulum cells. In addition, a typical pattern of alkaline phosphatase-positive fibroblastic reticulum cells is seen around the neoplastic T zones. These neoplastic areas are situated very near nonneoplastic B regions which sometimes contain germinal centers.

In high-grade malignant lymphomas, the microecological pattern of normal lymphoid tissue is usually not preserved.

The microecological pattern in Hodgkin's disease was first studied in so-called nodular paragranuloma (24, 37). Results of analyses with the immunoperoxidase technique, electron-microscopical investigations of the nodules, and clinical follow-up support the view that nodular paragranuloma is a tumor of B-lymphocyte origin and is related to progressively transformed germinal centers (22, 36).

Although other types of Hodgkin's disease have not been studied in detail in this respect some of the data in the literature (22) and our own findings indicate, that T zones are involved initially, at least in the nodular-sclerosis and mixed-cellularity types of Hodgkin's disease. The relationship between interdigitating reticulum cells and Sternberg-Reed cells or lacunar cells has not been clarified. In Hodgkin's disease it seems, however, that reticulum cells are involved in the neoplastic process, whereas they are not involved in non-Hodgkin's lymphomas.

SUMMARY

In normal human lymphoid tissue, four types of reticulum cell can be identified by ultrastructural and cytochemical criteria, viz.: fibroblastic, dendritic, histiocytic, and interdigitating reticulum cells. Ontogenetic studies and experimental data have indicated that fibroblastic and dendritic reticulum cells are probably locally derived from the mesenchyme, whereas histiocytic and interdigitating reticulum cells are derived from circulating precursors (e.g., monocytes). Thus, primarily fixed and secondarily fixed types of reticulum cells may be distinguished. Two of the types of reticulum cell occur exclusively in B or T-cell regions, viz.: dendritic reticulum cells in B regions and interdigitating reticulum cells in T regions. Fibroblastic reticulum cells are concentrated mainly at the borderline between T and B regions. Histiocytic reticulum cells are localized (a) in germinal centers, where they are also known as starry-sky cells (showing intrinsic phagocytosis), (b) interspersed among sinus endothelial cells in subsinusoidal areas, and (c) at the margins of T regions (at the last two sites the cells show extrinsic phagocytosis).

Specific reticulum cells are closely associated with the formation of B and T areas during ontogeny. The histotopographical relationship between the different fixed reticulum cells and various subpopulations of circulating lymphoid cells has been interpreted in a microecological concept of lymphoid tissue organization. This concept describes the cellular cooperation processes that are necessary as a basis for immunostimulation and immunoregulation.

The validity of the microecological concept has been assessed in a number of reactive changes in lymph node structure, sarcoidosis, and malignant lymphomas. Not only has the study of reticulum cells in lymphoid tissue provided basic information, but the microecological concept has proven to be of diagnostic help in the interpretation of histologic alterations in lymphoid tissue.

REFERENCES

1. Ackermann, G.A.: Developmental relationship between the appearance of lymphocytes and lymphopoetic activity in the thymus and lymph nodes of the fetal cat. Anat. Rec., 158:387–400, 1967.
2. Bailey, R.P., and Weiss, L.: Ontogeny of human fetal lymph nodes. Am. J. Anat., 142:15–28, 1975.
3. Bryant, B.J.: The histo- and morphogenesis of lymph nodes: An interpretation of some mechanisms. J. Reticuloendothel. Soc., 16:96–104, 1974.
4. Bryant, B.J., and Shifrine, M.: Histogenesis of lymph nodes during development of the dog. J. Reticuloendothel. Soc., 12:96–107, 1972.
5. Carr, I.: The macrophage. A review of ultrastructure and function. Academic Press, London-New York, 1973.
6. Daems, W.T., Korten, H.K., and Soranzo, M.R.: Differences between monocyte-derived and tissue macrophages. In: The reticuloendothelial system in health and disease. Adv. Exp. Med. Biol., vol. 73A, pp. 27–40, Reichard, S.M., Escobar, M.R., and Friedman, H., (eds.), Plenum Press, New York-London, 1976.
7. Drenkhahn, D.: personal communication, 1979.
8. Eikelenboom, P., Nassy, J.J.J., Post, J., Versteeg, J.C.M.B., and Langevoort, H.L.: The histogenesis of lymph nodes in rat and rabbit. Anat. Rec., 190:201–216, 1978.
9. Van Ewijk, W., Verzijden, J.H.M., Van der Kwast, T.H., and Luijcx-Meijer,

S.W.M.: Reconstitution of the thymus dependent area in the spleen of lethally irradiated mice. Cell Tiss. Res., 149:43–60, 1974.

10. Frieß, A.: Interdigitating reticulum cells in the popliteal lymph node of the rat. Cell Tiss. Res., 170:43–60, 1976.

11. Van Furth, R., Cohn, Z.A., Hirsch, J.G., Humphrey, J.H., Spector, W.G., and Langevoort, H.G.: The mononuclear phagocyte system: A new classification of macrophages, monocytes, and their precursor cells. Bull. Wld. Hlth. Org., 46:845–852, 1972.

12. Van Furth, R., Langevoort, H.L., and Schaberg, A.: Mononuclear phagocytes in human pathology—Proposal for an approach to improved classification. In: Mononuclear phagocytes in immunity, infection, and pathology, pp. 1–15., Van Furth, R., (ed.), Blackwell, Oxford-London-Edinburgh-Melbourne, 1975.

13. Gathings, W.E., Lawton, A.R., and Cooper, M.D.: Immunfluorescent studies of the development of pre-B cells, B lymphocytes and immunoglobulin isotype diversity in humans. Eur. J. Immunol., 7:804–810, 1977.

14. Von Gaudecker, B., and Müller-Hermelink, H.K.: Ontogenetic differentiation of epithelial and non-epithelial cells in the human thymus. In: Function and structure of the immune system. Adv. Exp. Med. Biol., vol. 114, pp. 19–23, Müller-Ruchholtz, W., and Müller-Hermelink, H.K., (eds.), Plenum Press, New York-London, 1979.

15. Hoefsmit, E.C.M.: Mononuclear phagocytes, reticulum cells, and dendritic cells in lymphoid tissues. In: Mononuclear phagocytes in immunity, infection, and pathology, pp. 129–146, Van Furth, R., (ed.), Oxford-London-Edinburgh-Melbourne: Blackwell 1975.

16. Hostetler, J.A., and Ackermann, G.A.: Lymphopoiesis and lymph node histogenesis in the embryonic and neonatal rabbit. Am. J. Anat., 124:57–75, 1969.

17. Izard, J., and DeHarven, E.: Increased numbers of characteristic type of reticular cell in the thymus and lymph nodes of leukemic mice: An electron microscope study. Cancer Res., 28:421–433, 1968.

18. Kaiserling, E., and Lennert, K.: Die interdigitierende Reticulumzelle im menschlichen Lymphknoten—Eine spezifische Zelle der thymusabhängigen Region. Virchows Arch. B., 16:51–61, 1974.

19. Kaiserling, E., Stein, H., and Müller-Hermelink, H.K.: Interdigitating reticulum cell in the human thymus. Cell Tiss. Res., 155:47–55, 1974.

20. Kamperdijk, E.W.A., Raamakers, E.M., de Leeuw, J.H.S., and Hoefsmit, E.C.M.: Lymph node macrophages and reticulum cells in the immune response. I. The primary response to paratyphoid vaccine. Cell Tiss. Res., 192: 1–23, 1978.

21. Lennert, K.: Lymphknoten. Diagnostik in Schnitt und Ausstrich. Bandteil A: Cytologie und Lymphadenitis. Handb. d. spez. path. Anat. u. Histol., vol. I/3A. Lubarsch, O., Henke, F., Rössle, R., and Uehlinger, E., (eds.), Springer, Berlin-Göttingen-Heidelberg, 1961.

22. Lennert, K., Kaiserling, E., and Müller-Hermelink, H.K.: Malignant lymphomas: Models of differentiation and cooperation of lymphoreticular cells. In: Differentiation of normal and neoplastic hematopoietic cells, Book B. Cold Spring Harbor Conferences on Cell Proliferation, vol. 5, pp. 897–913. Clarkson, B., Marks, P.A., and Till, J.E., (eds.), Cold Spring Harbor Laboratory, Cold Spring Harbor, 1978.

23. Lennert, K., and Niedorf, H.R.: Nachweis von desmosomal verknüpften Retikulumzellen im follikulären Lymphom (Brill Symmers). Virchows Arch., B., 4:149–150, 1969.

24. Lukes, R.J., Butler, J.J., and Hicks, E.B.: Natural history of Hodgkin's disease as related to its pathologic picture. Cancer, 19:317–344, 1966.
25. Markgraf, R., von Gaudecker, B., and Müller-Hermelink, H.K.: Ontogenetic study of human lymph node development. In preparation.
26. Milanesi, S.: Sulla presenza di dispositivi di giunzione tra le cellule dendritiche dei follicoli linfatici del linfonodo. Boll. Soc. ital. Biol. Sper., 41:1223–1225, 1965.
27. Mollo, F., Monga, G., and Stramignoni, A.: Dark reticular cells in human lymphadenitis and lymphomas. Virchows Arch. B, 3:117–126, 1969.
28. Mühlbach, H.: Histochemische Darstellung der alkalischen Phosphatase und der 5'-Nukleotidase in der menschlichen Gaumentonsille. Inaug. Diss., Kiel, 1977.
29. Müller-Hermelink, H.K.: Herkunft der Lymphozyten und Mikro-ökologie der lymphatischen Gewebe. Habilitationsschrift, Kiel, 1975.
30. Müller-Hermelink, H.K., and Caesar, R.: Elektronenmikroskopische Untersuchung der Keimzentren in menschlichen Tonsillen. Z. Zellforsch., 96:521–547, 1969.
31. Müller-Hermelink, H.K., and von Gaudecker, B.: Ontogenese des lymphatischen Systems. (Referat). Verh. Anat. Ges. (Jena), 74:in press.
32. Müller-Hermelink, H.K., Heusermann, U., Kaiserling, E., and Stutte, H.-J.: Human lymphatic microecology—Specificity, characterization and ontogeny of different reticulum cells in the B cell and T cell regions. In: Immune reactivity of lymphocytes. Adv. Exp. Med. Biol., vol. 66, pp. 177–182. Feldman, M., and Globerson, A., (eds.), New York-London: Plenum Press, 1976.
33. Müller-Hermelink, H.K., and Lennert, K.: The cytologic, histologic, and functional bases for a modern classification of lymphomas. In: Lennert, K., Malignant lymphomas other than Hodgkin's disease. Handb. d. spez. path. Anat. u. Histol., vol. I/3B, pp. 1–82. Uehlinger, E., (ed.), Springer, Berlin-Heidelberg-New York, 1978.
34. Nossal, G.J.V., Abbot, A., Mitchell, J., and Lummus, Z.: Antigens in immunity. XV. Ultrastructural features of antigen capture in primary and secondary lymphoid follicles. J. exp. Med., 127:277–290, 1968.
35. Papiernik, M.: Ontogeny of the human lymphoid system: study of the cytological maturation and the incorporation of tritiated thymidine and uridine in the foetal thymus and lymph node and in the infantile thymus. J. Cell. Phys., 80:235–242, 1972.
36. Poppema, S., Kaiserling, E., and Lennert, K.: Hodgkin's disease with lymphocytic predominance, nodular type (nodular paragranuloma) and progressively transformed germinal centres—A cytohistological study. Histopathology, 3:295–308, 1979.
37. Rappaport, H., Winter, W.J., and Hicks, E.B.: Follicular lymphoma. A reevaluation of its position in the scheme of malignant lymphoma, based on a survey of 253 cases. Cancer, 9:792–821, 1956.
38. Rausch, E., Kaiserling, E., and Goos, M.: Langerhans cells and interdigitating reticulum cells in the thymus-dependent region in human dermatopathic lymphadenitis. Virchows Arch., B, 25:327–343, 1977.
39. Schlaak, M., Schröder, P., and Wulff, J.C.: Cell cooperations in the mitogen-induced transformation of human blood lymphocytes in healthy persons and in Hodgkin's disease. In: Function and structure of the immune system. Adv. Exp. Med. Biol., vol. 114, pp. 401–405, Müller-Ruchholtz, W., and Müller-Hermelink, H.K., (eds.), Plenum Press, New York-London, 1979.

40. Schwarting, H., and Müller-Hermelink, H.K.: In-vitro studies on histiocytic and interdigitating reticulum cells of human lymphoid tissue. Submitted for publication.

41. Silberberg, I., Baer, R.L., and Rosenthal, S.A.: The role of Langerhans cells in allergic contact hypersensitivity. A review of findings in man and guinea pigs. J. invest. Dermatol., 66:210–217, 1976.

42. De Sousa, M.: Kinetics of the distribution of thymus and marrow cells in the peripheral lymphoid organs of the mouse: Ecotaxis. Clin. exp. Immunol., 9:371–380, 1971.

43. Stingl, G., Wolff-Schreiner, E., Pichler, W.J., Gschrait, F., Knapp, W., and Wolff, K.: Erstmaliger immunologischer Nachweis von Oberflächenrezeptoren an epidermalen Langerhanszellen (abstract). Münch. med. Wschr. 119:517, 1977.

44. Swartzendruber, D.C.: Desmosomes in germinal centers of mouse spleen. Exp. Cell. Res., 40:429–432, 1965.

45. Swartzendruber, D.C.: Observations on the ultrastructure of lymphatic tissue germinal centers. In: Germinal centers in immune responses, pp. 71–76. Cottier, H., Odartchenko, N., Schindler, R., and Congdon, C.C., Eds. Berlin-Heidelberg-New York: Springer, 1967.

46. Tew, J.G., Mandel, T., Burgess, A., and Hicks, J.D.: The antigen binding dendritic cell of the lymphoid follicles: Evidence indicating its role in the maintenance and regulation of serum antibody levels. In: Function and structure of the immune system. Adv. Exp. Med. Biol., vol. 114, pp. 407–410. Müller-Ruchholtz, W., and Müller-Hermelink, H.K., (eds.), New York-London: Plenum Press, 1979.

47. Veerman, A.J.P.: On the interdigitating cells in the thymus-dependent area of the rat spleen: A relation between the mononuclear phagocyte system and T-lymphocytes. Cell. Tiss. Res., 148:247–257, 1974.

48. Veldman, J.E.: Histophysiology and electron microscopy of the immune response. Ph.D.-Thesis. Groningen: N.V. Boekdrukkerij Dijkstra Niemeyer, 1970.

49. Veldman, J.E., Molenaar, I., and Keuning, F.J.: Electron microscopy of cellular immunity reactions in B-cell derived rabbits. Thymus derived antigen reactive cells, their micro-cnvironment and progeny in the lymph node. Virchows Arch., B, 28:217–228, 1978.

50. Wahl, S.M., Wilton, J.M., Rosenstreich, D.L., and Oppenheim, J.J.: Role of macrophages in the production of lymphokines by T and B lymphocytes. J. Immunol., 114:1296–1301, 1975.

6. HLA STUDIES IN MALIGNANT LYMPHOMAS

J.G. VAN DEN TWEEL

INTRODUCTION

The major stimulus for the investigation of the association between HLA and disease in man was the discovery by Lilly and coworkers (1) that the leukemogenic capacity of Gross virus in mice was influenced by the host's H-2 type (the analog of the human HLA system in mice). The subsequent demonstration by Amiel (2) that the 4c antigen was increased in patients with Hodgkin's disease, suggested that in the human situation also the development of malignant disease was influenced by this genetic predisposition, and that HLA studies would provide an insight into the role of genetic factors in the development of malignant disease.

Following Amiel's report, many other studies were performed in patients with Hodgkin's disease, leukemias and solid tumors. According to the 1979 data of the HLA and Disease Registry (a central organ compiling all information about HLA and disease), approximately 60 different forms of malignant disease have been studied up to now. These tumors include malignancies of the gastrointestinal tract, respiratory system, urogenital system in both men and women, the central and peripheral nervous system, the hematopoietic system, the lymphatic organs and the eyes. Only a few of the diseases studied, among these lymphomas and leukemias, show an increased frequency of one or more HLA antigens, and even these frequencies are not always significantly increased. In this paper we will discuss in two groups the malignant hematological diseases in which an alteration of HLA antigens is observed:

1) Malignant lymphomas
   a) Hodgkin's disease
   b) Non-Hodgkin lymphomas
2) Leukemias

J.G. van den Tweel et al. (eds.), Malignant Lymphoproliferative Diseases, 71–75
All rights reserved.
Copyright © 1980 by Martinus Nijhoff Publishers bv, The Hague/Boston/London.

THE MALIGNANT LYMPHOMAS

Hodgkin's disease

Hodgkin's disease was among the first diseases studied for the existence of an association between HLA and disease. A common pattern found in most studies is an increased frequency of HLA antigens of the old 4c system (B5, Bw35, B18 and B15) supporting the original findings of Amiel (2). Among those studies is an important one of Forbes and Morris (3). Increased frequencies of B7 (4) and of A1 and B8 have also been suggested in several studies; however, not all studies have revealed statistically significant alterations in gene frequencies. This might be due to the fact that in Hodgkin's disease four histological subtypes are recognized which occur with different frequency in different populations.

Graff and associates (5) studied the relationship between HLA antigens and the different histological subtypes in 103 Caucasian Hodgkin patients and found that only B5 was significantly more frequent in the total patient population, mainly because of a large proportion of patients with mixed cellularity and lymphocyte depletion types of Hodgkin's disease. B5 was not elevated in patients with nodular sclerosis. A1, B8 and B18 were significantly increased in mixed cellularity alone. In a study of 50 patients with nodular sclerosis and 25 patients with the mixed cellularity type of Hodgkin's disease at Los Angeles County Hospital, we found similar results (unpublished study).

An interesting study was published by Falk and Osoba (6). They were able to show an increased frequency of A1 and B5 irrespective of the disease duration, whereas B5 was increased only in those surviving for more than five years. Unfortunately, no histological subdivision was made in this study.

In family studies where two siblings were affected with Hodgkin's disease, an identical or haploidentical HLA type was always reported (7, 8). A potentially very important observation was recently published by Nuñez-Roldan and coworkers (9). They describe a family with seven children, three of which developed mixed cellularity Hodgkin's disease within a month. All of them possessed the same HLA genotype (A26–B18/A1–B5). The other four children had other genotypes. This observation suggests both an environmental and a genetic factor in the development of the disease.

In conclusion it seems that further studies of HLA antigens can unravel some of the many secrets that still surround Hodgkin's disease. There is certainly evidence that the clinical and pathological pattern of Hodgkin's disease is influenced by the HLA phenotype of the host. Also, the studies to date raise the question of whether Hodgkin's disease is really one disease entity. Further study of HLA may help answer this question.

Non-Hodgkin lymphomas

While the association between HLA and Hodgkin's disease has been studied by numerous investigators, the association between the HLA system and the non-Hodgkin lymphomas is a relatively unexplored area. This is mainly due to the fact that an accurate histological diagnosis for Hodgkin's disease, certainly in the past, was more readily available than for the other lymphomas.

Forbes and Morris (10) published one of the first papers on the association between HLA and non-Hodgkin lymphomas. In a study of 134 patients with follicular lymphoma, reticulum cell sarcoma and lymphosarcoma, they found a strong association between the group as a whole and HLA-B12 ($p < 0.005$). After dividing the population into the three diagnostic groups, it appeared that only the follicular lymphoma group demonstrated a significant association with the B12 antigen. In a retrospective study, Dick et al. (11) also detected an increased frequency of B12 in lymphoma patients.

Modern lymphoma classification as described in this book has facilitated more accurate histological typing of the non-Hodgkin lymphomas. Based on these new classifications a prospective study was started (12) with the aim of determining whether a correlation with HLA could be detected in the different histological subgroups. So far approximately 305 patients with malignant lymphoma (non-Hodgkin type) have been studied. The patient population comprises Blacks, Caucasians and Spanish-Americans. After dividing these groups into the diagnostic subclasses of the Lukes-Collins system, there were not enough of Spanish-Americans or Blacks to show any

Table 1. Comparison of some HLA types in Caucasian B-and T-cell lymphoma, preliminary data from USC-UCLA study.

		Frequency of positive cases (%)			
HLA antigen	Controls N = 558	B and T lymphomas N = 101	B-Cell lymphomas N = 81	T-Cell lymphomas N = 20	Small* cleaved FCC N = 31
Aw24	18	16	16	15	26
Aw33	2	9	9	5	6
B14	8	16	19	5	23

*Small cleaved follicular center cell lymphomas (a very frequent B-cell lymphoma).

clear correlations. The Caucasian B cell lymphoma group comprises 81 patients, all of which have been typed for the HLA-A, B and C antigens, and 59 of them also for the DR locus antigens. Among the elevated frequencies are Aw24, Aw33, and B14 (Table 1). The increases, however, are not statistically significant. Interestingly most increases only appear after accurate histological and immunological subdivision of the involved malignant lymphomas. DR typing so far reveals an increase of Dw7, especially if the small cleaved follicular center cell lymphomas are studied separately. More cases will have to be investigated to come to a definite conclusion as to whether there is an association between HLA and the different non-Hodgkin lymphomas in the different races. Studies so far, however, do not indicate that strong correlations as seen in many non-malignant diseases will be detected.

LEUKEMIAS

Many reports are now available on the association between HLA and acute lymphocytic leukemia. One of the first papers (13) showed an increased A2–B12 haplotype. Many of the other studies have confirmed the increased frequency of A2 (14) and also of Aw24. An interesting observation was made by Klouda et al. (15) who found that patients with the HLA antigen A9 had a high median survival time. Other studies, however, could not confirm the increased A9 frequency. An accurate study of the HLA antigens in T cell, B cell and null-cell leukemias is probably necessary to shed new light on these associations.

Only a few studies are available on HLA and chronic lymphocytic leukemias (CLL). A recent study (16) showed insignificant increased frequencies of A9, A28, and Aw30. The A9 association had previously been shown by Jeannet (17).

CONCLUSION

The search for associations between HLA and malignant diseases, so optimistically started after the discovery of an H-2 linked genetic predisposition for leukemogenic viruses in mice, has not brought the results that investigators hoped for.

Although numerous malignant diseases have been studied for a relation with the HLA complex only very few show a (significant) increase in certain HLA antigens. Malignant lymphomas, both the Hodgkin types and the non-Hodgkin types, are among the malignancies that tend to show an association. This association only appears after accurate histological subclassification of these tumors, indicating that we might be dealing with heterogeneous disease groups in malignant lymphoma.

REFERENCES

1. Lilly, F., Boyse, E.A., and Old, L.J.: Genetic basis of susceptibility to viral leukemogenesis. Lancet, 2:1207–1209, 1964.
2. Amiel, J.L.: Study of the leukocyte phenotypes in Hodgkin's disease. In: Histocompatibility Testing 1967, p. 79, Williams & Wilkins, Baltimore, 1967.
3. Forbes, J.F., and Morris, P.J.: Leukocyte antigens in Hodgkin's disease. Lancet, 2:849–851, 1970.
4. Van der Does, J.A., Elkerbout, F., D'Amaro, J., Van der Steen, G., Van Log-hem, E., Meera Khan, P., Bernini, L.F., Van Leeuwen, A., and Van Rood, J.J.: HL-A Typing in Dutch Patients with Hodgkin's Disease. Histocompatibility Testing p. 579, 1972.
5. Graff, K.S., Simon, R.M., Yankee, R.A., DeVita, V.T., and Rogentine, G.N.: HLA antigens in Hodgkin's disease: histopathologic and clinical correlation. J. Natl. Cancer. Inst., 52:1087–1090, 1974.
6. Falk, J., and Osoba, D.: HLA antigens and survival in Hodgkin's disease. Lancet, 2:1118–1121, 1971.
7. Maldonado, J.E., Taswell, H.F., and Kiely, J.M.: Familial Hodgkin's disease. Lancet, 2:1259, 1972.
8. Bowers, T.K., Moldow, Ch.F., Bloomfield, C.D., and Yunis, E.J.: Familial Hodgkin's disease and the major histocompatibility complex. Vox. Sang., 33:273–277, 1977.
9. Nuñez-Roldan, A., Martinez-Guibalalde, F., Gomoz-Garzia, P., Gomoz-Pereira, C., Nuñez-Ollero, G., and Torres-Gomez, A.: Possible HLA role in a family with Hodgkin's disease. Tissue Antigens, 13:377–378, 1979.
10. Forbes, J.F., and Morris, P.J.: Transplantation antigens and malignant lympho-mas in man. Follicular lymphoma, reticulum cell sarcoma and lymphosarcoma. Tissue Antigens, 1:265–269, 1971.
11. Dick, F.R., Fortuny, G., Athanasios, T., Greally, J., Wood, N., and Yunis E.J.: HLA and lymphoid tumors. Cancer Res., 32:2608–2611, 1972.
12. Van den Tweel, J.G., Dugas, D.J., and Loon, J.: HLA and malignant disease. Am. J. Clin. Pathol., in press.
13. Thorsby, E., Bratlie, A., and Lie, S.O.: HLA genotypes of children with acute leukemia. Scand. J. Haematol., 6:409–415, 1969.
14. Walford, R., Finkelstein, S., Neerhout, R., Konrad, P., and Shanbrom, E.: Acute childhood leukemia in relation to the HLA human transplantation genes. Nature, 225:461–462, 1970.
15. Klouda, P.T. Lawler, S.D., Till, M.M., and Hardisty, R.M.: Acute lymphoblas-tic leukemia and HLA: a prospective study. Tissue Antigens, 4:262–265, 1974.
16. Pollack, M.S., and Dubois, D.: Possible effects of non HLA antibodies in com-mon typing sera on HLA antigen frequency data in leukemia. Cancer, 39:2348–2354, 1977.
17. Jeannet, M., and Magnin, C.: HLA antigens in malignant disease. Transplant Proc., 3:1301–1303, 1971.

7. REGULATORY PROPERTIES OF T LYMPHOCYTES: IMPLICATIONS FOR STUDIES ON MALIGNANT LYMPHOID CELLS*

R.E. BALLIEUX

The immune system may be seen as a complex network comprising regulatory as well as effector cells. Whereas attention was formerly focused predominantly on the effector mechanisms of immune reactivity (antibodies, complement, lymphokines, cell mediated cytotoxicity, etc.), regulation of the immune response has become one of the leading subjects in present research in immunology. Great progress has been made in animal studies leading to the recognition of subsets of T lymphocytes exerting different regulatory functions (1). Thus, apart from T lymphocytes involved in the efferent phase of the immune response, antigen-specific regulatory T cells referred to as T helper (Th) and T suppressor (Ts) cells, can now be distinguished on a functional basis (Table 1). In mice, helper and suppressor activity is mediated by T-cell subsets which can be recognized by their surface phenotype. T-cells programmed for helper function are characterized by the Lyt 1^+, 23^- (Ia^+) alloantigens, whereas T-suppressor cells express the Lyt 1^-, 23^+ (Ia^+) phenotype (see also the contribution of E. Hensen in this volume). Elegant studies in mice established that the development of different T cell regulatory functions involve T-T cell interaction, thus supporting the concept of a cellular network maintaining homeostasis in the immune system (2, 3, 4) (Figure 1).

Analogous studies were undertaken in man, but in this field progress has been limited until recently due to two facts:

1) For ethical reasons the possibilities for experimental approach in man are very limited, and therefore most studies still have to be done in vitro using cell culture systems. Unfortunately, unlike the situation in the mouse, the induction and measurement of antibody response in human lymphoid cells in vitro is extremely difficult and has only recently become possible.
2) Surface markers, analogous to the Lyt system in the mouse, are lacking (or at least not known) in man.

*Part of the work described in this article has been subsidized by the Foundation for Medical Research Fungo (grant No. 13–40–91 and 13–40–31).

J.G. van den Tweel et al. (eds.), Malignant Lymphoproliferative Diseases, 77–83
All rights reserved.
Copyright © 1980 by Martinus Nijhoff Publishers bv, The Hague/Boston/London.

Table 1. Subsets of T-lymphocytes defined on the basis of function.

T$_{eff}$ (lymphokine) T$_{cytotox}$ (killer cell) T$_{ADCC}$ (antibody-dependent cytotoxicity) T$_{amplifier}$ (potentiates B-cell proliferation)	T helper T suppressor

Two important observations opened this field, however. The first concerns the finding by several groups that subsets of human T lymphocytes possess surface receptors for the Fc fragment of IgM (Tμ cells) and IgG (Tγ cells) (5, 6, 7). These surface receptors can be detected by a rosette test using ox erythrocytes (Eox) sensitized with anti-Eox immunoglobulin of IgM or IgG isotype, and thus may serve as a marker for a given subpopulation of T lymphocytes. Among the peripheral blood lymphocytes of healthy adults the majority of the T cells bear the receptor for IgM; the Tγ cells represent only a small fraction of the total T-cell population (Table 2).

Once the existence of Tμ and Tγ subsets was established, the question of the biological significance of the receptors for IgM and IgG became intriguing. It was not until 1976 that the first clue to the possible biological significance of the affinity of IgM molecules for T lymphocytes was found in the killing of IgM-coated tumor cells by T lymphocytes (6). However, a fundamental contribution in this field was made by Moretta et al. (7), who

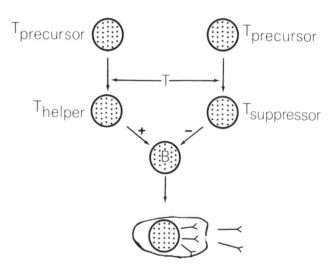

Figure 1. Positive regulation by T helper lymphocytes and negative regulation by T suppressor lymphocytes in the process of B-cell activation and differentiation into immunoglobulin synthesizing and secreting plasma cells. The generation of T-helper and T-suppressor cells by activation of the respective T-precursor lymphocytes by T-T interaction is represented schematically.

Table 2. Subsets of T-lymphocytes defined on the basis of the presence of Fc receptor (FcR).

$T\mu$ (60%)	:	FcR for IgM
$T\gamma$ (10%)	:	FcR for IgG
$T\mu, \gamma$ (5%)	:	FcR for IgM as well as IgG
$T\mu^-, \gamma^-$ (25%)	:	lacking detectable FcR

suggested that, in analogy with the Lyt system the mice, the surface receptors for IgM and IgG on human lymphocytes could lead to the recognition of helper and suppressor T cells in man.

Unfortunately, no experimental system was available at that time (1976) to measure antigen-specific helper and suppressor activity in human T lymphocytes. Therefore, instead of antigen, the B-cell mitogen pokeweed (PWM) was used. If human B cells are stimulated with PWM in culture, plasma cells develop, which synthesize and secrete immunoglobulin. Due to the non-antigen-specific stimulatory property of the mitogen, a polyclonal B-cell response is obtained. More important, however, is the fact that T cells are necessary to obtain B-cell activation by this mitogen. This was interpreted as a *helper effect* of T cells, and hence it was accepted that helper T cells could be recognized on a functional basis in the PWM system. Moretta, while working with Cooper, then established that in the PWM system T helper function was exerted by cells localized in the $T\mu$ fraction. He could also induce suppressor activity, as measured in the pokeweed system, and reported this activity to be linked to $T\gamma$ cells.

In the last two years this concept of human helper and suppressor T cells has been developed considerably. This progress is due to the fact that Dosch and Gelfand (8) were able to find the right conditions for the induction of a primary antibody response in vitro, using human peripheral blood lymphocytes (9). This development opened the way for studies that could establish whether the concept of "T help" was also valid in man with respect to an antigen-specific B-cell response.

It was again the group of Dosch and Gelfand (8) that showed the T-cell dependency of a specific antibody response in vitro for antigens such as ovalbumin (OA) and sheep erythrocytes (SE), which are known to be T-dependent antigens in the mouse. This original observation was confirmed and extended to other antigens such as haemocyanin (Hc) and DNP-OA by Heijnen et al. (10). The concept of antigen-specific T helper cells was thus firmly established in man (9, 11).

The next step included the search for the existence of antigenspecific suppressor cells in man. From studies in mice it was clear that T cells cultured in vitro with (relatively) high doses of protein antigens could be induced to exert antigen-specific suppression. Dosch and Gelfand (8) were the first to observe that the in vitro induction of antibody response in human blood lymphocytes by antigens such as OA and SE is abolished when a high dose of antigen is used in the culture system, and UytdeHaag et al. (12) showed that under these conditions antigen-specific T suppressor cells are induced. Thus, besides antigen specific helper activity, a distinct suppressive activity was established. Both regulatory functions were exerted by T cells. The question now arose as to whether these two different regulatory potentials were localized in separate T cell subsets, as suggested by the PWM experiments. It could indeed be shown by Heijnen et al. (10) that in man under certain in vitro culture conditions, helper activity is provided by $T\mu$ cells, while $T\gamma$ cells can be stimulated to express suppressor activity. In therefore seems permissible to superimpose the data obtained in the antigen-specific system on results obtained in the PWM system. This is important because in studies on the regulatory aspects of T lymphoma cells we are very probably dealing with a monoclonal proliferation of lymphoid cells. It is generally accepted that the recognition of antigen by immunocompetent lymphocytes is clonally restricted to one specificity. This implies that there is a very small change of finding the antigen that will correspond to the specific recognition site on a malignant lymphoid cell clone. Most studies on regulatory aspects of lymphoma T cells therefore make use of the PWM system, but important results have been obtained in spite of this restriction. This is illustrated by the following two examples.

Broder et al. (13) studied the capacity of leukemic cells from patients with the Sézary syndrome to regulate PWM-induced immunoglobulin synthesis by human peripheral B lymphocytes. As discussed above, the differentiation of B cells into immunoglobulin-producing plasma cells is T-cell dependent. Using the experimental design shown in Table 3, these authors demonstrated that in four of five patients the Sézary cells were able to provide "help" in the PWM system. Under the conditions used, no suppressive activity could be established. It was concluded from these findings that in these four patients the malignant lymphocytes represent neoplastic lymphocytes originating from the T-cell subpopulation programmed for helper function. These results strongly support the view that human helper T cells represent a distinct subset of T-lymphocytes. The fundamental question to be an-

Table 3. Immunoglobulin production by human B cells.

Cell source	Mitogen (PWM)	Ig production
B cells	−	−
B cells	+	−
B + $T_{norm.}$ cells	+	+
B + $T_{sézary}$ cells	+	+

Conclusion: Sézary cells reflect an exclusive expansion of helper T cells.

swered concerns the clonal character of the malignant helper-cell population. Broder et al. came to the conclusion that the absence of suppressive
activity that could be expected when increasing numbers of Sézary cells
were added to purified normal B cells, indicates that the Sézary T cell represents what these authors called a "homogeneous expansion of helper
cells". Solid data with respect to monoclonal expansion of antigen-specific
helper cells are, however, still lacking. In this respect it is of great interest
that virus-transformed mouse T cells of the leukemia line 485–2 express
antigen-specific helper activity (14). It is obvious that the crucial question to
be answered is whether the 485–2 cell line originated from a few transformed
T lymphocytes which by change were potential helper cells for the antigen in
question or whether endogeneous viruses generate receptor diversity in
lymphoid cells. Recently, Saxon et al. (15) made the interesting observation
that a monoclonal proliferation of neoplastic T lymphocytes in a patient
with ataxia telangiectasia was associated with both helper and suppressor
T-cell function. The malignant cells, that could be recognized by an abnormal 14-chromosome could be shown to contain a low percentage of $T\gamma$
cells, whereas roughly half of the neoplastic T-cells expressed Fc receptors
for IgM. Unfortunately, the functional proporties of purified neoplastic $T\mu$
and $T\gamma$ cells were not analyzed. It is conceivable, however, that the observed
helper and suppressor activities (as measured in the PWM system) were
exerted by T cells belonging the $T\gamma$ and the $T\mu$ subset respectively. If so,
the hypothesis can be put forward that the neoplastic transformation occurred at pre-T cell level without effecting the precursor's capacity to
mature into the two different subsets of helper and suppressor T-cells.
This area of research can now be explored more specifically, because techniques have become available for the in vitro induction and measurement
of antigen-specific helper and suppressor functions in man (16).

The second example concerns suppressor cell activity associated with
malignant T-lymphocytes. Han et al. (17) reported on five human leukemic
T-cell lines which, in co-culture experiments with normal lymphocytes in
the PWM system, suppressed Ig synthesis. It could be established that these
cells were actually suppressor-effector T cells. This is in contrast with the
findings of Broder et al. (18) concerning the necessity for neoplastic T cells
of a child with acute lymphoblastoid leukemia to interact with another T-cell
subset to obtain suppression. On the basis of their observations, a hypothetical interaction scheme for T-suppressor subsets, that would lead to Ts-
effector cells was formulated. In terms of these data and ideas, UytdeHaag
et al. (19) formulated a scheme for T-T interaction in the induction of
T-suppressor-effector cells under physiological conditions. This concept
seems valid, since UytdeHaag could establish that, very similar to the situation in the mouse, a suppressor T-precursor cell is activated by a T-suppressor-activator cell to become a T-suppressor-effector cell (Figure 2).

It is clear from the results discussed here, that studies on regulatory

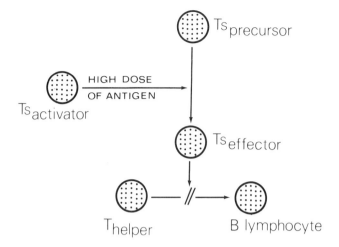

Figure 2. High doses of antigen induce T-suppressor-activator cells to generate T-suppressor-effector cells by activation of T-suppressor precursor cells. The Ts-effector cells prevent T-helper cells from successful interaction with B lymphocytes.

aspects of malignant T cells may contribute considerably to our scientific knowledge. There is an urgent need not only for careful clinical and pathological observations but in particular for extensive analyses of surface markers of malignant T cells, for careful analysis of their functional properties, and for a thorough analysis of a potential antigen-specific function of these cells in the regulatory circuit of the immune response.

REFERENCES

1. Cantor, H., and Boyse, E.: Regulation of the immune response by T cell subclasses. Cont. Top. Immunobiol., 7:47–73, 1977.
2. Eardley, D.D., Hugenberger, J., McVay-Bondrean, L., Shen, F.W., Gershon, R.K., and Cantor, H.: Immunoregulatory circuits among T cell sets. J. Exp. Med., 147:1106–1115, 1978.
3. Feldmann, M., Beverley, P.C.L., Woody, J., and McKenzie, I.F.C.: T-T interactions in the induction of suppressor and helper T cells: analysis of membrane phenotype of precursor and amplifier cells. J. Exp. Med., 145:793–801, 1977.
4. Tada, T., Taniguchi, M., and Okumura, K.: Regulation of antibody response by antigen specific T cell factors bearing I region determinants. Progress in Immunol., 3:369–377, 1977.
5. Ferrarini, M., Moretta, L., Abrile, R., and Durante, M.L.: Receptors for IgG molecules on human lymphocytes forming spontaneous rosettes with sheep red cells. Eur. J. Immunol., 5:70–72, 1975.
6. Gmelig Meyling, F., Ham, van der M. and Ballieux, R.E.: Binding of IgM by human T lymphocytes. Scand. J. Immunol., 5:487–495, 1976.
7. Moretta, L., Webb, S.R., Grossi, C.E., Lydyard, P.M. and Cooper, M.D.:

Functional analysis of two human T cell subpopulations: help and suppression of B cell responses by T cells bearing receptors for IgM and IgG. J. Exp. Med., 146:184–200, 1977.

8. Dosch, H.M., and Gelfand, E.W.: Generation of human plaque forming cells in culture: tissue distribution, antigenic and cellular requirement. J. Immunol., 118:302–308, 1977.

9. Ballieux, R.E., Heijnen, C.J., UytdeHaag, F., and Zegers, B.J.M.: Regulation of B cell activity in man: role of T cells. Immunol. Rev., 45:33–69, 1979.

10. Heijnen, C.J., UytdeHaag, F., Gmelig Meyling, F.H.J., and Ballieux, R.E.: Human B cell activation in vitro: localisation of antigen specific helper and suppressor function in distinct T cell subpopulations. Cell. Immunol., 43:282–292, 1979.

11. Dosch, H.M., and Gelfand, E.W.: Specific in vitro IgM responses of human B-cells: a complex regulatory network modulated by antigens. Immunol. Rev., 45:243:274, 1979.

12. UytdeHaag, F., Heijnen, C.J., and Ballieux, R.E.: Induction of antigen-specific human suppressor T lymphocytes in vitro. Nature, 271:556–559, 1978.

13. Broder, S., Edelson, R.L., Lutzner, M.A., Nelson, D.L., MacDermott, R.P., Durm, M.E., Goldman, C.K., Made, B.D., and Waldmann, T.A.: The Sézary syndrome: a malignant proliferation of helper T cells. J. Clin. Invest., 58:1297–1306, 1976.

14. Roder, J.C., Tyler, L., Singhal, S.K., and Ball, J.K.: Are T-cell lymphomas immunocompetent?. Nature, 274:540–541, 1978.

15. Saxon, A., Stevens, R.H., and Golde, D.W.: Helper and suppressor T-lymphocyte leukemia in ataxia telangiectasia. New. Engl. J. Med., 300:700–704, 1979.

16. Fauci, A.S., and Ballieux, R.E., (eds.). Antibody production in man: in vitro synthesis and clinical implications, Acad. Press, New York, U.S.A., 1979.

17. Han, T., Dadey, B., Nussbaum, A., Henderson, E.S., and Minowada, J.: Human leukemic T cell lines with suppressor activity on normal B cell differentiation. IRCS-Med. Sc., 6:535, 1978.

18. Broder, S., Poplack, D., Wang-Peng, J., Durm, M., Goldman, C., Muul, L., and Waldmann, T.A.: Characterization of a suppressor cell leukemia. Evidence for the requirement of an interaction of two T cells in the development of human suppressor effector cells. New. Engl. J. Med., 298:66–75, 1978.

19. UytdeHaag, F., Heijnen, C.J., Pot, C.H., and Ballieux, R.E.: T-T interactions in the induction of antigen specific human suppressor T lymphocytes in vitro. J. Immunol., 123:646–653, 1979.

8. IMMUNOLOGICAL APPROACH TO LYMPHOID NEOPLASMS

J.W. PARKER

INTRODUCTION

Characterization of non-Hodgkins lymphomas as B cell, T cell, or histiocytic type by immunological techniques is now widely accepted. A variety of procedures has been used for identifying these cell types, most involving the identification of surface receptors or antigens. Rosetting techniques using erythrocytes and other particles, and specific antisera labelled with fluorochromes, isotopes, or enzymes have been applied to the study of normal and neoplastic cells of human lymphoid tissues. Use of these techniques in conjunction with morphology and cytochemistry has resulted in lymphoma classifications which appear to relate more closely to our current understanding of the anatomy and function of the immune apparatus and thus are more appealing than previous classifications. The clinical value of these new classifications is under study, as we will hear in this course.

The prupose of this presentation is to review, in summary form, the immunological techniques used in discriminating between T and B lymphocytes—normal and neoplastic. Several excellent recent reviews provide details of methodology, interpretation, and clinical application (21, 25, 29, 40, 55, 77, 79, 90, 92).

The application of immunological techniques to lymphoma studies has already enhanced our understanding of these neoplasms. The next few years promise to be exciting ones as we see this understanding and our ability to manipulate the immune system and its neoplasms continue to unfold.

IDENTIFICATION OF T AND B LYMPHOCYTES AND MONOCYTES IN MAN

A range of identifers has been used for distinguishing T and B lymphocytes and monocytes (macrophages, histiocytes). The commonly used ones are listed in Table 1 (a more complete listing is given by Chess and Schlossman (21)). These may involve recognition of receptors on the cell surface detected by rosetting techniques or with specific antisera conjugated to a fluorochrome, enzyme, isotope or particle. In addition to the detection of

Table 1. Techniques most commonly used for identification of T cells, B cells and histiocytes.

	T cells	B cells	Histiocytes Monocytes
Rosette Methods			
E (SRBC)	+	−	−
EAC (IgM) (C$_3$ receptor)	(+)[1]	+	+
EA (IgG) (Fc receptor)	−	+	+
Surface Ig	(−)[2]	+	(+)[3]
Cytoplasmic Ig	−	+	−
Antisera			
HTLA	+	−	−
HBLA	−	+	−
Cytochemistry			
α-Naphthyl butyrase (NSE)	(+)[4]	−	+
Acid phosphatase	(+)	−	+
Tartrate-resistant acid phosphatase	−	(+)[5]	−
Muramidase (lysozyme)	−	−	+

Ig = immunoglobulin; HTLA = human T lymphocyte antigen; HBLA = human B lymphocyte antigen; NSE = nonspecific esterase.

Parentheses indicate that the finding lacks specificity, is controversial, or is only seen with certain types of lymphoma/leukemia.

[1] C$_3$ receptors on small population of normal T cells and convoluted T cell lymphoma/leukemia.

[2] T cells have a small amount of surface Ig not detected by immunofluorescent methods.

[3] Adsorbed via Fc receptors.

[4] Convoluted T cell lymphoma/leukemia.

[5] Hairy cell leukemia. Origin of cells (B cell vs histiocyte) controversial.

surface markers, which may be receptors and/or differentiation antigens, cytochemical procedures have been utilized, as have a range of in vitro essays for function. The most commonly used rosetting techniques, immunofluorescent and immunoparticle methods for detection of SIg, and the use of specific antisera for differentiation antigens will be considered here.

Although morphologically homogenous subpopulations of lymphocytes can be identified because of their surface properties, it should be remembered that as Taylor (80) has stated, "not all surface marker differences are indicative of the existence of separate functioning groups, for markers change during differentiation, maturation, and cell cycle, within a single cell line. In addition, not all the cells of a single functional group (as identified by surface markers) are morphologically monotonous (e.g., small T cells transforming to T immunoblasts-E rosette positive, yet morphologically diverse)."

Erythrocyte receptors

The E rosette method (3, 49) has been generally accepted as a major technique for the identification of both normal and neoplastic human T lymphocytes. It involves the spontaneous adherence of sheep erythrocytes (SRBC) to human T cells as illustrated in Figure 1. The determination that E rosette-forming cells are T cells has been based on the high percentage of rosettes in thymus cell suspensions and the fact that anti-human immunoglobulin sera do not inhibit E rosette formation, whereas anti-lymphocyte or anti-thymocyte sera do (77). However, the test is far from specific for T cells. Woda and colleagues (94) demonstrated that several human cell types formed E rosettes, including fibroblasts and parenchymal cells from liver, lung and parathyroid. This lack of specificity must be kept in mind when "poorly differentiated" neoplasms are studied.

The method is inherently simple, but in spite of recent attempts at standardization, technical modifications in various laboratories result in variable results. A range of factors may influence the results, some of them technical, e.g. the ratio of lymphoid cells to SRBCs, total concentration of cells, centrifugal force, the temperature and time of incubation during the rosette-forming period, the technique of resuspension and the method used for visual counting. E rosettes are fragile, the erythrocytes being only loosely attached to lymphocytes, and after incubation of erythrocytes and lymphocytes in a pellet, resuspension must be quite gentle (8). Too many red cells make it difficult to detect negative cells and falsely elevate the percentage of rosette-forming cells. Although we standardly use an overnight incubation period, the E rosette score appears to plateau after two hours at 4°C (56).

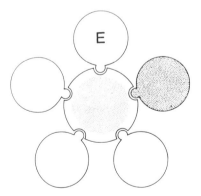

E = SHEEP ERYTHROCYTE
☐ – UNMODIFIED
☐ – NEURAMINIDASE TREATED

Figure 1. Sheep erythrocyte receptor (E rosettes).

Shorter incubation periods may detect a subset of strongly reacting cells which have been called "activated" rosettes (95). At 37°C normal peripheral blood lymphocytes show little evidence of rosette formation, although a small population does form rosettes (5). This may present a problem in interpretation of complement receptor results (performed at 37°C) in the study of neoplastic T cells, since they may form E rosettes at this temperature (73).

A variety of experimental manipulations have been reported which effect E rosette scores and interpretation. Enhancement is gained by performing the test in group AB human serum, in the presence of ficoll, or in fetal calf serum. We have found that ficoll produces an average elevation of E rosette score by three to five percentage points. Pretreatment of lymphocytes with neuraminidase (89) produces a consistently higher score, apparently by recruitment of SIg and Fc receptor-bearing cells. On the other hand, neuraminidase treatment of sheep erythrocytes also enhances rosette formation and reduces the differences observed when erythrocytes from different species are used. Although most E rosette studies of human lymphocytes employ SRBC, some investigators have demonstrated that human T cells will form rosettes with autologous and allogenic human red cells, but the score is lower (70). Murine erythrocytes differ in that they form rosettes with human B lymphocytes rather than T lymphocytes (18, 75).

Methodological modifications over the past several years have resulted in increasing E rosette percentages for normal human blood lymphocytes as reported from different laboratories (5%–15% in 1970 to 50%–80% in 1973) (77). It would appear that the suit has been tailored to fit the preconceived ideal figure. However, during this period it has also been learned that the physiological state of the individual influences his E rosette scores and that different lymphoid tissues contain varying percentages of E rosette-forming cells 95%–100% in post-natal thymus, 50%–80% in peripheral blood, and 20%–70% in lymph nodes (77). And, of course, various disease states have been reported to influence E rosette scores (30, 45). Inhibitory serum factors have been reported in patients with neoplasms (14) and Hodgkin's disease. Cytotoxic radiotherapy (32) and chemotherapy may produce an overall lowering of values (50), whereas other drugs such as levamisole enhance E rosette scores (88).

From the above we can see that although the technique for measuring E rosettes is simple, interpretation is colored by many factors. Consequently, over the past few years confusing information has been published. Much of this is indeed for technical and physiological reasons, but there is also a growing awareness that lymphocytes are part of a spectrum with T lymphocytes at one extreme, B lymphocytes at the other and a gray zone in between with cells less clearly B or T in origin. It has been suggested that some of this is due to double-marking cells which represent stages in the differentiation of T cells. As examples, human fetal thymocytes bear both complement receptors and sheep erythrocyte receptors at 12–22 weeks of gestation (76) and a small population of peripheral blood lymphocytes bears these same two receptors. However, another small population in man possesses both SIg and SRBC receptors (28, 52), and murine lymphocytes may also bear genuine B and T cell markers (SIg and θ antigen) (69). Lymphomas arising from these subpopulations will necessarily add to the confusion.

Percentages of E rosette-forming cells in a given cell suspension are generally determined by counting rosette-forming cells in liquid suspension. In such a preparation, it is difficult to determine which cell types are forming rosettes. Since nonlymphoid cells may form them, percentages alone are not sufficient. For this reason, particularly important in the study of lympho-proliferative disorders where it is necessary to know whether lymphoma cells or reactive T cells are forming rosettes, we routinely prepare stained preparations of the rosettes, using a cytocentrifuge. An even more valuable approach would be to apply the E rosette technique to tissue sections, but most investigators have reported little success with this.

Complement receptors

Human B cells and a minute population of T cells bear receptors for the products of activated C_3 (C_3b, C_3d) and C_4 (31, 70, 74). However other cells, i.e. erythrocytes, granulocytes, monocytes, eosinophils and basophils also possess complement receptors (13). Most investigators have used SRBC coated with rabbit antibody (IgM) to SRBC and nonlytic complement (mouse or human) to detect complement-receptor-bearing cells. This EAC (erythrocyte, antibody, complement) reagent is mixed with lymphocytes and 5%–25% of human peripheral blood lymphocytes from EAC rosettes (Figure 2). A problem presented by this method is that T lymphocytes may form rosettes with the "E" determinants on the sheep erythrocytes. This has been avoided by utilization of other species' red cells (22) and by incubation at 37°C, thereby inhibiting E rosette formation. The former approach has proved to be useful in another way since avian erythrocytes are nucleated and can be distinguished from SRBC in a double labelling of circulating lymphocytes which possess both sheep erythrocyte and complement receptors and identification of separate SRBC and C_3 receptor-bearing populations in the same suspension (Figure 3).

Another approach to identifying complement receptor-bearing cells has involved the use of zymosan beads (polysaccharide extract of yeast cell wall) coated with the C_3b component of human complement (Figure 4) (60, 61). Zymosan activates the complement system by an alternate pathway and thus antibody is not necessary. Any source of complement can be used since unlike SRBC, the zymosan particles are not lysed. This approach

J.W. PARKER

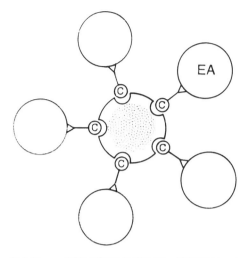

EAC = ERYTHROCYTE (SHEEP, CHICKEN)
+ ANTI-ERYTHROCYTE ANTIBODY
+ COMPLEMENT

COMPLEMENT = MOUSE SERUM OR
PURIFIED C3d OR C3b

Figure 2. Complement receptors (EAC rosettes).

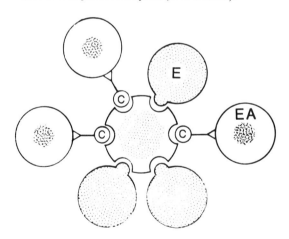

E = SHEEP ERYTHROCYTE

EAC = CHICKEN ERYTHROCYTE
+ ANTI-ERYTHROCYTE ab
+ COMPLEMENT

Figure 3. Combined markers (sheep receptor + complement receptor).

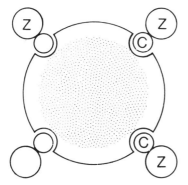

Z = ZYMOSAN PARTICLES
C = COMPLEMENT (C$_3$) ACTIVATED
    BY ZYMOSAN

Figure 4. Complement receptors (zymosan rosettes).

also provides a double-marking rosette method for detecting human T and B cells or double-marking cells in the same preparation.

Although it is readily apparent that the presence of complement receptors is not specific for B cells, the use of rosetting techniques to detect these receptors has provided some useful information. Shevach and colleagues (74) reported the adherence of EAC to frozen sections demonstrating complement receptors on lymphoid cells and macrophages. Stein (77) also using this approach, found that binding was primarily by lymphoid cells and that C$_3$d receptors could be detected on germinal center cells. C$_3$b receptors were also present on cells in the periphery of the follicle and in the interfollicular areas, suggesting a means of distinguishing between follicular B cells and B cells differentiating into plasma cells. This approach may prove useful in distinguishing follicular center cell lymphomas and plasmacytoid lymphocytic lymphomas.

The function of complement receptors is unknown, but it has been suggested that they may be sites for localization of antigen-antibody immune complexes which stimulate B cells to differentiate into antibody forming cells (71).

Fc receptors

Sheep erythrocytes coated with anti-sheep erythrocyte antibodies of the IgG type (EA rosettes (Figure 5) were originally reported to detect monocytes and macrophages bearing receptors for the Fc end of IgG. Later it was found that Fc receptors were also present on lymphocytes (4). The EA rosette technique has been commonly used in clinical studies, but Fc receptors are also detected with heat aggregated IgG tagged with a fluoro-

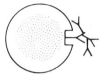

1. AGGREGATED IgG – FLUOROCHROME

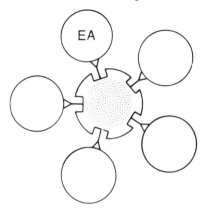

2. EA = Erythrocyte (Sheep, Human, Ox)
   + ANTIBODY (IgG) DIRECTED
   AGAINST ERYTHROCYTE

Figure 5. F_c receptors.

chrome or isotope (Figure 5). Binding of IgG-EA to lymphocytes by using human erythrocytes sensitized with high titer-anti-D serum (10) or ox erythrocytes sensitized with IgG antibodies (33) avoids the problem of spontaneous rosette formation (E) with SRBC, but the presence of Fc receptors on nonlymphoid cells including macrophages, granulocytes, cells from liver, kidney, breast, and various neoplastic cells (77) emphasizes the lack of specificity and thus limited value of Fc receptors as cell identifiers.

Some T cells also possess Fc receptors and a portion of "null" cells mediating antibody-dependent cellular cytotoxicity (ADCC) killer (K) cells, are also Fc receptor positive, leading to proposals that this receptor may function in immunoregulation, antigen localization and ADCC mediation. An interesting recent development is the observation that T cells which bear receptors for the Fc component of IgG, express suppressor activity in vitro, whereas another population of T cells with IgM-Fc receptors shows helper cell activity. These two populations have been isolated and characterized (45). However, since the cells bearing IgG receptors are phagocytic and NSE-positive, the possibility of origin from a lymphocyte-like monocyte progenitor remains.

Because the Fc receptor exists on other r hematologic cell types and is capable of adsorbing aggregated IgG and antigen-antibody complexes, it has created problems in evaluating surface immunoglobulin results as discussed below.

Surface immunoglobulin

Surface membrane immunoglobulin (SIg), by definition, refers to immunoglobulin manufactured by the lymphocyte and then bound to the cell membrane in contrast to immunoglobulin adsorbed onto the surface. This synthesized membrane SIg acts as a specific receptor for antigenic determinants and serves as the major mechanism for recognizing and binding antigen. SIg has proved to be the most reliable of markers for human B cells and can be detected using anti-immunoglobulin antibodies conjugated to fluorochromes, radioisotopes, peroxidase or particles (Figure 6). The methodology is straightforward, but subject to error through a variety of mechanisms and, of course, reliability is dependent on the sensitivity and specificity of the antisera used. The specificity of commercial reagents is not always assured and each lot of antiserum obtained commercially must be subjected to a rigorous assessment of sensitivity and specificity with reference to positive and negative controls. Blocking studies and immunodiffusion against purified light and heavy chain components from sources other than those used in the production of antisera should also be used. The dilution of an antiserum should be determined by titration to the "plateau end point", beyond which the percentage of SIg+ cells falls progressively with dilution (66, 79).

Precise cell identification in immunofluorescent preparations is generally difficult and differentiation from monocytes may present a major problem. For this reason, the use of immunoperoxidase (80) and immunomicrosphere methods (43, 81) offer distinct advantages since they allow examination of stained cells, permitting identification of the surface Ig-positive cells. The immunoperoxidase method is particularly useful of the detection of cytoplasmic immunoglobulin in paraffin sections, but small lymphocytes with easily detectable surface immunoglobulin show little cytoplasmic immunoglobulin (59). Thus cytoplasmic immunoglobulin cannot be demonstrated in most SIg-bearing cells. On the other hand, cells switching from synthesis of nonsecretory Ig (SIg) to synthesis of secretory Ig, e.g. immunoblasts and plasmacytoid lymphocytes, show cytoplasmic immunoglobulin, but relatively little surface immunoglobulin.

Adsorption of serum immunoglobulins by lymphocytes and monocytes presents a major problem. Mechanisms by which this occurs include nonspecific adsorption, particularly in hypergammaglobulinemia and hyperviscosity states and adsorption of IgG via Fc receptors (see Lukes et al. (56), for detailed discussion). Since granulocytes and monocytes also

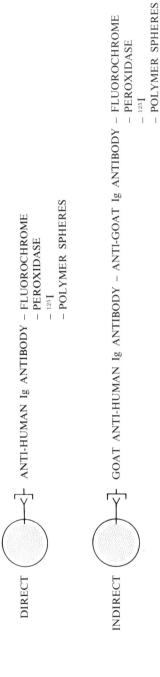

Figure 6. Cellular immunoglobulin (surface I$_g$—viable, unfixed cells: cytoplasmic I$_g$—fixed cells).

Table 2. T lymphocyte subpopulations*.

T_g cels	Fc receptor for IgG
	Large lymphocytes
	Marginated heterochromatin
	Cytoplasm 3+ (mitochondria, RER, Golgi)
	Azurophilic and electron dense granules
	NSE 0 − + (dispersed)
	Microvilli
	Phagocytosis of IgG coated erythrocytes
	Suppressor activity
T_m cells	Fc receptor for IgM
	Small to medium lymphocytes
	Cytoplasm + (few organelles)
	NSE 2 − 3 + (1-2 spots)
	Smooth plasma membrane
	No phagocytosis
	Helper activity

*Summarized from (45).

possess Fc receptors, they may show surface staining. In addition, receptors for the Fc fragment of other heavy chains exist (45), increasing this complication. Antilymphocyte or lymphoma antibodies may result in false positivity, or in the case of lymphomas and leukemias, mask a monoclonal population. Antibodies against immunoglobulins, e.g. rheumatoid factors, may result in binding to the SIg of B lymphocytes.

Much of this sort of interference can be eliminated by enzymatic stripping or incubation at 37°C for 2–24 hours during which immune complexes bound via Fc receptors are shed from the lymphocytes. SIG manufactured by the cell is not affected or resynthesized. Use of F(ab)$_2$ fragments of IgG molecules as antisera will avoid much of the problem caused by Fc receptor binding of aggregated IgG in the antisera.

Monoclonality

Lymphomas and leukemias of B cells are commonly referred to as "monoclonal" because the cells which possess detectable surface or cytoplasmic Ig bear only one or two heavy chains and one light chain, e.g. IgMκ, whereas a reactive or nonneoplastic lymphocyte population contains cells bearing the spectrum of heavy and light chains (polyclonal). Thus a monclonal pattern of surface or cytoplasmic Ig is relied upon as a powerful indicator of the neoplastic nature offthe proliferative process. Certain types of B cell proliferations, e.g. CLL and hairy cell leukemia, not infrequently show polyclonal SIg staining patterns. However, if the cells are incubated at 37°C and/or F(ab)$_2$ antisera are used, a monoclonal pattern emerges (Table 3). Whereas a monoclonal pattern is already apparent the figures do not change appreciably. Any residual polyclonality after incubation and F(ab)$_2$ use is

Table 3. Effect of incubation at 37°C and use of Fab antisera on surface Ig patterns*.

INCUBATION

Diagnosis	Specimen	Time incubated at 37°C	Specificity of antisera % cells stained						Staining Pattern
			IgA	D	G	M	κ	λ	
Reactive hyperplasia	Lymph node	45 min	14	48	50	33	24	33	Polyclonal
		overnight	16	30	26	18	25	14	Polyclonal
CLL	Spleen	45 min	26	2	36	42	41	22	Polyclonal
		overnight	4	1	40	16	32	0	G/Mκ
CLL	Blood	45 min	10	78	11	77	79	23	Polyclonal
		overnight	0	62	0	58	78	0	D/Mκ
Hairy cell leukemia	Spleen	45 min	15	56	3	20	40	0	Polyclonal
		overnight	4	57	1	26	51	0	D/Mκ
Hairy cell leukemia	Spleen	45 min	8	29	0	11	50	4	Polyclonal
		overnight	1	6	1	4	29	2	κ

ANTISERA

F(ab)₂

Diagnosis	Specimen	Antiserum	IgA	D	G	M	κ	λ	Staining Pattern
Reactive hyperplasia	Lymph node	Whole	4	20	6	19	19	9	Polyclonal
		F(ab)₂	10	11	4	13	17	5	Polyclonal
Reactive hyperplasia	Lymph node	Whole	2	10	5	9	14	3	Polyclonal
		F(ab)₂	1	13	10	16	11	7	Polyclonal
Large cleaved FCC	Blood	Whole	4	2	79	41	42	62	Polyclonal
		F(ab)₂	1	0	67	3	0	71	Gλ
Small cleaved FCC	Lymph node	Whole	4	1	2	47	54	0	Mκ
		F(ab)₂	9	0	0	48	53	0	Mκ
Small noncleaved FCC	Lymph node	Whole	14	15	11	70	62	4	Polyclonal
		F(ab)₂	25	0	1	68	65	2	A/Mκ

* A more detailed report is in preparation.

presumably due to nonneoplastic cells admixed with lymphoma/leukemia cells.

It is generally accepted that this monoclonality reflects the proliferative expansion of a clone of B cells arising from a single cell. The initial event may involve a single cell or several, but the end result is a dominant clone which expresses the Ig class of the parent cell. Observations that these cells may bear two heavy chains are compatible with studies which have demonstrated a sequential switch in the production of heavy chains, controlled at the gene level (C region genes). Lymphomas and leukemias bearing both IgM and IgD are not uncommon. However, the antigen combining site (hypervariable sequence of the V region of the Ig molecule — idiotype) is constant, and antibodies reacting only with the antigen combining sites of an Ig molecule (anti-idiotype antibodies) can be produced. It is this constancy of idiotypes produced by the neoplastic cells (35, 47) that holds great promise for answering basic questions about human lymphomas, i.e. the nature of so-called composite lymphomas (87) and the identification of neoplastic B cells otherwise undetected in a mixed population because of a lack of morphological identity. For example, the identification of circulating B lymphocytes bearing idiotypes common to those produced by plasma cells in multiple myeloma supports the idea that multiple myeloma is a neoplasm of B cells with cells in different stages of differentiation (47).

Rosetting methods for SIg

In addition to erythrocytes, a variety of particles have been used to detect the SIg of B lymphocytes. The principle is essentially the same as for other indicators, e.g. fluorochromes, enzymes, and radioisotopes, but with the added advantages that rosettes can be stained for standard light microscopic examination, the lymphocytes forming rosettes can be isolated by gradient centrifugation methods; and by using particles of varying size or appearance, multiple receptors can be identified simultaneously in the same cell preparation. The particle can be coated with anti-Ig antibodies to bind directly to the SIg-bearing lymphocyte or used in a "sandwich" technique.

Particles that have been used for these rosettes include polyacrylamide and other polymer beads (1, 43) and bacteria (58, 83). This binding may be part of a broader phenomenon since mouse erythrocytes also bind spontaneously to human B lymphocytes.

Differentiation antigens

Several investigators have reported the use of anti-T-cell and anti-B-cell antisera, raised against a range of antigen sources, including T-cell antisera made against fetal thymocytes, peripheral T cells, human brain, and T-cell lines; and B-cell sera directed against chronic lymphocytic leukemia cells, splenic lymphocyte membranes and B-cell lines (79a). It is readily apparent that these antisera recognize different antigens and presumably different subpopulations of cells. In addition, results with these antisera are frequently at variance with results from other techniques used to discriminate between T and B cells.

Initially T cell antisera were only used in cytotoxic assays, but more recently specific antisera have been developed for use in immunofluorescence and radioisotope-labelling procedures. In the case of human B-cell-associated antigens, antisera have been prepared against cell membrane antigens from human B-lymphoblastoid lines (48) and have been reported as specifically cytotoxic to B lymphocytes of peripheral blood, cells from B-lymphoblastoid lines and complement receptor-positive, SIg-negative (null) lymphocytes, but not to T lymphocytes or complement receptor-negative, null lymphocytes. One B-cell-associated antigen, a lipoprotein, designated P–23, 30 antigen by Chess and Schlossman (21), bears a close resemblance to murine Ia antigens. Others have detected antibodies with similar specificity in sera from pregnant women (93). Adsorption of a panel of the latter sera with appropriate platelets removed HLA-A and HLA-B antibodies and the resulting antisera reacted with non-T lymphocytes and monocytes. Similar antisera to human "B cell antigens" have been prepared by others (2, 6) and are also considered to be analogous to the Ia antigen of mice. These antigens are linked to the major histocompatibility locus and are expressed on B cells, closely linked to the HLA-D region determinants which control the mixed lymphocyte reaction, but are not on T cells (21), although reports of Ia determinants on subpopulations of mouse T cells have appeared (34). These Ia-like human B cell alloantigens have been found on cells from patients with CLL and ALL which are B cells (SIg), and on some non-marking ALL cells (35), but not on T-cell leukemias or lymphomas.

Data from studies using anti-T and anti-B antisera is accumulating, but is frequently conflicting and confusing because cells used for immunization and adsorption procedures, and species in which antisera are raised vary appreciably. Nevertheless, such information makes it increasingly clear that there is significant heterogeneity within the T and B lymphocyte classes. Subpopulations with different patterns (phenotypes) of membrane antigens are being identified and associated with funtion in vitro and, in the case of neoplasms, with clinical behavior. Chess and Schlossman (21) have studied human thymocyte differentiation using antisera (anti-HTL) prepared against E rosette positive acute lymphoblastic leukemia (T-ALL) cells, adsorbed with B lymphoblastoid cell lines. These react with thymocytes and leukemic cells from patients with T-ALL. Other antisera (anti-TH$_1$) prepared against highly purified peripheral T cells have provided evidence of differentiation of human T cells from thymocytes. Thymocytes bear receptors for sheep erythrocytes and both the HTL and TH_1 antigens, but with differentiation, the sheep cell receptor is retained and the HTL antigen lost. The TH_1 antigen is present on all thymocytes, but on only 40%–60% of the peripheral T cells.

Many workers have reported the existence of leukemia-associated antigens (see Taylor (79a, 79b), for a detailed account of these and differentiation antigens). Some are related to B cell alloantigens and others to thymic antigens. The clinical importance of these differentiation and leukemia-associated antigens lies in their use in identifying and clinically characterizing subtypes of lymphomas and leukemias, most extensively applied in ALL (9, 44).

Although this is a highly complex and fluid field at present, it holds promise for the identification, not only of functionally restricted subpopulations of normal lymphocytes, but of specific subtypes of leukemias or lymphomas within what otherwise appear to be morphologically homogenous groups.

Hybridomas

An intriguing approach to producing specific antisera against lymphoma-associated antigens involves the immunization of mice with whole lymphoma cells followed by in vitro hybridization of the murine antibody synthesizing spleen cells with mouse myeloma cells (63). Hybrid cells producing antibody against cellular antigens are cloned in soft agar and antibodies produced by a range of colonies are tested against a panel of target cells, normal and neoplastic, to detect clones with lymphoma specificity. Attractive features are the lack of necessity for extensive adsorption of antisera and the large quantities of monospecific antibodies produced in vitro by cloned cell lines or in vivo by mice transplanted with the hybrid clones.

Other identifying features

There are a range of other means by which T and B lymphocytes have been distinguished, some of them cytochemical, some functional. There is not the space to review these here and they have been listed by others (21, 79a, b). However, a few general comments are in order. The list by which the major populations of T and B lymphocytes can be distinguished is growing precipitously. As it lengthens it is apparent that a clearcut, distinct division between B and T lymphocytes is less easy than appeared at first. Nevertheless E rosettes, SIg and the enzymes, acid phosphatase and nonspecific esterase have proved to be relatively reliable markers for separating B and T lymphocytes and monocytes, and considering the complexities involved are surprisingly useful in distinguishing B and T and histiocytic lymphoma/ leukemias. Use of antisera directed against specific cell antigens would appear to offer even more precise distinctions, but these antisera have not been widely available. Other identifiers, particularly specific in vitro cell functions, are less useful clinically because of methodological complexity or lack of specificity, but hold promise as indicated by reports that specific types of lymphoma/leukemia cells manifest differentiated functions such as helper and suppressor activity (11, 12).

The DNA polymerase, terminal deoxynucleotidyl transferase (TdT) catalyzes the addition of deoxynucleotides to the 3'OH end of single stranded poly or oligo-deoxynucleotide primers without template direction. It has proved a useful biochemical marker because of its rather restricted distribution in cells of lymphoid tissues. This enzyme is present in T-blast cells and thymocytes and in cells from adult and childhood ALL, null or T-cell type. It is present in small quantities in normal bone marrow, but not in normal lymphoid tissues. TDT elevation in the cells of some patients with blast crisis in chronic granulocytic leukemias is unexplained. Antibodies to purified TdT have been prepared (20) and should prove useful in identifying positive cells in sections using immunoperoxidase cytochemistry.

LYMPHOMA STUDIES

USC lymphoma group

We began our studies with the point of view that cytomorphologic differences between lymphomas indicated their origin from T or B lymphocytes or nonmarking cells, and that this would be confirmed as the appropriate surface marker and cytochemical techniques were applied. As indicated above, none of these techniques provides absolute criteria for distinguishing cell types, and for that reason, it is important to use a panel of several methods for assessment of cell populations for the presence of T and B cells. Our studies involve lymphoid material obtained primarily from untreated patients, and include lymph nodes, spleens, bone marrow and peripheral blood as well as body fluids (spinal, peritoneal, pleural). Tissues are obtained from patients at the Los Angeles County-University of Southern California Medical Center and from approximately 20 participating hospitals of the Southern California Lymphoma Group. Essential to these studies is proper fixation and processing for preparing optimum paraffin sections. Zenkers or B-5 fixative is used and paraffin embedded tissues are sectioned at 4–6 microns. Sections are stained with hematoxylin and eosin (H&E) and methyl greenpyronin (MGP) (27) and cytoplasmic immunoglobulins and muramidase are identified by immunoperoxidase staining (78). Finely minced fragments of the same tissues are also fixed for transmission electron microscopy.

Once the material is fixed for diagnosis and electron microscopy, and cultured for microorganisms when indicated, cell suspensions of the lymphoid tissues are aseptically prepared by gently teasing through stainless steel wire mesh in RPMI 1640. Mononuclear cells are separated from peripheral blood, but not lymphoid tissue suspensions, on Ficoll/Hypaque. These cell suspensions are then utilized for marker studies — E rosettes, C_3 receptors, SIg. To reiterate, an important feature is the preparation of stained rosettes for morphologic identification of the rosette-forming cells, since each neoplastic lymphoid tissue contains residual T and B lymphocytes.

Surface immunoglobulin-bearing cells are detected with fluorescein isothiocyanate-labelled polyvalent and monospecific antiglobulin sera. Commercial antisera are used which have been checked for specificity by immunoprecipitation techniques and titered against a population bearing sufficient B lymphocytes (tonsil) to determine the "plateau end point" beyond which the percentage of SIg-positive cells falls progressively with dilution (66). The percentage of cells showing typical surface fluorescence is determined by counting 100–200 mononuclear cells. Phase optics are used to discriminate between mononuclear cells and granulocytes, but admittedly this is not always reliable. For every lymphoma from which there are sufficient cells, the cells are examined for heavy and light chains with monospecific antisera, to determine monoclonality. When too few cells are

Table 4. Immunological marker results on normal blood and reactive lymph nodes.

Parameter % cells bearing:	Peripheral blood Healthy donors Mean ± SD	Lymph nodes Reactive hyperplasia* Mean ± SD
SRBC receptors	68 ± 11	48 ± 20
Complement receptors	13 ± 10	22 ± 13
Surface Ig		
Total Ig	19 ± 8	26 ± 1
(polyvalent anti- serum)		
IgA	2 ± 2	3 ± 5
IgD	4 ± 3	10 ± 9
IgG	8 ± 5	8 ± 7
IgM	7 ± 3	15 ± 9
Igκ	9 ± 3	17 ± 11
Igλ	8 ± 5	13 ± 9

*This diagnosis includes both follicular and interfollicular hyperplasia, and the magnitude of the reaction varies widely.

available, staining for κ and λ chains alone indicates the presence or lack
of monoclonality. Problems produced by the nonspecific adsorption of Ig by
Fc receptors can generally be resolved by incubation of cells at 37°C and
use of F(ab)₂ antisera (Table 3).

Cytocentrifuge preparations are made from cell suspensions for cytochemical determinations as are touch imprints of the cut surface of the
lymphoid tissues. These preparations are routinely stained with Wright
stain, PAS, MGP, sudan black and for chloroacetate esterase, acid phosphatase (with and without tartrate) and nonspecific esterase activity.

Lymphoma cells and peripheral lymphocytes are used for HLA typing.
Whenever possible, marker results on cells obtained from a biopsy specimen are correlated with those on the peripheral lymphocytes and the
patients are followed throughout the course of the disease.

Results of studies of lymphoma/leukemia cells are compared with
studies on blood and lymph node lymphocytes from healthy donors and
patients with nonlymphoproliferative diseases (Table 4).

Current status, problems, and future

Utilization of techniques developed to distinguish B and T lymphocytes
in the study of disease has already contributed significantly to the understanding of a number of disorders, particularly the immune deficiencies. In
some instances these techniques may play a direct role in determining
prognosis and therapy. One area that has received much attention in recent
years is the application of B and T marker techniques to the study of human
lymphomas correlating markers with the morphological and clinical
features of specific lymphomas and leukemias. Many lymphomas and
leukemias can be characterized as for B- or T-cell origin on the basis of
morphology, and location within lymphoid tissues (follicular, paracortical,
etc.), confirmed by immunological markers. We are now in the phase of
further subdividing the major B- and T-cell classes into subpopulations as
they are identified by markers and specific functions. Some normal subpopulations reported include T lymphocytes which are antigen reactive
(23, 68), helper cells (45, 54, 64), killer cells (19, 42), and suppressor cells
(39, 45, 67). In the B-cell system there are antibody-synthesizing, surface
immunoglobulin-bearing cells (86), complement receptor cells and cytotoxic Fc receptor positive cells (ADCC) which may be immature or "null"
B cells (26). This means, of course, that we are in turn seeing lymphomas
and leukemias which appear to arise from some of these subclasses.

Nevertheless, it is also clear from increasing information about surface
determinants on subsets of T and B lymphocytes that one should not view
the separation of the B and T cells too rigidly. As Whiteside and Rowlands
(92) have discussed, most workers have been preoccupied with the differen-

ces in the B and T cell systems, having a rather restrictive view of this two component system. It should be remembered that T and B lymphocytes have a common origin and thus common genetic material. We do not know, as yet, whether the committment of B and T cells may not be reversible or that committed lymphocytes may express different surface determinants and functions under appropriate circumstances because of expression of normally repressed genetic material coding for these determinants or functions. This is particularly relevant in studies of neoplastic lymphocytes. Nonmarking or "null" cells (50) and lymphocytes with "double" markers (28) in healthy adults suggest that there is a small uncommitted lymphocyte pool of progenitor cells and the possibility remains that the B and T populations may be interchangeable under certain unusual circumstances. Considering the abnormal state of the cells in lymphoproliferative disorders, we must keep an open mind in evaluating surface marker studies of lymphomas and leukemias. For example, we have recently studied three cases of lymphoma which appear to be composed of both T and B neoplastic cells as determined with E rosettes and SIg. Does this represent two distinct neoplastic clones arising independently, i.e. a true composite lymphoma, or one clone with genetic derepression of a marker which is normally not expressed in the differentiated state? Or does it reflect excessive production of T cell "immunoglobulin", normally undetectable by immunofluorescence? The evidence for immunoglobulinlike antigen receptors on T cells (41, 46, 57, 91) and the report by Gatien and colleagues (38) that cells in the fetal thymus in the 9–10th week of gestation possess SIg suggests that the latter is not implausible.

With these reservations, it still appears that the heterogeneity of the B- and T-cell populations, which at first glance is confusing, may prove to be of significant clinical use in lymphoma studies. Since there is already abundant evidence that lymphomas may retain the markers and functions of the normal cell counterparts from which they arise, the ability to identify subtypes of lymphomas within the major morphological classes may turn out to be a belssing in disguise. Careful correlation of morphology with markers may well allow recognition of morphological subtypes based on subtle, previously unrecognized features. Of even more importance, the receptor/antigen patterns or "phenotypes" of different lymphomas and leukemias may be associated with distinctive clinical features and different responses to therapeutic regimens. This has already been demonstrated in acute lymphocytic leukemia of childhood in which patients with leukemic cells expressing surface markers have a poorer prognosis and require more intensive therapy than those with nonmarking or null cells (84).

The problems encountered now relate to the infancy of our knowledge of "differentiation antigens", whether they be receptors, enzymes or other functioning proteins. We know little about the few such antigens recognized in humans — their functions, relation to cell cycle, and specificity for certain cell types or stages in the development of one cell type. For example, does the antigen-marking pattern of a T-cell lymphoma reflect its stage of differentiation or the part of the cell cycle most of the cells are in? Most surely the pattern is a reflection of both, and a composite picture reflecting a spectrum of cells at different stages of differentiation and cell cycle is seen. A relatively synchronized population with few leaders and stragglers will naturally present the cleanest pattern. As this information is collected our understanding of the immune system and in turn lymphomas grows.

In spite of all the confusion, complexity, and problems in methodology and interpretation, it is apparent that empirical studies of lymphoma and leukemia cells by a wide range of identifiers will continue to enhance our understanding of the biology of lymphoproliferative disorders and lead to increasingly more rational evaluations of prognosis and selection of therapy. This can only be accomplished by the study of large numbers of cases with examples of each of the types of lymphomas and leukemias included. The cells must be well characterized morphologically and by a battery of marker techniques, and the results correlated with long range clinical evaluations. These studies are underway at several centers, and as the papers in this volume illustrate, a great deal of progress has already been made.

SUMMARY

As neoplasms of the immune system, lymphomas can be characterized by a variety of immunological techniques. These techniques, used in conjunction with morphology and cytochemistry, have promoted the development of lymphoma classifications which relate more closely to our current understanding of the anatomy and function of the immune system than earlier classifications. Immunological techniques used in the study of lymphomas are reviewed in terms of their value, problems and future applications.

ACKNOWLEDGEMENTS

The studies described are the results of a collaborative effort by the Lymphoma Group of the University of Southern California Cancer Center, Los Angeles, which includes Doctors A.D. Cramer, T.L. Lincoln, R.J. Lukes, P.R. Meyer, J.W. Parker, P.K. Pattengale, and C.R. Taylor, and D. Dugas. Expert technical assistance has been provided by M.J. Cain, P. Lee, M. Clarke, R. Scroggs and J. Steiner. The program is supported by NIH grant CA 19449.

REFERENCES

1. Ammann, A.J., Borg, D., Kondo, L., and Wara, D.W.: Quantitation of B cells in peripheral blood by polyacrylamide beads coated with anti-human chain antibody. J. Immunol., Methods, 17:365–371, 1977.
2. Arbeit, R.D., Sachs, D.H., Amos, D.B., and Dickler, H.B.: Human lymphocyte alloantigen(s) similar to murine Ir region-associated (Ia) antigens. J. Immunol., 115:1173–1175, 1975.

3. Bach, J.-F., Judet, C., Arce, S., and Dormont, J.: Exploration de la fonction thymique chez l'homme. (Exploration of thymic function in man. II. The sheep red cell rosette phenomenon, a T cell marker in man). Nouv. Presse Med., 3:655–660, 1974.

4. Basten, A., Miller, J.F.A.P., Sprent, J., and Pye, J.: A receptor for antibody on B lymphocytes. I. Method of detection and functional significance. J. Exp. Med., 135:610–626, 1972.

5. Berger, B.M., Schuman, R.M., Daniele, R.P., and Nowell, P.C.: E rosette formation at 37°C: A property of mitogen-stimulated human peripheral blood lymphocytes. Cell. Immunol., 26:105–113, 1976.

6. Billing, R., Rafizadeh, B., Drew, I., Hortman, G., Gale, R., and Terasaki, P.: Human B lymphocyte antigens expressed by lymphocytic and myelocytic leukemia cells. I. Detection by rabbit antisera. J. Exp. Med., 144:167–178, 1976.

7. Binz, H., and Wigzell, H.: Similar or identical idiotypes on IgG molecular and T cell receptors with specificity for the same alloantigens. In: Membrane receptors of lymphocytes, pp. 101–116, Preud'homme, L., Seligmann, M., and Kourilsky, F.M., (eds.), North Albany, New York, 1975.

8. Birnbaum, G.: Numbers of rosette forming cells in human peripheral blood. Cell. Immunol., 21:371–378, 1976.

9. Borella, L., Sen, L., and Casper, J.T.: Acute lymphoblastic leukemia (ALL) antigens detected with antisera to E rosette-forming and non-E rosette-forming ALL blasts. J. Immunol., 118:309–315, 1977.

10. Brain, P., and Marston, R.H.: Rosette formation by human T and B lymphocytes. Eur. J. Immunol., 3:6–9, 1973.

11. Broder, S., Edelson, R.L., and Lutzner, M.A., et al: The Sézary syndrome: a malignant proliferation of helper T cells. J. Clin. Invest., 58:1297–1306, 1976.

12. Broder, S., Mann, D., and Waldmann, T.A.: Pro-suppressor T-cell leukemia. Clin. Res., 26:374 A, 1978.

13. Brown, G., and Greaves, M.F.: Enumeration of absolute numbers of T and B lymphocytes in human blood. Scand. J. Immunol., 3:161, 1974.

Browne, O., Bell, J., Holland, P.D.J., and Thornes, R.P.: Plasmapheresis and immunostimulation. Lancet, 2:96, 1976.

15. Cantor, H.: T cells and the immune response, Prog. Biophys. Mol. Biol., 25:73–82, 1972.

16. Cantor, H., and Boyse, E.A.: Functional subclasses of T lymphocytes bearing different Ly antigens. I. The generation of functionally distinct T-cell subclasses is a differentiative process independent of antigen. J. Exp. Med., 141: 1376–1389, 1975.

17. Cantor, H., and Boyse, E.A.: Functional subclasses of T lymphocytes bearing different Ly antigens. II. Cooperation between subclasses of Ly + cells in the generation of killer activity. J. Exp. Med., 141:1390–1399, 1975.

18. Catovsky, D., Cherchi, M., Okos, A., Hegde, U., and Galton, D.A.G.: Mouse red-cell rosettes in B-lymphoproliferative disorders. Br. J. Heamatol., 33:173–177, 1976.

19. Cerottini, J.-C., Nordin, A.A., and Brunner, K.T.: Cellular and humoral response to transplantation antigens. I. Development of alloantibody-forming cells and cytotoxic lymphocytes in the graft-versus-host reaction. J. Exp. Med., 134:553–564, 1971.

20. Chan, J.Y., and Srivastava, B.I.S.: Antigenic relationships in calf thymus and human leukemic cell terminal deoxynucleotidyl transferase. Biochim. Biophys. Acta, 447:353–359, 1976.

21. Chess, L., and Schlossman, S.F.: Human lymphocyte subpopulations. Adv. Immunol., 25:213–241, 1977.

22. Chiao, J.W., Pantic, V.S., and Good, R.A.: Human peripheral lymphocytes bearing both B cell complement receptors and T cell characteristics for sheep erythrocytes detected by a mixed rosette method. Clin. Exp. Immunol., 18:483–490, 1974.

23. Cone, R.E., Sprent, J., and Marchalonis, J.J.: Antigen-binding specificity of isolated cell-curface immunoglobulin from thymus cell activated to histocompatibility antigens. Proc. Natl. Acad. Sci., U.S.A., 69:2556–2560, 1972.

24. Cooper, M.D.: Immunodeficiency with special reference to molecular defects. In: VII Immunopathology Symposium, Schwaben, West Germany, June, 1976.

25. Cooper, M.D., and Lawton, A.R.: Development of lymphoid tissue. In: The immunopathology of lymphoreticular neoplasms, pp. 1–21, Twomey, J.J., and Good, R.A., (eds.), Plenum Medical Books, New York/London, 1978.

26. Cordier, G., Samarut, C., Brochier, J., and Revillard, J.C.: Antibody dependent cell cytotoxicity (ADCC): Characterization of "killer" cells in human lymphoid organs. Scand. J. Immunol., 5:233–242, 1976.

27. d'Alblaing, G., Rogers, E.R., Parker, J.W., and Lukes, R.J.: Laboratory suggestion: A simplified and modified methyl green pyronin stain. Am. J. Clin. Pathol., 54:667–669, 1970.

28. Dickler, H.B., Adkinson, N.F., Jr., and Terry, W.D.: Evidence for individual human peripheral blood lymphocytes bearing both B and T cell markers. Nature, 247:213–215, 1974.

29. Dwyer, J.M.: Identifying and enumerating human T and B lymphocytes. Prog. Allergy, 21:178–260, 1976.

30. Eastham, R.J., Mason, J.M., Jennings, B.R., Belev, P.W., and Maguda, T.A.: T-cell rosette test in squamous cell carcinoma of the head and neck. Arch. Otolaryngol., 102:171–175, 1976.

31. Eden, A., Miller, G.W., and Nussenzweig, V.: Human lymphocytes bear membrane receptors for C3b and C3d. J. Clin. Invest., 52:3239–3242, 1973.

32. Facchini, A., Maraldi, N.M., Bartoli, S., Farulla, A., and Manzoli, F.A.: Changes in membrane receptors of B and T human lymphocytes exposed to ^{60}Co Gamma Rays. Radiation Res., 68:339–348, 1976.

33. Ferrarini, M., Moretta, L., Abrile, R., and Durante, M.L.: Receptors for IgG molecules on human lymphocytes forming spontaneous rosettes with sheep red cells. Eur. J. Immunol., 5:70–72, 1975.

34. Frelinger, J.A., Niederhuber, J.E., and Shreffler, P.C.: Effects of anti-Ia sera on mitogenic responses. III. Mapping the genes controlling the expression of Ia determinants on concanavalin A-reactive cells to the I-J subregion of the H-2 gene complex. J. Exp. Med., 144:1141–1146, 1976.

35. Fu, S.M., Winchester, R.J., and Kunkel, H.G.: The occurrence of the HL-B alloantigens on the cells of unclassified acute lymphoblastic leukemias. J. Exp. Med., 142:1334–1338, 1975.

36. Fu, S.M., Chiorezzi, N., Kunkel, H.G., Halper, J.P., and Harris, S.R.: Induction of in vitro differentiation and immunoglobulin synthesis of human leukemic B lymphocytes. J. Exp. Med., 148:1570–1578, 1978.

37. Fuks, Z., Glatstein, E., and Kaplan, H.S.: Patterns of presentation and relapse in the non-Hodgkin's lymphomata. Br. J. Cancer 31, Suppl., 2:286–297, 1975.

38. Gatien, J.G., Schneeberger, E.E., and Merler, E.: Analysis of human thymocyte subpopulations using discontinuous gradients of albumin: Precursor lymphocytes in human thymus. Eur. J. Immunol., 5:312–317, 1975.

39. Gershon, R.K.: T cell control of antibody production. Contemp. Top. Immunobiol., 3:1–40, 1974.
40. Gershon, R.K., and Metzler, C.M.: Regulation of the immune response. In: The immunopathology of lymphoreticular neoplasms, pp. 23–51, Twomey, J.J., and Good, R.A., (eds.), Plenum Medical Books, New York/London, 1978.
41. Goldschneider, I., and Cogen, R.B.: Immunoglobulin molecules on the surface of activated T lymphocytes in the rat. J. Exp. Med., 138:163–175, 1973.
42. Goldstein, P., Wigzell, H., Blomgren, H., and Svedmyr, E.A.J.: Autonomy of thymus-processed lymphocytes (T cells) for their education into cytotoxic cells. Eur. J. Immunol., 2:489–501, 1972.
43. Gordon, I.L., Lukes, R.J., O'Brien, R.L., Parker, J.W., Rembaum, A., Russell, R., and Taylor, C.R.: Visualization of surface immunoglobulin of human B lymphocytes using microsphere-immunoglobulin conjugated in Giemsa-stained preparations. Clin. Immunol. Immunopathol., 8:61–63, 1977.
44. Greaves, M.F., Janossy, G., Roberts, M.: Membrane phenotyping: Diagnosis, monitoring and classification of acute "lymphoid" leukemias. In: Immunological diagnosis of leukemias and lymphomas, pp. 61–75, Theirfelder, S., Rodt, H., and Thiel, E., (eds.), Springer-Verlag, New York, 1977.
45. Grossi, C.E., Webb, S.R., Zicca, A., Lydyard, P.M., Moretta, L., Mingari, C., and Cooper, M.D.: Morphological and histochemical analyses of two human T-cell subpopulations bearing receptors for IgM or IgG. J. Exp. Med., 147:1405–1417, 1978.
46. Haustein, D., Marchalonis, J.J., and Harris, A.W.: Immunoglobulin of T lymphoma cells. Biosynthesis, surface representation, and partial characterization. Biochemistry, 14:1826–1834, 1975.
47. Holm, G., Mellstedt, H., Pettersson, D., and Biberfeld, P.: Idiotypic immunoglobulin structure on blood lymphocytes in human plasma cell myeloma. Immunol. Rev., 34:139–163, 1977.
48. Humphreys, R.E., McCune, J.M., Chess, L., Herrman, H.C., Malenka, D.J., Mann, D.L., Parham, P., Schlossman, S.F., and Strominger, J.L.: Isolation and immunologic characterization of human, B-lymphocyte-specific, cell surface antigen. J. Exp. Med., 144:98–112, 1976.
49. Jondal, M., Klein, E., and Yefenof, E.: Surface markers on human B and T lymphocytes. VII. Rosette formation between peripheral T lymphocytes and lymphoblastoid B-cell lines. Scand. J. Immunol., 4:259–266, 1975.
50. Jønsson, V.: Technical aspects of the rosette technique for detecting human circulating B and T lymphocytes. Normal values and some remarks on null lymphocytes. Scand. J. Heamatol., 13:361–369, 1974.
51. Jønsson, V.: Influence of prednisone and cytostatics on human blood B-, T- and O-lymphocytes in diseases. Scand. J. Heamatol., 15:109–116, 1975.
52. Kaplan, M.E., and Clark, C.: An improved rosetting assay for detection of human T lymphocytes. J. Immunol. Methods, 5:131–135, 1974.
53. Katz, D.H., and Benacerraf, B.: The regulatory influence of activated T cells on B cell responses to antigen. Adv. Immunol., 15:1–94, 1972.
54. Kontiainen, S., and Andersson, L.C.: Antigen-binding T cells as helper cells. Separation of helper cells by immune rosette formation. J. Exp. Med., 142:1035–1039, 1975.
55. Loor, F.: Structure and dynamics of the lymphocyte surface. Prog. Allergy, 23:1–153, 1977.
56. Lukes, R.J., Parker, J.W., Taylor, C.R., Tindle, B.H., Cramer, A.D., and

Lincoln, T.L.: Immunologic approach to non-Hodgkin lymphomas and related leukemias. Analysis of the results of multiparameter studies of 425 cases. Semi. Hematol., 15:322–351, 1978.

57. Marchalonis, J.J., Cone, R.E., and Atwell, J.L.: Isolation and partial characterization of lymphocyte surface immunoglobulins. J. Exp. Med., 135:956–971, 1972.

58. Mayer, E.P., Bratescu, A., Dray, S., and Teodorescu, M.: Ennumeration of human B lymphocytes in stained blood smears by their binding of bacteria. Clin. Immunol. Immunopathol., 9:37–46, 1978.

59. Melchers, F., and Andersson, J.: IgM in bone marrow-derived lymphocytes. Changes in synthesis, turnover and secretion, and in numbers of molecules on the surface of B cells after mitogenic stimulation. Eur. J. Immunol., 4:181–188, 1974.

60. Mendes, N.F., Tolnai, M.E.A., Silveira, N.P.A., Gilbertsen, R.B., and Metzgar, R.S.: Technical aspects of the rosette tests used to detect human complement receptor (B) and sheep erythrocyte-binding (T) lymphocytes. J. Immunol., 111:860–867, 1973.

61. Mendes, N.F., Mihi, S.S., Peixinho, Z.F.: Combined detection of lymphocytes by rosette formation with sheep erythrocytes and zymosan-C_3 complexes. J. Immunol., 113:531–536, 1974.

62. Miller, J.F.A.P.: The cellular basis of immune responsiveness. In: Clinics in haematology, vol. 6, Disorders of lymphopoiesis and lymphoid function, pp. 277–298, Fundenberg, H.H., (ed.). W.B. Sanders Co., London/Philadelphia/Toronto, 1977.

63. Milstein, C., Adetugbo, K., Cowan, N.J., Kohler, G., Secher, O.S., and Wilde, C.D.: Somatic cell genetics of antibody-secreting cells: Studies of clonal diversification and analysis by cell fusion. Cold Spring Harbor Symp. Quant. Biol, 41:793–803, 1977.

64. Mitchison, N.A., Rajewsky, K., and Taylor, R.B.: Cooperation of antigenic determinants and of cells in the induction of antibodies. In: Developmental aspects of antibody formation and structure, pp. 547–564, Sternbak, R.A., and Riha, T., (eds.), Academic Press, New York, 1970.

65. O'Brien, R.L., Parker, J.W., and Dixon, J.F.: Mechanisms of lymphocyte transformation. In: Progress in molecular and subcellular biology, vol. 6, pp. 201–270, Hahn, F.E., (ed.). Springer-Verlag, Heidelberg, 1978.

66. Preud'homme, J.L., and Labaume, S.: Immunofluorescent staining of human lymphocytes for the detection of surface immunoglobulins. Ann. N.Y. Acad. Sci., 254:254–261, 1975.

67. Rich, R.R., and Pierce, C.W.: Biological expressions of lymphocyte activation. II. Generation of a population of thymus-derived suppressor lymphocytes. J. Exp. Med., 137:649–659, 1973.

68. Roelants, G.E., Ryden, A., Hägg, L.B., and Loor, F.: Active synthesis of immunoglobulin receptors for antigen by T lymphocytes. Nature, 247:106–108, 1974.

69. Roelants, G.E., Loor, F., von Boehmer, H., Sprent, J., Hägg, L.B., Mayor, K.S., and Ryden, A.: Five types of lymphocytes ($Ig^-\theta^-$, $Ig^-\theta^+$ weak, $Ig^-\theta^+$ strong, $Ig^+\theta^-$ and $Ig^+\theta^+$) characterized by double immunofluorescence and electrophoretic mobility organ distribution in normal and nude mice. Eur. J. Immunol., 5:127–131, 1975.

70. Ross, G.D., Rabellino, E.M., Polley, M.J., and Grey, H.M.: Combined studies of complement receptor and surface immunoglobulin-bearing cells and sheep

erythrocyte rosette-forming cells in normal and leukemic human lymphocytes. J. Clin. Invest., 52:377–385, 1973.

71. Ross, G.D.: Lymphocyte complement receptors and their relationship to other membrane receptors. In: Clinical evaluation of immune function in man, pp. 27–45, Litwin, S.D., Christian, C.L., and Siskind, G.W., (eds.), Grune and Stratton, New York, 1976.

72. Sachs, L.: Control of normal cell differentiation and the phenotypic reversion of malignancy in myeloid leukemia. Nature, 274:535–539, 1978.

73. Sen, L., Mills, B., and Borella, L.: Erythrocyte receptors and thymic-associated antigens on human thymocytes, mitogen-induced blasts, and acute leukemia blasts. Cancer Res., 36:2436–2441, 1976.

74. Shevach, E.M., Jaffe, E.S., and Green, I.: Receptors for complement and immunoglobulin on human and animal lymphoid cells. Transplant. Rev., 16:3–28, 1973.

75. Stathopoulos, G., and Elliott, E.V.: Formation of mouse or sheep red-blood-cell rosettes by lymphocytes from normal and leukaemic individuals. Lancet, 1:600–601, 1974.

76. Stein, H., and Müller-Hermelink, H.K.: Simultaneous presence of receptors for complement and sheep red blood cells on human fetal thymocytes. Br. J. Haematol., 36:227–233, 1977.

77. Stein, H.: The immunologic and immunochemical basis for the Kiel Classification. In: Malignant lymphomas other than Hodgkin's disease, pp. 529–657, Lennert K., (ed.), Springer-Verlag, Berlin, Heidelberg, New York, 1978.

78. Taylor, C.R.: An immunohistological study of follicular lymphoma, reticulum cell sarcoma and Hodgkin's disease. Eur. J. Cancer, 12:61–75, 1976.

79. Taylor, C.R.; Hodgkin's Disease and the Lymphomas, Annual Research Reviews. Horrobin, D.F., (ed.), Eden Press, Montreal, and Churchill, Longman, Livingston, Edinburgh/London (79a: vol. 2, 1978; 79b: vol. 3, 1979.)

80. Taylor, C.R.: Immunocytochemical methods in the study of lymphoma and related conditions. J. Histochem. Cytochem., 26:495–512, 1978.

81. Taylor, C.R., Gordon, I.L., Rembaum, A., Russell, R., Parker, J., O'Brien, R.L., and Lukes, R.J.: Human B lymphocytes in Giemsa stained preparations. J. Immunol. Methods, 17:81–89, 1978.

82. Teodorescu, M., Mayer, E.P., and Dray, S.: Simultaneous identification of T and B cells in blood smears using antibody coated bacteria. Cell. Immunol. 24:90–96, 1976.

83. Teodorescu, M., Mayer, E.P., and Dray, S.: Enumeration and identification of human leukemic lymphocytes by their natural binding of bacteria Cancer Res., 37:1715–1718, 1977.

84. Tsukimoto, I., Wong, K.Y., and Lampkin, B.C.: Surface markers and prognostic factors in acute lymphoblastic leukemia. New Engl. J. Med., 294:245–248, 1976.

85. Uhr, J.W., and Möller, G.: Regulatory effect of antibody on the immune response. Immunology, 8:81–127, 1968.

86. Unanue, E.R., Grey, H.M., Rabellino, E., Campbell, P., and Schmidtke, J.: Immunoglobulins on the surface of lymphocytes. II. The bone marrow as the main source of lymphocytes with detectable surface-bound immunoglobulin. J. Exp. Med., 133:1188–1198, 1971.

87. van den Tweel, J.G., Lukes, R.J., and Taylor, C.R.: Pathophysiology of lymphocyte transformation. A study of so-called composite lymphomas. Am. J. Clin. Pathol., 71:509–520, 1979.

88. Verhaegen, H., De Cree, J., De Cock, W., and Verbruggen, F.: Restoration by levamisole of low E-rosette forming cells in patients suffering from various diseases. Clin. Exp. Immunol., 27:313–318, 1977.

89. Warner, N.L.: Membrane immunoglobulins and antigen receptors on B and T lymphocytes. Adv. Immunol., 19:67–216, 1974.

90. Weissman, I.L., Warnke, R., Butcher, E.C., Rouse, R., and Levy, R.: The lymphoid system: Its normal architecture and the potential for understanding the system through the study of lymphoproliferative diseases. Human Pathol., 9:25–45, 1978.

91. Whiteside, T.L., and Rabin, B.S.: Surface immunoglobulin on activated human blood thymus-derived cells. J. Clin. Invest., 57:762–771, 1976.

92. Whiteside, T.L., and Rowlands, D.T., Jr.: T-cell and B-cell identification in the diagnosis of lymphoproliferative disease. Am. J. Pathol., 88:754–790, 1977.

93. Winchester, R.J., Fu, S.M., Wernet, P., Kunkel, H.G., Dupont, B., and Jersild, C.: Recognition by pregnancy serums of non-HL-A alloantigens selectively expressed on B lymphocytes. J. Exp. Med., 141:924–929, 1975.

94. Woda, B.A., Fenaglio, C.M., Nette, E.G., and King, D.W.: The lack of specificity of the sheep erythrocyte—T lymphocyte rosetting phenomenon. Am. J. Pathol. 88:69–80, 1977.

95. Wybran, J., and Fudenberg, H.: How clinically useful is T and B cell quantitation: Ann. Intern. Med., 80:765–767, 1974.

9. IMMUNOPEROXIDASE TECHNIQUES IN LYMPHOMA RESEARCH

C.R. TAYLOR

BACKGROUND

Immunoperoxidase methods have much in common with established immunofluorescence procedures. Both have the potential for specific demonstration of cell and tissue antigens, with similar limitations demanding rigorous control of specificity.

Immunofluorescence

With the introduction of stable compounds of fluorescein isothiocyanate (FITC) Coons and colleagues were able to prepare conjugates of FITC with antibody, and the fluorescent antibody technique was born (5, 6). Over the succeeding years immunofluorescence methods found wide application, and the demonstration of the tissue or cellular localization of specific antigens or antibodies provided impetus for major advances in immunology and immunopathology.

Most studies of tissue immunoglobulin by immunofluorescence utilized fresh or specially processed tissues, for, until recently, it was generally held that immunoglobulins do not survive fixation with formalin or processing to paraffin blocks: "Antigen and antibody activity is inactivated by conventional methods" (27). Also, immunofluorescence methods were considered unsuitable for the study of formalin-fixed tissues per se, due to the excitation of marked autofluorescence. The fallacy of these assumptions was revealed by some of the initial studies leading to the use of immunohistologic methods in routinely fixed tissues (3). Further refinements of immunofluorescence techniques applied to fixed embedded tissues have been reported by Knowles et al. (14), Huang et al. (12) and Denk et al. (7, 8). In these studies tissue was subjected to partial proteolytic digestion with trypsin or pronase prior to immunological staining. The papers by Knowles and colleagues (14) and Warnke and colleagues (40) described the current state of the art in relation to the study of lymphocytes and malignant lymphomas (see also Taylor, (35)).

Paradoxically, the overall success of fluorescent antibody methods in-

J.G. van den Tweel et al. (eds.), Malignant Lymphoproliferative Diseases, 111–131

creased the demand for a satisfactory alternative labeling system, principally to avoid the disadvantages of the impermanence and poor morphology of immunofluorescence preparations, and the requirements for fresh or specially processed tissues.

Alternative to immunofluorescence

The availability of enzyme-labeled antibodies (22, 1, 28) provided an alternative to the immunofluorescence method. A number of modifications of enzyme labeling methods have been described—enzyme bridge method (19), the PAP procedure (28)—and may properly be included under the general title of immunoperoxidase techniques (Figure 1). The crucial step in rendering this method more generally useful to the practicing pathologist was its application to "routine" formalin-fixed paraffin-embedded tissues (36, 30, 20). Two principal advantages accrued. First, morphology was excellent, equivalent to haematoxylin and eosin stained material; second, retrospective studies were possible on stored material from the "files" of routine diagnostic laboratories. Thus a wealth of material was available for immediate study.

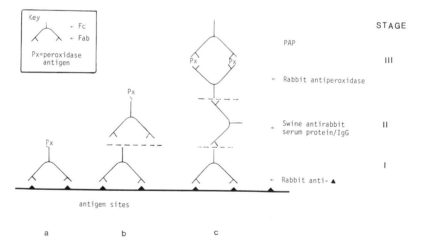

Figure 1. Immunoperoxidase procedures.
a) Peroxidase antibody conjugate, direct;
b) Peroxidase antibody conjugate, indirect;
c) Peroxidase-anti-peroxidase (PAP) immune complex method.

Methods have wide applicability, limited only by availability of specific antisera (stage I). Sequence of staining tissue antigen (▲): stage I, primary specific antiserum—rabbit anti- ▲; stage II, swine anti-rabbit serum protein/IgG; stage III, rabbit anti-peroxidase as separate reagent or as part of PAP complex. In each instance site of localization of peroxidase is demonstrated by means of chromogenic substrate, often diaminobenzidine with hydrogen peroxide.

Immunoperoxidase vs. immunofluorescence procedures

The various procedures utilizing labeling by horseradish peroxidase should be considered as alternatives to orthodox immunofluorescence methods, and should be employed in preference to immunofluorescence methods only on the basis of certain demonstrable advantages for specific projects, not merely because of the novelty of the immunoperoxidase procedure. The principal advantages of the immunoperoxidase method are:

1) Specialized microscopy is required for the examination of immunofluorescence preparations, while immunoperoxidase preparations are examined by orthodox light microscopy.
2) Preparations stained by immunoperoxidase methods are permanent.
3) The colored reaction products of substrates, such as diaminobenzidine, which gives a clear brown color, are compatible with the usual histological stains, and allow assessment of morphology by traditional criteria.
4) The requirement for fresh (or specially processed) tissue is avoided, and the method is thus suitable for use by the diagnostic pathologist who is usually in receipt of tissues which have been formalin-fixed and paraffin-embedded when the need for immunological studies becomes apparent.

Immunoperoxidase methods

Several variations offthe immunoperoxidase method have been described (review Taylor (32)), each using the enzymatic activity of horseradish peroxidase with a chromogenic substrate as a visual marker. Those most commonly employed are summarized in Figure 1.

Conjugate methods (Figure 1, a and b)

Peroxidase conjugated antibody methods, by direct or indirect techniques, are strictly analogous to comparable immunofluorescence methods. In the direct method the antibody conjugate has specificity directed against the antigen under study. In the indirect method a primary antiserum having specificity against the antigen is applied initially, followed by a peroxidase/antibody conjugate from a second species, directed against the immunoglobulin components of the primary antiserum. This indirect, or sandwich, method has certain advantages in that it is more sensitive than the direct method, is more versatile by substitution of primary antisera against a wide variety of antigens, and can be subjected to additional specificity controls by replacement of the primary antiserum by other antisera of the same origin but irrelevant specificity.

Nonconjugate procedures (Figure 1, c)

The enzyme bridge method and the PAP method were designed particularly to circumvent some of the disadvantages inherent in conjugation procedures in which there may be denaturation of antibody, inactivation of enzyme, aggregation of unlabeled or partly labeled antibody, residual free enzyme, and residual free unlabeled antibody. Clearly, free antibody, or antibody conjugated to inactivated enzyme, will bind competitively with active conjugate so reducing sensitivity, while denatured antibody, free enzyme, and aggregates will contribute to nonspecific staining.

The enzyme bridge method (19, 10) utilizes a three layer antibody technique, with the final stages involving the addition of antibody to horseradish peroxidase and then free horseradish peroxidase. In principle this resembles the PAP method, which is now more commonly used, principally for reasons of convenience and enhanced sensitivity.

The PAP method

The PAP method (peroxidase-anti-peroxidase—Figure 1, c) (28, 30, 31, 32, 33) was initially introduced by Sternberger and colleagues (29) as an alternative to peroxidase conjugate and immunofluorescence procedures, with an additional advantage of enhanced sensitivity (estimated at 100–1000 times that of immunofluorescence (28)). As in the enzyme bridge method, this technique depends upon the addition of an excess of swine anti-rabbit immunoglobulin (Figure 1c, stage II) to bind the rabbit immunoglobulin of the PAP immune complex (consisting of rabbit antibody to horseradish peroxidase and horseradish peroxidase antigen) (Figure 1, stage III) to the primary rabbit antiserum (Figure 1, stage I). The method was subsequently adapted for use on fixed paraffin-embedded tissues (30, 32) where its sensitivity has significant advantages in the demonstration of residual antigens that survive the fixation-embedding process.

Modes of application of immunoperoxidase procedures

Immunoperoxidase procedures have been used for the detection and demonstration of cell surface antigens, intracellular antigens, and antigens distributed in the extracellular space of tissues. The detection of antigen in different localizations (e.g. cell membrane versus cell cytoplasm) is dependent upon the mode of exposure of the cell population to the immunoperoxidase system. For example, living cells exclude immunoglobulin from the cytoplasm and any antiserum applied to viable cells in suspension will detect surface antigens only. Following fixation, varying degrees of penetration of labeled antisera into cells (or into tissue sections) occur, determined by the nature of fixation, the extent of disruption of the cell membrane, and the molecular size of the largest component of the immunoperoxidase detection system (16, 9, 21).

Only studies of cytoplasmic immunoglobulins in fixed paraffin sections will be described here. Cell surface antigens (such as surface immunoglobulin) present in small amounts are not well visualized in fixed sections, due to the fact that free immunoglobulin in the tissue fluids cannot be washed from the cells, so precluding the development of sufficient contrast for reliable demonstration of the relatively small amounts of immunoglobulin at the B-cell surface. (To demonstrate surface immunoglobulin in suspension cells must be washed thoroughly to free them of adsorbed serum or tissue fluid immunoglobulin.)

Control and standardization

A system dependent upon the detection of antigen by specific antibody is only as good as the antibody or antibodies employed in the methodology (25). Many commercially available reagents give apparently specific reactions when assayed by precipitation-diffusion techniques; however, it must be remembered that techniques for studies of surface immunoglobulin are considerably more sensitive than immunodiffusion, and may reveal the presence of unwanted specificities that may not be detectable by the former method. Similarly, immunoperoxidase procedures such as the PAP method, with its exquisitie sensitivity, may detect trace specificities in tissue staining, requiring the use of antisera at higher dilutions in order to eliminate this unwanted staining. Hence the need for biological positive and negative controls. Optimal dilutions of all antisera should be determined by chequer board titrations with increasing dilutions of antisera (32). One solution to this form of "nonspecific" staining lies in utilizing highly purified mono-specific* antisera, and in the use of good "biological controls". The most useful controls are known positives and known negatives of the tissue/antigen system under study. Controls are readily available for cytoplasmic immunoglobulin studies, in normal and neoplastic plasma cell populations: myeloma cells are usually demonstrably monoclonal for κ and for λ, and for heavy chain classes. Other controls include the use of antisera directed against an irrelevant specificity; e.g. rabbit anti-human lysozyme or rabbit anti-human albumin antibodies provide good controls for rabbit antihuman immunoglobulin components and the various anti-immunoglobulin sera (anti-κ, anti-λ, anti-γ, anti-α, anti-μ, etc.) provide intrinsic controls one

---

*In monospecific antiserum several species of immunoglobulin are present with varying affinities for the antigenic determinant in question (25). In addition, many "monospecific" antisera in fact contain antibodies of different specificities, directed against two or more separate antigenic determinants in the molecule used as immunogen.

against the other. Recently Isaacson and Wright (13) have proposed the sue of antiserum against J chain as an additional control, reasoning that positive J chain staining should be observed only in cells synthesizing immunoglobulin, and not in cells taking up immunoglobulin from the environment.

MATERIALS AND METHODS

The basic case populations reviewed here have been described previously (Oxford cases, Taylor (30, 31); Los Angeles cases, Taylor (33), though the numbers have changed in some categories by accrual of selected new cases. The results and observations are included in summary form to provide a basis for discussion of the practical usefulness of the method in lymphoma research and diagnosis. Studies from other laboratories are cited in the text. The methodology used is based upon the principles discussed above. The PAP method was employed with diaminobenzidine/hydrogen peroxide as substrate. The sequence of staining and the dilutions used are summarized in Table 1. Optimal dilutions were determined. Sections were pretreated with normal swine serum to reduce background staining and with methanol/hydrogen peroxide to abolish endogenous peroxidase activity according to principles described elsewhere (32).

The case population studied is shown in Table 2. Tissue was obtained in the form of paraffin blocks; fixation was in formalin, Zenker's or B-5 fixative, though in some cases details of fixation and processing were unknown. Cases of reactive lymphadenopathy, secondary carcinoma, and anaplastic tumour of uncertain type were included for comparative purposes.

Antisera and PAP reagent were obtained from Dakopatts (A.S., Copenhagen; Dako, 22 N. Milpas, Santa Barbara, Calif. USA) Antisera were

Table 1. Immunoperoxidase procedure for demonstrating cytoplasmic immunoglobulin in paraffin sections: peroxidase-anti-peroxidase (PAP) immune complex method (Figure 1, c).

1. Paraffin sections—xylol-alcohol.
2. Block endogenous peroxidase with methanol containing 0.3% hydrogen peroxide, 30 min.
3. Normal swine serum 1/20, 10 min.
4. Rabbit antiserum to human immunoglobulin components,* 30 min.
5. Swine anti-rabbit serum protein 1/20, 30 min.
6. PAP 1/100, 30 min.
7. Diaminobenzidine reaction, counterstain with haematoxylin, dehydrate, and mount in D.P.X.

The reactions are carried out in Tris buffer (pH 7.6), with washes after stages 3, 4, 5 and 6 in Tris saline (a dilution of Tris buffer 1/10 in normal saline).

*Dilutions according to chequer board titration: anti-κ, anti-λ 1/2000, anti-γ 1/400, anti-α, anti-μ 1/300.

Table 2. Lymphomas and related conditions studied by immunoperoxidase methods.

Immunoblastic sarcoma	148
Follicle center cell lymphoma	132
Small cleaved 55	
Small noncleaved 16	
Large cleaved 26	
Large noncleaved 35	
Plasmacytoid lymphocytic lymphoma	39
Multiple myeloma[1]	71
Small lymphocytic/CLL	4
Convoluted lymphocytic lymphoma	6
Lymphoepithelioid cell lymphoma	6
Hodgkin's disease	87
Anaplastic tumor[2]	38
Secondary carcinoma	12
Reactive lymphadenopathy[3]	72
Hairy cell leukaemia (spleen)	6
"Reticulum cell sarcoma" of brain	24
	645

[1] Includes 33 Oxford cases (37) and 29 previously published cases from Los Angeles series (38).

[2] Includes cases of uncertain histologic designation, in which a diagnostic distinction between carcinoma and lymphoma or other sarcoma was not possible on pathological grounds.

[3] Includes nonspecific lymphadenitis, immunoblastic lymphadenopathy, and cases of lymphadenopathy with a known aetiology (e.g. toxoplasmosis, infectious mononucleosis).

checked for specificity by two dimensional immunodiffusion with monoclonal myeloma proteins.

Diaminobenzidine (DAB, 3, 4, 3′, 4′ tetra-amino-biphenyl hydrochloride)-hydrogen peroxide, using the method of Graham and Karnovsky (11), was employed as substrate. DAB is a potential carcinogen and should, therefore, be used with full precautions. The reaction with DAB produces a crisp, brown color which does not fade and which contrasts well with haematoxylin or haematoxylin-eosin counterstains.

RESULTS

Immunoperoxidase studies—the case population

This paper summarizes the application of immunoperoxidase techniques to the study of 500 cases of lymphoma and related conditions (Table 2), with particular reference to defining and refining existing morphological criteria for cell and tumour identification. Correlations with surface marker studies are also reported in cases where they serve to elucidate the immunohistologic findings. For B cells the principal surface marker was detection of surface immunoglobulin by direct immunofluorescence, utilizing goat antisera specific for human light and heavy chains, and scored in suspension following initial incubation in serum-free medium to remove adsorbed immunoglobulin. E rosette formation (spontaneous nonimmune rosettes with sheep red cells) was employed as a T cell marker. Preparations were also examined using a cytocentrifuge to assess the morphology of the rosetting cells, with reference to determining whether or not recognizable neoplastic cells formed E rosettes. Details of the surface marker methods and their interpretation have been given elsewhere (reviews, Taylor (35); Lukes et al. (17, 18); see also Parker J.W. and Lukes R.J. in this volume).

Diagnostic groups

Case material studied by immunoperoxidase methods is listed by diagnosis in Table 2; results are summarized in Tables 3 and 4.

Multiple myeloma

Case material from patients with myeloma of documented light and heavy chain type provides a control population of immunoglobulin-containing tissues of known light and heavy chain type. In most studies the pattern of immunohistologic staining of myeloma cell populations has been found to be consistent with the serum monoclonal protein type (37, 24). The demonstration of a monoclonal pattern (exclusively one light chain and one heavy chain) gives grounds for suspecting multiple myeloma even in cases where the histologic criteria set out by Canale and Collins (4) are not fulfilled. Benign monoclonal gammopathy does not show a clear monoclonal pattern of staining in the marrow plasma cell infiltrate. It must, however, be noted that anomalous (nonmonoclonal) immunohistologic patterns have been observed in a small number of cases, principally those lacking histologic "differentiation" (poorly differentiated myeloma) or those failing to secrete light or heavy chain or both (32). The explanation for these anomalous patterns, whether technical or biological, is not yet clear. In the present series less than 15% of myeloma cases showed anomalous patterns. Pinkus and Said (24) saw no such cases.

Non-Hodgkin lymphomas

In the first instance, case material from non-Hodgkin lymphomas was examined in order to study the pattern of immunoglobulin staining in the cytoplasm of individual lymphoma cells, with reference to developing concepts of the origin of these tumors from the lymphocyte and the possible

Table 3. Results of immunoperoxidase studies in non-Hodgkin lymphomas.

	Total	Tumor cell Ig negative[1]	Tumor cell Ig positive[1]			
			Definite Monoclonal	Probable Monoclonal	Anomalous[2] Pattern	Poor Quality[3]
Immunoblastic sarcoma (IBS)[4]	148	72	38	9	15	24
(B cell)	(59)	(5)	(31)	(8)	(9)	(6)
(T cell)	(52)	(43)	(1)	(1)	(3)	(4)
Follicle center cell lymphoma	132	58	29	15	11	19
Plasmacytoid lymphocytic lymphoma	39	2	21	5	5	6
Myeloma	71	1	54	1	10	5
"Reticulum cell sarcoma" brain	24	5	8	3	2	6
Lymphoepithelioid lymphoma	6	6	0	0	0	0
Convoluted lymphoma	6	6	0	0	0	0
Secondary carcinoma/anaplastic tumor	40	22	0	2	5	11
Reactive lymphadenopathy	72	(variable numbers of plasma cells with polyclonal pattern, three possible monoclonal)				
Total	538					

[1] Ig positive reactive plasma cells are present in almost all cases, together with variable proportions of immunoglobulin positive immunoblasts in some cases. These stain with a polyclonal pattern and serve as a valuable intrinsic control. Their presence makes the detection of an associated underlying monoclonal population difficult or impossible in some cases.

[2] Pattern of tumor cell staining not consistent with usual concepts of monclonality (see text).

[3] Includes cases in which there were inadequate numbers of cells for study, or in which fixation was apparently poor. In some cases this could be attributed to necrosis or extensive autolysis, in others the nature of the fixation process was unknown.

[4] B- and T-cell subtypes of immunoblastic sarcoma defined by morphologic criteria. These subtype designations confirmed by surface marker studies in 20 cases (13 T-cell IBS, 7 B-cell IBS).

Table 4. Summary of combined immunoperoxidase and surface marker studies showing marking of recognizable tumor cells.

Classification category (Table 2)	No.	Ig in Cytoplasm			Surface Ig			E rosette Positive[3]
		Neg.	Monoclonal[1]	Polyclonal	Monoclonal[1]	Polyclonal or low[2]	Neg.	
Small lymphocyte - B	8	7	1	0	7	1	0	0
Follicle center cell lymphoma	57	26	28	3	38	19	0	0
Plasmacytoid lymphocytic lymphoma	12	0	11	1	10	2	0	0
Immunoblastic sarcoma—B	7	0	7	(1)[4]	5	1	1	0
Immunoblastic sarcoma—T	13	11	1	1	0	10	3	13
Immunoblastic sarcoma—nonmarking	2	1	0	1	0	2	0	0

[1] Monoclonal: cases in which the tumor cell population stained exclusively for one light chain and one heavy chain.

[2] Polyclonal or low: cases in which the SIg pattern was not obviously monoclonal, including those cases with very low percentages of SIg positive tumor cells.

[3] Lymphomas were designated E rosette positive when lymphoma cells formed spontaneous rosettes with sheep erythrocytes as viewed in stained cytocentrifuge preparations.

[4] One "monoclonal" case had an anomalous neoplastic cell component—see text.

relationship of the different histological types of lymphoma to the process of lymphocyte transformation (30). In every case the pattern of immuno-peroxidase staining with each of the different primary anti-immunoglobulin sera was assessed for intensity and number of positive cells, and for morpho-logy of negative or positive-staining cells, in an attempt to define precisely the pattern of immunoglobulin staining of the cells comprising the B lym-phocyte series. Immunoglobulin was observed principally in plasma cells and in immunoblasts outside the germinal follicles, but varying preparations of large cleaved and noncleaved follicle center cells also showed definite evidence of immunoglobulin formation in the perinuclear space and in the cytoplasm. Similar findings in relation to immunoglobulin and the morpho-logic phases of B-cell development were described by Kojima and Tsunoda (15). The results of later studies are summarized in Tables 3 and 4.

Immunoblastic sarcoma

Immunohistological studies were performed on 148 cases of immuno-blastic sarcoma (IBS). In 22 of these cases fresh tissue was available, and sufficient cells were extracted for surface marker studies (Table 4), thus allowing comparison of the results of immunoperoxidase and surface marker studies, and correlation of both these parameters with the morphological features. Of the 13 cases classified as immunoblastic sarcoma of T-cell type (T-IBS) all, by definition, showed positive E rosette formation by neoplastic cells. In eleven cases there was no detectable cytoplasmic immunoglobulin in recognizable neoplastic immunoblasts (Table 4), though apparently mature plasma cells intermingled with the immunoblasts were clearly positive. In the remaining two cases a small number of immunoglobulin-positive immunoblasts were present, and the immunoglobulin staining pattern in tissue sections of one was thought possibly to be monoclonal; interpretation was difficult due to the presence of many "reactive" "mature" plasma cells (immunoblasts). The immunoblasts of T-IBS were also negative for lysozyme, though in half the cases large numbers of lysozyme-positive histiocytes were distributed diffusely throughout the lesion.

Of the seven cases of B-IBS with marker studies (Table 4), six showed a pattern of staining compatible with usual concepts of monoclonality (ex-clusively κ or λ, with one heavy chain class, see Taylor (33)). In the seventh case the majority of the neoplastic immunoblasts showed a monoclonal staining pattern, but bizarre polyploid immunoblasts interspersed through-out the section stained with both anti-κ and anti-λ sera; heavy chain staining was monoclonal for γ chain. In none of the seven cases were E rosettes observed in relation to the neoplastic cells, and in five cases surface im-munoglobulin showed a clear-cut monoclonal pattern. In the sixth case the surface immunoglobulin staining suggested nonspecific absorption of polyclonal serum immunoglobulin (see Lukes et al. (17)), and in the seventh case the polyvalent antiserum gave negative results, and insufficient material was available for the full surface immunoglobulin panel.

In the remaining two cases for which a full panel of surface marker studies was available neither the morphologic appearances nor the immunologic findings permitted classification into T- or B-cell subtypes.

Using morphologic criteria derived from study of these 22 cases, it was possible to subclassify most of the 126 remaining cases of IBS as of B- or T-cell type on the basis of morphology only (full surface marker panels had not been performed in these cases). Thus a total of 148 cases were examined by immunohistologic methods, and upon morphologic review, 59 were judged to be of B-cell and 52 of T-cell type (Table 3). The morphologic criteria employed to make this distinction will be described in the discussion of these results.

In the remaining 37 cases the diagnosis of immunoblastic sarcoma was upheld, but subclassification into B- or T-cell type was not possible on morphologic grounds.

Of the 59 B-IBS cases (as defined by morphology), 48 showed immunoglobulin within the cytoplasm of recognizable neoplastic immunoblasts. In 31 the pattern was clearly monoclonal, and in a further eight suggestively so (giving a total of 39 with a monoclonal pattern). In most cases of B-IBS the plasma cells included both "mature" and "immature" forms. Such cells showed a monoclonal staining pattern matching that of the predominant immunoblasts, emphasizing the wide spectrum of morphological appearances of the neoplastic clone. In nine cases a monoclonal pattern was not apparent. In four of these cases there appeared to be a mixed population of cells, some containing κ chain and some λ chain, with an admixture of heavy chain types, predominantly γ and μ (polyclonal). In five cases, part of the neoplastic cell population, comprised of immunoblasts and plasmacytoid cells, appeared monclonal, while large bizarre polyploid cells interspersed throughout the tumor showed double (anomalous) staining of individual cells for both κ and λ lights chains and often for two or more heavy chains.

In the T-IBS group only two of 52 cases showed a possible "monoclonal B cell type" immunoglobulin staining pattern.

Of the 37 cases of morphologically indeterminant T or B cell subclass, six showed a pattern of staining consistent with a monoclonal B-cell origin, three showed anomalous patterns, 24 were negative for cytoplasmic immunoglobulin and 14 were impossible to interpret for technical reasons.

Follicle center cell lymphoma

One hundred and thirty-two cases (Table 3) were examined for cytoplasmic immunoglobulin by immunoperoxidase methods. Surface marker studies were carried out in 57 of these cases and served to confirm the B-cell origin of this tumor (Table 4). In most cases (67%) surface immunoglobulin was monoclonal, though some showed a "pseudo-polyclonal" pattern, believed to represent absorption of serum immunoglobulin by the Fc receptor of the neoplastic cells, thus giving a false impression of polyclonicity (35, 17, 18).

Immunoperoxidase staining revealed a monoclonal pattern of cytoplasmic immunoglobulin in tumour cells of 33% of the total cases (44 of 132) and 49% of the cases with surface marker studies (28 of 57). In 44% (58 of total 132) of cases immunoglobulin was not detectable in the neoplastic follicle center cells, or was present in such a small proportion of cells that it was not possible to make a judgment of clonicity.

The staining patterns of the histological subgroups of 113 follicle center cell lymphomas are summarized in Table 5. In tumors classified as of small cleaved type, according to the predominat form of the neoplastic cell, positive cytoplasmic immunoglobulin staining was usually observed only in the minor population of large cleaved or large noncleaved cells present in such tumors. In addition, in a few cases large numbers of plasmacytoid cells withing the tumor showed a monclonal pattern matching that of the follicle center cells staining within the neoplastic follicles.

In E rosette cytocentrifuge preparations recognizable neoplastic cells from these cases did not form rosettes.

Plasmacytoid lymphocytic lymphoma

Thirty-nine plasmacytoid lymphocytic lymphomas were examined, and surface marker studies were performed in 12 of these. Twenty-six of the 39 cases (67%, Table 3) showed a pattern of staining consistent with the usual concepts of monoclonality. In five cases (13%) a monoclonal staining pattern was not observed; in three a polyclonal pattern was present and in two individual cells appeared to contain both light chains or two or more heavy chains—anomalous pattern. In two of the "polyclonal" cases a "biclonal gammopathy" was also present in the serum, $\lambda\gamma$–$\kappa\gamma$ in one, $\kappa\gamma$–$\lambda\mu$ in the other. In the monoclonal immunoglobulin-positive cases the majority of immunoglobulin-containing cells were of plasmacytoid type, though the proportion of such cells varied greatly in different tumors. In some cases monoclonal staining of a minor immunoblastic cell component was also observed, again emphasizing the range of morphologic forms within the monoclonal population. Positive staining of small lymphocytes was not observed, though forms with intermediate morphology showed staining. In some cases interpretation of clonality was difficult due to the possible presence of an infiltrate of reactive plasma cells and immunoblasts having a polyclonal pattern. Surface marker studies revealed a monoclonal SIg pattern of 10 of the 12 cases studied (Table 4).

Table 5. Results of immunoperoxidase studies of cytoplasmic immunoglobulin in follicle center cell (FCC) lymphomas (132 cases)[1].

	Total	Tumor Cells Ig Negative[2]	Tumor Cells Ig Positive[3]		
			Definite Mono-clonal	Possible Mono-clonal	Anomalous patterns
Small cleaved—follicular	30	16	8	4	2
Small cleaved—diffuse	20	14	1	4	1
Small noncleaved—follicular	3	2	0	0	1
Small noncleaved—diffuse	11	8	2	1	0
Large cleaved—follicular	6	2	3	1	0
Large cleaved—diffuse	12	6	5	1	0
Large noncleaved—follicular	10	4	2	2	2
Large noncleaved—diffuse	21	6	8	2	5
Total	113	58	29	15	11

[1] Eleven cases of sclerosing FCC are excluded, together with eight other cases in which material studied was inadequate or of poor quality.

[2] No evidence of Ig in recognizable tumor cells—positive plasma cells present in all cases (intrinsic control), though often in small numbers.

[3] Ig present in a variable proportion of recognizable neoplastic cells of the defined morphologic type, or in intermediate forms with plasmacytoid features judged to form part of a spectrum with the neoplastic follicle center cell. Infiltration by reactive plasma cells made interpretation difficult in some cases.

Small lymphocytic B-cell lymphoma

Tissue sections were examined in eight cases of CLL/small lymphocytic lymphoma. Immunoperoxidase methods revealed no cytoplasmic immunoglobulin, other than that present in scattered apparently reactive plasma cells, in most cases. In one case the immunoglobulin-containing cells accounted for about 15% of the total cell population, but were plasmacytic in form, rather than small lymphocytic; this was not appreciated on morphologic examination prior to the performance of immunoperoxidase studies. Even in retrospect this case was not readily distinguishable from the other seven cases on histological grounds. It represents a small lymphocytic lymphoma with an immunoglobulin-containing monoclonal cell component showing plasmacytoid features.

"Reticulum cell sarcoma" of the brain

Material from the 24 cases of primary CNS lymphoma examined for the presence of cytoplasmic immunoglobulin revealed a pattern of staining akin to that observed in lymphomas occurring systemically. The findings have been described elsewhere (33).

Hodgkin's disease

Eighty-seven cases of Hodgkin's disease were studied. Immunoglobulin was demonstrated within Reed-Sternberg cells of some cases as described elsewhere (30, 31) and alluded to in later parts of this volume.

DISCUSSION

Interpretation of results

Results of immunohistologic studies must always be interpreted in relation to positive and negative control preparations. A clear-cut monoclonal pattern in neoplastic cells presents no problem in interpretation. Weak or equivocal staining is best ignored; there is growing evidence that trypsinisation of formalin fixed tissues may enhance specific staining so resolving some of these problems (Dr. R. Cardiff, Sacramento, California, personal communication).

Clear polyclonal staining showing the presence of more than one cell population is, by implication, evidence of a nonneoplastic state. Yet some lesions that morphologically are indistinguishable from immunoblastic sarcomas, appear to show true polyclonal staining. The significance of this observation in relation to the biology of neoplasia or in relation to the utilization of this technique remains uncertain.

Polyclonal staining should be distinguished from "anomalous" staining in which a population of cells shows double staining of individual cells (e.g. individual cells react with both anti-κ and anti-λ sera). In cases of IBS, cells with anomalous staining appear on morphologic grounds to be part of the neoplastic process; they are usually large and bizarre with polyploid nuclei and prominent nucleoli. Several interpretations have been offered; more than one may apply: synthesis of more than one light chain type by individual bizarre tumor cells; failure of antisera to discriminate between light chain components in early stages of immunoglobulin synthesis within the cell; adsorption of immunoglobulin via Fc receptor activity; passive absorption of serum components, including immunoglobulin, by degenerating cells; active phagocytosis; adsorption of antibody as a result of specific host immune response against tumor cells.

Fixation and processing

That formalin fixation and embedding in paraffin by routine procedures might be less than catastrophic, at least with respect to certain antigens, was first revealed by preliminary studies of immunoglobulin distribution in plasma cells of formalin-fixed paraffin-embedded tissues (36). One major concern, of course, was that although immunoglobulin was detectable in formalin paraffin sections, it might represent only a small fraction of that originally present, and the sensitivity of the method might be so low as to render it of little practical value. A somewhat crude study comparing the demonstration of immunoglobulin-containing plasma cells in cryostat sections, in Sainte-Marie cold ethanol paraffin sections, and in formalin paraffin sections, of adjacent tissue blocks, by both immunofluorescence and immunoperoxidase procedures, went someway toward allaying these fears (3). The detection of immunoglobulin-containing cells by the immunoperoxidase conjugate procedure in formalin paraffin sections compared well to that of immunofluorescence on cryostat sections. It was also interesting to note that the immunofluorescence method worked quite well on formalin paraffin sections, in that plasma cells were clearly demonstrable, although the ability to identify the types of cells was much less than in corresponding immunoperoxidase preparations. Subsequently other reports have described the demonstration of a variety of antigens by immunofluorescence in pretreated (partially digested with trypsin or pronase) formalin paraffin sections (23, 7, 8, 12, 26).

Clearly, however, not all antigens will survive the process of formalin fixation and paraffin embedding to a useful degree. Antigens which do survive and can be demonstrated include immunoglobulin, lysozyme, lactoferrin, ferritin, haemoglobin A and F, α-foetoprotein, testosterone, HBsAg, α-1-antitrypsin, ACTH, STH, HCG, and gastrin (32, 33). Nonetheless, the studies of Warnke and colleagues (40, 41) and of Banks (Z) reveal that various fixation/processing procedures have adverse effects úpon the antigenicity of immunoglobulins. Variations in fixation may partially explain some of the anomalous findings described above, at least with regard to the demonstration of immunoglobulin.

Morphology

The major advantage of the immunoperoxidase procedure is that it provides excellent morphological detail and permits the correlation of histological and cytological features with the pattern of immunoglobulin staining of the neoplastic cells of a variety of B-cell-derived neoplasms. The findings are of some value in the differential diagnosis and classification of B-lymphocyte-derived neoplasms (Table 6).

The observation of a monoclonal pattern of immunoglobulin staining (exclusively one light chain and one heavy chain), as opposed to a polyclonal pattern, in the cytoplasm of the cells of a putative neoplasm, provides evidence not only of the lymphocytic origin of the cell population under examination, but also its neoplastic nature. This is of particular value in distinguishing some cases of follicle center cell lymphoma, immunoblastic

Table 6. Interpretation of immunoperoxidase studies—typical examples of diagnostic categories.

	κ	λ	γ	*Antisera* α	μ	δ	$M\chi$
Reactive plasma cells	+ + + +	+ + +	+ + + +	+ +	+ +	+	−
Multiple myeloma	+ + + +	±	±	+ + + +	±	±	−
Plasmacytoid lymphocytic lymphoma	±	+ + + +	±	±	+ + + +	±	−
CLL (MLWD)	−	−	−	−	−	−	−
Follicular lymphoma	±+	±	±+	±	±	±	−
IBS-B	+ + + +	±	+ + + +	±	±	±	−
IBS-T	±	±	±	−	−	−	(+)
Reactive granuloma (histocytes)	±	±	±	−	−	−	+ +
Histiocytic sarcoma	±	±	±	±	±	±	+ + +
Anaplastic carcinoma	±	±	±	−	−	−	−

− → + + + + Semi-quantitative score of number of positive cells.
IBS Immunoblastic sarcoma (B- or T-cell type)
MLWD Malignant lymphoma lymphocytic well differentiated
Mx Anti muramidase (lysozyme)
Note: In the B-cell series the pattern of staining of the neoplastic cell, e.g. myeloma cell: plasma cell, large amount of cytoplasmic immunoglobulin; CLL lymphocyte: small lymphocyte little or no detectable cytoplasmic immunoglobulin, though surface immunoglobulin is present.

sarcoma (of B-cell type), plasmacytoid lymphocytic lymphoma, plasmacytoma, and multiple myeloma, from various forms of reactive hyperplasia and plasmacytosis in lymph node, bone marrow and tissue biopsies,
which may otherwise present diagnostic problems. Banks and associates
have reported similar findings using immunoperoxidase methods in the
study of lymphoma (2). By use of this method anaplastic tumors may occasionally be related to the B-cell series by their content of monclonal
immunoglobulin, and various morphologically disparate forms of lymphoma may be seen possibly to have an unsuspected common lineage
(composite lymphomas). The demonstration of diverse morphologic forms
of the B-cell series (cleaved and noncleaved follicle center cell cells,
immunoblasts, plasma cells) within a monoclonal population as revealed by
immunoperoxidase staining is clearly relevant to those observations. This
aspect is discussed more fully in a separate chapter in this volume dealing
specifically with the interrelations of B-cell lymphomas (see also Taylor
(35)).

B-IBS—immunoblastic sarcoma

On the basis of the studies described here, B-IBS appears typically to be
monoclonal immunoglobulin-positive (Table 4). It is characterized by a
diffuse proliferation of large cells with basophilic cytoplasm. The nucleus
is usually large, round and regular, with a distinct nuclear membrane and
usually a prominent single central nucleolus. Plasmacytoid features are
usually present and sometimes obvious.

Immunoglobulin negative tumors, T-IBS

Clearly, not all immunoglobulin-negative tumors are examples of T-IBS
(Table 6). Immunoglobulin-negative tumors might result from artifactual
loss of immunoglobulin during processing, or the method might be insufficiently sensitive to detect low levels of immunoglobulin present in some
tumors. Alternatively, immunoglobulin-negative cells might represent B
cells in a nonsynthetic phase of the cell cycle, or T cells, or any other cell
type. However, the conjunction of immunoperoxidase staining with E
rosette studies has permitted a preliminary definition of the morphology
of the T immunoblast and the corresponding neoplasm (T-immunoblastic
sarcoma, T-IBS). T-IBS appears to be characterized by a diffuse proliferation of cells which resemble B immunoblasts to some extent, except that
usually they have extensive cytoplasm that is not basophilic. The nuclear
membrane is usually less distinct, and the nuclear outline often irregular or
complexly folded. The nucleoli are less conspicuous and sometimes multiple, and the chromatin is usually finely dispersed throughout the nucleus,

rather than clumped at the nuclear membrane as is typical of B-IBS. The process, like B-IBS, is diffuse, but often seems initially to involve the T cell zone of the lymph nodes (paracortex), sparing the follicles in early stages.

While the morphologic features described here show overlap in individual cases, taken together they permit the B-IBS/T-IBS distinction to be made in approximately 75% of cases of IBS.

CONCLUSION

Immunoperoxidase methods allow the general pathologist to apply specific immunocytochemical techniques to tissues for the purposes of further diagnosis, or for research and investigation. Though the technique in formalin fixed tissues was first worked out with regard to the identification of immunoglobulin in lymphoma and myeloma, the main uses of the method are now perhaps to be found in relation to the identification of a range of other cell products, including cell and tumor-associated antigens, hormones and hormone receptors (34, 35). Within haematopathology the method has a role, as indicated in Table 6, in the differential diagnosis of lymph node and bone marrow biopsies and when a neoplasm of B-cell nature is suspected. In research the possibilites are largely untapped, awaiting only the availability of specific antisera to normal and neoplastic lymphocyte products (antigens). The recent report of staining of J chain (a possible marker of immunoglobulin synthesising cells) and α_1 anti-trypsin (a possible marker of cells of the histiocyte series) (13) serves merely to remind us of the as yet undiscovered applications of this versatile method. It is time for an assessment of possibilites. In the use of this method we stand not at the beginning, nor at the end, but perhaps at the end of the beginning.

REFERENCES

1. Avrameas, S., and Uriel, J.: Methode de marquage d'antigenes et d'anticorps avec des enzymes et son application en immunodiffusion. C.R. Acad. Sci., 262:2543–2545, 1966.
2. Banks, P.M.: Diagnostic applications of an immunoperoxidase method in hematopathology. J. Histochem. Cytochem., in press.
3. Burns, J., Hambridge, M., and Taylor, C.R.: Intracellular immunoglobulins: A comparative study on three standard tissue processing methods using horseradish peroxidase and fluorochrome conjugates. J. Clin. Pathol., 27:548–557, 1974.
4. Canale, D.D., and Collins, R.D.: Use of bone marrow particle sections in the diagnosis of multiple myeloma. Am. J. Clin. Pathol., 61:382–392, 1974.
5. Coons, A.H., Creech, H.J., and Jones, R.N.: Immunological properties of an

antibody containing a fluorescent group. Proc. Soc. Exp. Biol., 47:200–202, 1941.

6. Coons, A.H., and Kaplan, M.H.: Localization of antigens in tissue cells: II. Improvement in a method for the detection of antigen by means of fluorescent antibody. J. Exp. Med., 91:1, 1950.

7. Denk, H., Radaszkiewicz, T., and Witting, C.: Immunofluorescence studies of malignant lymphomas in formalin fixed material. Z. Krebsforsch., 88:101–102, 1976.

8. Denk, H., Radaszkiewicz, T., and Witting, C.: Immunofluorescence studies on pathologic routine material: application to malignant lymphomas. Beitr. Pathol., 159:219–225, 1976.

9. Feltkamp-Vroom, T.M.: Preparation of tissues and cells for immuno-histochemical processing. Ann. N.Y. Acad. Sci., 254:21–26, 1975.

10. Ford, P.M. and Stoward, P.J.: The detection of autoantibodies with an enzyme bridge method. J. Clin. Pathol., 27:118–121, 1974.

11. Graham, R.C., Jr., and Karnovsky, M.J.: The early stages of absorption of in-jected horseradish peroxidase in the proximal tubules of mouse kidney: Ultra-structural cytochemistry by a new technique. J. Histochem. Cytochem., 14:291–302, 1966.

12. Huang, S.N., Minassian, H., and More, J.D.: Application of immunofluorescent staining on paraffin sections improved by trypsin digestion. Lab. Invest., 35:383–390, 1976.

13. Isaacson, P., and Wright, D.H.: Anomalous staining patterns in immuno-histologic studies of malignant lymphoma. J. Histochem. Cytochem., in press.

14. Knowles, D.M. II, Winchester, R.J., and Kunkel, H.G.: A comparison of peroxidase- and fluorochrome-conjugated antisera for the demonstration of surface and intracellular antigens. Clin. Immunol. Immunopathol., 7:410–425, 1977.

15. Kojima, M., and Tsunoda, R.: Localization of immunoglobulins in germinal centers of human tonsils. In: The reticuloendothelial system in health and disease: Immunologic and pathologic aspects, p. 77, Friedman, H., Escobar, M.R., and Reichard, S.M., (eds.), Plenum Publishing, New York, 1976.

16. Kraehenbuhl, J.P., and Jamieson, J.D.: Localization of intracellular antigens by immunoelectron microscopy. Int. Rev. Exp. Pathol., 13:1–53, 1974.

17. Lukes, R.J., Taylor, C.R., Parker, J.W., Lincoln, T.L., Pattengale, P.K., and Tindle, B.H.: A morphologic and immunologic surface marker study of 299 cases of non-Hodgkin's lymphomas and related leukemias. Am. J. Pathol., 90:461–486, 1978.

18. Lukes, R.J., Parker, J.W., Taylor, C.R., Tindle, B.H., Cramer, A.D., and Lincoln, T.L.: Immunologic approach to non-Hodgkin's lymphoma and rela-ted leukemias. An analysis of the results of multiparameter studies of 425 cases. Semin. Hematol., 15:322–351, 1978.

19. Mason, T.E., Phifer, R.F., Spicer, S.S., Swallow, R.A., and Dreskin, R.B.: An immunoglobulin-enzyme bridge method for localizing tissue antigens. J. Histochem. Cytochem., 17:563–569, 1969.

20. Mason, D.Y., and Taylor, C.R.: The distribution of muramidase (lysozyme) in human tissues. J. Clin. Pathol., 28:124–132, 1975.

21. Nakane, P.K.: Recent progress in the peroxidase-labeled antibody method. Ann. N.Y. Acad. Sci., 254:203–210, 1975.

22. Nakane, P.K., and Pierce, G.B., Jr.: Enzyme-labeled antibodies: Preparation and application for the localization of antigens. J. Histochem. Cytochem., 14:929–931, 1966.

23. Kayak, N.C., and Sachdeva, R.: Localization of hepatitis B surface antigen in conventional paraffin sections of the liver. Am. J. Pathol., 81:479–492, 1975.

24. Pinkus, G.S., and Said, J.W.: Profile of intracytoplasmic lysozyme in normal tissues, myeloproliferative disorders, hairy cell leukemia, and other pathologic processes. An immunoperoxidase study of paraffin sections and smears. Am. J. Pathol., 89:351–366, 1977.

25. Ploem, J.S.: Fifth international conference on immunofluorescence and related staining techniques. General introduction. Ann. N.Y. Acad. Sci., 254:4–20, 1975.

26. Portmann, B., Galbraith, R.M., Eddleston, A.L.W.F., Zuckerman, A.J., and Williams, R.: Detection of HB_sAg in fixed liver tissue: Use of a modified immunofluorescent technique and comparison with histochemical methods. Gut., 17:1–9, 1976.

27. Sainte-Marie, G.: A paraffin embedding technique for studies employing immunofluorescence. J. Histochem. Cytochem., 10:250–256, 1962.

28. Sternberger, L.A.: Immunocytochemistry. Prentice-Hall, Englewood Cliffs, N.J.: Inc., 1974.

29. Sternberger, L.A., Hardy, P.H., Cuculis, J.J., and Meyer, H.G.: The unlabeled antibody enzyme method of immunohistochemistry. J. Histochem. Cytochem., 18:315–333, 1970.

30. Taylor, C.R.: The nature of Reed-Stenrberg cells and other malignant cells. Lancet, 2:802–807, 1974.

31. Taylor, C.R.: An immunohistological study of follicular lymphoma, reticulum cell sarcoma and Hodgkin's disease. Eur. J. Cancer, 12:61–75, 1976.

32. Taylor, C.R.: Immunoperoxidase techniques: practical and theoretical aspects. Arch. Pathol. Lab. Med., 102:113–121, 1978.

33. Taylor, C.R.: Immunocytochemical methods in the study of lymhoma and related conditions. J. Histochem. Cytochem., 6:495–512, 1978.

34. Taylor, C.R.: Immunohistological approach to tumor diagnosis. Oncology, 35:189–197, 1978.

35. Taylor, C.R.: Hodgkin's Disease and the Lymphomas. vol. III. Annual Research Review 1978. Eden Press, Montreal, Canada, and Churchill Longman Livingstone, Edinburgh/London, 1979.

36. Taylor, C.R., and Burns, J.: The demonstration of plasma cells and other immunoglobulin containing cells in formalin-fixed, paraffin-embedded tissues using peroxidase labelled antibody. J. Clin. Pathol., 27:14–20, 1974.

37. Taylor, C.R., and Mason, D.Y.: Immunohistological detection of intracellular immunoglobulin in formalin-paraffin sections from multiple myeloma using the immunoperoxidase technique. Clin. Exp. Immunol., 18:417–429, 1974.

38. Taylor, C.R., Russell, R., and Chandor, S.: An immunohistologic study of multiple myeloma and related conditions, using an immunoperoxidase method. Am. J. Clin. Pathol., 70:612–622, 1978.

39. Taylor, C.R., Russell, R., Lukes, R.J., and Davis, R.L.: An immunohistological study of immunoglobulin content of primary CNS lymphomas. Cancer, 41:2197–2205, 1978.

40. Warnke, R., Pederson, M., Williams, C., and Levy, R.: A study of lymphoproliferative diseases comparing immunofluorescence with immunohistochemistry. Am. J. Clin. Pathol., 70:867–875, 1978.

41. Warnke, R.: Alteration of immunoglobulin-bearing lymphoma cells by fixation. J. Histochem. Cytochem., in press.

10. IMMUNOFLUORESCENCE METHODS

W. HIJMANS

Application of the immunofluorescence method is still increasing, but its possibilities are often not fully exploited, perhaps because many investigators are insufficiently informed about the theoretical background and the technical aspects of this method.

Its widespread use can be explained by the high sensitivity and the high specificity of the method and by the possibility to localize and identify antigens on the microscopical level. The high sensitivity is the result of the principle of fluorescence. This means wave length transformation on excitation, whereby the fluorescent dye emits light. The amount of emitted light is a function of the amount of light absorbed by the dye. This principle should be compared with the principle of absorption microscopy on which standard microscopy is based. In the latter case high concentrations of a given substance in the specimen lead to a high degree of absorption, which means that the observer sees less. In immunofluorescence the dye has been coupled to an antibody that can combine with a given antigenic substance in the substrate. This results in a degree of specificity of an antigen-antibody reaction, and thus makes it possible to locate and identify antigens with the microscope.

In this chapter some theoretical and practical aspects of the microscope, the reagents, and the substrate will be discussed. Many additional details have recently been published elsewhere (2).

THE MICROSCOPE

Originally a routine microscope with transmitted light was used in this method, which was introduced by Coons in 1941. The standard condensor was then replaced by a dark-field condensor, which greatly decreased the amount of excitation light leaking through the filters. This gave a great improvement in color contrast.

In 1967, Ploem described his system of epi-illumination (Figure 1) in which a light beam is directed, via an interference dividing plate, to the specimen, which then emits the fluorescent light. Filters are inserted in the excitation and the emission pathways to remove unwanted light. This sys-

J.G. van den Tweel et al. (eds.), Malignant Lymphoproliferative Diseases, 133–136
All rights reserved.
Copyright © 1980 by Martinus Nijhoff Publishers bv, The Hague/Boston/London.

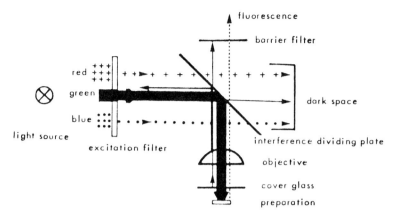

Figure 1. The system of epi-illumination according to Ploem.

tem is so much superior to the system with dia-illumination, that only the former will be discussed here.

The major components of this system are the light source, the filters, and the optics.

1) The usual light source is a high-pressure mercury lamp. The efficiency of a given light source should be judged on the basis of its brilliancy, that is, the amount of energy emission per surface area, rather than on the basis of the total energy output.

Quantitative assessments have shown the relative values of the different light sources. The 50 and the 200 watt mercury lamps are about equal and the 100 watt type is 5 to 8 times superior but requires a highly stabilizing DC power supply. The cheap 50 watt mercury lamp is therefore a good second choice.

2) Filters present problems because they are never ideal and the terminology is confusing. It is not generally realized that filters often also transmit some light in the wavelength region they are supposed to block. For highly efficient fluorescence systems the permissible transmission in the regions may have to be as low as 10^{-8}. The terminology of filters is less confusing if a distinction is made between the colored glass filters, which consist of glass mixed with different organic salts, and the interference filters, which consist of a glass base on which multiple layers of dielectric materials have been deposited.

From a functional point of view, one can distinguish filters which transmit light of a wavelength longer than a given value. These are called long-wavelength pass (LP) filters in contrast to those which do the reverse, i.e., the short-wavelength pass (SP) filters (in German *Kurz Pass*: KP). In addition, there are filters with a narrow band pass (BP).

3) The optics. Eyepieces enlarge, which leads to a magnification of the image. The total amount of light, however, does not increase, and this means less light per surface area. Increasing of the magnification of the eyepiece therefore results in a decreased brightness of the image; therefore, low-power eyepieces should be used for immunofluorescence work.

The situation with respect to the choice of the objective is different. In fluorescence microscopy with epi-illumination the amount of emitted light is determined by the amount of light received by the specimen per unit of surface area. This amount is a function of the collecting power of the objective, expressed in the value of the numerical aperture. Classically, a high numerical aperture (N.A.) meant a high magnification, but fortunately the optical industry is now manufacturing objectives which combine a relatively low magnification with a high N.A. value, especially for fluorescence microscopy with epi-illumination. It has been possible to determine the brightness quantitatively, and it could be shown that doubling of the N.A. led to a sixteenfold increase in brightness.

An additional advantage of epi-illumination is that it can be easily combined with phase contrast microscopy.

THE REAGENTS

There are two fluorochromes which are suitable for routine use: fluorescein isothiocyanate and tetramethylrhodamine isothiocyanate. The former compound has a higher efficiency. Both can easily be conjugated to proteins and the dye-to-protein ratio can be monitored. Antisera are rarely mono-specific and absorption is almost always necessary. This should be done with solid adsorbents to avoid the presence of immune complexes in the solution. The preparation of $F(ab')_2$ fragments of the immunoglobulin molecules has been advocated to prevent the formation of complexes composed of aggregated molecules and adherence of these aggregates, via Fc receptors, to cell membranes, but the contribution of $F(ab')_2$ fragments to specificity has been overemphasized.

The user should be in a position to judge the reagents so that he can apply them intelligently. The basic information that should be supplied by the manufacturer is summarized in Table 1. Final assessment should be done by performance testing, in which the reagent is used in the test for which it is intended. These tests can be carried out in various modifications, such as the direct test in which the antiserum preparation has been conjugated or the indirect test which makes use of a fluorochrome conjugated anti-immunoglobulin reagent. The former is a one-layer method and suffers less from specificity pitfalls; it is easier to manipulate and takes less time than the indirect method, but it is less sensitive and therefore consumes more of the often precious antisera.

Table 1. Antisera and conjugates: basic information required.

1) The species of animal immunized
2) The source and method of preparation of the antigen
3) The immunizing schedule, route, and adjuvant
4) The absorbent and absorption procedure, and evidence of specificity before and after absorption
5) The immunoglobulin separation process or other chemical treatment applied, particularly the preservative used and any other dilutions or additions such as proteins used for stabilization
6) Specificity as determined by reproducible standard tests
7) Some indication of the potency of the antiserum, with a guideline for a working dilution
8) Fluorochrome used, with F/P ratio
9) The lot number

THE SUBSTRATE

One can distinguish three kinds of substrate, each with its own problems.

1) Suspensions, for which the cells can be washed or treated in other ways to remove any bound antibodies except those resulting from cell-membrane antigen-antibody interaction. Such suspensions can be stained directly for the detection of surface markers, or cytocentrifuge slides can be prepared. The cytocentrifuge method provides enriched slides of well-presented washed cells. If suspensions are used, the phase contrast equipment often provides essential information on the morphology of the cells.
2) Cryostat sections can be excellen for the study of cytoplasmic antigens, but if cell surface-associated antigens are being investigated, background values should be minimal. This is the case when the antigen is surface specific, such as for instance a T-cell antigen, or if the extracellular content is very low, for instance in the case of IgD.
3) Sections of fixed material are usually not suitable for immunofluorescence.

REFERENCES

1. Faulk, W.F., and Hijmans, W.: Progr. Allergy, 16:9, 1972.
2. Hijmans, W., Haaijman, J.J., and Schuit, H.R.E.: Immunofluorescence. In: Immunology of ageing, vol. V of the Uniscience series, Methods in ageing research, Adler, W.H., and Nordin, A.A., (eds.), C.R.C. Press, W. Palm Beach, Fla. 1980.
3. Seligman, M., Preud'homme, J.L., and Kourilsky, J., (eds.): Membrane receptors of lymphocytes, North Holland Publ., Amsterdam, 1975.

11. CYTOCHEMICAL METHODS

E.-W. SCHWARZE

INTRODUCTION

The cytochemical techniques mentioned below are standard methods. They are used for the detection of intracellular substrates or the indirect demonstration of enzymes. The demonstration of hydrolases is based on the following principle: endogenous enzymes split a substrate that has been dissolved in an incubation medium; one or more of the resulting products react with a coupling salt (coupler) also present in the solution, to give a chromogenic reaction. Oxidoreductases are demonstrated with hydrogen acceptors, e.g. benzidine, which in a reduced form, are insoluble chromogenic conjugates.

In our laboratory the methods described here are routinely applied to air-dried tissue imprints, blood and bone marrow smears, and cytocentrifuge sediments of cell suspensions (the last in cases studied with Dr. G. Tolksdorf). The cytochemical staining patterns obtained with some of the methods are, to a variable degree, suitable for characterizing different functional variants of lymphoid cells and distinguishing lymphoid cells from nonlymphoid cells. Thus, we use these methods in a functional approach to, and the diagnosis of, malignant lymphomas, especially non-Hodgkin's lymphomas (NHL).

METHODS

Periodic acid Schiff (PAS) reaction (modification of the methods of McManus and Hotchkiss—cf. 46).

After fixation with methanol-formalin (9:1 vol/vol) for 10 sec at 4°C, slides are washed in tap water for 10 min and air-dried. Slides are then placed in 1% periodic acid solution for 10 min, quickly washed in distilled water, placed in Schiff's reagent for 45–50 min, and washed once in SO_2-water for 5 min and three times in distilled water for 10 min.

Counterstaining is performed with Mayer's hemalum for this and all the following reactions.

J.G. van den Tweel et al. (eds.), Malignant Lymphoproliferative Diseases, 137–148.
All rights reserved.
Copyright © 1980 by Martinus Nijhoff Publishers bv, The Hague/Boston/London.

Nonspecific α-naphthyl acetate esterase reaction (pH 7.5) (azo dye method—5, 16, 31, 34)

Fixation: none. Slides are incubated at 20°C for 30 min in a filtered mixture of stock solutions A and B. Stock solution A: 10mg α-naphthyl acetate dissolved in 0.8ml acetone. Stock solution B: hexazotized pararosaniline according to Davis and Ornstein (12), i.e., 1 drop of 4% solution of pararosaniline mixed for 60 sec with 1 drop of 4% solution of sodium nitrite and then diluted with 25 ml phosphate buffer (pH 7.5).

Acid nonspecific α-naphthyl acetate esterase reaction pH 5.8 (modification of the methods of Mueller et al. (40) and Kulenkampff et al. (27)).

Fixation: none. Slides are incubated for 2–2½ hours in a filtered mixture of stock solutions A and B. Stock solution A: 10 mg α-naphtyl acetate dissolved in 0.4ml acetone. Stock solution B: hexazotized pararosaniline, i.e., 25 drops of 4% solution of pararosaniline mixed for 60 sec with 25 drops of 4% solution of sodium nitrite and diluted with 40 ml Sörensen buffer (pH 5.8); pH is adjusted to 5.8 with 2 N NaOH.

Acid phosphatase reaction (azo dye method—17, 38, 31, 34)

Fixation: none. Slides are incubated at 20°C for 4 hours in a filtered mixture of stock solutions A and B. Stock solution A: 10mg naphthol-AS-BI phosphate dissolved in 1 ml dimethyl formamide or 2 ml dimethyl sulfoxide. Stock solution B: hexazotized pararosaniline, i.e., 6 drops of 4% solution of pararosaniline mixed for 60 sec with 6 drops of 4% solution of sodium nitrite and then diluted with 30ml veronal-acetate buffer (pH 7.62); pH is adjusted to 5.0–5.1 with 2 N HCl.

Tartrate-resistant acid phosphatase reaction (34, 66)

Fixation:none. Same substrate and incubation as for acid phosphatase, but without 2N HCl; 225 mg tartaric acid (L(+) – tartrate) is added to stock solution B and pH is adjusted to 5.0–5.1 with 1N NaOH.

Alkaline phosphatase reaction (azo dye method, Kaplow's technique—22, 23, 31, 34)

Method 1: Fixation for 30 sec. at 4°C in methanol-formalin (9:1 vol/vol). Slides are incubated at 20°C for 30 min in a filtered mixture of stock solutions A and B. Stock solution A: 5mg naphthol-AS-BI phosphate dissolved in

0.25 ml dimethyl formamide. Stock solution B: 30mg fast red violet LB salt dissolved in 40 ml propane diol buffer (pH 9.75).

Method 2: No fixation. Slides are incubated at 20°C for 60 min in a filtered mixture of stock solutions A and B. Stock solution A: 10 mg naphthol-AS-BI phosphate dissolved in 0.4 ml dimethyl formamide. Stock solution B: hexazotized Astra-Neufuchsin, i.e., 1 drop of 4% solution of Astra-Neufuchsin ($C_{22}H_{24}ClN_3$; Merck, Germany) mixed for 60 sec with 3 drops of 4% solution of sodium nitrite and then diluted with 40 ml propane diol buffer (pH 9.75); pH is adjusted to 8.6–8.8 with 2N HCl.

Naphthol-AS-D-chloroacetate esterase reaction (Leder's stain—29, 31, 34)

Fixation for 30–60 sec in methanol-formalin (9:1 vol/vol). Slides are incubated at 20°C for 30 min in a filtered mixture of stock solutions A and B. Stock solution A: 10 mg naphthol-AS-D- chloroacetate dissolved in 1 ml dimethyl formamide. Stock solution B: hexazotized pararosaniline, i.e. 1 drop of 4% solution of pararosaniline mixed for 60 sec with 1 drop of 4% solution of sodium nitrite and then diluted with 30 ml veronal-acetate buffer (pH 7.62); pH is adjusted to 6.3 with 2 N HCl.

Peroxidase reaction (benzidine technique—1, 24, 31, 34)

Fixation for a few seconds at 4°C in methanol- formalin (1:10 vol/vol). Slides are incubated at 20°C for 10 min in a filtered mixture of solutions A and B. Solution A: 0.08 ml H_2O_2. Solution B: 200 mg benzidine dissolved in 4 ml acetone, mixed well with 4 ml dimethyl sulfoxide and diluted with 32 ml bidistilled water.

Note: For all reactions, the slides should be shaken well during incubation.

RESULTS AND COMMENTS

Periodic acid Schiff reaction (46)

The PAS reaction product is pink, red, or violet. PAS[+] lymphoma cells (Figure 1) may contain small or medium-sized granules disseminated in the cytoplasm (pattern a), solitary or multiple intracytoplasmic and/or intranuclear globules (b), or coarse blocks (c), or may show a diffuse cytoplasmic staining (d).

PAS reaction patterns b and d are of significant and diagnostic value. Diastase-resistant PAS[+] globules represent immunoglobulin (Ig) (13, 14, 58) and characterize a lymphoma as a B-cell neoplasm capable of secretory

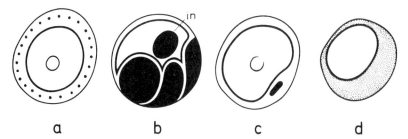

Figure 1. Periodic acid Schiff (PAS) reaction patterns. (a) Small to medium-sized granules disseminated in the cytoplasm. (b) Solitary or multiple intracytoplasmic and/or intranuclear (in) globules. (c) Coarse block(s) in the cytoplasm. (d) Diffuse cytoplasmic staining.

Ig production, viz.: lymphoplasmacytic/lymphoplasmacytoid lymphoma (LP immunocytoma), germinal center cell lymphomas, and B-immunoblastic lymphoma (36). Diffuse cytoplasmic PAS⁺ staining is seen more often in lymphoid cells of LP immunocytoma than in cells of chronic lymphocytic leukemia (CLL); in particular, lymphoplasmacytoid cells and plasma cells show this PAS reaction pattern.

Disseminated PAS⁺ granules (pattern a) which are mostly glycogen, have less value for the differential diagnosis, since this pattern is observed with variable frequency in various types of NHL and nonlymphoid neoplasias, and cannot be considered to be a discriminative marker of B- or T-cell neoplasms. It is notable that a majority of the cases of CLL show a negative reaction in lymph-node imprints, even when blood smears reveal PAS⁺ CLL cells.

Pattern c is not a reliable criterion for the lymphoid origin of tumor cells in the differential diagnosis of, for example, acute lymphoblastic leukemia (ALL), since coarse PAS⁺ blocks are also seen in acute myeloid leukemia (AML), acute myelomonocytic leukemia (AMML), and erythroleukemia (3, 32, 34, 54). There is apparently no significant correlation between the morphologic and immunologic subtypes of ALL and this PAS reaction pattern (6, 7, 10).

α-Naphthyl acetate esterase (αNAE) reaction (pH 7.5) (5, 16, 31)

α NAE⁺ lymphocytes and lymphoma cells contain one or more medium-sized or small, spotlike, brownish-red granules or disseminated small or medium-sized granules. A diffuse cytoplasmic staining is not typical of lymphoid cells. In contrast, monocytic and histiocytic cells show diffuse α NAE activity and usually α NAE⁺ granules as well. Reticulum cells, e.g., dendritic reticulum cells in B regions of lymphoid tissue, and endothelial cells of epithelioid venules are also αNAE⁺; these cells show both diffuse staining and small cytoplasmic granules.

The αNAE reaction is of diagnostic value for the recognition of AMML, immature histiocytic neoplasias, and other nonlymphoid tumors that must be considered in the differential diagnosis of certain types of NHL. The nonspecific esterase reaction at a neutral or alkaline pH is of no, or only little value for discriminating B and T cells and their neoplasias, unless one uses α-naphthyl butyrate at pH 8.0 as substrate (19), which results in a reaction pattern comparable to that of acid nonspecific esterase (see below). In three cases of T-CLL, however, we found an αNAE reaction pattern that we had never seen in a case of B-CLL: in one case of T-CLL, about 90% of the lymphocytes in a lymph-node imprint showed a few distinct medium-sized αNAE$^+$ granules in the cytoplasm; in the second case, about 90% of the leukemic cells (on blood smears) showed mainly small or medium-sized granules; and in the third case, about 70% of the leukemic cells chiefly revealed two small or medium-sized αNAE$^+$ granules, but no spotlike activity.

The published data on the αNAE reaction pattern in hairy-cell leukemia are not uniform (cf. (43)).

Acid α-naphthyl acetate esterase (AαNAE) reaction (pH 5.8) (27, 28, 40, 64)

AαNAE$^+$ lymphocytes and lymphoma cells (Figure 2) contain one or occasionally two spotlike granules (pattern a) or medium-sized and smaller granules either accumulated in a focal area of the cytoplasm (b) or, more often, distributed throughout the cytoplasm (c$_1$), sometimes with a semi-circular accentuation (c$_2$). Aα NAE$^+$ granules are always distinct in lymphocytes. The Aα NAE reaction pattern in monocytic and histiocytic cells is comparable to their α NAE reaction pattern (see above).

The Aα NAE reaction is significant because of the spotlike pattern typical of (resting) T cells (20, 25, 27, 40, 45, 48, 50, 57), particularly helper cells (18). It has become evident, however, that this AαNAE reaction pattern is not constantly displayed by T cells. It is not seen in all T cell subsets (18),

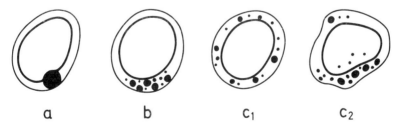

Figure 2. Acid α-naphthyl acetate esterase reaction patterns. (a) One or two spotlike granules. (b) Medium-sized and smaller granules accumulated in a focal area of the cytoplasm, (c$_1$) disseminated in the cytoplasm, or (c$_2$) with a semicircular accentuation.

and in the case of stimulated T cells (20, 25, 64) the number of $A\alpha NAE^+$ cells is reduced, although this varies with the mitogen used (cf. (64)), and such cells may even be $A\alpha NAE^-$. When stimulated T cells (T blasts) re-transform into resting (secondary) T lymphocytes, however, they regain the $A\alpha$ NAE marker (64). On the other hand, when human lymphocytes were exposed to the substrate for 4–21 hours, up to 20% of the cells that did not form rosettes with sheep erythrocytes were found to express spotlike $A\alpha$ NAE activity (27, 44, 49). Only some of the medium-sized postnatal thy-mocytes show spotlike $A\alpha$ NAE activity (25, 49, 54). A detailed description of the immunologic and cytochemical features of prethymocytes, prothy-mocytes, and mature thymocytes is given elsewhere in this book (see chapter by Stein, Tolksdorf and Lennert).

In imprints from a case of lymphoblastic lymphoma of the convoluted-cell type, probably of the peripheral T-cell subtype defined by Stein et al. (60), most of the blast cells contained a spotlike $A\alpha$ NAE reaction product or focal aggregations of accumulated large granules. In other words, the blast cells from this patient displayed the $A\alpha$ NAE reaction pattern of peripheral T (helper) lymphocytes. A comparable pattern was described by Knowles et al. (25) in blast cells from a case of T-ALL.

Most of the leukemic cells that we observed on blood smears and/or imprints in three cases of T-CLL, three cases of T-prolymphocytic leu-kemia, and two cases of Sézary's syndrome, exhibited a granular $A\alpha$ NAE reaction pattern, whereas only a relatively small number of the cells showed spotlike activity (pattern a), with a maximum of about one-third of the leukemic cells on blood smears. In one case of T-CLL, however, there was a quite large number (about 60%) of cells with large $A\alpha NAE^+$ granules (it is not always possible to make a clear distinction between large granules and "spots").

It is remarkable that a positive $A\alpha$ NAE reaction has been found in stimulated B cells (50, 54, 64), and a spotlike reaction pattern has been observed in cells of cell lines from human B-cell lymphomas, in cells in biopsy specimens from patients with myeloma (61), and constantly in rat B cells (15). However, none of the $A\alpha NAE^+$ B-cell lymphomas we have studied so far expressed a pronounced spotlike pattern. Most of the leuke-mic cells in a cytocentrifuge sediment from a patient with B-prolymphocytic leukemia contained chiefly small to medium-sized $A\alpha NAE^+$ granules dis-seminated in the cytoplasm. We observed a somewhat similar pattern in a variable number of cells in imprints from about one-third of the 30 cases of B-CLL we have analyzed so far and from a few cases of LP immunocy-toma. Hairy cells in imprints from the spleen of one patient with hairy-cell leukemia displayed disseminated $A\alpha NAE^+$ granules and a diffuse cytoplas-mic staining. In imprints from the spleens of two other patients with hairy-cell leukemia, the hairy cells showed small to medium-sized or large granules disseminated in the cytoplasm, but often with a semicircular distribution in part of the cytoplasm (pattern c_2). This pattern appears to be characteristic of hairy cells (cf. (63)).

Acid phosphatase (AcP) reaction (2, 17, 31, 38)

AcP^+ lymphocytes and lymphoma cells (Figure 3) contain one or more small spotlike reddish-brown granules (pattern a) or multiple small to medium-sized granules either accumulated in the Golgi area (b) or disseminated in the cytoplasm in a circular (c_1) or semicircular pattern (c_2). The AcP reaction product in lymphocytes and lymphoid cells is usually not as distinct as their $A\alpha NAE^+$ granules. Monocytic and histiocytic cells are characterized by a granular AcP reaction and, simultaneously, diffuse cytoplasmic staining. In a few cases of malignant histiocytic neoplasia the diffuse staining is confined to a variable-sized area of the cytoplasm. Focally pronounced, diffuse AcP reactivity is also seen in interdigitating reticulum cells in T regions of lymphoid tissue.

Two AcP reaction patterns in lymphoid cells, namely, pattern b and pattern c_2, are of special interest and have some diagnostic significance. A predominantly focal, often tightly packed accumulation of granules (pattern b) makes up the AcP reaction pattern of lymphoblastic lymphoma of the convoluted-cell type (35, 59) and has been applied as a marker for T-lymphoblastic lymphoma since the publications of Catovsky and co-workers ((8, 11); cf. (52)). This AcP reaction pattern was described by Leder (30) in cases of acute leukemia that we would presently interpret as T-ALL, spec. a (tumor-forming) leukemia of T-precursor cells according to Stein et al. (59). Immunologic findings and the AcP reactivity in pre-thymocytes, prothymocytes, and mature thymocytes are described elsewhere in this volume (Stein, Tolksdorf and Lennert). Strong focal AcP reactivity is indeed characteristic of T lymphoblasts and may be regarded

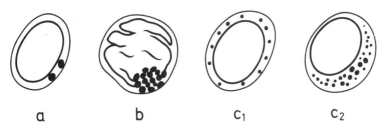

a   b c_1 c_2

Figure 3. Acid phosphatase reaction patterns. (a) One or more small spotlike granules. (b) Multiple, small to medium-sized granules accumulated in the Golgi area, (c_1) distributed in a circular pattern around the nucleus, or (c_2) arranged in a semicircular pattern in a more or less expanded part of the cytoplasm.

as a definite indication of the T-cell nature of a lymphoblastic lymphoma or ALL in cases showing the constellation of a thymic or mediastinal mass with convoluted-cell type cytology and occuring in a child (boys preponderate). In such cases one may dispense with immunologic techniques. It is important to realize, however, that focally pronounced AcP reactivity is not specific or restricted to T-lymphoblastic lymphoma, and in the convoluted-cell type it varies in intensity and somewhat in pattern as well.

Focal AcP reactivity has been observed in less than 10% of the cases of non-B/non-T-ALL studied by Seligmann et al. ((56); cf. (21, 65)) and also in a few cases of nonlymphoid immature leukemia (3, 9, 34, 54). We have seen a spotlike AcP reaction product in a case of B-immunoblastic lymphoma and disseminated, focally pronounced AcP reactivity in a plasmablastic lymphoma, but no such pattern in a case of T-immunoblastic lymphoma (55).

Among the low-grade malignant NHL we studied there were three cases of T-prolymphocytic leukemia; lymph-node imprints and blood smears from these patients revealed small spotlike AcP^+ granules (pattern a) in only up to 20% of the cells. A granular AcP reaction was evident in more than 90% of the leukemic cells from three cases of T cell and in about 90% of the infiltrating cells on imprints available from one of these cases. Only one of the three cases of T-CLL, however, showed a pattern of small spotlike granules (in about 25% of the leukemic cells), and none of these cases exhibited a pattern resembling spotlike AαNAE activity or the AcP reaction pattern seen in T-lymphoblastic lymphoma. A few cases of various types of low-grade malignant NHL of the B-cell type, namely, polymorphic immunocytoma and germinal center cell lymphoma, displayed a focal reaction (pattern b).

A semicircular distribution of medium-sized AcP^+ granules (pattern c_2) is characteristic of B cells, such as lymphoplasmacytoid cells and plasma cells. Plasma cells often display a focal accumulation of granules in addition to the semicircular distribution. Thus, this AcP reaction pattern is characteristic of LP immunocytoma and NHL with components of immunocytoma. We have also seen a case of B-prolymphocytic leukemia in which the cells exhibited a semicircular pattern of AcP^+ granules, sometimes combined with focally pronounced AcP activity.

Tartrate-resistant acid phosphatase (AcP/T^+) reaction (34, 66)

Most cases of hairy-cell leukemia and some cases of B- and T-prolymphocytic leukemia show AcP/T^+ activity. Thus, this test is of high diagnostic value, even though a few cases of various other types of NHL, such as the B-immunoblastic lymphoma mentioned above, are also AcP/T^+.

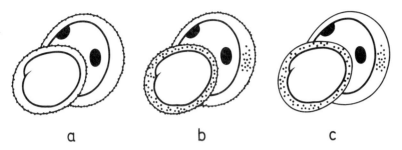

a   b   c

Figure 4. Alkaline phosphatase reaction patterns. (a) Small granules at the cell membrane. (b) Membrane-bound granules and intracytoplasmic granules as well. (c) Intracytoplasmic granules alone.

Alkaline phosphatase (AlkP) reaction (22, 23, 30)

AlkP$^+$ lymphoma cells (Figure 4) display predominantly small, brown or reddish-brown granules at the cell membrane (pattern a). Lymphoid cells rarely contain intracytoplasmic AlkP$^+$ granules, either in addition to the surface activity (pattern b) or alone (pattern c).

A significant finding is that the AlkP$^+$ malignant lymphomas (37) found so far in humans were exclusively NHL of the B-cell type (cf. (41, 47, 53, 54)) and were mostly derived from, or related to, germinal center cells (4, 42, 53, 54); most of them were of low-grade malignancy, and the number of AlkP$^+$ cells varied from case to case (53). Leder (33) described a case of AlkP$^+$ prolymphocytic leukemia with enzyme-positive cells in imprints from infiltrated lymph-nodes but AlkP$^-$ leukemic cells in blood smears.

It should also be mentioned that the cytochemical investigation of Schaefer and Fischer (51) indicated that T-lymphocytes of bank voles (a type of rodent) are AlkP$^+$. AlkP can also be demonstrated by biochemical methods on the surface of lymphocytes from patients with T-CLL and cells from patients with acute T-cell leukemia (26).

Naphthol-AS-D-chloroacetate esterase (NASDCAE) reaction (29, 31, 39) *and peroxidase (POX) reaction* (1, 24, 34)

Lymphocytes and other lymphoid cells are always NASDCAE$^-$ and POX$^-$. Cells of the myeloid and myelomonocytic cell series normally show a granular reaction product with both methods. Tissue mast cells are also NASDCAE$^+$.

The NASDCAE and POX reactions are of diagnostic value in the identification of immature myeloid and myelomonocytic cells and tissue mast cells. The POX reaction is more sensitive than the NASDCAE reaction, and should therefore be applied in all NASDCAE$^-$ cases in order to have an adequately reliable cytochemical basis for the diagnosis or exclusion of a myeloid neoplasia. An NASDCAE⁻ or POX⁻ reaction does not, however, exclude the myeloid nature of a neoplasia. This means that the differential diagnosis of AML, ALL, and stem-cell leukemia in a given case by cytochemical methods is difficult or even impossible, since PAS⁺ granules or blocks may be found in all of these immature cell neoplasias (see above). Furthermore, other enzyme reactions may not show the characteristic patterns described above. In such cases, immunologic and/or electron-microscopical analyses are necessary for definite classification.

SUMMARY

A few cytochemical reaction patterns have proved to be useful in the diagnosis and functional characterization of some types of non-Hodgkin's lymphoma and in the differential diagnosis between these lymphomas and other neoplasias.
1) Intracytoplasmic and/or intranuclear PAS⁺ globules, which represent stored immunoglobulin, are an indication of the B-cell nature of a lymphoid cell or a lymphoma that shows synthesis of secretory immunoglobulin.
2) Simultaneously diffuse and granular staining with nonspecific esterase at a neutral pH is, like other esterase reactions, suitable for recognizing monocytic and histiocytic cells and their neoplasias.
3) A spotlike acid nonspecific esterase reaction product is, at present, the most reliable cytochemical marker of the helper cell subtype of T cells and T-cell lymphomas. T-lymphocytic lymphomas typically show a repetitative pattern of distinct granules, with a spotlike reaction product in only a minority of the cells. Hairy cells appear to have a fairly typical granular acid nonspecific esterase reaction pattern.
4) Even though a strong, focally pronounced acid phosphatase reaction is neither exclusively nor constantly seen in T-lymphoblastic lymphoma, when such an enzyme pattern is associated with typical cytologic and clinical features, it is highly characteristic of this lymphoma subtype and its T-cell nature.
    When acid phosphatase staining reveals a semicircular pattern of positive granules, this is an indication of B cells, such as lymphoplasmacytoid cells and plasma cells. Thus, such an acid phosphatase reaction pattern is a marker of LP immunocytoma and other non-Hodgkin's lymphomas with components of immunocytoma. Tartrate-resistant acid phosphatase-positive granules are highly characteristic of hairy-cell leukemia and are also often found in prolymphocytic leukemia of the B and T types.
5) Predominantly membrane-bound alkaline phosphatase activity has proved to be a characteristic feature of B cells in lymphoid follicles and of malignant lymphomas that are composed of or derived from germinal center cells, e.g., some cases of centroblastic/centrocytic lymphoma, centrocytic lymphoma, and others.
6) and 7) The naphthol-AS-D-chloroacetate esterase and peroxidase reactions are cytochemical aids in the identification or exclusion of immature myeloid neoplasias that have to be considered in the differential diagnosis of some types of non-Hodgkin's lymphoma.

REFERENCES

1. Adler, R.: Hoppe-Seylers Z. Physiol. Chem., 41:59, 1904.
2. Barka, T., and Anderson, P.J.: J. Histochem. Cytochem., 10:741, 1962.
3. Bennett, J.M., and Reed, C.E.: Blood Cells 1:101, 1975.

4. Berard, C.W., Jaffe, E.S., and Braylan, R.C. et al.: Cancer (Philad.), 42:911, 1978.
5. Braunstein, H.: J. Histochem. Cytochem., 7:202, 1959.
6. Brouet, J.-C., and Seligmann, M.: Cancer (Philad.), 42:817, 1978.
7. Brouet, J.-C., Valensi, F., and Daniel, M.-Th. et al.: Brit. J. Haematol., 33:319, 1976.
8. Catovsky, D.: Lancet, 11:327, 1975.
9. Catovsky, D.: cited by Pangalis et al. (24), 1976.
10. Catovsky, D., and Enno, A.: Lymphology, 10:77, 1977.
11. Catovsky, D., Galetto, J., and Okos, A. et al.: J. Clin. Pathol., 27:767, 1974.
12. Davies, B.I., and Ornstein, L.: J. Histochem. Cytochem., 1:469, 1959.
13. Diebold, J., Zittoun, R., and Fine, J.M. et al.: Nouv. Rev. Franc. Hémat., 11:429, 1971.
14. Dutcher, T.F., and Fahey, J.L.: Proc. Soc. Exp. Biol. Med., 103:452, 1960.
15. Fossum, S.: Scand. J. Immunol., 8:273, 1978.
16. Gömöri, G.: Int. Rev. Cytol., 1:323, 1952.
17. Goldberg, A.F., and Barka, T.: Nature (London), 195:297, 1962.
18. Grossi, C.E., Webb, S.R., and Zicca, A. et al.: J. Exp. Med., 147:1405, 1978.
19. Higgy, K.E., Burns, G.F., and Hayhoe, F.G.J.: Scand. J. Haematol., 18:437, 1977.
20. Horwitz, D.A., Allison, A.C., and Ward, P. et al.: Clin. Exp. Immunol., 30:289, 1977.
21. Huhn, D., Rodt, H., and Thiel, E.: In: Thierfelder, S. et al., see (35), pp. 169–170, 1977.
22. Kaplow, L.S.: Blood, 10:1023, 1955.
23. Kaplow, L.S.: Amer. J. Clin. Path., 39:439, 1963.
24. Kaplow, L.S.: Blood, 26:215, 1965.
25. Knowles, D.M., Hoffman, T., and Ferrarini, M., et al.: Cell Immunol., 35:112, 1978.
26. Kramers, M.T.C., Catovsky, D., and Foa, R.: Brit. J. Haematol., 40:11, 1978.
27. Kulenkampff, J., Janossy, G., and Greaves, M.F.: Brit. J. Haematol., 36:231, 1977.
28. Lake, B.D.: J. Clin. Path., 24:617, 1971.
29. Leder, L.-D.: Klin. Wschr., 42:553, 1964.
30. Leder, L.-D.: Klin. Wschr., 43:795, 1965.
31. Leder, L.-D.: Der Blutmonocyt. Springer Verlag, Berlin-Heidelberg-New York, 1967.
32. Leder, L.-D.: Acta Histochem., Suppl. IX:141, 1971.
33. Leder, L.-D.: Klin. Wschr., 56:313, 1978.
34. Leder, L.-D., and Stutte, H.J.: Verh. Dtsch. Ges. Path., 59:503, 1975.
35. Lennert, K.: In: Malignant lymphoma (slide seminar), Lukes, R.J., and Lennert, K., 10th. Int. Congr. Acad., Path., Hamburg, 1974.
36. Lennert, K.: in collaboration with Mohri, N., Stein, H., Kaiserling, E., and Müller-Hermelink, H.K.: Malignant lymphomas other than Hodgkin's Disease. Springer Verlag, Berlin-Heidelberg-New York, 1978.
37. Lennert, K., Löffler, H., and Leder, L.-D.: Virchows Arch. Path. Anat., 334:399, 1961.
38. Löffler, H., and Berghoff, W.: Klin. Wschr., 39:1220, 1962.
39. Moloney, W.C., McPherson, K., and Fliegelman, L.: J. Histochem. Cytochem., 8:200, 1960.

40. Mueller, J., Brun del Re, G., and Buerki, H. et al.: Eur. J. Immunol., 5:270, 1975.
41. Nanba, K., Itagaki, T., and Iijima, S.: Beitr. Path., 154:233, 1975.
42. Nanba, K., Jaffe, E.S., and Braylan, R.C. et al.: Am. J. Clin. Path., 68:535, 1977.
43. Nanba, K., Jaffe, E.S., and Soban, E.J. et al.: Cancer (Philad.), 39:2323, 1977.
44. Obrist, K., Albrecht, R., and Nagel, G.A.: Experientia, 34:660, 1978.
45. Pangalis, G.A., Waldman, S.R., and Rappaport, H.: Am. J. Pathol., 69:314, 1978.
46. Pearse, A.G.E.: Histochemistry. Theoretical and applied, vol I. Churchill, Livingstone, London, 1968.
47. Poppema, S., Halie, R., and Elema, I.B.: Z. Immun.-Forsch., 154:351, 1978.
48. Rajvanshi, V., Peter, H.H., and Avenarius, H.J.: Z. Immun.-Forsch., 155:330, 1979.
49. Ranki, A.: Clin. Immun. Immunopath., 10:47, 1978.
50. Ranki, A., Tötterman, T.H., and Häyry, P.: Scand. J. Immunol., 5:1129, 1976.
51. Schaefer, H.-E., and Fischer, R.: Verh. Dtsch. Ges. Path., 57:293, 1973.
52. Schwarze, E.-W.: Lancet, 11:1264, 1975.
53. Schwarze, E.-W.: Verh. Dtsch. Ges. Path., 63:488, 1979.
54. Schwarze, E.-W: Habilitation thesis, University of Kiel, 1979.
55. Schwarze, E.-W., and Tolksdorf, G.: Verh. Dtsch. Ges. Path., 62:513, 1978.
56. Seligmann, M., Brouet, J.-C., and Preud'Homme, J.-L.: In: Thierfelder, S. et al., see 35., pp. 1–15, 1977.
57. Sher, R., Golver, A., and Fripp, P.J.: South Afr. Med. J., 50:1009, 1976.
58. Stein, H., Lennert, K., and Parwaresch, M.R.: Lancet, 11:855, 1972.
59. Stein, H., Petersen, N., and Gaedicke, G. et al.: Int. J. Cancer, 17:292, 1976.
60. Stein, H., Tolksdorf, G., and Burkert, M. et al.: In: Crowther, D.G. (ed.): Leukemia and non-Hodgkin lymphoma. Adv. Med. Oncol. Res. Educ., 7:144–152, Pergamon Press, Oxford-New York, 1979.
61. Sundström, C., Nilsson, K., and Ranki, A. et al.: Scand. J. Haemat., 21:47, 1978.
62. Thierfelder, S., Rodt, H., and Thiel, E., (eds.): Immunological diagnosis of leukemias and lymphomas. Haematology and blood transfusion, vol. 20 (see (10), and (29)), Springer-Verlag, Berlin-Heidelberg-New York, 1977.
63. Tolksdorf, G., and Stein, H.: Blut, 39:165, 1979.
64. Tötterman, T.H., Ranki, A., and Häyry, P.: Scand. J. Immunol., 6:305, 1977.
65. Wehinger, H., and Möbius, W.: Acta Haemat., 56:129, 1976.
66. Yam, L.T., Li, C.Y., and Lam, K.W.: New Engl. J. Med., 284:357, 1971.

ACKNOWLEDGEMENT

The author wishes to thank Mrs. M. Soehring for translating and preparing the manuscript.

12. ELECTRON MICROSCOPY IN THE STUDY OF HUMAN LYMPHOMAS

J.W. PARKER

In general the ultrastructural characteristics of human lymphomas confirm light microscopic (LM) impressions. However, additional information is obtained since subtle nuclear or cytoplasmic features are not always apparent with the light microscope. For example, minor degrees of nuclear irregularity in "cleaved" and "convoluted" cells are easily seen by EM, but may be missed in paraffin sections. Cytoplasmic features indicating plasmacytoid differentiation (well-developed rough endoplasmic reticulum (RER)) and the microvilli of hairy cells are also better appreciated with EM. Thus EM examination of lymphomas may assist the pathologist in determining the cell type, and further, may provide a means for studying the interrelationships between lymphoma cells and other cells of the lymphoid tissues, e.g. stromal elements.

In another sphere, the use of EM in the differential diagnosis of poorly differentiated neoplasms involving lymphoid tissues may be of significant clinical value. The presence of identifying features such as specific granules, melanosomes, desmosomes and other organelles may be quite helpful.

A major problem in the use of EM by the pathologist relates to sample size. Specimens are by necessity quite small and are only representative of the lymphomatous process if there is diffuse and extensive involvement of the tissue studied or, if not, there is adequate sampling.

The use of immunocytochemical techniques with labels such as peroxidase or ferritin, enzyme cytochemistry using electron dense reaction products, and rosette methods has increased the value of EM in lymphoma studies, particularly since the same techniques are used for LM. The purpose of this paper is to briefly discuss some of the techniques used in the EM study of human lymphomas and to describe the ultrastructural features of the various lymphoma cell types in the Lukes/Collins classification.

SAMPLING: A PROBLEM

The degree of involvement of a lymphoid organ by a lymphomatous process may be minimal or extensive, focal or diffuse. If diffuse, adequate sampling for EM study presents little difficulty. However, if a node is only partially

J.G. van den Tweel et al. (eds.), Malignant Lymphoproliferative Diseases, 149–174.
All rights reserved.
Copyright © 1980 by Martinus Nijhoff Publishers bv, The Hague/Boston/London.

or focally involved, adequate sampling is essential. The conventional approach, in order to assure proper fixation of tissues, is to finely mince the tissue into 1–2mm blocks. Once embedded in a resin, 1–2μm sections are prepared for LM. These may be trimmed to a still smaller size to select a particular area for EM examination. The relative sample sizes are indicated in Figure 1 in which the size of standard resin-embedded section for EM is compared to a paraffin section. Different approaches are used to resolve this sampling problem. One is to take multiple samples from several parts of the lymph node, hoping to hit the involved areas, but this is generally impractical because of the large number of blocks that must be examined. Another approach is to embed a 1–2mm thick section of lymph node with a large surface area in epoxy resin and then section this with a special microtome to produce 1–2 μm sections for LM evaluation. The appropriate areas identified in this section can be reembedded, cut-out, and ultra-thin sections prepared for EM. This same approach can be used to provide sections for cytochemical or immunocytochemical staining from selected embedding media followed by identification of areas where staining is observed for EM examination.

SPECIAL EM TECHNIQUES

The principle involved in using cytochemical techniques which will specifically identify and localize a cellular component or product in an electron micrograph is that the end or reaction product, either because of its electron density or configuration, is sufficiently distinctive to be distinguished from other parts of the cell which are stained by fixative (OsO_4) or counterstains and thus are also electron dense. The specificity of a method depends, of course, on the specificity of the antibody (immunocytochemistry), the substrate (enzyme cytochemistry) or the chemical reaction between stain and cellular component.

Cytochemistry

Certain cytochemical reactions performed routinely for LM can be adapted for EM. The stain or reaction product must have sufficient electron density to make it apparent against a background of lesser densities in counterstained or unstained sections. An example of this is the PAS reaction which can be used for EM by the addition of silver methenamine (1). The reaction lacks specificity, but may be useful in examining lymphomas since immunoglobulin is stained. Since silver is in the reaction product, the end result is a highly dense, "stained" area. A variety of other stains have been used to

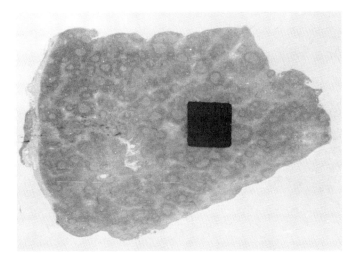

Figure 1. Relative areas sampled with paraffin 1–2 µm epoxy sections. Epoxy-embedded material (black) is trimmed even further for ultra-thin sectioning.

detect other cellular and intercellular components in EM using reagents which contain copper, lead and other metals.

Enzyme cytochemistry

The principles regarding reaction conditions and enzyme specificity are in general the same for EM as for LM with the exception that the reaction product must be electron dense. The limitation of the light microscope in the accurate localization of enzyme activity within the cell is avoided in EM where the exact location of an enzyme within an organelle is possible. A wide spectrum of enzymes (phosphatases, dehydrogenases, glycosidases, transaminases, etc.) can be demonstrated if the reaction conditions and fixation are appropriate for the preservation of both enzyme activity and fine structure (6). Aldehydes generally preserve enzyme activity better than other fixative and gluteraldehyde is the most widely used.

The ultrastructural localization of phosphatase activity has been widely studied and involves the precepitation of metal salts, primarily lead and calcium. Phosphate ions liberated from organic phosphate substrates form insoluble precipitates with the metal cations. These are opaque to electrons, and if various diffusion and absorption artifacts are avoided the precipitates are restricted to those areas of the cell where phosphatase activity resides.

Because of problems inherent in metal-salt precipitation methods, alternative methods have been developed using azo dyes. These methods depend

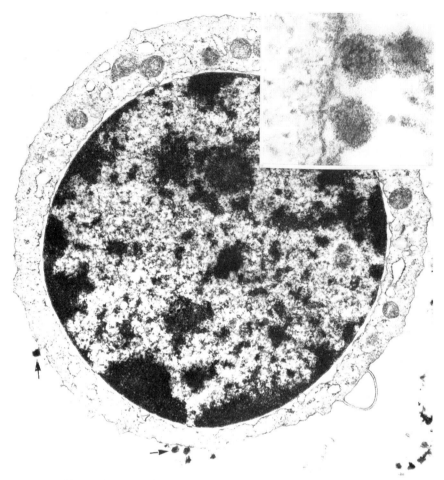

Figure 2. Chronic lymphocytic leukemia, B cell. Methacrylate-methacrylic acid immuno-spheres (arrows) attached to surface Ig. Anti-Ig antibody is conjugated to microspheres.
× 11,160: insert × 72,000.

on the precipitation of a naphthol or substituted naphthol, enzymatically released, by a diazonium salt. The electron density of the precipitate is enhanced by using diazonium salts of large molecular weight, coupling the dye with a metal containing diazonium salt, or by using a crystalline azo dye (6).

Application of enzyme cytochemistry to the ultrastructural study of lymphomas has been relatively limited, although methods for detecting 5-nucleotidase and ATPase ultrastructurally have been used in differentiating the different types of stromal cells in normal lymphoid tissue and lymphomas (12).

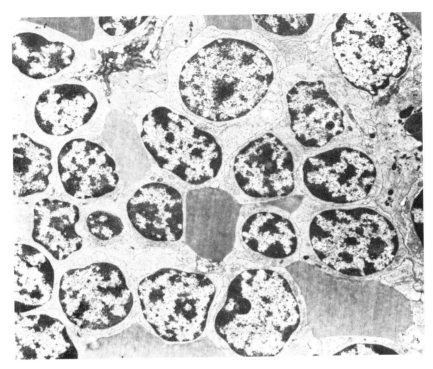

Figure 3. Small lymphocytic lymphoma, B cell, spleen. Most cells are small lymphocytes with peripheral condensed heterochromatin. The larger partially transformed lymphocytes have nucleoli, more dispersed heterochromatin, a few strands of RER, and scattered ribosomes and polyribosomes. × 3,600.

Inherent limitations in metal-salt and azo dye techniques make an immunological method for localizing enzymes quite attractive. Immunocytochemical techniques with their exquisite senitivity and specificity render it possible to localize enzymes in cells as long as specific antibodies are available.

Immunocytochemistry

This approach employs the specificity of antibodies for the demonstration of cell components that have antigenic determinants. The indicators or labels used, unlike fluorescein, are materials which can be localized at the site of antigen-antibody reaction by EM because they are inherently electron dense (metals), have a distinct configuration (ferritin, hemocyanin, tobacco mosaic virus, microspheres, etc.), or because they can produce an electron dense reaction product (enzymes). Horseradish peroxidase, as an example of the latter, has proved to have broad application, because it can

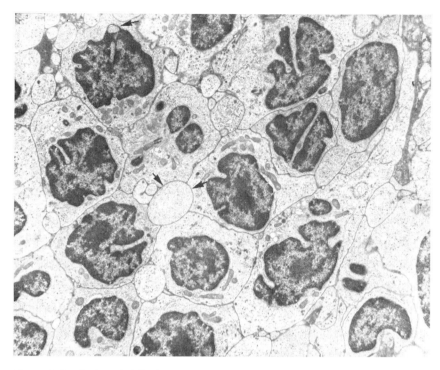

Figure 4. Small cleaved follicular center cell lymphoma (FCC), lymph node. Nuclei are irregular with deep indentations. The heterochromatin is condensed marginally and centrally. Nuclear envelopes or blebs (arrow) are uncommon, but are frequently seen in large cleaved FCC. Cytoplasm is abundant and some cells are elongated. Long cytoplasmic processes and round "fingers" of cytoplasm, cross sectioned (arrows), indicate intertwined cytoplasmic projections and a cohesive cell population with extensive intercellular contact.

be used for both LM and EM (21). Other enzymes such as phosphatases can also be used, but the peroxidase label in conjunction with a chromogenic substrate such as diaminobenzidine, which is rendered electron opaque by treatment with OsO_4, provides an excellent visual marker for both LM and EM. Taylor has used this approach to advantage in the LM study of lymphomas (23).

Pre- or post-embedding immunoperoxidase staining may be applied to the ultrastructural localization of antigens. In the former, thick frozen sections of fixed tissues are stained by the immunoperoxidase technique prior to post-fixation, embedding and ultra-thin sectioning. With this method penetration into the thick sections is a limiting factor due to the large molecular size of the antibody or antibody-peroxidase conjugate, but the use of $F(ab')_2$ and peroxidase fragments helps to resolve the problem (16, 10). Post-embedding staining involves staining antigens at the surface

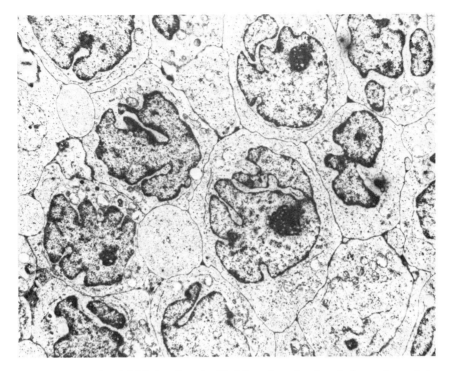

Figure 5. Large claved FCC, lymph node. Nuclei are irregular, but the heterochromatin is more dispersed than in small cleaved FCC. Nucleoli are prominent with well-defined nucleo-nemata. The abundant cytoplasm with scattered strands of REP and ribosomes again shows evidence of extensive cellular interaction. × 2,400.

of ultra-thin sections of the resin-embedded tissue. Since the antigen is at the surface, penetration may not be a problem, but the effect of dehydrating agents and embedding resins on different antigens is unpredictable.

The perfusion barriers presented by the plasma membrane and membranes surrounding intracellular compartments in fixed cells, particularly those cross-linked by fixatives such as glutaraldehyde, make it difficult to obtain penetration by particle or enzyme-labeled antibodies. In spite of the diffusion problems encountered in the use of the immunoperoxidase method in EM, it is significantly less a problem than that encountered with particle tracers such as ferritin. Again, antibody or enzyme fragments can by used effectively or the membrane barriers mechanically disrupted by freezing or altered with membraneactive agents such as detergents (for an excellent review see Kraehenbuhl and Jamieson (10)).

In the case of lymphomas, the antigens or receptors of interest may be either intracellular or on the cell membrane. For the latter, penetration is

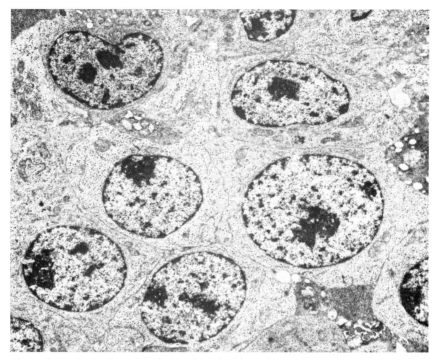

Figure 6. Small noncleaved FCC, lymph node. The uniform round and oval nuclei contain prominent nucleoli. Clumps of heterochromatin are small and generally dispersed. Profiles of RER and polysomes are fairly numerous. Nuclei and cytoplasm are much more uniform than in the cleaved cell lymphomas. × 3,600.

not a problem, but the cells must be stained in suspension for detection of surface determinants (19).

The major advantage of enzyme labels in immunocytochemistry far out-strips the disadvantages. The reaction of enzyme with substrate yields a large number of visible product molecules per single molecule of antibody and sensitivity is thus greatly increased. Methodological and immunological nonspecificity presents problems, but these generally can be resolved as discussed by Taylor (23).

Rosetting techniques

A variety of types and sizes of particles have been used to detect surface antigens or receptors on cells in suspension, examined by either light or electron microscopy. The particles used include erythrocytes of different species, ferritin, distinctive viral particles, or microspheres (3) (Figure 2). The advantage of using smaller particles such as polymeric micro-

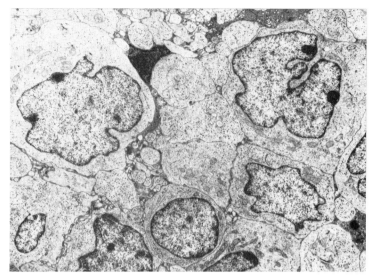

Figure 7. Large noncleaved FCC, lymph node. These nuclei are somewhat irregular but not to the degree seen in cleaved cells, and the chromatin is fine and dispersed. Nucleoli are small and situated in contact with the nuclear membrane. The cytoplasm is abundant, containing scattered polyribosomes and rare profiles of RER. The presence of some cleaved cells helps differentiate this lesion from IBS. × 1,650.

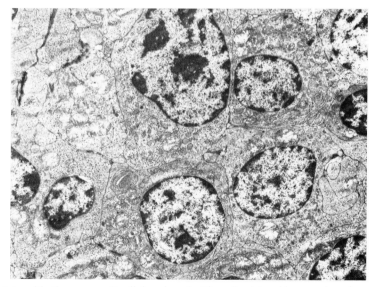

Figure 8. Immunoblastic sarcoma, B cell, lymph node. The cells pictured here are in various stages of transformation, but all show many profiles of RER, frequently dilated and containing a homogenous electron dense material (immunoglobulin). The large immunoblast possesses prominent nucleoli and shows some margination of heterochromatin. Polysomes are numerous and mitochondria swollen. × 1,920.

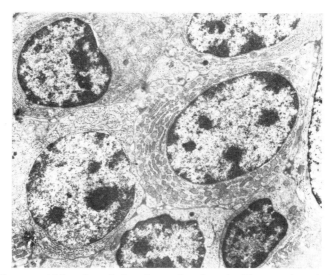

Figure 9. Plasmacytoid lymphocytic lymphoma, lymph node. The cytoplasm is definitely plasmacytoid with well developed RER with dilated cysternae containing immunoglobulin. The nuclei are round or oval and contain scattered clumps of heterochromatin still retaining a lymphocyte appearance. × 5550.

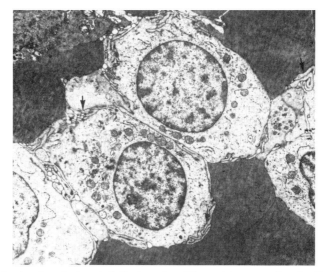

Figure 10. Leukemic reticuloendotheliosis, spleen. The nuclei are round and uniform with a minor degree of margination of heterochromatin. The abundant cytoplasm contains scattered strands of RER, a few ribosomes and several mitochondria. Interdigitating cytoplasmic processes (arrows), representing microvilli, may be quite prominent as in this case, but are not always apparent. Nuclei in circulating cells in the peripheral blood have a different appearance, frequently showing deep central indentations dividing the nucleus in half. In these peripheral blood cells bundles of cytoplasmic fibrils may ring the nucleus and penetrate into the nuclear cleft. In some cases mitochondria form a halo around the nucleus as well. × 5550.

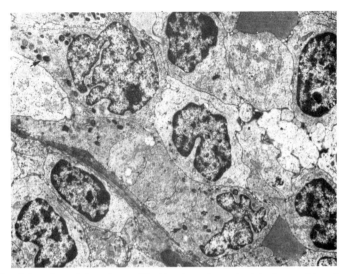

Figure 11. Small lymphocytic lymphoma, T cell, spleen. In contrast to the small lymphocytic lymphoma of B-cell type, the nuclei are irregular and show slightly less condensation of heterochromatin. The cytoplasm is also more irregular and in the larger cells there are scattered dense bodies (lysosomes) presumably representing azurophilic granules (arrows). The larger of the two cells with the markedly irregular nuclei possesses a prominent nucleolus. This degree of nuclear irregularity is not seen in all cases of T-CLL, and in fact T- and B-cell CLL may be indistinguishable morphologically. × 3,600.

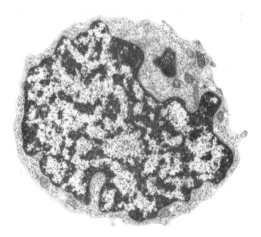

Figure 12. Convoluted T cell lymphoma, peripheral blood. More important than the nuclear irregularity seen in this lesion is the chromatin pattern. In paraffin sections it appears fine and stippled. In electron micrographs as illustrated here it has a speckled or "salt and pepper" appearance.

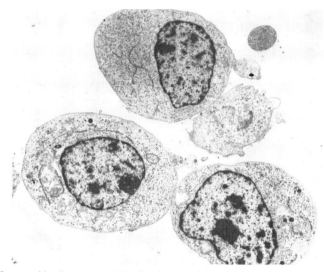

Figure 13. Immunoblastic sarcoma, T cell. These nuclei are oval and only slightly irregular with distinct nucleoli at the nuclear membrane or centrally. The heterochromatin is condensed in small clumps, but with little nuclear membrane margination. A few strands of RER are present, but show no dilitation and no indication of organization, unlike those seen in a typical **B-IBS**. Polyribosomes are numerous but scattered and swollen mitochondria and lipid vacuoles are present. × 3,600.

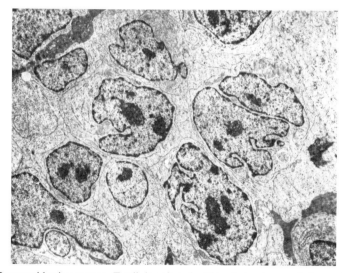

Figure 14. Immunoblastic sarcoma, T cell, lymph node. This photomicrograph demonstrates the nuclear irregularity which may be seen in this lesion. Some of the cells show deep nuclear indentations producing marked irregularity. The heterochromatin is dispersed and generally fine and nucleoli large and prominent. There are several strands of RER, but no dilitation and the cytoplasm does not have a plasmacytoid appearance. × 3,600.

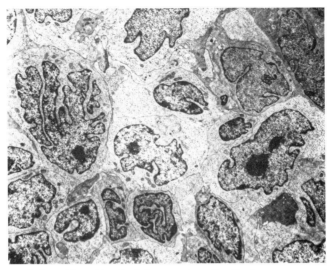

Figure 15. Mycosis fungoides, skin. Both large and small cells show pronounced nuclear irregularity. There is some marginal heterochromatin, but in general the chromatin is dispersed. Nucleoli are prominent in the larger cell and cytoplasm is abundant but contains few organelles. The large markedly irregular nucleus reflects the convolutions which in three dimensions would give it a cerebriform appearance. × 2,700.

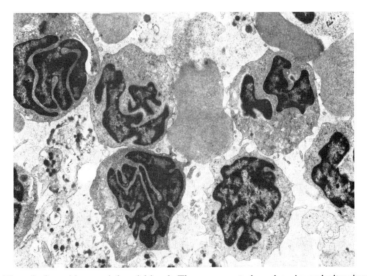

Figure 16. Mycosis fungoides, peripheral blood. The exaggerated nuclear irregularity gives a serpentine appearance reflecting the cerebriform nature of the nuclei. The cells show more condensation of heterochromatin at the nuclear membrane, obscuring the nucleoli, than in Figure 15. The cytoplasm shows a few microvilli, but relatively few organelles.

162 J.W. PARKER

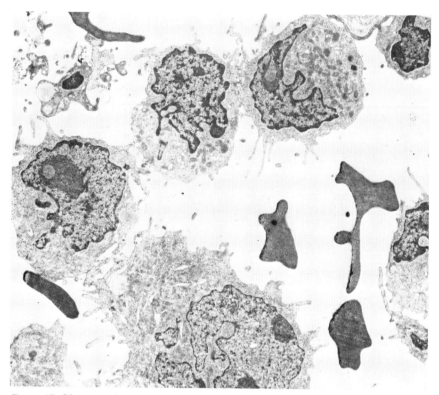

Figure 17. Sézary syndrome, cultured cells. Peripheral blood cells stimulated in vitro with concanavalin A, after three days in culture. Cells are larger and with more prominent nucleoli than in cells prior to culture or in control cultures. × 4,050.

spheres lies in the potential for large numbers of spheres to attach to each cell. In addition, polymers offer a great deal of chemical versatility. They may be derivatized to react with proteins or their composition altered to include heavy metals, radioisotopes, fluorescent dyes, etc. An example of this is seen in our use of microspheres containing iron to selectively identify subpopulations of lymphocytes and remove them in a magnetic field. An added advantage is that the same microspheres may be phagocytized by nonlymphoid cells in suspension, and by combining particles of different sizes or configurations in the same suspension more than one receptor or antigen on a given cell may be identified by EM.

These approaches to the specific identification of lymphoma cell types have not been widely used in ultrastructural studies and deserve more attention. However, even without them certain distinctive features seen in both light and electron microscopy have allowed pathologists to categorize lymphomas based on cytological differences correlated with immunological and cytochemical characteristics.

MATERIALS AND METHODS

We have described our morphological, immunological, and cytochemical studies of several hundred cases of lymphomas and leukemias (14). From this group a large number of speciments (lymph nodes, spleens, bone marrow aspirates, peripheral blood) were also examined ultrastructurally. For this, solid tissues were minced while immersed in Karnovsky's fixative (5), as soon as possible after surgical removal. Cell suspensions and buffy coats were similarly fixed and the specimens were processed for EM as previously described (18).

RESULTS

The major morphological features of the different types of lymphoma in the Lukes/Collins classification are summarized in Table 1, and electron micrographic examples of each are provided (Figures 1–17). These examples are selected from over 500 cases of lymphoma examined ultrastructurally over the past five years. Since they are selected to illustrate typical features, they naturally do not reflect the spectrum of cells present in any given specimen.

DISCUSSION

As a diagnostic tool electron microscopy is of limited value in the diagnosis of lymphomas. It is largely confirmatory, but may be of some value because subtle changes, difficult to appreciate on light microscopy, are obvious with EM (cleaved cells, convoluted cells, pasmacytoid cells). And, just as with light microscopy, enzyme and immunocytochemical procedures may assist in differentiating cell types. As yet, these approaches have not been widely used in lymphoma studies.

Henry (7) has described some of the advantages of the use of EM in studying lymphomas. These include its use in the differential diagnosis of lymphoma (i.e. distinction of lymphomas and carcinomas); identification of the lymphoma cell type and degree of differentiation; and demonstration of inclusions, organelles, and cell-to-cell contact as useful markers. Examples given are the identification of dendritic cells because of the presence of desmosomes (9, 12); the use of desmosomes to identify metastatic carcinomas; plasmacytoid differentiation; and distinction between neoplastic

Table 1. Morphologic features of lymphomas.[1]

Camera Lucida Drawing	Light Microscopy	Electron Microscopy	Comment
B CELL LYMPHOMAS (1) SMALL LYMPHOCYTIC LYMPHOMA–B CELL	Diffuse proliferation of noncohesive small lymphocytes. Uniform, round nuclei with basophilic compact chromatin and inconspicuous nucleoli. Narrow rim of pale cytoplasm. Large transformed lymphocytes and mitoses rare.	Generally uniform population of cells with round or oval nuclei with one inconspicuous nucleolus and perinuclear heterochromatin. Blocks of heterochromatin at nuclear membrane. Scanty cytoplasm containing few mitochondria and lysosomes and small Golgi apparatus. Ribosomes, but few polyribosomes. Rare strands of ER. Surface generally smooth but occasional microvilli. Occasional case with inclusions—crystalline or homogenous immunoglobulin inclusions in RER or perinuclear space; ribosome-lamellae complex. Partially or fully transformed lymphocytes generally uncommon, but variable—dispersed chromatin; prominent nucleolus, ring shaped or with compact nucleolonemata; ribosomes and polyribosomes; Golgi occasionally well developed; Mitochondria swollen and pale; lysosomes uncommon; occasional strands ER and RER. (Figure 3.)	Lymphocytes usually indistinguishable from normal lymphocytes, but may be smaller with less cytoplasm. Ribosome-lamellae complex not limited to CLL, more common in hairy cell leukemia.
 (2) FCC–SMALL CLEAVED	Wide range of cell sizes, but small cells predominate. Nuclei have basophilic compact chromatin and many show deep cleavage planes. Nucleoli are inconspicuous and cytoplasm is indistinct or scanty. Transformed lymphocytes present in small numbers, but occasionally 10%–20%. Mitoses rare. Small cleaved cells in follicles, interfollicular	Irregular nuclei with one or more deep indentations. Condensed marginal heterochromatin, inconspicuous nucleoli. Nuclear envelopes uncommon. Ribosomes moderate to numerous, ER sparse, Golgi poorly developed, few lysosomes, mitochondria variable. (Figure 4.)	Small cleaved cells predominate, but range from small lymphocytes to larger cleaved cells and noncleaved cells not uncommon. Occasional cases show plasmacytoid cytoplasm with RER and occasionally, Ig inclusions. Associated fibroblastic reticulum cells, phagocytic histiocytes, dentritic reticulum cells in varying numbers. Nuclear irregu-

larity may be so marked as to suggest a convoluted T-cell lymphoma, but latter has more dispersed, "stippled" chromatin pattern.

Noncleaved cells (transformed lymphocytes) may be numerous. Cytoplasmic Ig may give signet ring appearance.

Phagocytic histiocytes with phagocytized cellular debris and intact lymphocytes (emperipolesis) common. Vacuoles contain lipid.

Nuclei irregular, some with deep indentations. Heterochromatin may be condensed at nuclear membrane, but generally is more dispersed and in smaller aggregates than small cleaved cells. Nucleoli with nucleonemata larger than in SC cells. Nuclear envelopes fairly common and occasionally bizarre. Few strands RER, moderate ribosomes and polyribosomes. Mitochondria may be numerous, Golgi moderately developed, lysosomes variable. Cytoplasmic inclusions in a few cases. (Figure 5.)

Nuclei round or oval, but shallow indentations not infrequent. May have nuclear envelopes (blocks). Heterochromatin at nuclear membrane in small clumps. Interchromatin selectively clear. Nucleoli large with visible nucleonemata. Large number polyribosomes, few RER profiles. Mitochondria few, but large. Vacuoles common. Tubular inclusions nonspecific. (Figure 6.)

tissues and capsule. 75% are follicular, remainder diffuse.

Nuclei larger than nuclei of reactive histiocytes. Prominent nuclear irregularity. Occasional large nuclei with exaggerated cleaved planes may resemble Reed-Sternberg cells. Mitoses variable and related to number of noncleaved cells. Cytoplasm moderate and pyroninophilic. Frequent association with intercellular material and sclerosis. Small cleaved and noncleaved cells generally present in small numbers. Predominance of large cleaved cells determines cell type. Occasional case with cytoplasmic Ig inclusions (a).

Cells resemble small transformed lymphocytes. Nuclei round but variable in size (by definition do not exceed size of histiocyte nucleus). Nuclear chromatin finely dispersed. 1-3 small nucleoli. Moderate amount

(3)
FCC—LARGE CLEAVED

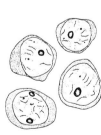

(4)
FCC—SMALL NON-CLEAVED

Table 1. (continued)

Camera Lucida Drawing	Light Microscopy	Electron Microscopy	Comment
	of pyroninophilic cytoplasm with cohesive cell borders. "Starry sky" reactive histiocytes common. When nuclei uniform in size and configuration and nucleoli small, fulfill criteria for Burkitt lymphoma. When more nuclear variation and prominent nucleoli, Burkitt-like or non-Burkitt lymphoma (seen in U.S.). Minimal follicular pattern in 10%. Generally diffuse, obliterating lymph node architecture.		
 (5) FCC-LARGE NON-CLEAVED	Similar to small noncleaved but cells and nuclei larger. More cytoplasm but lightly stained. Nuclei round or oval, but irregular forms often present. Nucleoli prominent—frequently two at the nuclear membrane on short axis of an oval nucleus, a characteristic feature. Mitoses numerous. Individual cell necrosis and necrotic zones common. A minor proportion of accompanying small and large cleaved cells	Large transformed lymphocytes (blast cells) with one or more prominent nucleoli typically at nuclear membrane of round or oval nuclei. Mild nuclear irregularity not uncommon. Heterochromatin fine and dispersed. Few RER profiles, moderate Golgi, large swollen mitrochrondria. May show nuclear envelopes. Moderate to many polyribosomes. No plasmacytoid cytoplasmic features. (Figure 7.)	Differences from B-IBS include lack of plasmacytoid differentiation and presence of cleaved cells. Resemble blast cells seen in mitogen stimulated cultures.

and lymphomatous follicles indicates FCC nature. Follicular in 10% of cases.

(6)
IMMUNOBLASTIC SARCOMA-B CELL

Cells resemble large non-cleaved FCC, but more deeply staining amphophilic and pyroninophilic cytoplasm. Often plasmacytoid features. Cleaved cells and follicular pattern not present. Presents as relatively monomorphous collections of large abnormal immunoblasts, sometimes in background of severe, abnormal immunoblastic reaction. Initial involvement of node is frequently partial, later may totally replace node. Differentiated from T-IBS by plasmacytoid features, pyroninophilia, and cytoplasmic Ig. Nucleoli often central and prominent. Nucleus appears vesicular owing to margination of chromatin with resultant thick nuclear membrane.

Large nuclei, central large nucleoli with prominent nucleonemata. Dispersed, fine heterochromatin but some nuclear membrane margination. Many polyribosomes and generally well developed RER. Occasional globular Ig inclusions in cytoplasm. Mitochondria variable, Golgi moderately developed. (Figure 8.)

Not distinguishable from T-IBS unless plasmacytoid cytoplasm (well-developed RER) and/or monoclonal Ig in cytoplasm.

(7)
PLASMACYTOID LYMPHOCYTIC LYMPHOMA

Similar to small lymphocytic lymphoma, but has abnormal plasmacytoid cell component of variable prominence. These cells possess cytoplasm resembling plasma cell, but nucleus more like lymphocyte. Some cells have

Blocks of heterochromatin at nuclear membrane and around inconspicuous nucleolus. Well developed, abundant RER may contain immunoglobulin in dilated cisternae. Latter may contain globular Ig inclusions. Ig in perinuclear space may invaginate nucleus producing an inclusion. Some cases with large transformed lymphocytes resembling large noncleaved cells

Lymphocytes with plasmacytoid differentiation in contrast to a primary plasma cell neoplasm (Multiple myeloma). Degree of differentiation and number of transformed cells quite variable.

Table 1. (continued)

Camera Lucida Drawing	Light Microscopy	Electron Microscopy	Comment
(8) LEUKEMIC RETICULOENDOTHELIOSIS (HAIRY CELL LEUKEMIA)	PAS-positive supranuclear structures (Dutcher bodies). In tissue sections cells appear medium sized with abundant pale cytoplasm and round to oval nuclei with finely granular chromatin. In well-fixed material cell borders are sharply demarcated and interlocking with prominent acidophilic intercellular zone. In smears and imprints cytoplasm abundant, finely granular, and margin poorly defined or with hairlike processes.	or immunoblasts, may possess well developed RER, but generally not. (Figure 9.) Nuclei oval, but frequently indented in peripheral blood. Nucleolus small, heterochromatin dispersed as small clumps with some nuclear membrane margination. Cytoplasm abundant and electron luscent in tissue, less so in blood. Mitochondria frequently numerous and may ring nucleolus as do bundles of fibrils which may penetrate, with cytoplasm, into nuclear indentation. Vesicles variable. Microvilli long and branching in peripheral blood cells, not always apparent in tissues, but may be seen as interdigitating cytoplasmic processes. Ribosomes and polyribosomes variable. Few strands RER. Mitochondria frequently swollen, may be misshapen. Ribosome-lamellae complexes occasionally present. (Figure 10.)	Cells primarily in sinuses in lymph nodes and in Bilroth's cords in the spleen. Possess features of both histiocytes and lymphocytes. Evidence for immunoglobulin synthesis is strong, but cells also phagocytic in vitro. Cell of origin unknown. Tartrate resistant acid phosphatase granules in cytoplasm. NSE negative.
T CELL LYMPHOMAS (1) SMALL LYMPHOCYTIC LYMPHOMA–T CELL	Cells resemble those of small lymphocytic lymphoma, B-cell type. Nuclei with compact chromatin. Small rim of pale cytoplasm. Nuclei occasionally irregular. Azurophilic granules may show acid phosphatase activity.	Cells may be indistinguishable from B-cell type, but some cases show nuclear irregularity with degree and number of such cells variable. Chromatin as in B-cell type. Amount of cytoplasm variable. May be clusters of small dense lysosomes (azurophilic granules). Moderate numbers of ribosomes, few polyribosomes. May be deposits of cytoplasmic glycogen. Surface smooth or with short microvilli. Transformed lymphocytes uncommon. Some cases with occasional cells with convoluted or even cerebriform nuclei. Parallel tubules arranged in cytoplasm not uncommon (Figure 11).	Nuclear irregularity generally minor and less than in convoluted T-cell lymphoma. Heterochromatin more blocklike in contrast to stippled chromatin of convoluted cells. Interdigitating reticulum cells may be present in small T-cell lymphoma, but not in convoluted lymphomas.
	Diffuse proliferation of "primitive" noncohesive cells, occurring as infil-	Markedly irregular nucleus with deep indentations to the point of apparent segmentation in cross section. Finely dispersed, "stippled" chromatin.	Nuclear indentations not always easily seen by light microscopy. Stippled chroma-

trative masses in partially or totally involved nodes. Cells have scanty cytoplasm, range in size from small lymphocytes to 4 times that size. Nuclear chromatin finely stippled and evenly distributed. Nucleolus inconspicuous. Nuclei of smaller cells are round, while nuclei of larger cells appear "convoluted" because of dense irregular lines penetrating into nucleus from surface and subdividing it. Proportion of small and large cells varies with case. Mitoses numerous. "Starry sky" phagocytes occasionally present.

Usually one inconspicuous nucleolus. Ribosomes and polyribosomes present, but rare RER. Golgi well developed. Lysosomes and multivesicular bodies. Golgi and lysosomes may nestle in nuclear indentation. Cytoplasmic glycogen occasional. Plasma membrane smooth. (Figure 12.)

tin important differentiation feature. Large acid phosphatase globules localized in Golgi area. PAS positive globules common in cytoplasm and may ring nucleus.

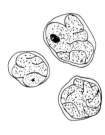

(2) CONVOLUTED T-CELL LYMPHOMA

Admixture of lymphocytes with small irregular, contorted nuclei and transformed lymphocytes. Latter predominate and resemble lymphocytes transformed in vitro In sections they have pale, water-clear cytoplasm with well-defined interlocking plasma membranes giving a cohesive appearance. Nucleus round or oval with fine evenly distributed chromatin and one or more small but distinct nucleoli. Diffuse involvement of node, initially in paracortical areas. Reactive histiocytes may be present in large numbers.

Dispersed, fine heterochromatin with little peripheral margination. Nucleoli distinct but small—central or at nuclear membrane, compact or with visible nucleonemata. Ribosomes and polyribosomes frequently sparse giving cytoplasm a relatively electron-luscent appearance. RER uncommon, Golgi moderate, lysosomes infrequent. Mitochondria may be swollen. Some cells with irregular, even cerebriform nuclei. (Figure 13, 14.)

Differentiating features seen by light microscopy not as apparent with EM. Lack of RER and cytoplasmic Ig only features reliable in distinguishing from B-IBS on EM.

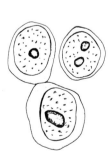

(3) IMMUNOBLASTIC SARCOMA T-CELL

Table 1. (continued)

Camera Lucida Drawing	Light Microscopy	Electron Microscopy	Comment
  (4) MYCOSIS FUNGOIDES AND SÉZARY CELL	Cells 2-3× diameter of small lymphocyte. Linear subdivisions in nuclei frequently indistinct in early disease, but in late aggressive stages nuclei large and quite irregular with prominent subdivisions. In comparison with convoluted lymphocytic lymphoma, MF/Sézary cells have more compact chromatin and fewer mitoses.	Characteristic cells in both entities essentially the same ultrastructurally. Diagnostic (Lutzner) cell, whether small, medium or large, characterized by a deeply indented convoluted nucleus with maximum degree of irregularity producing a cerebriform nucleus which, in cross section, is serpentine in appearance. Heterochromatin is clumped at the nuclear membrane. Medium size cells may show less irregularity than small. Cytoplasm of either may vary in electron density, some with ribosomes others with polyribosomes. Few RER profiles, Golgi moderately developed, few lysosomes and vesicles. Dermal infiltrates may contain small lymphocytes with little cytoplasm and large MF cells with typical nuclei and resemble immunoblasts. In the tumor stage of MF with involvement of skin and lymph node, predominant cells may be large blast cells with many polyribosomes and irregular cerebriform nuclei. Cells in Sézary syndrome essentially same as Lutzner cells. Nucleoli are not prominent, cytoplasm contains ribosomes but few polyribosomes and very little RER. Lysosomes and vesicles are frequent. Glycogen collections in the cytoplasm seen in some cases. May also be smaller lymphocytes with less nuclear irregularity. Interdigitating reticulum cells in some cases. Cerebriform cells and transformed lymphocytes may be seen in peripheral blood of both MF and Sézary syndrome. (Figures 15, 16, 17.)	Cerebriform nuclei not specific for MF/Sézary cells. Have been reported in lichen planus, various non-lymphomatous dermatological conditions and are seen in mitogen stimulated lymphocytes in vitro. Lutzner cells also present in lymph nodes in T-cell areas in dermatopathic and other forms of lymphadenitis. Cerebriform cells persist in culture and appear to be stimulated by mitogens to transform.

[1]Modified and reproduced with permission of the publisher from Seminars in Hematology 15:322–351, 1978.

large lymphocytes and histiocytes. However, as Henry indicates, these advantages are of rather limited value. For example, desmosomes within lymph nodes are not limited to dendritic cells, but are also found between endothelial cells and fiber-forming reticular cells. He also indicates that in a series of cases in which the diagnosis made on paraffin sections was modified by subsequent EM, the diagnoses did not differ appreciably from those made on 1–2 μm epoxy sections. Thus, although there are some advantages and some forms of information are provided that cannot be obtained by light microscopy, most diagnoses are made by the pathologist on the basis of well-fixed 4–6 μm paraffin sections or 1–2 μm epoxy-embedded material with the former having the advantage of greater sample size.

Lymphomas that have received some attention from electron microscopists are the nodular or follicular lymphomas. Their relationship to counterparts in reactive lymph node follicles or germinal centers has been described ultrastructurally by several workers (2, 13, 9); however, some differences in the role of dendritic cells and the presence of desmosomes are noted. Kojima et al. (9) regarded dendritic cells as lymphoid cell precursors and nodular lymphomas as dendritic cell neoplasms. Levine and Dorfman (13) found no desmosomes between lymphoid cells and determined that the dendritic cells made up a very small portion of the total lymphoma population. They concluded that the cell is nothing more than a residual marker cell of a preexisting germinal center. Lennert and Niedorf (12) described dendritic cells with long cytoplasmic processes and prominent desmosomes in nodular lymphomas, whereas Glick et al. (2) observed similar cells, associated with collagen fibers, in lymphomas with both nodular and diffuse growth patterns. Lennert and coworkers (12) have more recently made the point that the stromal cells of lymphoid tissues are useful in differential diagnosis with an association between dendritic reticulum cells and follicular lesions. Interdigitating reticulum cells are associated with some T zone lymphomas. Our own experience has been that the specificity of these associations is not sufficient to be more than supportive in diagnosis. Nevertheless, these relationships may become more readily apparent by combining morphology with enzyme and immunoelectron microscopy. Their importance lies in largely unexplored indications that stromal cells may play a role in immunoregulation.

Another example of the type of information that can be obtained by EM with more clarity than with LM is seen in the following. In the Lukes/ Collins concept of follicular center cell transformation, the sequence is: small lymphocyte → cleaved cell → noncleaved cell → immunoblast → plasma cell; whereas in the Lennert scheme it is seen as small lymphocyte → centroblast (large noncleaved cell) → centrocyte (cleaved cell) → plasma cell. Based on electron micrographs from a small number of our cases of small cleaved FCC lymphoma in which many of the predominant cells show

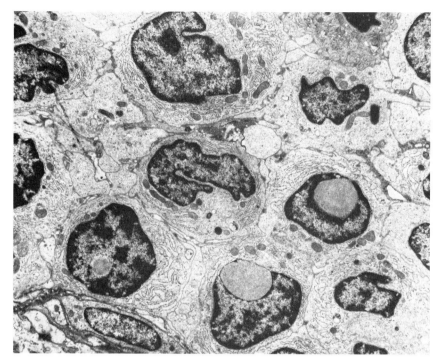

Figure 18. Small cleaved FCC with plasmacytoid features, conjunctiva. This lesion was a typical small cleaved FCC showing marked nuclear irregularity in most areas, but in some areas the cells, as seen here, showed not only nuclear irregularity, but definite plasmacytoid features, i.e., well organized, dilated profiles of RER and nuclear immunoglobulin inclusions. × 3,600.

nuclear immunoglobulin inclusions (Dutcher bodies) and a plasmacytoid cytoplasm (Figure 18), it would appear that the more likely sequence is that described by Lennert and colleagues.

For the pathologist the electron microscope is an extension of the light microscope. It provides information not made available by LM, and, as with cytochemistry, it may assist in the diagnosis of difficult cases. The application of newer enzyme and immunolgical techniques to EM provides another dimension which may or may not be of significant value in diagnosis, but surely promises to provide valuable information about the biology of lymphomas.

ACKNOWLEDGMENT

Electron micrographs were prepared by R. Wong and D. Anderson. Their expert technical assistance is gratefully acknowledged.

REFERENCES

1. de Martino, C., and Zamboni, L.: Silver methanamine stain for electron micros-copy. Ultrastructural Res., 19:273–282, 1967.
2. Glick, A.D., Leech, J.H., and Waldron, J.A., et al.: Malignant lymphomas of follicular center cell origin in man. II. Ultrastructural and cytochemical studies. J. Natl. Cancer Inst., 54:23–36, 1975.
3. Gordon, I.L., Dreyer, W.J., Yen, S.P.S., and Rembaum, A.: Light microscope identification of murine B and T cells by means of functional polymeric micro-spheres. Cell. Immunol., 28:307–324, 1977.
4. Gordon, I.L., Lukes, R.J., O'Brien, A.L., Parker, J.W., Rembaum, A., Russell, R., and Taylor, C.R.: Visualization of surface immunoglobulin of human B lymphocytes using microsphere-immunoglobulin conjugate in Giemsa-stained preparations. Clin. Immunol. Immunopathol., 8:51–63, 1977.
5. Graham, R.C., Jr. and Karnovsky, M.J.: The early stages of absorption of injected horseradish peroxidase in the proximal tubules of mouse kidney: ultrastructural cytochemistry by a new technique. J. Histochem. Cytochem., 14:291–302, 1966.
6. Hayat, M.A.: Electron Microscopy of Enzymes. Principles and methods, vol. 1, pp. 1–149, Von Nostrand Rheinhold Company, New York, 1973.
7. Henry, K.: Electron microscopy in the non-Hodgkin's lymphomata. Br. J. Cancer 31, Suppl., 2:73–93, 1975.
8. Izard, J. and de Harven, E.: Increased numbers of a characteristic type of reti-cular cell in the thymus and lymph nodes of leukemic mice—an electron microscopic study. Cancer Res., 28:421, 1968.
9. Kojima, M., Imai, Y. and Mori, N.: A concept of follicular lymphoma—a proposal for the existence of a neoplasm originating from the germinal center. Gann Monograph on Cancer Research No. 15. University of Tokyo Press, Tokyo, 1973, pp. 195–202.
10. Kraehenbuhl, J.P., and Jamieson, J.P.: Localization of intracellular antigens by immunoelectron microscopy. Int. Rev. Exp. Pathol., 13:1–53, 1974.
11. Lennert, K.: Malignant lymphomas other than Hodgkin's disease. Springer-Verlag, Berlin, Heidelberg, New York, 1978.
12. Lennert, K. and Niedorf, H.R.: Nachweis von desmosomes verknufften Reticulumzellen in follicularen Lymphom. Virchows Arch. [Zellpathol.], 4:148–150, 1969.
13. Levine, G.D., and Dorfman, R.F.: Nodular lymphoma: an ultrastructural study of its relationship to germinal centers and a correlation of light and electron microscopic findings. Cancer, 35:148–164, 1975.
14. Lukes, R.J., Parker, J.W., Taylor, C.R., Tindle, B.H., Cramer, A.D., and Lincoln, T.L.: Immunologic approach to non-Hodgkin's lymphoma and rela-ted leukemias. An analysis of the results of multiparameter studies of 425 cases. Semin. Hematol., 15:322–351, 1978.
15. Mason, D.Y., and Taylor, C.R.: The distribution of muramidase (lysozyme) in human tissues. J. Clin. Pathol., 28–124–132, 1975.
16. Nakane, P.K.: Recent progress in the peroxidase-labelled antibody method. Ann. N.Y. Acad. Sci., 254:203–211, 1975.
17. Nossall, G.J.V., Abbot, A., Mitchell, J., and Lummus, Z.: Ultrastructural features of antigen capture in primary and secondary follicles. J. Exp. Med., 127:277, 1968.

18. Parker, J.W., Royston, A.I., and Pattengale, P., et al.: Morphological differences between cultured human B and T lymphoblastoid cell lines: a light
    and electron microscopic and cytochemical study. J. Natl. Cancer Inst.,
    60:59–68, 1978.
19. Reyes, F., Lejone, J.L., Gourdin, M.F., Mannoni, P., and Dreyfus, B.: The
    surface morphology of human B lymphocytes as revealed by immunoelectron
    microscopy. J. Exp. Med., 141:392–410, 1975.
20. Rosenthal, N.: The lymphomas and leukemias. Bull. N.Y. Acad. Med., 30:583,
    1954.
21. Sternberger, L.A.: Enzyme immunocytochemistry. In: Electron microscopy of
    enzymes, vol. 1, pp. 150–191, Hayat, M.A., (ed.), van Nostrand Rheinhold Co.,
    New York, 1973.
22. Taylor, C.R.: An immunohistologic study of follicular lymphoma, reticulum
    cell sarcoma and Hodgkin's disease. Eur. J. Cancer, 12:61–75, 1976.
23. Taylor, C.R.: Immunoperoxidase techniques: practical and theoretical
    aspects. Arch. Pathol. Lab. Med., 102:113–121, 1978.
24. van den Tweel, J.G., Taylor, C.R., and Parker, J.W. et al.: Immunoglobulin
    inclusions in non-Hodgkin's lymphomas. Am. J. Clin. Pathol., 69:306–313,
    1978.

13. CHANGING CONCEPTS IN THE CLASSIFICATION OF LYMPHOMA

C. R. TAYLOR

Nowhere in pathology has a chaos of names so clouded clear concepts as in the subject of lymphoid tumours.

R. Willis (20)

INTRODUCTION

For those histopathologists deeply involved in the study of malignant lymphomas the recognition and diagnosis of any particular disease process has always been a very personal thing, and the nomenclature applied has not always been uniform even in single institutions. The problems arising from the use of these diverse personalized systems of nomenclature were well illustrated by Wallhauser who, in 1933, was able to collect 51 separate alternate names for Hodgkin's disease without recourse to direct translation from other languages.

With respect to Hodgkin's disease, the widely recognized subclassifications of Jackson and Parker (4), and subsequently of Lukes, Butler and Hicks (7), have undoubtedly resulted in a more uniform standard of nomenclature and diagnosis. However, the position regarding nomenclature of other lymphomas, the so-called non-Hodgkin lymphomas, is less favorable, and there is at present no general agreement upon classification of these morphologically diverse tumors.

PRINCIPLES AND RATIONALE OF CLASSIFICATION

Omnis cellula e cellula. Virchow

In the beginning diseases were described and named according to some combination of their clinical manifestations and their gross features at autopsy. Diagnosis was made absolute at the autopsy table and, as such, fell unchallenged into the realm of the early pathologist.

The first of the first great classifiers of disease was Carl Linné (Linnaeus, 1707–1778) who devised a classification of plants based on the "sexual

J.C. van den Tweel et al. (eds.), Malignant Lymphoproliferative Diseases, 175–184.
All rights reserved.
Copyright © 1980 by Martinus Nijhoff Publishers by, The Hague/Boston/London.

system" (*Species Plantarum*–1753). Ten years later, armed with an M.D. degree, Linnaeus launched the classification of diseases (*Genera Morborum*– 1763). From that time on physicians have scarcely paused to look back. Classifications devised subsequently have been based upon various criteria, although the "sexual system" has been found wanting in relation to the classification of lymphomas. Classifications of diseases of man, in the time of Linnaeus as now, have followed faithfully the concepts of the causation of disease. One early theory considered diseases to result from an imbalance of the bodily humors, as for example a surfeit of black bile (melancholia). All this was, of course, in the dark ages before the dawn of histopathology. The publication, in the mid 19th century, of Virchow's *Cellularpathologie* effectively laid to rest the "humoral concept" of disease. Coupled with the concurrent advances in light microscopy, including tissue sectioning and staining techniques, *Cellularpathologie* provided the impetus and foundation for more or less rational systems of nomenclature and classification based upon histological criteria.

HISTORICAL ASPECTS OF LYMPHOMA CLASSIFICATION

> Tumors are classified like normal tissues on a histologic basis. . . . The type of cell is the one important element in every tumor. From it the tumor should be named.
>
> Mallory, 1914

> There occur tumours corresponding to almost all kinds of normal tissues, and clearly our classification of tumours will run parallel with our classification of normal tissues.
>
> Willis, (20)

In the past proposed classification of lymphoreticular neoplasms or lymphomas have generally developed from concepts of the reticuloendothelial or lymphoid system current at the time. The concepts in turn have been influenced by the development and application of new laboratory techniques, exemplified by the use of the microtome, simple stains, special stains, electron microscopy, immunologic methods, and so on.

Malignant lymphoma, a term first used by Billroth (2), was adopted more recently by Gall and Mallory, and subsequently by others, as an alternative to the terms "reticulosis' and "reticulosarcoma". Malignant lymphoma, therefore, is a collective term for an ill-defined group of lymphoreticular neoplasms, including some part of both the "reticulosis" and "reticulosarcoma" groups. The terms reticulosis and reticulosarcoma themselves reflect the three basic divisions of lymphadenopathy proposed by Robb-Smith

(13) and reviewed by Lennert as late as 1966:

We differentiate according to Robb-Smith and in analogy to Ewing, three categories of lymphadenopathy: 1) reactive hyperplasia, 2) sarcomas of lymphoreticular tissue, 3) a group of diseases lying between (7).

Many of the early attempts at classification of lymphoreticular tumors followed naturally upon Aschoff's definition of the reticuloendothelial system and upon Maximow's concept of the reticulum cell as some sort of shadowy ancestral haemopoietic cell (1, 8). Pullinger (10) adopted Maximow's theory of the reticulum cell as a central multipotent stem cell element and suggested that:

A group of diseases of the reticulum exists in which proliferation is possible into one or several of the possible cell progeny (10).

Thus developed the "reticulosis"–"reticulum cell sarcoma" concept that is still not extinct in the minds of men everywhere.

For twenty years classifications rose and classifications fell, yet all reflected this concept of the reticulum cell as the mother lode of the lymphoid tissues. Within this concept a number of pathologists favored a dynamic view of lymphoreticular neoplasia:

They are all mesenchymal tumors which vary only in degree and type of differentiation . . . —a striking fluidity of histologic pattern with transitions and combinations (3).

Adherence to this essentially unitarian concept of lymphoreticular neoplasia constituted the "fluid lymphoma school" (14). Standing in oppostion to the "fluid lymphoma school" were those pathologists who subscribed to the view that lymphomas were constant and immutable—the "fixed entity hypothesis".

THE HISTIOCYTE DYNASTY

The publication of Rappaport's classification in 1956 (12, 11) (Table 1) represented a major shift of opinion and had two major consequences. It sounded the death knell of the reticulum cell, and it portended the eclipse of the "fluid lymphoma school". Lymphomas came to be regarded as fixed immutable entities, distinct and distinguishable from one another, and of lymphocytic, histiocytic or mixed cell derivation. The Rappaport classification soon found favor among pathologists for its relative simplicity and ease of application. Clinicians gave their approval as clinical-pathologic

Table 1. Classification of non-Hodgkin lymphomas[1] (Modified from (16)).

Traditional Terminology	Rappaport	Lukes-Collins	Lennert (Kiel)	WHO[2]
Nodular (Follicular)	Lymphocytic W.D.	Small cleaved	Centrocytic = cleaved [3]	Lymphosarcoma (Nodular) Prolymphocytic
Follicular lymphoma	Lymphocytic P.D. Mixed	Small noncleaved, Large cleaved	Centroblastic = noncleaved [3]	Lymphoblastic
	Histiocytic	Large noncleaved		
Diffuse	Lymphocytic W.D.	Small lymphocytic	Lymphocytic	Lymphosarcoma (Diffuse) Lymphocytic Lymphoplasma-cytic
		Plasmacytic Lymphocytic	Lymphoplasmacytoid (Immunocytoma)	
Lymphosarcoma*	Lymphocytic P.D.* Mixed	Small cleaved	Centrocytic [3]	Prolymphocytic
		Large cleaved		

			Centroblastic [3]	Immunoblastic
Reticulum cell sarcoma	Histiocytic	Large noncleaved	Immunoblastic Sarcoma (B or T cell)	
		Immunoblastic Sarcoma (B or T cell)		
		Histiocytic	Lymphoblastic Burkitt*	Burkitt*
Burkitt's	Undifferentiated	Small noncleaved*		
		Convoluted*	Convoluted*	Lymphoblastic*

Interrupted line separates good histology from bad in the Kiel classification, and may be extended across the other classification,s the principal exception being that convoluted lymphoma makes up part of the lymphosarcoma and lymphocytic P.D. groups.*

Entries enclosed in boxes in the Lukes-Collins and Kiel classifications designate follicular center cell tumors.

[1] Shows approximate correspondence of cytologic types—precise matching is not feasible.

[2] This classification also includes reticulosarcoma and plasmacytoma groups. Plasmacytoma//myeloma is not included in other classifications.

[3] In the Kiel classification most follicular center cell tumors in fact fall into a "centrocytic-centroblastic" category, that overtly recognizes the fact that most of these tumors are composed of a mixture of the two cell types.

correlations were established, and the system entered general use. As such it endures to the present day as the only scheme almost universally recognized, if not universally understood, by clinicians and pathologists alike. Recently, however, many institutions have introduced modifications to the original proposal; these in a sense have devalued the Rappaport classification, for many of the modifications (e.g. Jaffe et al., intermediate cell type (5); Nathwani et al., lymphoblastic type (9)) have not received a consensus of approval.

A NEW ERA DAWNS

Since Rappaport formulated his classification there have been radical changes in our understanding of the function and morphology of the "reticuloendothelial" system. As a direct consequence of advances in basic immunology the lymphocyte has emerged as a distinct cell type, with a previously unsuspected wide range of functional and morphological expressions. Following the precepts of Mallory and Willis, that the classification of tumors parallels the classification of normal tissues, this realization has had profound effects upon concepts of classification of the tumors of the lymphoid system. The recent epidemic of new classifications (Table 2) represents the attempts of the current generation of pathologists to incorporate these new ideas into a traditional morphologic framework.

Table 2. An epidemic of lymphoma classifications for references see Annual Research Reviews (15, 16, 18).

Bennet et al.	1974
Chelloul	
Diebold	
Dorfman	
Hamilton-Fairly & Freeman	
Lennert et al.	
Lukes & Collins	
Mathé & Belpomme	
Tubiana & LeBourgeois	
Beard	1975
Burg & Braun-Falco	
Schnitzer	
Bryon et al.	1976
Mathé, Rappaport (WHO)	
Jaffe et al.	1977

Most of the new immunologically based classifications of lymphoma embrace two separate realizations (16, 17):

1) The morphologically monotonous small lymphocyte conceals at least two distinct functional cell populations (B lymphocytes and T lymphocytes); 2) The small lymphocyte is not an end stage cell, but has the potential for radical morphological and functional change upon exposure to antigen. (Transformation occurs with progressive morphologic change to a large primitive-appearing cell, the transformed lymphocyte or immunoblast.)

Other aspects of normal lymphocyte behavior such as lymphocyte circulation and lymphocyte homing have received less attention from the pathologist, and have proved more difficult to incorporate into classification schemes. Nevertheless, if neoplastic lymphocytes indeed mimic their normal counterparts, then they might also be expected to show a propensity to circulate and to home to specific regions in the peripheral lymphoid organs, the so-called B- and T-cell areas.

In addition, the translation of the methods of the immunologist into clinical pathology has furthered the study of human lymphoproliferative diseases, for it has permitted critical examination of the biologic validity of recently proposed classifications. Some broad conclusions may be drawn from the immunological/morphological studies described elsewhere in this volume (H. Stein; K. Lennert; J.W. Parker). Upon these we should base any reappraisal of the value of current classification schemes.

These basic studies and the conclusions drawn from them did not occur in logical orderly sequence. Nevertheless, they may be arranged in such a way in an attempt to summarize the general course of events that has led to the immunologic/morphologic concepts under discussion at this Boerhaave Course in Lymphomas.

MALIGNANT LYMPHOMAS—TOWARDS AN "IMMUNE BASED" CLASSIFICATION

1) The development of cellular immunology has led to a new understanding of the potentialities of the small lymphocyte; radical changes in behavior, surface markers, and morphology occur as intrinsic parts of differentiation in the embryo and of transformation following antigenic stimulation after birth.

2) As a result, previous concepts have been overthrown; the concept of the reticulum cell as the central stem cell of the haemopoietic system can no longer be maintained, and the large "primitive" appearing cell of lymphoid tissues appears to be neither reticulum cell nor histiocyte, but rather transformed lymphocyte or immunoblast.

3) Obeying the usual precept that neoplastic cells resemble and mimic normal cells, the idea that "lymphomas" may be lymphocytic, mixed, or histiocytic in origin now seems illogical. All 'lymphomas" must be considered to be of lymphocytic lineage.

4) The application of immunological methods to the study of lymphocytic leukaemia and malignant lymphoma has resulted in an improved understanding of the genesis and origin of these lymphocyte-derived neoplasms and basically supports the belief that most of the principal forms of malignant lymphoma can indeed be related to demonstrable subclasses or subtypes of the lymphocyte.

5) Some of the variations and differences among neoplastic lymphocyte populations reflect the heterogeneity of normal lymphocyte populations:

a) The variation in morphologic and immunologic expressions occurring during transformation;

b) The different behavioral patterns manifested by lymphocyte circulation and homing;

c) The division into two or more major functional subclasses (B cells, T cells and possibly null cells);

d) The existence of further functional or maturational subgroups within the major B- and T-cell classes (some of these subclasses may reflect phases of lymphocyte differentiation in the embryo or foetus).

6) Recognition of the above aspects of normal lymphocyte behavior created a critical need for a change in terminology of the corresponding neoplasms to reflect these concepts; the basic concepts underlying several of the new classification schemes are somewhat similar, but the usage and definition of various terms within the classification schemes show little correspondence (Table 1). The problem of classification is inextricably interwoven with that of terminology.

7) Though many new classification schemes reflect these immunologic concepts, they are nevertheless firmly based upon the "old-fashioned" histologic precepts that neoplastic cells are monomorphous, are distinguishable from nonneoplastic cells by morphologic criteria, and reproduced by division of recognizable neoplastic cells. Physicians and pathologists who have embraced the immunologic concepts outlined above will readily see that these basic beliefs are incompatible with current knowledge of lymphocyte proliferation, involving the physiologic process of transformation with the accompanying radical changes in morphology and immunologic expression (16, 17).

8) Several of the "histologic types" of lymphoma, currently regarded as distinct and separate, may be more closely related than is presently supposed, for they share a common derivation from the lymphocyte. Thus the differences in histologic appearance must be explained on some basis other than differences in lineage. Through careful attention to the lessons of cellu-

lar immunology regarding the "metamorphosis" (change in morphology) of the lymphocyte in transformation, it is possible to attain some glimmerings of understanding relation changes in histologic appearance to changes in the proportion of lymphocytes at different phases of the transformation-maturation process. This concept is discussed more fully in a companion paper—"The Interrelations of B-Cell Lymphomas" (Taylor, in this volume).

CONCLUSION

It seems that we are upon the threshold of achieving a classification of lymphoma that is both scientifically accurate and clinically acceptable. Residual problems can only be resolved by open discussion and by continuing attention to developing knowledge of normal lymphocyte form and function. There is a need for continuing morphologic/immunologic/clinical studies to establish the validity and value, if any, of an immunologic approach to lymphoma diagnosis. Real attempts must be made to translate this new information into a form that is acceptable and useful to practicing pathologists and clinicians. For example, a new classification of lymphoma might be scientifically accurate, yet might be completely inapplicable in clinical practice, due to a lack of such ancillary aids as multiple surface marker studies, lymphocyte function assays (transformation assays, helper cell assays, suppressor cell assays, etc.) and cytochemical panels.

Alternatively a scheme might be both scientifically accurate and applicable by the pathologist in practice, yet it might have no value to the clinician in determing prognosis or therapy. The proposed classifications of lymphoma that are immune based are at present subject to increasing clinical scrutiny, and rightly so. Upon the results of this scrutiny, in the final analysis, they will stand or fall.

SUMMARY

Lymphocytic leukaemias and malignant lymphomas are composed of neoplastic lymphocytes and their morphologic and behavioral characteristics are reflections of the morphology and behavior of the normal lymphoid progenitor cells. Any consideration of lymphocytic leukaemias and malignant lymphomas according to current immunologic principles must therefore take account of the biology of the normal lymphocyte.

This paper seeks to reexamine some of the established morphologic concepts of lymphoma with reference to the results of studies attempting to correlate the morphologic and immunologic characteristics of the neoplastic cells. The relationship of the various neoplastic cell types to current knowledge of the variation in form and function of the lymphocyte, according to its state of physiological activation, is given particular emphasis.

REFERENCES

1. Aschoff, L.: Das reticulo-endotheliale System. Ergeb. inn. Med. Kinderheilk., 26:1–118, 1925.
2. Billroth, T.: Wien. med. Wochenschr., 21:1065, 1871.
3. Custer, R.P., and Bernhard, W.G.: The interrelationship of Hodgkin's disease and other lymphatic tumors. Am. J. Med. Sci., 216:625–642, 1948.
4. Jackson, H., Parker, F.: Hodgkin's disease and allied disorders. Oxford University Press, New York, 1947.
5. Jaffe, E.S., Braylan, R.C., Nanba, K., Frank, M.M., and Berard, C.W.: Functional markers: a new perspective on malignant lymphomas. Cancer Treat. Rep., 61:953–962, 1977.
6. Lennert, K.: Classification of malignant lymphoma (European concept). In: Progress in lymphology, Ruttiman, A., (ed.), G. Thieme, Stuttgart, 1966.
7. Lukes, R.J., Butler, J.J., and Hicks, E.B.: Natural history of Hodgkin's disease as related to its pathologic picture. Cancer, 19:317–344, 1966.
8. Maximow, A.: Relation of blood cells to connective tissue and endothelium. Physiol. Rev., 4:533–563, 1924; and also in: Special cytology, Cowdry, E.V., (ed.), Hoeber, New York, 1928, 1932.
9. Nathwani, B.N., Kim, H., and Rappaport, H.: Malignant lymphoma, lymphoblastic. Cancer, 38:964–983, 1976.
10. Pullinger, B.D.: Histology and histogenesis. In: Rose research on lymphadenoma, p. 117, John Wright & Sons, Bristol, England, 1932.
11. Rappaport, H.: Tumours of the hematopoietic system. Atlas of Tumour Pathology, section 3, fasc. 8, AFIP, 1966.
12. Rappaport, H., Winter, W.J., and Hicks, E.B.: Follicular lymphoma: A reevaluation of its position in the scheme of malignant lymphoma, based on a survey of 253 cases. Cancer, 9:792–821, 1956.
13. Robb-Smith, A.H.T.: Hyperplasia and neoplasia of lymphoreticular tissue. M.D. Thesis, London, 1936. Published in part in J. Pathol. Bact., 47:457–480, 1938.
14. Robb-Smith, A.H.T.: The interrelationship of lymphoreticular hyperplasia and neoplasia. In: The effects of environment on cells and tissues, p. 165. Proceedings of the IX World Congress of Anatomic and Clinical Pathology, Excerpta Medica, Amsterdam, 1975.
15. Taylor, C.R.: Hodgkin's disease and the lymphomas, vol. 1. Annual Research Review 1976, Horrobin, D.F., (ed.), Eden Press, Montreal, 1977.
16. Taylor, C.R.: Hodgkin's disease and the lymphomas, vol. 2. Annual Research Review 1977, Horrobin, D.F., (ed.), Eden Press, Montreal, and Churchill Longman Livingstone, Edinburgh/London, 1978.
17. Taylor, C.R.: Classification of lymphomas: "new thinking" on old thoughts. Arch. Pathol. Lab. Med., 102:549–554, 1978.
18. Taylor, C.R.: Hodgkin's disease and the lymphomas, vol. 3. Annual Research Review 1978, Horrobin, D.F., (ed.), Eden Press, Montreal, and Churchill Longman Livingstone, Edinburgh/London, 1979.
19. Wallhauser, A.: Hodgkin's disease. Arch. Path., 16:522–562, 672–712, 1933.
20. Willis, R.A.: Pathology of tumours. Butterworths, London, 1948.

B-CELL LYMPHOMAS

14. THE FUNCTIONAL APPROACH TO THE PATHOLOGY OF MALIGNANT LYMPHOMAS*

R. J. LUKES

INTRODUCTION

The malignant lymphomas for decades have languished in the dark ages of medical understanding as a result of the lack of fundamental knowledge of immunology and lymphopoiesis. There has been remarkable recent progress in the investigation of these areas that has led to the recognition of the development and function of the T- and B-lymphocytic systems in both animals and man. The range of morphologic expressions of the lymphocyte has been broadened through the study of both smears and histologic sections of lymphocytes transformed in vitro by mitogens.

In a series of presentations and papers since 1971, we have attempted to relate the morphologic and functional expressions of malignant lymphoma to our modern understanding of immunology (32–38). We have proposed that the malignant lymphomas are neoplasms of the immune system and involve immune defective cells as counterparts of normal cells. A functional approach using multiparameter definitional studies and an immunologic or functional classification were outlined (32–34). The classification was based on the T- and B-cell systems and the proposal that the lymphomas of large cells principally involve transformed lymphocytes rather than histiocytes or reticulum cells as believed in the past (32-38, 45). Since our original proposal, numerous reports, including our own, have appeared in the literature in support of our proposals and the T- and B-cell nature of the malignant lymphomas (1, 5–7, 9–11, 13, 15, 17, 19, 23, 25, 36–38, 41, 43, 54, 57, 64).

In this presentation the essential features of our approach will be reviewed briefly along with a consideration of the results of our multiparameter studies, the clinical pathologic correlations, the prelymphomatous states and the clinical relevance of the new functional approach.

* This investigation was supported by Grant Number CA19449, awarded by the National Cancer Institute, the Department of Health, Education, and Welfare, of the U.S.A.

J.G. van den Tweel et al. (eds.), Malignant Lymphoproliferative Diseases, 187–211
All rights reserved.

BASIC CONCEPTS OF THE FUNCTIONAL APPROACH

The basic concepts of our approach have been presented in detail previously (33–38), and the immunologic basis is reviewed elsewhere in this volume by my colleague, Dr. John W. Parker. The essential features, therefore, only will be considered.

Our interest in an immunologic approach for the malignant lymphomas was stimulated by the remarkable progress in the understanding of immunology and the recognition of malignant lymphomas developing in patients with congenital immune defects (18). The approach is based on three principles that we have interrelated with our morphologic observations. In a series of papers beginning in 1971 we presented our new approach on the basis of the following proposals: 1) malignant lymphomas involve the T- and B-cell systems and rarely the histiocyte-monocyte system; 2) lymphomas commonly develop from alterations in lymphocyte transformation either as a block or "a switch on" (derepression) with the various cytologic types of lymphoma representing positions in the T- and B-cell transformation sequence; and 3) the follicular center is a B-cell area and the interfollicular or paracortical area is a T-cell zone. In addition, it seemed likely that lymphomas might develop from defects in development at various levels, from the lymphoid precursor cell to the functioning small lymphocyte effector cell. The multiparameter approach for the characterization of T- and B-cell types, derived from experimental animal studies, was proposed (33–34). It included the special collection system of biopsy specimens for refined morphologic studies, cytochemistry, ultrastructural studies, and immunologic surface marker techniques. Subsequently, it has been expanded to include immunoperoxidase stains for cytoplasmic immunoglobulin and muramidase (lysozyme), cell kinetics, and chromosomal studies.

The understanding of the immunologic approach to malignant lymphomas requires an appreciation of the morphologic expressions of in vitro lymphocyte transformation in both smears and histologic sections. Unfortunately, few pathologists have had exposure to such material since the discovery of the phenomenon in 1960 (49). This lack of familiarity through the decades accounts for the traditional view that lymphomas of large cells were of reticulum cell or histiocytic type and variants of lymphocytes were always small. From our investigative morpholigic studies of in vitro lymphocyte transformation, we became aware of the remarkable change of lymphocytes exposed to mitogens from a small lymphocyte to the so-called hyperbasophilic blast cell or transformed lymphocyte. We suggested that the small lymphocyte represented the dormant form of the lymphocyte and the transformed lymphocyte, the metabolically active dividing form (33–38). Because of the bidirectional nature of in vitro lymphocyte transformation, it seems most appropriate to regard the in vivo lymphocyte transformation phenomenon as modulation rather than lymphocyte differentiation. From this consideration, the term "lymphoblast" seems incorrect since the primitive-appearing lymphocyte is essentially the dividing form of the lymphocyte and not a precursor cell. Thus, it appears that during antigenic stimulation the small lymphocyte changes into a transformed or the dividing lymphocyte form with the production of daughter cells; these eventually revert back to small dormant lymphocytes when the antigenic stimulus sub- sides. Thus, the small lymphocyte and the transformed lymphocyte appear to represent dormant and dividing kinetic states rather than mature and precursor forms as traditionally believed. From this consideration there appear to be three basic forms of lymphocytes: 1) the dormant small lymphocyte of T cell, B cell, and the lymphoid precursor cell; 2) the transformed or dividing form; and 3) the functional expressions in both T- and B-cell systems, e.g., the plasma cell of the B-cell system.

From my experience with human malignant lymphomas, the process commonly appears to develop as either a block or a "switch on" in lympho- cyte transformation. According to this view, the small lymphocytes in chronic lymphocytic leukemia (CLL) of either B- or T-cell types accumulate from a block in lymphocyte transformation and represent a disorder of low aggressiveness. On the other hand, the lymphomas of the transformed lymphocyte, the dividing form of the lymphocyte, are highly aggressive, high turnover rate processes and seem to develop possibly from a "switch on" (derepression) of lymphocyte transformation. In the latter process there seems to be an inability to revert to the small dormant lymphocyte or to "switch off" the lymphocyte transformation mechanism. We have also observed intermediate forms composed of partially transformed lympho- cytes in both T- and B-cell systems. In addition, lymphomas of small lymphocytes of either T- and B-cell type have varying tendencies in the course of the disease to change into lymphomas of transformed lymphocytes apparently through a "switch on" of the lymphocyte transformation mechanism. This morphologic transformation is associated with a parallel change in the clinical manifestations of the process from a low aggressive to a highly aggressive process. In the past the occurrence of two distinctive cyto- logic types in a patient was designated as a composite lymphoma (12). From our appreciation of lymphocyte transformation, the composite lymphomas of the past involve most commonly two expressions of a lymphocyte, the small lymphocyte and the transformed lymphocyte, and with few exceptions do not represent two different types of lymphomas (63).

The morphologic features of in vitro transformed lymphocytes in histo- logic sections demonstrated a striking similarity to the large pyronino- philic cytoplasmic cells in normal reactive follicular centers. This similarity suggested that the follicular center, as a B-cell region, might represent the site of B-cell transformation and the large pyroninophilic cytoplasmic cell, the transformed B cell. Camera lucida studies of normal follicular center cells (FCC) suggested that there were two cell types: 1) cleaved cells and 2) the noncleaved cells in addition to the phagocytic starry-sky histiocytes, and the dendritic reticulum cells. A wide range in the size of the cleaved and noncleaved FCC was noted. The follicular center was proposed as a site of B-cell transformation with the cellular sequence illustrated schematically in Figure 1.

In this proposal there are two types of B-cell transformation, the intrafollicular which is apparently related to the primary reaction and the post-follicular, to the secondary reaction. In our follicular center cell concept of the primary reaction, the small B lymphocyte from the follicular lymphocytic mantle is induced to undergo transformation in the follicular center under the influence of antigen on the surface of the dendritic reticulum cell to form the large noncleaved FCC type, with intermediate stages. In the initial stage, the small lymphocyte develops nuclear cleavage as the small cleaved FCC. It gradually enlarges to the large cleaved cell as it acquires pyroninophilic cytoplasm. In the next sequence, the nucleus rounds up and the cytoplasm becomes more pyroninophilic as it becomes a small noncleaved FCC. With further enlargement of the nucleus, there is an increase in number and prominence of nucleoli on the nuclear membrane, and

SCHEMATIC REPRESENTATION OF TRANSFORMATION
OF FOLLICULAR CENTER CELLS IN STAGES

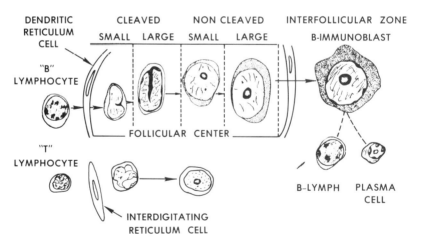

Figure 1. The proposed sequence of transformation in the follicular center and B cells is compared with the interfollicular sequence in T cells. From Lukes, R.J., et al.: An immunologic approach to classification of malignant lymphomas: a cytokinetic model of lymphoid neoplasia. In: Differentiation of normal and neoplastic hematopoietic cells., p. 940. Cold Spring Harbor Laboratories, 1978. By permission.

acquisition of more pyroninophilic cytoplasm as the large noncleaved or fully transformed FCC is formed. The small and large cleaved cells seem to be essentially nondividing cells, while the small and large noncleaved FCC are the dividing cells of the follicular center. In light microscopy sections, the large noncleaved cell at times appears to be moving out of the follicular center into the lymphocytic mantle and the interfollicular tissue where it is designated the B immunoblast. This observation is supported by the recent ultrastructural studies of Kojima and Tsunoda (24) in which cytoplasmic immunoglobulin, demonstrated by the immunoperoxidase technique, labels the large noncleaved cells. These cells, in the view of Kojima and Tsunoda (24), seem to be passing through channels in the lymphocytic mantle into the interfollicular tissue. The B immunoblast of the interfollicular tissue is a dividing cell and the immediate precursor of the plamsa cell. It continues to divide and form daughter cells and, ultimately, plasma cells as required. Finally, it reverts to the small lymphocyte. This memory lymphocyte in the secondary reaction is capable of prompt reactivation to form the immuno-blast directly on subsequent exposure to this antigen. The sequence of trans-formation in the FCC concept is acknowledged to be in conflict with the generally held view of germinal cell development. Our view is based upon the acknowledged in vitro change, from the small lymphocyte to the large trans-formed lymphocyte, and upon our observations of the evolutionary stages in FCC lymphomas. This is supported by the immunoperoxidase studies of Taylor (60) in which a gradual increase in cytoplasmic immunoglobulin was demonstrated in normal FCC, from the large cleaved FCC stage through the noncleaved FCC to the interfollicular immunoblast and plasma cell. Lymphocyte transformation in the T-cell system appears to occur in a parallel fashion in the interfollicular tissue without the formation of plasma cells or cleaved nucleated cells.

Camera lucida studies of the cells of nodular lymphomas demonstrated that they were composed of cleaved and noncleaved FCC of varying size and closely resembled cleaved and noncleaved FCC of the normal follicular center (32–35). Support for this observation was provided by the ultrastruc-tural study of Glick et al. (17) and Levine and Dorfman (30). The cytologic types of malignant lymphoma all can be related to positions in T- or B-cell transformation with the exception of three T-cell types: the convoluted lymphocyte which is proposed as a pre-T cell (57); the cerebriform cell of Sézary's syndrome and mycosis fungoides; and the lymphoepithelioid cell type which is found in association with epithelioid clusters of histiocytes (26–27). It seems likely that the latter two types are the result of proliferative expansion of functional effector T cells rather than representative of a stage in T-cell transformation. The B-cell lymphomas are explicable on the basis of an alteration in B-cell transformation. With a block in transformation at the position of the small lymphocyte, for example, these cells accumulate in great numbers; small cleaved FCC and follicles are lacking and plasma cells are essentially absent. These findings are typical of chronic lymphocytic leukemia (CLL) in which there is poor antibody production and hypogammaglobulinemia is common. A hypothetical block in transformation in the next sequence in the FCC hypothesis at the small cleaved FCC position would be association with a predominance of small cleaved FCC cells and commonly follicle formation to some degree. At the next position, the large cleaved FCC is associated with follicle formation, but often it is accompanied by sclerosis similar to that described by Bennett and associates (4). The next positions the small and large noncleaved FCC are associated with numerous mitoses and apparently a high proliferative rate. Follicle formation is infrequent and occurs in approximately 10% of each type in our recent study. The small noncleaved FCC includes both the Burkitt and so-called non-Burkitt lymphomas. The follicular center cell origin of the Burkitt lymphomas has been supported by the results of the recent study of Mann and colleagues (42). Immunoblastic sarcoma occupies the postfollicular position of the transformed lymphocyte and, with the noncleaved FCC, seems to result from the "switch on" of the transformation mechanism. Its development in abnormal immune B-cell processes will be discussed in the section on Prelymphomatous States. The final position in the B-cell sequence is the post-follicular area in the sequence from which we hypothesize the development of the plasmacytoid lymphocytic lymphoma. This lymphoma resembles the small lymphocytic type but possesses plasmacytoid cytoplasm. From our experience, it includes cases of Waldenström's syndrome, also those with elevated serum IgG and IgA, and many without evident gammopathy (29).

Table 1. Immunologic classification.

U CELL (Undefined)	
T CELL	B CELL
Small lymphocyte	Small lymphocyte
Convoluted lymphocyte	Plasmacytoid lymphocyte
Cerebriform cell of Sézary's	Follicular center cell (FCC) types
and mycosis fungoides	Follicular, follicular and diffuse,
Lymphoepithelioid cell	diffuse, and with and without
	sclerosis
	Small cleaved
	Large cleaved
	Small noncleaved
	Large noncleaved
Immunoblastic sarcoma	Immunoblastic sarcoma
HISTIOCYTIC	
CELL OF UNCERTAIN ORIGIN	
Hodgkin's disease	
UNCLASSIFIABLE (for technical reasons)	

FUNCTIONAL CLASSIFICATION

Our functional classification initially was presented in 1972 and 1973 before the use of the multiparameter technical approach (33–35) and included five major groups: 1) U cell (undefined); 2) T cell; 3) B cell; 4) Histiocytic; and 5) Unclassifiable for technical reasons. In the updated version, listed in Table 1, a sixth group, Cell of Uncertain Origin, has been added and includes Hodgkin's disease. In the original classification Hodgkin's disease was listed in a questionable position in the T-cell group because the T cells in this disorder seem to be fundamentally abnormal. We have proposed that the Reed-Sternberg cell may involve a polyploid transformed lymphocyte (2, 62), and this is supported by the demonstration of cytoplasmic immunoglobulin by Taylor (61). This view, however, has been challenged, and the precise nature of the Reed-Sternberg cell remains unsettled. Three new cytologic types have been added to the immunologic classification as a result of our multiparameter studies (36–38): 1) the small lymphocyte of T cells; 2) immunoblastic sarcoma of T cells; and 3) a distinctive type of T cell, the lymphoepithelioid cell type, which previously was included in the heterogeneous group of disorders described by Lennert (26) under the term epithelioid type of lymphogranulomatosis.

The U cell (undefined) was created for primitive-appearing cellular proliferations that lacked distinctive morphologic features and also failed to mark specifically with existing techniques. This group currently includes the so-called non-B, non-T cell, or null cell type of acute lymphocytic leukemia that is possibly the precursor cell or stem cell of lymphopoiesis. Recently, Schlossman et al. (55) and Winchester et al. (65), using highly specific B-cell antisera, presented evidence that this process involves special B lymphocytes. In our multiparameter studies of large case series (36–38), the cases which fail to mark by the various techniques are classified according to their morphologic features and are not placed in the U cell (undefined) group since they exhibit distinctive morphologic features.

In the updated version of the immunologic classification, shown in Table 1, the T- and B-cell groups both include a small lymphocytic type and a fully transformed lymphocytic type, immunoblastic sarcoma (IBS). Within the T-cell group there are lymphocytes with remarkable nuclear configurational figures: 1) the cerebriform cells of Sézary's syndrome and mycosis fungoides; 2) the primitive convoluted lymphocyte that is typically encountered as a lymphoma-leukemia process and interrelates with T-cell ALL (3, 5, 7); and 3) the lymphoepitheloid cell of Lennert (27) in which a distinctive medium-size lymphocyte is associated with clusters of epithelioid histiocytes of reactive type. The B-cell group, as noted above, also includes small lymphocytic and immunoblastic sarcoma (IBS) types. There are also the plasmacytoid lymphocytic type and the follicular center cell (FCC) types which are plasma cell precursors. Each of the FCC types may be observed in follicular, follicular and diffuse, diffuse histologic patterns, and with and without sclerosis.

The appropriate position for the neoplasms of "true" histiocytic type is uncertain at the present time. Establishment of the diagnosis of histiocytic lymphoma as a neoplasm of phagocytes, in our view, requires the demonstration of specific macrophage enzyme markers, preferably by the α-naphthol butyrate on tissue imprints or frozen tissue sections (66) and also by the immunoperoxidase stain for cytoplasmic muramidase (lysozyme) in paraffin section (60). In the future it seems likely that the term lymphoma will be reserved for neoplasms with varied expressions of lymphocytes, whereas the histiocytic malignancies as tumors of macrophages will be included most appropriately with the monocyte macrophage group of neoplasms.

The unclassifiable group allows for categorization of those processes that are technically unsatisfactory for precise cytologic classification but sufficient for identification of the process as lymphomatous. Hodgkin's disease, which is included in the group, Cell of Uncertain Origin, is sub-

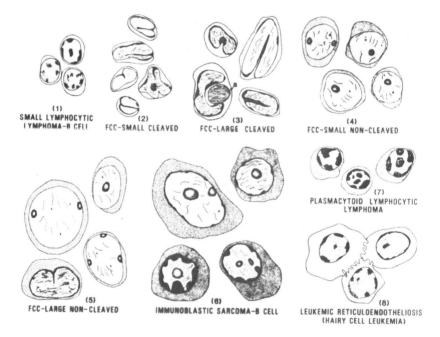

Figure 2. Camera lucida drawings of the cytologic types of B-cell lymphomas. From Lukes, R.J., et al.: The pathology of lymphoreticular neoplasms. In: The immunopathology of lymphoreticular neoplasms, p. 247 Twomey, J.J., and Good, R.A., (eds.), Plenum, New York, 1978. By permission.

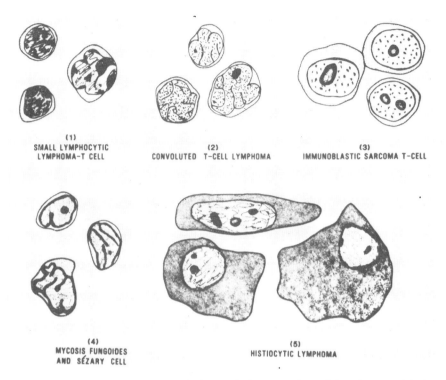

(1)
SMALL LYMPHOCYTIC
LYMPHOMA-T CELL

(2)
CONVOLUTED T-CELL LYMPHOMA

(3)
IMMUNOBLASTIC SARCOMA T-CELL

(4)
MYCOSIS FUNGOIDES
AND SÉZARY CELL

(5)
HISTIOCYTIC LYMPHOMA

Figure 3. Camera lucida drawings of the cytologic types of T-cell lymphomas, with the exception of the recently observed lymphoepithelioid cell type. A drawing of cells from our single proven case of histiocytic type is included for comparison. From Lukes, R.J., et al.: The pathology of lymphoreticular neoplasms. In: The immunopathology of lymphoreticular neoplasms, p. 246, Twomey, J.J., and Good, R.A., (eds.), Plenum, New York, 1978. By permission.

classified according to the four types of the Rye modification of the Lukes-Butler classification (40): 1) lymphocyte predominance; 2) nodular sclerosis; 3) mixed cellularity; and 4) the lymphocyte depletion.

The morphologic features of the T- and B-cell types are illustrated in Figures 2 and 3 in the camera lucida drawings of cases proven by our multiparameter studies (36–38). A detailed morphologic description of the cytologic types has been presented previously (36–38). The camera lucida drawings dramatically illustrate the relative size, the variations in quantity of cytoplasm and nuclear configuration, and the differences in the character of the nuclear chromatin in the various T- and B-cell subtypes. For example, comparison of the lymphomas of large transformed lymphocytes, including the large noncleaved FCC and IBS of B-cell and IBS of T-cell types, reveals considerable differences in appearance. Immunoblastic sarcoma of B-cell type is large and has prominent nucleoli, abundant amphophilic cytoplasm and even plasmacytoid features. The large noncleaved FCC has smaller nucleoli and little cytoplasm which is less intensely stained; it also lacks plasmacytoid features. Immunoblastic sarcoma of T-cell type typically exhibits a wide range of cell size, pale staining, water-clear cytoplasm with interlocking cell borders. The nucleus may be similar to the other two types of transformed lymphocytes.

RESULTS OF MULTIPARAMETER STUDIES

A multiparameter technical approach has been employed for the redefinition of the cytologic types of malignant lymphomas. These include special morphology, cytochemistry, electron microscopy, and immunologic surface marker studies. In addition, we frequently employ immunoperoxidase stains on paraffin sections for the demonstration of cytoplasmic immunoglobulin and muramidase. In vitro lymphocyte transformation studies, at times, also are used to evaluate lymphocyte capability. More recently, cell kinetic studies have been added to define the proliferative characteristics of the lymphoma cells. The essential battery of characterizing techniques is listed in Table 2. The spontaneous sheep erythrocyte technique (E) is an

Table 2. Techniques most commonly used for identification of T and B cells and histiocytes.

Technique	T Cells	B Cells	Histiocytes, Monocytes
Sheep erythrocyte rosettes			
E (spontaneous)	+	—	—
EAC (IgM) (complement)	(+)	+	+
EA (IgG) (Fc receptor)	—	+	+
Surface Ig	—	+	(+)
Cytoplasmic Ig	—	+	—
Antisera			
HTLA	+	—	—
HBLA	—	+	—
Cytochemistry			
α-naphthyl butyrase (NSE)	(+)	—	+
Acid phosphatase	(+)	—	—
Tartrate-resistant acid phosphatase	—	(+)	—
Muramidase (lysozyme)	—	—	+

(+)–Lacks specificity, is controversial, or is seen only with certain types of lymphoma-leukemia.
EAC–Erythrocyte-antibody-complement complex. EA-Erythrocyte-antibody complex.
T cells have a small amount of SIg that is not detected by immunofluorescent methods.
HTLA–Human T-lymphocyte antigen. HBLA-Human B-lymphocyte antigen.

effective marker of T cells. The demonstration of surface immunoglobulin is a useful indicator of B cells, but it may result from nonspecifically adsorbed immunoglobulin which obscures the identity of cells. Histiocytes and monocytes are most ideally characterized by the cytochemical technique, α-napthyl butyrate on tissue imprints or frozen tissue (66), and by the immunoperoxidase technique for muramidase (60). Highly specific antisera (HTLA for T cells and HBLA for B cells) may prove to be the most effective identifying techniques. Currently, however, it is difficult to produce such antisera with ideal specificity. The immunoperoxidase technique for the detection of cytoplasmic immunoglobulin in paraffin sections has proven to be extremely helpful in a significant proportion, but not all, of B-cell cases. The combined results of parallel studies carried out at both of the above institutions on 384 cases of non-Hodgkin's lymphomas and related leukemias were reported (36). We published the results of our multiparameter studies on two large series of 299 and 425 cases along with a critical analysis of the technical problems encountered (37, 38). As of June 30, 1979, we have completed studies on 653 cases of non-Hodgkin's disease and related leukemias and the results are essentially similar to those of the above reports. A large number of reports of similar findings have appeared in the literature confirming the T- and B-cell nature of non-Hodgkin's lymphomas and related leukemia (1, 6, 7, 9, 11, 13, 15, 19, 23, 25, 43, 57).

The results from the above studies all indicate that malignant lymphomas commonly mark as T- or B-cell types, with the exception of the rare histiocytic type and the unmarked portion of ALL. Of the 653 cases, 72% were classified morphologically in the B-cell group, 21% in the T-cell, 6.7% in the U-cell, and 0.2% (1 case) in the histiocytic group. The large number of cases of Hodgkin's disease investigated by these techniques are not included in this data.

A significant proportion of the cases of each cytologic type included in the B-cell group marked in a monoclonal fashion with surface immunoglobulin (SIg). However, in each of the B-cell types, several cases possessed only a small percentage of cells with SIg, and a variable proportion of cases of each type exhibited a polyclonal type of SIg, even through the morphologic features of the cases were typical of the cytologic type. Of the 24 cases interpreted as hairy cell leukemia, only 10 have marked monoclonally with SIg. In our combined report (36), three of Dr. Collins' cases resynthesized the immunoglobulin after initial stripping with trypsin. The monoclonal nature of the SIg on each of the cytologic types of B-cell lymphomas provides strong support for the B-cell nature of cytologic types, but it is acknowledged that immunoglobulin synthesis by the lymphoma cells provides the most ideal evidence. Those cases that are morphologically characteristic of each of the B-cell types, but fail to mark typically with SIg, represent a significant problem. The cases with few cells having detectable SIg are likely to be biologically different B cells, presenting upon the surface little SIg which is difficult to detect unless the antisera is exquisitely sensitive. Polyclonal SIg appears to be the result of a technical problem involving nonspecific adsorption of immunoglobulin or an avid Fc receptor on the B-cell surface. In the past year we have used $F(ab')_2$ reagent nonspecific antisera for the determination of SIg. This technical change along with prior incubation of the cell suspension of $37°C$ for 45 minutes has eliminated the problem of polyclonicity of B-cell lymphomas. Of the lymphomas interpreted morphologically as B cell cytologic subtypes, 70% marked in a monoclonal fashion and the remainder were either low marking or non-marking with SIg.

Immunologic confirmation of the T-cell nature of the cytologic types of lymphomas classified morphologically in this study is based on the morphologic demonstration of E-rosette formation about the lymphoma cells in cytocentrifuge preparations, without the demonstration of surface immunoglobulin and in the absence of cytochemical evidence of histiocytes or monocytes. Determination of the frequency of E rosettes alone is not believed to be a reliable determinant of a T-cell lymphoma because of the frequent admixture of nonlymphomatous T-cells. Only the morphologic identification of lymhpoma cells forming valid E rosettes in cytocentrifuge preparation is regarded as the essential proof.

The convoluted T-cell lymphoma (50 cases) was the most common type in the T-cell group. It exhibited a wide range in the frequency of E rosettes, with only 13 cases having E rosettes in excess of 50%. The four cases of the lymphoepithelioid cell type, the newly recognized T-cell lymphoma, which is associated with clusters of reactive epithelioid histiocytes all demonstrated a high frequency of E-rosette formation. Of the 16 cases interpreted as IBS of T cells, all had sufficient cells for study. There was a wide range of E-rosette formation with a median of 51%, and all were shown to form E rosettes morphologically. The histiocyte group contained only a single case (0.2%). The lymphoma cells in this case were demonstrated to be positive with α-naphthyl butyrate and also for muramidase by the immunoperoxidase technique. In addition, this case presented recognizable morphologic features of histiocytes, distinctive from the T- and B-cell types of lymphomas.

From the results of our multiparameter prospective study of 49 cases of lymphomas and leukemias of childhood (64) and the morphologic retrospective evaluation of 114 cases of childhood lymphomas (56), the B- and T-cell neoplasms in this age group are basically lymphoma-leukemic processes with evidence of both processes appearing in the course of the disease in most cases. The convoluted T-cell process, which we decribed (3, 33–35) presents outside the marrow in peripheral lymph nodes, with or without mediastinal masses, while the small noncleaved FCC Burkitt-like B-cell type primarily presents in the abdomen and, less frequently, in the nasopharynx, paranasal sinuses, or orbital tissues (56). Both processes in our experience frequently develop a diffuse leukemic marrow involvement in the course of the process and commonly relapse in the central nervous system. In the past, these processes have been classified either as a leukemia or a lymphoma, depending upon whether the initial presentation was in the marrow or peripheral blood or as a mass, such as in the mediastinum. We have observed a similar process in adults, but in considerably lower frequency (54).

It was difficult to obtain viable cells on the lymphomas of large cells, such as B-cell IBS and large noncleaved FCC, apparently because of the fragility of these high proliferative rate type processes. Similarly, attempts to separate viable cells in sclerosing lymphomas or cutaneous masses were generally not effective.

The findings in the above studies are sufficient to indicate that the lymphomas can be classified principally as subtypes of the T- and B-cell systems and that the terminology of the past, which lacks immunologic connotations, is incorrect. The diffuse histologic types, such as the histiocytic and poorly differentiated lymphocytic types of Rappaport (51), are heterogeneous and include both T- and B-cell types. The morphologic features of the cytology of lymphomas are predictive of their T- and B-cell nature if the histologic material is optimal and the observer is experienced.

CLINICAL-PATHOLOGIC CORRELATIONS

The functional approach to lymphomas, which combines morphologic observations and the multiparameter technical studies, has permitted the identification of homogeneous cellular proliferations of the T- and B-cell systems. The cytologic types of the past each subtype have been demonstrated to include T- and B-cell subtypes and are, therefore, heterogeneous. The homogeneity of the immunologic-cytologic types appears to represent newly emerging lymphoma entities, such as the convoluted T cell, IBS of B and T cells, plasmacytoid lymphocytic type, the four follicular center cell types, and the small T- and small B-lymphocytic types associated with CLL. Identification of the cerebriform cell of the well-known entities, Sézary's syndrome and mycosis fungoides, has brought greater understanding and unity to these disorders (41). Eventually, it seems likely that these new entities will have well-established characteristic presentations, sites of dissemination, functional expressions, and rates of progression. All of these features reflect the histologic behavior of the T- and B-cell subtypes of lymphomas that are counterparts of normal immune cells.

The anatomic presentation of lymphomas as a possible site of origin of the process may relate to the T- and B-cell nature of the process. The B-cell lymphomas dominantly involve the gastrointestinal tract including the tonsils, and the nasopharynx. In our experience, they also essentially account for all the lymphomas arising in patients with abnormal disorders that are discussed in the section on Prelymphomatous States. These lymphomas are usually of IBS B-cell type and at times seem to arise at the site of abnormal immune proliferations, such as the thyroid in Hashimoto's disease (46), and the salivary gland in Sjögren's syndrome (59). Lymph node presentation in the B-cell lymphomas is most common in the FCC types and often produces lymphomatous follicles which are B-cell structures. In the T-cell group of lymphomas, the convoluted T cell commonly presents in the anterior mediastinum in the region of the thymus or in the lower cervical lymph nodes in the paracortical or T-cell region. The cerebriform cell of Sézary's Syndrome and mycosis fungoides has a predilection for the skin, but it is uncertain whether or not it arises primarily in this tissue.

There is accumulating evidence of the affinity of lymphoma cells of T- and B-cell types for selective anatomic sites as they disseminate. In the T-cell group, the cerebriform cell has a well-known affinity for the skin, especially the superficial dermis, and even a tropism for the epidermis. It is uncertain whether the skin is a primary site or a tissue of dissemination. The convoluted T cell, following the initial manifestation in the mediastinum or lymph node, may be observed extending into the pleural fluid or disseminating to the bone marrow in a diffuse leukemic manner. The central nervous system also is a common site of dissemination. In the B-cell group, three types of spread are evident: 1) to regional lymph nodes in IBS from primary sites, such as the GI tract; 2) generalized spread, such as in the small cleaved FCC type, to the Malpighian bodies in the spleen, the portal areas of the liver, and the peritrabecular regions in the bone marrow; and 3) in the small lymphocytic B-cell type to the marrow and peripheral blood as part of the CLL process.

Our understanding of the functional expressions of the T- and B-cell entities is extremely limited and only a few examples are known or suspected. In the T-cell group the cerebriform cell in Sézary's syndrome is associated with damage and erythematous alteration of the skin, possibly as the result of a cytotoxic lymphokine produced by the lymphoma cells. The cerebriform cell also has been shown to have a helper cell role in enhancing immunoglobulin production (8). A suppressor role has also been observed in ALL of T cells. In the B-cell type knowledge of their functional role primarily relates to immunoglobulin production. This is well known in the processes related to the plasmacytoid lymphocytic type (29). The same monoclonal type of immunoglobulin has been demonstrated in the cytoplasm, on the surface of the lymphoma cells, and in the serum. Similarly, we have found monoclonal immunoglobulin in the cytoplasm and on the surface of the large non cleaved FCC type and the IBS of B-cell type, usually in smaller quantities, but not rarely in the serum (31, 36–38).

The rate of progression and the evolution of the process can be related to the cytologic type of malignant lymphoma. The evolution of the cytologic types of T- and B-cell lymphomas is illustrated schematically in Table 3 in relationship to the clinical aggressiveness of the process. The lymphomas of small T- and B-cell types, in general, have few or rare mitoses and represent low proliferative rate lymphomas. In Table 3 they are listed in the low aggressive clinical group. The lymphomas of large T- and B-cell types are associated with numerous mitoses and represent the high proliferative rate lymphomas. With the exception of the convoluted T cell, they consist of transformed lymphocytic types, IBS of T- and B-cell types, and the noncleaved FCC types. All of these types are listed in the high aggressive clinical group in Table 3. From a review of Table 3, it is apparent that all of the small T- and B-cell types in the low aggressive group may evolve eventually into a highly aggressive cytologic type. The frequency of this change varies widely with the cytologic type. For example, the small cleaved FCC commonly changes ($> 40\%$) in the course of the disease to the large noncleaved FCC. The small B-lymphocytic type of CLL, on the other hand, rarely changes to IBS in Richter's syndrome. This change in aggressiveness is

Table 3. Evolution of cytologic types of malignant lymphoma in relation to aggressiveness.

Low Aggressiveness	*High Aggressiveness*
T CELL	*CONVOLUTED LYMPHOCYTE*
Small lymphocyte	
Cerebriform lymphocyte	IBS (T cell)
Lymphoepithelioid cell	
B CELL	
Small lymphocyte — rare	
Plasmacytoid lymphocyte	IBS (B cell)
(Myeloma) — rare	
Small cleaved FCC ═ ─ ─ ? ─ ─ ─ ─ ─ ─ → common	Small noncleaved FCC
Large cleaved FCC	Large noncleaved FCC

IBS–Immunoblastic sarcoma
FCC–Follicular center cell
Most cases of IBS (immunoblastic sarcoma) of B-cell type evolve from previous non-neoplastic abnormal immune states.
From Lukes, R.J.: Lymphoma; The functional approach to the pathology of malignant lymphoma. In Clinical lymphography. p. 154 Clouse, M.E., (ed.), Williams & Wilkins, Baltimore, 1977. by permission.

interpreted as a "switch on" (derepression) of the lymphocyte transformation mechanism in each of the T- and B-cell types. The conditions influencing this change in aggressiveness are unknown. Each of the transformed lymphocytic types in the high aggressive clinical group may have its initial presentation as IBS of T- or B-cell type or as a noncleaved FCC, without evidence of a preceding low aggressive type of process. In this situation it is uncertain whether or not the small lymphocytic variants are obscured by the highly aggressive cellular proliferations. Unquestionably, biopsy of multiple sites at presentation or in sequence with relapse will permit the recognition of these evolutionary changes in the process. It should be emphasized that the evolution of lymphomas from the small lymphocytic variants to transformed lymphocytic types is in parallel to the development of lymphomas of IBS type in the abnormal immune disorders.

PRELYMPHOMATOUS STATES

Malignant lymphomas traditionally have been considered to occur randomly in humans. Beginning in the past decade, however, there were scattered reports of lymphomas occurring in congenital immune defects (18), a small series reported by Talal in Sjögrens' syndrome (59), a collected case series by Penn in the immunosuppressed graft rejection patients (50), and, more recently, multiple case series in Mediterranean malabsorption syndrome, also known as alpha-chain disease (52). For the most part, these cases have been reported as examples of reticulum cell sarcoma apparently because of the large size of the proliferating cell. In our earlier reports on the functional approach we emphasized the similarity of in vitro transformed lymphocytes to lymphomas of large cell type, often interpreted in the past as histiocytic lymphoma or reticulum cell sarcoma. Our experience during recent years with lymphomas arising in these above disorders indicates that they are indistinguishable morphologically from in vitro transformed

Table 4. Prelymphomatous states.

1. Congenital immune deficiencies
2. Immunosuppressed graft rejection state
3. Sjögren's syndrome
4. Autoimmune states
5. Systemic lupus erythematosus
6. Rheumatoid arthritis
7. Immunoblastic lymphadenopathy
8. Hashimoto's disease
9. Gluten sensitive enteropathy
10. α-chain disease
11. Senescence

lymphocytes, usually with features of immunoblastic sarcoma of B-cell type (32–34). Using the immunoperoxidase technique, Dr. Clive Taylor of our group has demonstrated monoclonal cytoplasmic immunoglobulin often in the cytoplasm of these cases and a lack of the histiocyte enzyme, muramidase (lysozyme) (37–38). Subsequently, in a new hyperimmune B-cell disorder, immunoblastic lymphadenopathy (IBL), we observed 10% of the cases evolving during the course of the disease to IBS of B-cell type (39). In our more recent experience with a much larger series of IBL cases, the incidence may reach at least 20% of the cases. Nathwani et al. (48) have reported a similar experience with the closely related disorder, angioimmunoblastic lymphadenopathy. Thus, IBL appears to be the prototype of a group of pre-lymphomatous conditions and has a lifelong vulnerability of the development of malignant lymphoma of IBS B-cell type.

In the past few years we have observed malignant lymphomas of transformed lymphocytic type, usually IBS of B-cell type, developing in a variety of abnormal immune states which are listed in Table 4. Senescence is included as an abnormal immune state since there is accumulating evidence of the loss of immune capability in a significant portion of the population with advancing age. It is unquestionably important to recognize the senescent group because of the expanding size of this age group in our population. In addition, many of our cases of IBS B-cell type are observed in the elderly population without any other evidence of immunologic abnormality. Recently, we have had the opportunity to study the so-called primary lymphomas of the thyroid and demonstrated the high frequency (81%) of morphologic evidence of Hashimoto's disease and the increased clinical aggressiveness of immunoblastic sarcoma over large noncleaved FCC in the thyroid (46). We also have had the opportunity to study morphologic material from a small case series in each of the other prelymphomatous states. Unfortunately, few of the cases have been characterized with our multiparameter approach, and it is uncertain how the patients who develop lymphoma differ immunologically from the typical patients who remain free of lymphoma. The development of malignant lymphoma of transformed lymphocytes, usually IBS B-cell type, in abnormal immune or prelymphomatous states raises the question of an alteration in the control mechanism of lymphocyte transformation in these conditions, possibly a loss of suppressor cell activity that permits the development of the lymphoma. It is important to emphasize that IBS of T-cell type arises above *de novo* or from another T-cell type, as shown in Table 3, possibly also from a "switch on" or lack of control of the transformation mechanism.

The development of a lymphoma, reported as the malignant histiocytosis type, in patients with malabsorption in adult coeliac disease recently was published by Isaacson and Wright (21–22). Identification of the cells as neoplastic histiocytes was based on the observation of erythrophagocytosis by the tumor cells and the demonstration of muramidase by the immuno-peroxidase technique (60). This observation differs from our experience with this disorder in which the lymphomas of IBS type have been encountered usually with plasmacytoid features. It should be emphasized that the term "malignant histiocytosis" is generally reserved for a systemic proliferation of malignant histiocytes rather than malignant lymphoma. A comparison study of a larger series of cases is necessary to resolve this discrepancy.

Clinical relevance of the functional classification

Evidence of the clinical significance of our immunologic cell types is becoming dramatically apparent. The clinical distinctness of the cytologic types of the Lukes-Collins classification has been confirmed by a number of studies (3, 6, 29, 31, 46, 54, 56, 63, 64). Furthermore, their prognostic value has been shown to be enhanced by immunologic surface marker studies when the lymphoma cells fail to mark, apparently reflecting biologic differences within the cell types (6).

The identification of homogeneous cytologic B- and T-cell subtypes has resulted in the recognition of distinctive new clinico-immuno-pathologic entities such as the convoluted T cell (3), immunoblastic sarcoma of T or B cells (31), the plasmacytoid lymphocytic type (29), and the follicular center cell types. Their biologic significance and clinical relevance is expanded by the recognition of the abnormal immune prelymphomatous states of immunoblastic sarcoma and the appreciation of the evolution in varying frequency of the low aggressive T- and B-cell type, shown in Table 3 through the lymphocyte transformation mechanism, to the high aggressive types without a fundamental change in cell type.

The clinical value claimed for the Rappaport classification (51) is limited largely to the reported prognostic value of the nodular forms of lymphomas when compared to their diffuse expressions. The published data, however, is derived from invalid comparisons of nodular lymphomas which we now recognize to be fairly homogeneous follicular center cell types, with heterogeneous diffuse cytologic types. Each diffuse cytologic type of Rappaport (51) is now acknowledged to include three to five B- and T-cell subtypes. For example, the diffuse histiocytic type of Rappaport includes the large cleaved FCC, the large noncleaved FCC, IBS of B cells, IBS of T cells and a true histiocytic of macrophage type. Such heterogeneity in each of the Rappaport cytologic types (51) invalidates most of the claimed clinical relevance of the Rappaport classification (51). It is important to emphasize that the British (4) and the Dorfman (14) classifications are modifications of the Rappaport classification (51), though both recognize the follicular nature of nodular lymphomas and Dorfman adds our convoluted lymphocytic and undefined cytologic types as well as several nonspecific types such as the large lymphoid (pyroninophilic) type. In addition, Rappaport has acknowledged the need for change by adding the terms convoluted, cerebriform and Burkitt's types of lymphoma as well as recognizing the follicular nature of nodular lymphoma (53).

The WHO classification (44) which retains the traditional terms lymphosarcoma and reticulosarcoma while including a long list of synonyms seems completely inappropriate since lymphoma experts acknowledge that the traditional terms have lost their morphologic meaning and therefore their clinical relevance.

The Kiel classification (16, 28) is quite similar to our classification but fails to recognize the T- and B-cell nature of lymphomas as do the other three classifications. Many of the terms in the Kiel classification (16) are similar or readily translated to our terminology. The centrocytic and centroblastic terms are intended to be synonymous with cleaved FCC and noncleaved FCC. However, it is not clear whether or not these types are equivalent in application. Separation of the lymphomas into two grades of clinical progression is similar to our low and high aggressive groups, shown in Table 3. In his recent book, Professor Lennert (28) has added several more terms which bring his classification in closer alignment with our classification, shown in Table 1. Review of the other terms employed in the British (4), Dorfman (14) and Rappaport (51) classifications reveals that they are not relevant for a modern understanding of immunology or lymphopoiesis and therefore obviously will have limitations in clinical relevance.

DISCUSSION

The results of the immunologic approach for malignant lymphomas have demonstrated the heterogeneity of the cytologic types of the past and permitted recognition of a number of new clinical morphologic entities. Both situations have numerous immediate and future implications. Morphologic identification of our cytologic types of T- and B-cell lymphomas can be achieved effectively by a pathologist experienced with the functional approach without the use of multiparameter techniques. The approach, however, requires detailed cytologic evaluation and, therefore, careful attention to fixation and processing of the tissue and thin (4 micron) sections. The immediate implication for pathologists of the immunologic approach is the need for special collection and handling and processing of lymph nodes and related tissues, particularly the cutting of fresh thin tissue blocks, to achieve ideal fixation. In my view, some variation of Zenker's fixative produces the most ideal cytologic details for evaluation.

The heterogeneity of the cytologic types of the past has immediate implications in therapy which are already being appreciated clinically. We have proposed that the histiocytic lymphoma of Rappaport (51) includes five cytologic types of lymphoma: 1) the large cleaved FCC; 2) the large non-cleaved FCC; 3) IBS of B cells; 4) IBS of T cells; and 5) the rare true histiocytic lymphoma. We have indicated that this heterogeneity may account for the diversity of clinical expressions and the variability in response to MOPP therapy in which a significant proportion of patients respond, but many fail. The recent report of Strauchen et al. (58) has provided dramatic support for our view. In their study a series of cases, classified as histiocytic lymphoma, were clinically staged and treated in a uniform fashion. The histologic material was classified also in a manner similar, though not identical, with our approach. Three distinctively different responses to therapy were observed. The large cleaved FCC type responded effectively with an almost 80% survival, while the group related to IBS responded poorly and had only a 20% survival. The group equivalent to the large noncleaved FCC exhibited an intermediate response with a 40% survival. This wide range in therapeutic responsiveness using a uniform therapeutic regimen is a dramatic verification of the importance of recognizing heterogeneity within the cytologic types of the past. The heterogeneity of ALL also has been appreciated recently (20). In the past, ALL included T-cell ALL (20%–25%), B-cell ALL (1%–5%), the so-called null cell type (70%–75%), and also the pre-T and pre-B cell types. The high incidence of relapse of the T-cell and B-cell types of ALL on conventional ALL therapy is now generally acknowledged and is forcing an alteration in the therapeutic approach to ALL.

The future implications of the functional approach to malignant lymphomas involve the question of reliability of morphologic interpretation in the diagnosis and whether or not special techniques will be required for accurate identification of the T- and B-cell subtypes of lymphoma. The results of our multiparameter studies on large numbers of cases (36–38) have demonstrated that the morphologic findings were more reliable in recognizing the T- and B-cell types of lymphoma because of the technical problems inherent in these techniques. This observation has been supported by the study of Bloomfield et al. (6). If the histologic material is properly prepared, an experienced pathologist will be able to classify the lymphomas effectively. Admittedly there will be situations where the differential diagnosis is difficult and a high degree of precision is required. The precise diagnosis of the convoluted T cell, also designated lymphoblastic convoluted by Nathwani et al. (47), may be confirmed by the demonstration of an acid phosphatase positive globule in the Golgi region (11, 57) and E-rosette formation about the lymphoma cells in centrifuge preparations. In our experience, however, delay in fixation of air dried smears or imprints for 24 hours or more is necessary to achieve ideal results with the acid phosphatase stain. Examination of the spinal fluid from patients with the convoluted T-cell type, using concentrated specimens and the E-rosette technique is an essential component case evaluation in this disorder and has permitted the identification of CNS involvement even when the spinal fluid cell count was less than five. In such clinically critical situations a special regional referral laboratory which performs selected procedures may be essential.

The multiparameter studies from many centers have resolved the majority of the cytologic characterization problems. For example, nodular lymphomas have been clearly demonstrated to be lymphomatous follicles (17, 23, 30), and our proposal that Burkitt's lymphoma has a follicular origin has been supported by the observations of Mann and colleagues (42). Only the debate over the differentiation of the large cells, particularly between the IBS of B and T cells, remains. Unquestionably, resolution of this problem requires the multiparameter study of the larger series of cases than is currently available. In our recently completed study of functionally evaluated large cell lymphomas, using multiple pathologists in a blind study, we were able to distinguish all the cytologic types. The major difficulty encountered was the differentiation of T-cell IBS and the large noncleaved FCC types.

For us, the quest continues in search of a more fundamental understanding of the biology of lymphomas and their relationship to their normal cellular counterparts. Ultimately, a more ideal understanding of the immunology of normal and lymphoma cells will permit the completion of the definition of the new entities and lead to a redesign of therapy on a sound biologic basis.

SUMMARY

The malignant lymphomas are now acknowledged to be neoplasms of the immune system, and involve the T- and B-cell systems; and the large cells, regarded as histiocytes or reticulum cells in the past, essentially are accepted as transformed lymphocytes of either T or B cells. Numerous multiparameter definitional studies have supported the T- and B-cell nature of lymphomas and have permitted the identification of homogeneous cytologic types that are emerging as distinctive clinical entities, such as the convoluted T cell and immunoblastic sarcoma. They have demonstrated the heterogeneity of all the diffuse cytologic types of lymphoma of the past and also acute lymphocytic leukemia and accounted for the diversity of their clinical expressions and responses to therapy. The functional approach has allowed the recognition of abnormal immune states with a variable predisposition for malignant lymphoma in which there is evolution to immunoblastic sarcoma. It also has permitted the appreciation that the change from low to high aggressive lymphomatous states involves lymphocyte transformation from a small T- or B-cell type to its large transformed expression without a fundamental change in cell type. The biologic and clinical relevance of the new cytologic types is now becoming apparent.

REFERENCES

1. Aisenberg, A.D., and Long, J.C.: Lymphocyte surface characteristics in malignant lymphoma. Am. J. Med., 58:300–306, 1975.
2. Anagnostou, D., Parker, J.W., Taylor, C.R., Tindle, B.H., and Lukes, R.J.:

Lacunar cells of nodular sclerosing Hodgkin's disease. Cancer 39:1032–1043, 1977.

3. Barcos, M.P., and Lukes, R.J.: Malignant lymphoma of convoluted lymphocytes: A new entity of possible T-cell type. In: Conflicts in childhood cancer, p. 147, Sinks, L.F., and Godden, J.E., (eds.), Alan R. Liss, New York, 1975.

4. Bennett, M.H., Farrer-Brown, G., Henry, K., and Jelliffe, A.M.: Classification of non-Hodgkin's lymphomas. Lancet 2:405, 1974.

5. Berard, C.W., Gallo, R.C., Jaffe, E., Green, I., and DeVita, V.T.: Current concepts of leukemia and lymphoma: Etiology, pathogenesis and therapy. Ann. Intern. Med. 85:351–366, 1976.

6. Bloomfield, C.D., Gajl-Peczalska, K.J., Frizzera, G., Kersey, J.H., and Goldman, A.I.: Clinical utility of lymphocyte surface markers combined with the Lukes-Collins histologic classification in adult lymphoma. N. Engl. J. Med., 301–512–518, 1979.

7. Braylan, R.C., Jaffe, E.S., and Berard, C.W.: Malignant lymphomas: Current classification and new observations. In: Hematologic and lymphoid pathology decennial 1966–1975, Sommers, S.C., (ed.). Appleton-Century-Crofts, New York, 1975.

8. Broder, S., Edelson, R.L., Lutzner, M.A., Nelson, D.L., MacDermott, R.P., Durm, M.E., Goldman, C.K., Meade, B.D., and Waldmann, T.A.: The Sézary syndrome—A malignant proliferation of helper T cells. J. Clin. Invest., 58:1297–1306, 1976.

9. Brouet, J., Flandrin, G., and Seligmann, M.: Thymus-derived nature of the proliferating cells in Sézary's syndrome. N. Engl. J. Med., 289:341–344, 1973.

10. Brouet, J., Labaume, S., and Seligmann, M.: Evaluation of T and B lymphocyte membrane markers in human non-Hodgkin's malignant lymphomas. Br. J. Cancer 31, Suppl. II:121–127, 1975.

11. Catovsky, D., Galetto, J., Okos, A., Milliani, E. and Galton, D.A.G.: Cytochemical profile of B and T leukaemic lymphocytes with special reference to acute lymphoblastic leukaemia. J. Clin. Pathol., 27:767–771, 1974.

12. Custer, R.P., and Bernhard, W.G.: Interrelationship of Hodgkin's disease and other lymphatic tumors. Am. J. Med. Sci., 216:625–642, 1948.

13. Davey, F.R., Goldberg, J., Stockman, J., and Gottlieb, A.J.: Immunologic and cytochemical cell markers in non-Hodgkin's lymphomas. Lab. Invest. 35:430–438, 1976.

14. Dorfman, R.F.: Classification of non-Hodgkin's lymphomas. Lancet 1:1295, 1974.

15. Gajl-Peczalska, K.J., Bloomfield, C.D., Coccia, P.F., Sosin, H., Brunning, R.D., and Kersey, J.H.: B and T cell lymphomas. Am. J. Med., 59:674–685, 1975.

16. Gerhard-Marchant, R., Hamlin, I., Lennert, K., Rilke, F., Stansfield, A.G., and VanUnnik, J.A.M.: Classification of non-Hodgkin's lymphomas. Lancet 2:405, 1974.

17. Glick, A.D., Leech, J.H., Waldron, J.A., Flexner, J.M., Horn, R.G., and Collins, R.D.: Malignant lymphomas of follicular center cell origin in man. II. Ultrastructural and cytochemical studies. J. Natl. Cancer Inst. 54:23–36, 1975.

18. Good, R.A. and Finstad, J.: The association of lymphoid malignancy and immunologic functions. In: Proceedings of the international conference on leukemia-lymphoma. Zarafonetis, C.J.D., (ed.), Lea and Febiger, Philadelphia; 1968.

19. Green, I., Jaffe, E., Shevach, E.M., Edelson, R.L., Frank, M.M., and Berard,

C.W.: Determination of the origin of malignant reticular cells by the use of surface membrane markers. In: The reticuloendothelial system, International Academy of Pathology monograph no. 16. p. 282, Rebuck, J.W., Berard, C.W., Abell, M.R., (eds.), Williams and Wilkins, Baltimore, 1975.

20. Haegert, D.G., Stuart, J., and Smith, J.L.: Acute lymphoblastic leukaemia: A heterogeneous disease. Br. Med. J., 2:312–314, 1975.

21. Isaacson, P., and Wright, D.H.: Intestinal lymphoma associated with malabsorption. Lancet 1:67–70, 1978.

22. Isaacson, P., and Wright, D.H.: Malignant histiocytosis of the intestine; Its relationship to malabsorption and ulcerative jejunitis. Human Pathol., 9:661–677, 1978.

23. Jaffe, E.S., Shevach, E.M., Frank, M.M., Berard, C.W., and Green, I.: Nodular lymphoma; Evidence for origin from follicular B lymphocytes. N. Engl. J. Med., 290:813–819, 1974.

24. Kojima, M., and Tsunoda, R.: Localization of immunoglobulins in germinal centers of human tonsils. In: The reticuloendothelial system in health and disease: Immunologic and pathologic aspects. p. 77, Freidman, H., Escobar, M.R., Reichard, S., (eds.), Plenum, New York, 1976.

25. Leech, J., Glick, A., Horn, R., and Collins, R.: Immunologic histochemical and ultrastructural studies of malignant lymphomas presumed to be of follicular center cell origin. J. Natl. Cancer Inst., 54:11–21, 1975.

26. Lennert, K., and Mestdagh, J.: Lymphogranulomatosen mit konstant hohem epitheloidzellgehalt. Virchows Arch. Path. Anat., 344:1–20, 1968.

27. Lennert, K., Mohri, N., Stein, H., and Kaiserling, E.: Histopathology of malignant lymphomas. Br. J. Haematol., 311:193–203, 1975.

28. Lennert, K.: Malignant lymphomas other than Hodgkin's disease. Berlin. Springer-Verlag, 1978.

29. Levine, A.M., Lichtenstein, A., Gresik, M.V., Taylor, C.R., Feinstein, D.I., and Lukes, R.J.: Clinical and immunologic spectrum of plasmacytoid lymphocytic lymphoma without serum monoclonal IgM. Brit. J. Haematol., in press.

30. Levine, G.D., and Dorfman, R.F.: Nodular lymphomas: An ultrastructural study of its relationship to germinal centers and a correlation of light and electron microscopic findings. Cancer 35:148–164, 1975.

31. Lichtenstein, A.K., Levine, A.M., Lukes, R.J., Taylor, C.R., Cramer, A.D., Lincoln, T.L., and Feinstein, D.I.: Immunoblastic sarcoma: A clinical description. Cancer 43:343–352, 1979.

32. Lukes, R.J., and Collins, R.D.: New observations on follicular lymphoma. In: GANN monograph on cancer research 15, Malignant diseases of the hematopoietic system, p. 209, Akazaki, K., Rappaport, H., Berard, C.W., Bennett, J., Ishikawa, E., (eds.), University Park Press, Baltimore, 1973.

33. Lukes, R.J., and Collins, R.D.: Immunologic characterization of human malignant lymphomas. Cancer 34:1488–1503, 1974.

34. Lukes, R.J., and Collins, R.D.: A functional approach to the classification of malignant lymphoma. Recent Results Cancer Res. 46:18–30, 1974.

35. Lukes, R.J., and Collins, R.D.: New approaches to the classification of the lymphomata. Br. J. Cancer 31, Suppl., II:1–28, 1975.

36. Lukes, R.J., and Collins, R.D.: The Lukes-Collins classification and its significance. Cancer Treat Rep. 61:971–979, 1977.

37. Lukes, R.J., Taylor, C.R., Parker, J.W., Lincoln, T.L., Pattengale, P.K., and Tindle, B.H.: A morphologic and immunologic surface marker study of 299

cases of non-Hodgkin's lymphomas and related leukemias. Am. J. Pathol., 90:461–485, 1978.

38. Lukes, R.J., Parker, J.W., Taylor, C.R., Tindle, B.H., Cramer, A.D., and Lincoln, T.L.: Immunologic approach to non-Hodgkin's lymphomas and related leukemias. Analysis of the results of multiparameter studies of 425 cases. Semin. Hematol. 15:322–351, 1978.

39. Lukes, R.J., and Tindle, B.H.: Immunoblastic lymphadenopathy. A new hyperimmune entity resembling Hodgkin's disease. N. Engl. J. Med. 292:1–8, 1975.

40. Lukes, R.J., Craver, L.L., Hall, T.C., Rappaport, H., and Ruben, P.: Hodgkin's disease, report of Nomenclature Committee. Cancer Res. 26:1311, 1966.

41. Lutzner, M., Edelson, R., Schein, P., Green, I., Kirkpatrick, C., and Ahmed, A.: Cutaneous T cell lymphoma: The Sézary syndrome, mycosis fungoides and related disorders. Ann. Intern. Med. 85:534–552, 1975.

42. Mann, R.B., Jaffe, E.S., Braylan, R.C., Nanba, K., Frank, M.M., Ziegler, J.L., and Berard, C.W.: Non-endemic Burkitt lymphoma, a B-cell tumor related to germinal centers. N. Engl. J. Med., 295:685–691, 1976.

43. Mathé, G., Belpomme, D., Dantchev, D., Khalil, A., Afifi, A.M., Taleb, N., Pouillart, P., Schwarzenberg, L., Hayat, M., DeVassal, F., Jasmin, C., Misset, J.L., and Musset, M.: Immunoblastic lymphosarcoma, a cytological and clinical entity? Biomedicine 22:473–488, 1975.

44. Mathé, G. and Rappaport, H.: Histological and cytological typing of neoplastic diseases of haematopoietic and lymphoid tissues, International Histological Classification of Tumours no. 14. World Health Organization, Geneva, 1976.

45. Maurer, R., and Lukes, R.J.: Eine neue funktionelle interpretation maligner lymphome. Die Lukes-Collins Klassifikation und ihre Grundlagen. Schweiz. med. Wschr. 109:76–86, 1979.

46. Maurer, R., Taylor, C.R., Terry, R. and Lukes, R.J.: Non-Hodgkin lymphomas of the thyroid. Virchows Arch. Path. Anat. 383:293–317, 1979.

47. Nathwani, B.N., Kim, H., and Rappaport, H.: Malignant lymphoma, lymphoblastic. Cancer 38:964–983, 1976.

48. Nathwani, B.N., Rappaport, H., Moran, E.M., Pangalis, G.A. and Kim, H.: Malignant lymphoma arising in angioimmunoblastic lymphadenopathy. Cancer 41:578–606, 1978.

49. Nowell, P.C.: Phytohemagglutinin: An initiator of mitosis in cultures of normal human leukocytes. Cancer Res. 20:462–466, 1960.

50. Penn, I.: Malignant tumors in organ transplant recipients. In: Recent results in cancer research. Springer-Verlag, New York, 1970.

51. Rappaport, H.: Tumors of the hematopoietic system, Atlas of tumor pathology, section III-fasc. 8. Armed Forces Institute of Pathology, Washington, D.C., 1966.

52. Rappaport, H., Ramot, B., Hulu, N., and Park, J.K.: The pathology of so-called Mediterranean abdominal lymphoma with malabsorption. Cancer 29: 1502–1511, 1972.

53. Rappaport, H.: Discussion II: Roundtable discussion of histopathologic classification. Cancer Treat. Rep. 61:1037–1048, 1977.

54. Rosen, P.J., Feinstein, D.I., Pattengale, P.K., Tindle, B.H., Williams, A.H., Cain, M.J., Bonorris, J.B., Parker, J.W., and Lukes, R.J.: Convoluted lymphocytic lymphoma in adults. Ann. Int. Med. 89:319–324, 1978.

55. Schlossman, S.F., Chess, L., Humphreys, R.E., and Strominger, J.L.: Distribution of Ia-like molecules on the surface of normal and leukemic human cells. Proc. Natl. Acad. Sci. USA 73:1288–1292, 1976.

56. Schneider, B.K., Higgins, G.R., Swanson, V., Isaacs, H., Tindle, B.H., and Lukes, R.J.: Malignant lymphomas of childhood. Submitted for publication.
57. Stein, H., Peterson, N., Gaedicke, G., Lennert, K., and Landberg, C.: Lymphoblastic lymphoma of convoluted or acid phosphatase type; A tumor of T precursor cells. Int. J. Cancer 17:292–295, 1976.
58. Strauchen, J.A., Young, R.C., DeVita, V.T., Jr., Anderson, T., Fantone, J.C., and Berard, C.W.: Clinical relevance of the histopathological subclassification of diffuse "histiocytic" lymphoma. N. Engl. J. Med. 299:1382–1387, 1978.
59. Talal, N. and Bunim, J.: The development of malignant lymphoma in the course of Sjögren's syndrome. Am. J. Med. 36:529–540, 1964.
60. Taylor, C.R.: Immunoperoxidase techniques: Theoretical and practical aspects. Arch. Pathol. Lab. Med., 102:113–121, 1978.
61. Taylor, C.R.: An immunohistological study of follicular lymphoma, reticulum cell sarcoma and Hodgkin's disease. Eur. J. Cancer 12: 61–75, 1976.
62. Tindle, B.H., Parker, J.W., and Lukes, R.J.: "Reed-Sternberg cells" in infectious mononucleosis? Am. J. Clin. Pathol. 58:607–617, 1972.
63. van den Tweel, J.G., Lukes, R.J. and Taylor, C.R.: Pathophysiology of lymphocyte transformation. A study of so-called composite lymphomas. Am. J. Clin. Pathol. 71:509–520, 1979.
64. Williams, A.H., Taylor, C.R., Higgins, G.R., Quinn, J.J., Schneider, B.K., Swanson, V., Parker, J.W., Pattengale, P.K., Chandor, S.B., Powars, D., Lincoln, T.L., Tindle, B.H. and Lukes, R.J.: Childhood leukemia and lymphoma. I. Correlation of morphology and functional studies. Cancer 42:171–181, 1978.
65. Winchester, R.J., Fu, S.M., Wernet, P., Kunkel, H.G., Dupont, B., and Jersild, C.: Recognition by pregnancy serums of non-HL-A alloantigens selectively expressed on B lymphocytes. J. Exp. Med. 141:924–929, 1975.
66. Yam, L.T., Li, C.Y. and Crosby, W.H.: Cytochemical identification of monocytes and granulocytes. Am. J. Clin. Pathol. 55:283–290, 1971.

15. GERMINAL CENTER CELL LYMPHOMAS AND THE KIEL CLASSIFICATION

K. LENNERT

INTRODUCTION

As Table 1 shows, the Kiel classification and Lukes' classification are quite similar. The terms differ, but the entities are mostly the same. There are some differences, however, especially among the germinal center cell (GCC) or follicular center cell (FCC) tumors, which I shall discuss briefly after I have presented the principles of the Kiel classification.

There are two main groups, namely, low-grade and high-grade malignant lymphomas (top and bottom of Table 1, respectively). The low-grade group is made up of lymphocytic, lymphoplasmacytic/lymphoplasmacytoid, plasmacytic, centrocytic, and centroblastic/centrocytic lymphomas. The high-grade group includes centroblastic, lymphoblastic, and immunoblastic lymphomas. Some of the lymphomas are subclassified into subtypes, but I shall not discuss these in detail here, since I wish to concentrate on the differences between the two classifications.

The first difference concerns what is called T-zone lymphoma and the T-immunoblastic lymphoma of the Kiel classification. The former is designated T-cell immunoblastic sarcoma by Lukes, and is the same as the tumor Collins and co-workers described as T-cell node-based lymphoma or peripheral T-cell lymphoma (5). The T-immunoblastic lymphoma of the Kiel classification is, however, a subtype of immunoblastic lymphoma consisting only of T immunoblasts, whereas T-zone lymphoma is composed mainly of T lymphocytes, but also has a variable number of T immunoblasts.

Another difference might lie in the polymorphic subtype of lymphoplasmacytic/-cytoid lymphoma. Some cases of this subtype would perhaps be classified by Lukes as B-cell immunoblastic sarcoma.

The main differences are found in the group of tumors that are to be discussed in this paper, namely the GCC lymphomas. As shown in Table 2, Lukes and Collins distinguish between cleaved FCC and non-cleaved FCC, which correspond to the centrocytes and centroblasts, respectively, of the Kiel nomenclature. Furthermore, Lukes and Collins distinguish a small-cell and a large-cell variant of both types of FCC. In the original Kiel classification, this distinction either was not made (as in the case of centro-

Table 1. The Kiel classification of non-Hodgkin's lymphomas in comparison with Lukes' classification.

Kiel classification	Equivalent in Lukes' classification
Lymphocytic	
CLL of B type	B cell, small lymphocyte
CLL of T type	T cell, small lymphocyte
Hairy cell leukemia	Hairy cell leukemia
Mycosis fungoides and	Cerebriform lymphocyte (mycosis
Sézary's syndrome	fungoides, Sézary)
T-zone lymphoma	T cell, immunoblastic sarcoma
Lymphoplasmacytic/-cytoid	
lymphoplasmaytic	
lymphoplasmacytoid	B cell, plasmacytoid lymphocyte
polymorphic	B cell, immunoblastic sarcoma (?)
Plasmacytic	—
Centrocytic	
Centroblastic/centrocytic	B cell, FCC, small and large cleaved
Centroblastic	B cell, FCC, large noncleaved
Lymphoblastic	
B-lymphoblastic, Burkitt	
type and others	B cell, FCC, small noncleaved
T-lymphoblastic,	
convoluted-cell type	
and others	T cell, convoluted lymphocyte
unclassified	U cell (undefined) and unclassifiable
Immunoblastic	Immunoblastic sarcoma
with plasmablastic/	
plasmacytic differen-	
tiation (B)	B cell, immunoblastic sarcoma
without plasmablastic/	
plasmacytic differen-	T cell, immunoblastic sarcoma
tiation (B or T)	and others (?)
(Reticulosarcoma, malignant	
histiocytosis)	Histiocyte

Table 2. Germinal center cell lymphomas in the classification of Lukes and Collins in comparison with the Kiel classification

Lukes and Collins	Equivalent in the Kiel classification
FCC, cleaved (small and large)	Centrocytic Centroblastic/centrocytic
FCC, noncleaved	
small	B-lymphoblastic, mainly Burkitt type
large	Centroblastic

cytic and centroblastic/centrocytic lymphoma) or was reflected by other terms (B-lymphoblastic versus centroblastic).

There are various reasons for excluding Burkitt's tumor from the GCC lymphomas, the most important being the lack of definitive proof that Burkitt's tumor is derived from germinal centers. Centroblastic lymphoma and large noncleaved FCC lymphoma are, however, probably almost identical.

In contrast, there is an essential difference between centrocytic and centroblastic/centrocytic lymphoma on the one hand and the cleaved FCC lymphoma of Lukes and Collins on the other hand. Whereas Lukes says that all cleaved FCC lymphomas consist of a mixture of cleaved and noncleaved FCC, we apply the term centrocytic lymphoma only to tumors that are exclusively composed of centrocytes. We explicitly separate centroblastic/centrocytic lymphoma from such tumors. In centroblastic/centrocytic lymphoma, centrocytes predominate but there are also a few (basophilic) centroblasts. We do not consider it justifiable to equate all tumors containing centrocytes, as is done in Lukes' and Collins' classification. There are various reasons for making a distinction between centrocytic lymphoma and centroblastic/centrocytic lymphoma (see Lennert and Mohri (6)). The strongest argument has been provided by immunologic investigations: Tolksdorf et al. (4) have shown that centroblastic/centrocytic lymphoma always contains a relatively large number of T lymphocytes (25% or more), whereas centrocytic lymphoma shows only a few T lymphocytes (5% or less).

Many people may be surprised or confused by the large number of new and unusual terms given in Table 1. The situation is similar in many other fields of medicine, however. Two examples would be glomerulonephritis and glioma. The number of entities of glomerulonephritis and glioma is also very high. This is tolerated, however, because it is of clinical relevance. The same is probably true in the case of malignant lymphoma. Furthermore, one should remember that the lymphoid tissue is always in motion, with cellular modulation and transformation occurring constantly. Thus, it is reasonable to expect that the large number of cell variants will be reflected in their neoplasms. If one can prove that the tumor variants are of clinical relevance, then, in my opinion, these variants should be included in our classifications.

Malignant lymphoma, centrocytic

The various types of GCC lymphoma as defined by the Kiel classification will be discussed in more detail in the following sections. The first type is centrocytic lymphoma. This tumor does not contain any centroblasts (noncleaved FCC), and the general impression is relatively monotonous. Many tumor cells have cleaved nuclei. It is important to realize that the cytoplasm is not visible with Giesma staining. Thus, the nuclei appear to be naked. Nucleoli are small and often multiple. In the anaplastic variant of centrocytic lymphoma, the cells are somewhat larger and more pleomorphic. There is sometimes high mitotic activity; in other cases, there are only a few mitotic figures.

If one looks at the first stage of centrocytic lymphoma, one may find that it occurs in the B area, particularly the lymphocytic mantle of germinal centers. A nonneoplastic germinal center is then surrounded by neoplastic centrocytes. One can readily imagine that the lymphoma will show a nodular growth pattern for a while.

The fiber pattern in centrocytic lymphoma is usually characteristic: the centrocytes stick together, and there are large fibers between complexes of tumor cells. The growth pattern is generally diffuse; only occasionally is there a somewhat nodular pattern.

With the acid phosphatase reaction, one can recognize a moderate or large number of histiocytic reticulum cells. These are distributed quite uniformly throughout the tumor.

Imprints reveal a very typical, homogeneous picture. The nuclear cleavage is not as obvious as it is in sections, but identations of the nuclei are sometimes visible. One can recognize that the nucleoli are small and not basophilic. Cytoplasm is sparse to moderately abundant and light bluish gray.

The tumor cells bear a large amount of immunoglobulin (Ig) on their surface, with pronounced capping (3). This is also recognizable on electron microscopy (1). In addition, Kaiserling (1) showed that many cases of centrocytic lymphoma contain dendritic reticulum cells connected by desmosomes. This is another argument in favor of interpreting centrocytic lymphoma as a GCC tumor.

Malignant lymphoma, centroblastic/centrocytic

The second type of GCC lymphoma in the Kiel classification is centroblastic/centrocytic lymphoma, which used to be known as Brill-Symmers disease, follicular lymphoma, or nodular lymphoma. We call it centroblastic/centrocytic lymphoma, because we define all lymphomas according to their cellular composition and not on the basis of their growth pattern. We do add an adjective, however, to specify the growth pattern as follicular, follicular and diffuse, or diffuse. We consider the term nodular to be misleading, because it is based on the concept that every type of lymphoma can show either a nodular or a diffuse growth pattern. It is now time to drop this concept which was advocated by Rappaport for years and is widely accepted.

A "nodular" pattern is seen only in non-Hodgkin's lymphomas of GCC. This fact should be made explicit by using the restrictive term follicular.

The relative frequencies of the three types of growth pattern have been determined in two series. In the second series, 55% of the cases of centro-blastic/centrocytic lymphoma were purely follicular, 40% were follicular and diffuse, and only 5% were diffuse.

In addition to the growth pattern, we specify whether sclerosis is present or absent. Sclerosis is least common in cases with a follicular growth pattern (17%), more frequent in the follicular and diffuse type (70%), and always present in cases with a diffuse growth pattern.

Enzyme histochemical staining sometimes reveals the growth pattern of centroblastic/centrocytic lymphoma particularly clearly. The nonspecific esterase reaction demonstrates not only the histiocytic and dendritic reticu-lum cells, but also the epithelioid venules in the interfollicular areas. The latter are definitely T zones, which contain not only interdigitating reticulum cells, but also numerous T lymphocytes. This feature distinguishes centro-blastic/centrocytic lymphoma from centrocytic lymphoma.

On electron microscopy, dendritic reticulum cells with desmosome-like connections are seen in the neoplastic areas.

Imprints reveal centroblasts with sparse basophilic cytoplasm and medium-sized nucleoli, and numerous centrocytes. Lymphocytes are also visible, many of them are T lymphocytes. One may find GCC in the patient's peripheral blood as well; these are often cleaved.

We have made some special observations in centroblastic/centrocytic lymphoma. In follicular cases we have found PAS-positive cells which were actually centrocytes. In imprints, these cells sometimes showed a violet cytoplasm, and some cells contained intranuclear inclusions. The PAS-positive inclusions in the cytoplasm and nucleus were apparently Ig deposits. It is evidently important to realize that not only plasma cells, but also centrocytes may contain Ig. Intranuclear PAS-positive inclusions are found in about 2–3% of the cases. The inclusions are green with Goldner staining, and are thus probably IgM.

Another new variant was described by Kim, Dorfman, and Rappaport (2) as "signet ring cell lymphoma". This is actually a form of centroblastic/centrocytic lymphoma that shows a large number of Ig deposits in the lymphoma cells.

The age distribution of centroblastic/centrocytic lymphoma shows a peak between the ages of 50 and 60 years. Centrocytic lymphoma, on the other hand, has its peak occurrence about 10 years later in life. In my opinion, an important feature of centroblastic/centrocytic lymphoma is the slight predominance of females. In contrast, centrocytic lymphoma shows a 2.5:1 preponderance of males. This difference in sex distribution is another argument in favor of distinguishing between these two types of GCC lymphoma. Furthermore, there is a quite obvious difference in prognosis between the two types of lymphoma, that of centroblastic/centrocytic lymphoma being more favorable.

The incidence of centroblastic/centrocytic and centrocytic lymphoma evidently differs from country to country. In the U.S.A., centroblastic/centrocytic lymphoma shows a very high relative frequency (> 50%), whereas centrocytic lymphoma accounts for only about 5% of the cases of non-Hodgkin's lymphoma. In Kiel, we have about 25% centroblastic/centrocytic lymphomas, but 10% centrocytic lymphomas. Among the cases collected in Milan, Italy, I diagnosed centrocytic lymphoma in about 25% and centroblastic/centrocytic lymphoma in only about 15%.

Malignant lymphoma, centroblastic

The third type of GCC lymphoma is centroblastic lymphoma, which belongs to the group of high-grade malignant lymphomas. In rare cases, this neoplasm shows a follicular growth pattern. In most cases, however, the growth pattern is purely diffuse. The tumor cells are basophilic. Nucleoli are medium-sized and often situated at the nuclear membrane. These cells may be interpreted as centroblasts. In some cases there is a more polymorphic picture, with some cells that look like immunoblasts; but most of the cells are centroblasts. There may be some anaplastic centrocytes as well.

Centroblastic lymphoma can occur as the primary tumor; but it can also develop secondarily from a centroblastic/centrocytic lymphoma. This development may take only a few weeks, or it may last many years. Of the cases of centroblastic/centrocytic lymphoma in our autopsy collection, 40% had evolved into centroblastic lymphoma. It is remarkable that centrocytic lymphoma never develops into centroblastic lymphoma. This is another argument in favor of distinguishing between centroblastic/centrocytic lymphoma and centrocytic lymphoma.

REFERENCES

1. Kaiserling, E.: Ultrastructure of non-Hodgkin's lymphomas. In: Malignant lymphomas other than Hodgkin's disease, pp. 471–528, Lennert, K., Springer-Verlag, New York, Heidelberg and Berlin, 1978.
2. Kim, H., Dorfman, R.F., and Rappaport, H.: Signet ring cell lymphoma: A rare morphologic and functional expression of nodular (follicular) lymphoma. Am. J. Surg. Pathol., 2, 1978.
3. Stein, H.: The immunologic and immunochemical basis for the Kiel classification. In: Malignant lymphomas other than Hodgkin's disease, pp. 529–657, Lennert, K., Springer-Verlag, New York, Heidelberg and Berlin, 1978.
4. Tolksdorf, G., Stein, H., Lennert, K.: Morphological and immunological definition of a malignant lymphoma derived from germinal center cells with cleaved nuclei (centrocytes). Br. J. Cancer., in press.

5. Waldron, J.A., Leech, J.H., Glick, A.D., Flexner, J.M., Collins, R.D.: Malignant lymphoma of peripheral T-lymphocyte origin. Cancer, 40:1604–1617, 1977.
6. Lennert, K., and Mohri, N.: Histopathology and diagnosis of non-Hodgkin's lymphomas. In: Malignant lymphomas other than Hodgkin's disease, pp. 111–469, Lennert, K., Springer-Verlag, New York, Heidelberg and Berlin, 1978.

16. MALIGNANT LYMPHOMAS OF GERMINAL CENTER CELL ORIGIN: PREVALENCE, TYPE OF PRESENTATION, STAGES, AND SURVIVAL (PRELIMINARY DATA)

F. RILKE, R. CANETTA AND M.R. CASTELLANI

In clinical use the term nodularity, when applied to a malignant non-Hodgkin's lymphoma, is almost synonymous with favorable histology. Whereas in the classical Rappaport classification (17, 18) nodularity has been considered as a mere architectural variant — the opposite of diffuseness — of the basic cytologic types of malignant lymphoma, the more recent classificatory approaches (1, 5, 15) tend to separate malignant lymphoma with a nodular structure.

Although nodular malignant lymphomas have been recognized in recent years to represent malignant neoplasms derived from the cells of the center of the secondary follicles (2, 8, 9), this cytogenealogic identification has found its way into only some of the currently available classification schemes of malignant lymphomas, and specifically the Kiel classification (7) and that proposed by Lukes and Collins (14). In the latter, malignant lymphomas of follicular center cell origin are classified according to nuclear size (small and large) and shape (cleaved or noncleaved), architectural pattern (follicular or diffuse), and the presence or absence of sclerosis. Furthermore, the diagnosis is made according to the predominance of the cell type, i.e., the presence of a small percentage of large cells does not exclude the diagnosis small follicular center cell lymphoma.

In the Kiel classification the low-grade malignant lymphomas were subdivided into four groups (a fifth, the plasmocytic, was added later) two of which refer to a malignant lymphoma of germinal center cell origin, namely the centrocytic and the centroblastic/centrocytic malignant lymphoma. Only the latter is recognized as able to produce a follicular pattern, being composed of cells which are the malignant counterpart of the normal lymphatic cellular constituents of the secondary follicle, namely the centroblasts and the centrocytes. The diagnosis of this entity is not substantially affected by the ratio of the large to the small cells, except for those rare cases in which an almost pure follicular proliferation of large cells is evident. However, centroblastic-centrocytic malignant lymphoma may also show either a partially obscured follicular pattern with diffuse areas of a purely diffuse type of proliferation. The latter has been reported to be

J.G. van den Tweel et al. (eds.), Malignant Lymphoproliferative Diseases, 221–227

much more rare than the follicular pattern (12). Pure centrocytic malignant lymphoma on the contrary does not show any follicularity. The growth pattern is diffuse, but there may be a certain degree of nodularity which is reminiscent of primary rather than secondary lymphocytic follicles. Among the neoplastic centrocytes, centroblastlike cells may occasionally be encountered, particularly in imprint preparations, and are thought to represent modulation changes of single centrocytes rather than primary constituents of the tumor.

It therefore seems evident that the Kiel classification only provides different categories for centrocytic and centroblastic-centrocytic diffuse malignant lymphoma, which would be classified together according to any other scheme. For this reason, the present preliminary data can hardly be compared with well-documented studies (11, 29).

High-grade malignant centroblastic lymphomas are made up exclusively, or to a very large extent, of large cells of the secondary follicle, which are sufficiently distinctive morphologically to be recognized as such. However, diffuse centroblastic proliferations are not infrequently mixed with cells that are very similar to the large basophilic immunoblasts. Furthermore, it seems that centroblastic malignant lymphoma can be subdivided into *de novo* and so-called "secondary" cases. The latter are essentially represented by centroblastic proliferations that occur in the course of centroblastic-centrocytic malignant lymphomas, for which sequential biopsy specimens are available. and these have been thought to be the most common type of centroblastic malignant lymphoma. In the classification on the material presented here, no provision was made for these two subgroups.

Three hundred and forty-three consecutive untreated patients with malignant lymphoma were evaluated between 1970 and 1975. From all of them at least one biopsy had been obtained from either superficial lymph nodes or clinically prominent extranodal sites. The site of the biopsy did not necessarily correspond to the site of the main clinical presentation. For the discussion of these preliminary data, the relevance of the distinction between malignant lymphoma originating in lymph nodes and primary malignant lymphoma in extranodal sites (10) will not be taken into consideration.

The histologic examination yielded the diagnosis shown in Table 1 in terms of the Kiel classification. Low-grade malignant lymphomas were diagnosed in 192 cases and high-grade malignant lymphomas in 146 cases. The only slight preponderance of low-grade malignant lymphomas over high-grade malignant lymphomas makes this series quite different from other reported series (13, 16). On the other hand, a high incidence of "histiocytic" malignant lymphoma has already been reported for the material observed in our institute (21). Three cases of Lennert's malignant lymphoma and one case of composite malignant lymphoma combining Hodgkin's disease and centroblastic-centrocytic malignant lymphomas are listed separately. One additional case remained unclassified.

Among the low-grade malignant lymphomas, those of germinal center cell origin have been subdivided into centrocytic; centroblastic-centrocytic follicular; centroblastic-centrocytic follicular and diffuse; and centro-blastic-centrocytic diffuse malignant lymphoma. Along the lines expressed in the paper by Warnke et al. (22), for the further evaluation of the case material, the groups centroblastic-centrocytic follicular and centroblastic-centrocytic follicular and diffuse were combined. Centrocytic malignant lymphomas were diagnosed in 89 cases, i.e. 25.9% of the whole series or 46.3% of the low-grade malignant lymphomas. This was the largest group in the series. Centroblastic-centrocytic follicular, and follicular and diffuse were diagnosed in 46 cases (13.4% of the whole group or 23.9% of the low-grade malignant lymphomas) and centroblastic-centrocytic diffuse in 20 (5.8% of the entire group and 10.4% of the low-grade malignant lymphomas). Centroblastic malignant lymphoma was diagnosed in 46 cases, i.e. 13.4% of the whole series and 31.5% of the high-grade malignant lymphomas. It should be noted that centroblastic and immunoblastic malignant lymphoma together (108 cases) represent 31.5% of the whole series, and almost all of these cases had been diagnosed previously also as "histiocytic" (predominantly diffuse) malignant lymphoma when the Rappaport classification was

Table 1. Distribution of 343 patients (1970–75) according to the Kiel classification.

	No.	%
Low-grade malignant lymphoma		
Lymphocytic, CLL	5	1.5
Lymphocytic, other	4	1.2
Lymphoplasmacytoid	25	7.3
Plasmacytic	2	0.6
Centrocytic (Cc)	89	25.9
Centroblastic-centrocytic, follicular (Cb-cc, f)	21	6.1
Centroblastic-centrocytic, follicular & diffuse (Cb-cc, f + d)	25	7.3
Centroblastic-centrocytic, diffuse (Cb-cc, d)	20	5.8
Low-grade malignant, unclassified	1	0.3
High-grade malignant lymphoma		
Centroblastic (Cb)	46	13.4
Lymphoblastic, Burkitt's type	6	1.7
Lymphoblastic, convoluted cell type	14	4.3
Lymphoblastic, other	15	4.3
Immunoblastic	62	18.0
High-grade malignant, unclassified	3	0.9
Lennert's lymphoma	3	0.9
Malignant lymphoma, unclassified	1	0.3
Composite lymphoma (HD* + Cb-cc, f)	1	0.3

*HD, Hodgkin's disease.

Table 2. Germinal center cell lymphomas: stage, sex, and age.

	Cc	*Cb-cc, f & f + d*	*Cb-cc, d*	*Cb*
I	4 (3)	8	5	3 (2)
I E	9 (4)	2	1 (1)	7 (1)
II	3	4	3 (1)	5
II E	18 (5)	6 (2)	4 (1)	8 (2)
III	6	8	—	5
III E	12 (2)	2	—	2
IV	37	16	7	16
Total	89 (14)	46 (2)	20 (3)	46 (5)
M/F	58/31	25/21	11/9	22/24
Age: Mean	53.98	53.79	53.65	48.73
(Range)	(19–84)	(30–75)	(31–77)	(12–80)

*In parentheses, clinical stage.

applied. A total of 201 cases of malignant lymphomas of germinal center origin were thus evaluated.

Pathologic staging was available for all patients except 24 who had clinical staging only (chest x-ray, lymphangiogram, and bone marrow biopsy or aspiration). Pathologic staging included closed liver biopsy, laparoscopy with biopsies of the liver and the spleen, and classical staging laparotomy procedure including splenectomy. The distribution according to the Ann Arbor staging classification modified for non-Hodgkin's malignant lymphomas is shown in Table 2. Centrocytic malignant lymphomas showed a definite predominance in males, whereas all other groups were represented almost equally. Centrocytic malignant lymphomas occurred in a larger age group than centroblastic malignant lymphoma but was not seen in childhood. Centroblastic malignant lymphoma was diagnosed in one child.

Clinical presentation (Table 3) was predominantly nodal in 15% of the

Table 3. Germinal center cell lymphomas: type of presentation.

	Cc	*Cb-cc, f & f + d*	*Cb-cc, d*	*Cb*
Nodal presentation	13 (15%)	20 (43%)	8 (40%)	13 (28%)
Extranodal presentation	39 (44%)	10 (22%)	5 (25%)	17 (37%)
Stage IV	37 (41%)	16 (35%)	7 (35%)	16 (35%)
Total	89	46	20	46
Multiple extranodal sites	28 (31%)	9 (20%)	5 (25%)	8 (17%)
Bulky disease*	7 (8%)	2 (8%)	7 (35%)	16 (35%)

*7 × 7 cm or more.

cases of centrocytic malignant lymphomas, in 43% of centroblastic-centrocytic follicular and follicular and diffuse; in 40% of centroblastic-centrocytic diffuse; and in 28% of centroblastic malignant lymphomas, whereas it was predominantly extranodal (Waldeyer's ring, skin, stomach, etc.) in 44% of centrocytic lymphomas, in 22% of centroblastic-centrocytic follicular and follicular and diffuse, in 25% of centroblastic-centrocytic, diffuse; and in 37% of centroblastic malignant lymphomas.

Stage IV at onset was diagnosed in 41% of the centrocytic groups and 35% of all other groups. Multiple extranodal sites of primary involvement were found in 31% of centrocytic malignant lymphomas and in a lower percentage of the other types of malignant lymphoma. Large tumor masses (more than 7 cm in diameter) were found in 35% of both centroblastic-centrocytic diffuse and centroblastic malignant lymphomas. Bulky disease was noted in a small number of cases of centrocytic and centroblastic-centrocytic follicular and follicular and diffuse.

Multiple biopsy specimens and endoscopic samples revealed a rather frequent involvement of Waldeyer's ring in centrocytic malignant lymphomas, almost twice that found for all other categories considered (Table 4). Bone marrow invasion was a comparatively infrequent finding, probably because of inadequate sampling at that time. In a more recent, selected series, the incidence of involvement was found to be higher (4).

The data on survival rates are preliminary and the subdivision into stages is not taken into consideration. Furthermore, in the course of the years considered in the present study, several and different therapeutic regimens were employed. The main qualitative and quantitative differences in the treatment procedures consisted in the various combinations of chemo- and radiotherapy. Their influence on the survival was slightly less than 50% at 36 months for centrocytic malignant lymphomas and similar to that of centroblastic malignant lymphomas. Centroblastic-centrocytic follicular, and follicular and diffuse malignant lymphomas did not diverge substantially from centroblastic-centrocytic diffuse malignant lymphomas either as to overall survival or the disease-free survival rate at 36 months (about 50%).

The disease-free survival rate at 36 months for centrocytic malignant lymphomas was again closer to that of centroblastic malignant lymphomas

Table 4. Germinal center cell lymphomas: documented involvement of sites.

	Cc		Cb-cc, f & f + d		Cb-cc, d		Cb	
Waldeyer's ring	41	(46%)	10	(22%)	5	(25%)	9	(20%)
Spleen	20	(22%)	13	(28%)	2	(10%)	8	(17%)
Liver	18	(20%)	12	(26%)	2	(10%)	5	(10%)
Stomach	9	(10%)	4	(9%)	5	(25%)	5	(10%)
Bone marrow	9	(10%)	4	(9%)	2	(10%)	3	(6%)

than to that of centroblastic-centrocytic follicular and follicular and diffuse, and of centroblastic-centrocytic diffuse.

These preliminary findings obtained in a cooperative clinicopathologic correlative study presently in progress at the Instituto Nazionale Tumori of Milan indicate that centrocytic malignant lymphoma should be correctly identified histologically, since its biological and clinical behavior is quite peculiar and shows some similarities to high-grade malignant lymphomas. A less favorable prognosis for centrocytic malignant lymphomas than for the other low-grade forms has already been reported by Brittinger et al. (3), Dühmke (6), and Meugé et al. (16). The existence of a large-cell subtype of centrocytic malignant lymphomas has been previously recognized histologically, and cell kinetic studies have shown that large cell centrocytic malignant lymphomas have a higher degree of proliferation than do the small cell type (19). Whether this subtype of centrocytic malignant lymphomas may influence the data presented and, if so, to what extent, will be further investigated.

REFERENCES

1. Bennett, M.H., Farrer-Brown, G., Henry, K., and Jelliffe, A.M.: Classification of non-Hodgkin's lymphomas (Letter). Lancet, 2:405–406, 1974.
2. Braylan, R.C., Jaffe, E.S., and Berard, C.W.: Malignant lymphomas: current classification and new observations. Pathol. Annu., 10:213–270, 1975.
3. Brittinger, G., Bartels, H., Bremer, K., Burger, A., Dühmke, E., Gunzer, U., König, E., Stacher, A., Stein, H., Theml, H., and Waldner, R.: Retrospektive Untersuchungen zur klinischen Bedeutung der Kiel-Klassifikation der malignen Non-Hodgkin-Lymphome. Strahlentherapie, 153:222–228, 1977.
4. Castellani, R., Bonadonna, G., Spinelli, P., Bajetta, E., Galante, E., and Rilke, F.: Sequential pathologic staging of untreated non-Hodgkin's lymphomas by laparoscopy and laparotomy combined with marrow biopsy. Cancer, 40:2322–2328, 1977.
5. Dorfman, R.F.: Classification of non-Hodgkin's lymphomas (Letter). Lancet, 1:1295–1296, 1974.
6. Dühmke, E.: Zur klinischen Relevanz der histologischen Differenzierung maligner Non-Hodgkin-Lymphome nach der "Kiel-Klassifikation." Strahlentherapie, 152:129–139, 1976.
7. Gerard-Marchant, R., Hamlin, I., Lennert, K., Rilke, F., Stansfeld, A.G., and van Unnik, J.A.M.: Classification of non-Hodgkin's lymphomas (Letter). Lancet, 2:406–408, 1974.
8. Jaffe, E.S., Shevach, E.M., Frank, M.M., Berard, C.W., and Green, I. Nodular lymphoma—evidence for origin from follicular B lymphocytes. New Engl. J. Med., 290:813–819, 1974.
9. Jaffe, E.S., Shevach, E.M., Sussman, E.H., Frank, M.M., Green, I., and Berard, C.W.: Membrane receptor sites for the identification of lymphoreticular cells in benign and malignant conditions. Br. J. Cancer, 31 (2):107–120, 1975.

10. Johnson, R.E., DeVita, V.T., Kun, L.E., Chabner, B.R., Chretien, P.B., Berard, C.W., and Johnson, S.K.: Patterns of involvement with malignant lymphoma and implications for treatment decision making. Br. J. Cancer, 31 (2): 237–241, 1975.
11. Jones, S.E., Fuks, Z., Bull, M., Kadin, M.E., Dorfman, R.F., Kaplan, H.S., Rosenberg, S.A., and Kim, H.: Non-Hodgkin's lymphomas. IV. Clinico-pathological correlation in 405 cases. Cancer, 31:806–823, 1973.
12. Lennert, K., Mohri, N., Stein, H., and Kaiserling, E.: The histopathology of malignant lymphoma. Br. J. Haematol., suppl., 31:193–203, 1975.
13. Lennert, K., and Stein, H.: Personal points of view on the Kiel classification. Recent Results Cancer Res., 64:31–37, 1978.
14. Lukes, R.J., and Collins, R.D.: Immunologic characterization of human malignant lymphomas. Cancer, 34:1488–1503, 1974.
15. Mathé, G., Rappaport, H., O'Conor, G.T., and Torloni, H.: Histological and Cytological Typing of Neoplastic Diseases of Haematopoietic and Lymphoid Tissues, p. 28. World Health Organization, Geneva, 1976.
16. Meugé, C., Hoerni, B., De Mascarel, A., Durand, M., Richaud, P., Hoerni-Simon, G., Chauvergne, J., and Lagarde, C.: Non-Hodgkin malignant lymphomas. Clinico-pathologic correlations with the Kiel classification. Retrospective analysis of a series of 274 cases. Eur. J. Cancer, 14:587–592, 1977.
17. Rappaport, H.: Tumors of the hematopoietic system (Atlas of tumor pathology, section 3, fasc. 8). Armed Forces Institute of Pathology, Washington, D.C., 1966.
18. Rappaport, H., Winter, W.J., and Hicks, E.B.: Follicular lymphoma. A re-evaluation of its position in the scheme of malignant lymphoma, based on a survey of 253 cases. Cancer, 9:792–821, 1956.
19. Silvestrini, R., Piazza, R., Riccardi, A., and Rilke, F.: Correlation of cell kinetic findings with morphology of non-Hodgkin's malignant lymphomas. J. Natl. Cancer Inst., 58:499–504, 1977.
20. Van Unnik, J.A.M., Breur, K., Burgers, J.M.V., Cleton, F., Hart, A.A.M., Kroese, W.F.S., Somers, R., and van Turnhout, J.M.M.P.M.: Non-Hodgkin's lymphomata: clinical features in relation to histology. Br. J. Cancer, 312:201–207, 1975.
21. Veronesi, U., Musumeci, R., Pizzetti, F., Gennari, L., and Bonadonna, G.: The value of staging laparotomy in non-Hodgkin's lymphomas (with emphasis on the histiocytic type). Cancer, 33:446–459, 1974.
22. Warnke, R.A., Kim, H., Fuks, Z., and Dorfman, R.F.: The coexistence of nodular and diffuse patterns in nodular non-Hodgkin's lymphomas. Significance and clinicopathologic correlation. Cancer, 40:1229–1233, 1977.

17. IMMUNOGLOBULIN EXPRESSION IN B-CELL LEUKEMIAS AND B-CELL LYMPHOMAS

B. CHRISTENSSON, G. BIBERFELD AND P. BIBERFELD

INTRODUCTION

Several functional and immunological markers for human B and T lymphocytes have been described and used for the study of lymphoproliferative diseases. The production of immunoglobulin is at present the most reliable B-cell marker. Accordingly, B-cell derived malignancies have been extensively studied with regard to surface and cytoplasmic immunoglobulin expression. Results of such studies have given a basis for a functionally-oriented classification of immunoproliferative disorders. Although the biological significance of these functional markers in the various histological types of human lymphomas is not clear, recent studies have shown the prognostic value of such an immunological classification.

METHODOLOGY

Immunofluorescence (IFL) is currently the most widely used method for the demonstration of membrane-bound and cytoplasmic immunoglobulin in B lymphocytes and B-cell lymphomas. However, the possibility of several types of false positive results should be kept in mind when using IFL for quantification of truly immunoglobulin positive cells (1). Cytophilic IgG may be one source of possible error; another is the adsorption of IgG, particulary when aggregated or complexed with antigen by Fc receptors for IgG on moncytes/macrophages and some lymphocytes. Some patients may develop auto-antibodies reactive with lymphocyte membrane antigens (2a, 2b). Thus Ig-positive cells must be identified as of lymphocytic origin and surface bound Ig to be of endogenous origin.

Extrinsic, absorbed Ig on lymphocytes can be removed by preincubation at 37°C (3) or by trypsinization followed by incubation at 37°C, allowing for the re-expression of endogenous Ig. Fc receptor binding can also be eliminated by the use of $F(ab)^2$ fragments of antibody (1).

For the detection and characterization of cytoplasmic Ig, we have mainly made use of immunofluorescent staining of washed cells on cytosmears.

The development of immunoperoxidase methods and the PAP technique (4) has also made it possible to demonstrate the occurrence of immuno-globulin isotypes of cytoplasmic Ig in formalin-fixed tissue sections (4). This latter technique has the added advantage of great sensitivity and of permitting simultaneous immunologic and morphologic characterization of malignant cells.

Demonstration of light-chain restriction (either κ or λ) is usually consi-dered reliable proof of monoclonality, whereas simultaneous expression of several Ig classes may also be seen in clonal proliferation.

In cases of both chronic lymphocytic leukemia (CLL) and myeloma, antisera specific for the variable part of the monoclonal Ig molecule (anti-idiotypic sera) have been used to quantify and characterize cells of malig-nant (myeloma) clones (5, 6). Such studies have revealed that the myeloma cells (clones) are represented by cells with widely different morphologic differentiation (7).

FINDINGS

CLL

In most cases of CLL the tumor cells bear monoclonal surface Ig, although occasionally biclonal cases have been found (8, 9, 10). Variations in the expression of immunoglobulin classes as well as other B-cell markers have been observed (11, 12, 13a, b). Further evidence for clonal proliferation in

Table 1. Ig heavy and light chain classes in CLL.

Study	Ig+/total	μ	δ	$\mu + \delta$	Comments
		κ/λ	κ/λ	κ/λ	
Preud'homme et al. (8)	18/20	2/1	0/0	10/5	Two cases both $\kappa + \lambda$
Kubo et al. (15)	6/7	1/0	1/0	3/1	one case not tes-ted light chains
Fu et al. (13a)	14/14	4	3	7	Light chains not tested
Stein and Bruhn (60)	12/12	0	2	10	Light chains not tested
Christensson et al. (43)*	7/7	2/1	1/0	1/2	Lymph node cells in CLL
Total	57/60	$\mu = 11/57$ $\kappa/\lambda = 5/2$	$\delta = 7/57$ $\kappa/\lambda = 2/0$	$\mu + \delta = 39/57$ $\kappa/\lambda = 14/8$	

*IFL on frozen sections.

CLL has been provided by results obtained with the use of anti-idiotypic sera with CLL cells (5, 14).

Simultaneous expression of both IgM and IgD on the same CLL cells has been frequently shown with double-labeling methods (13, 14, 15).

The results of various studies on the expression of immunoglobulin isotypes in CLL are shown in Table 1. The vast majority (>95%) of CLL cases express Ig and are evidently of B-cell origin. In a few CLL cases it has been claimed that the CLL cells were expressing both B- and T-cell markers (16, 17). However, the possibility of false positive reactions was not completely excluded.

A few cases of true T-lymphocytic CLL have also been reported (18). The cells of these patients were shown to lack surface Ig, even after in vitro culture, to form E rosettes and to react with antisera against peripheral T cells and in some cases also with antisera against thymocytes and brain antigen (16).

The most frequently expressed heavy chain on the surface of CLL cells was μ, usually in association with δ (Table 1), and cytoplasmic Ig was usually lacking. This pattern of Ig expression is similar to that of B cells in early stages of differentiation (see below). Accordingly, it has been proposed that CLL's are neoplasms of B cells "frozen" in an early stage of differentiation (19, 20a).

However, the concept of a block in differentiation in B cells might not hold in all cases. Recent observations seem to indicate that CLL cells from a number of patients can be stimulated to blast transformation and Ig production by polyclonal B-cell activators (20b). Other cases were unresponsive, thus suggesting the occurrence of CLL types with different functional characteristics.

Prolymphocytic leukemia

A rare variant of the B-CLL type is called prolymphocytic leukemia. The cells are usually larger and cytologically show features of incompletely activated mature lymphocytes. As in typical B-CLL cases, the predominant surface immunoglobulin class is IgM, often associated with IgD, but the cells of the prolymphocytic type usually stain more strongly for surface membrane Ig than cells of the more common CLL type (21).

In about 20% of the CLL cases a serum monoclonal spike can also be found. In most cases the Ig class of the serum M-component is identical to the Ig class on the surface of the CLL cells. Production and secretion of such monoclonal Ig would suggest a further maturation of at least some of the CLL cells. Such cases may represent a transitional form between CLL and Waldenström's disease (22, 23). Unlike those in CLL, the monoclonal cells in Waldenström's disease show a more pleomorphic character, ranging from small lymphocytes to more lymphoplasmacytoid cells but express the same monoclonal surface membrane IgM, identical to that of the serum M-component (22, 24).

Heavy-chain disease

Since the first report of diseases with isolated γ-chain production given in 1964 by Franklin et al. (25), several cases with isolated heavy-chain production have been reported (26). These diseases have been considered in most cases as lymphoplasmacytic neoplasms, although the neoplastic nature of the disease in some cases has been disputed. The α chain disease is the most common and therefore the best studied variant. It is usually located primarily in the gastrointestinal tract and is usually associated with a serum α chain M-component. The α chains are not associated with light chains, although in some reported cases, light chains of one subtype have been demonstrated on the surface of the IgA-bearing cells. In the late course of the disease, there may arise an immunoblastic lymphoma with cells bearing α chains but not light chains on their membranes (27). Production of α chains but not light chains has also been demonstrated by in vitro biosynthetic assays (28). Although monoclonality cannot be proved by light-chain restriction in most cases, it has been suggested by the finding of restrictions in heavy-chain structures (29).

Waldenström's disease

In contrast to heavy-chain diseases, the proliferating lymphocytes in Waldenström's disease carry monoclonal light chains. Although IgM is the predominant heavy-chain class, both IgM and IgD can be found on the malignant cells. The amount of IgD appears to decrease with increasing maturation within the clone (30). Cases of more pleomorphic lymphoid proliferations with serum M-component and cell-bound monoclonal IgG and IgA have also been reported (22). Often, a proportion of cells with lymphoplasmacytoid morphology and cytoplasmic Ig are found in these cases of pleomorphic B-cell proliferation. Also, cases with lymphoplasmacytoid morphology but lacking serum M-component, probably reflecting an impaired secretory mechanism, have been described (31).

Multiple myeloma

In multiple myeloma the malignant monoclonal population consists mainly of plasmacytoid cells with cytoplasmic M-protein, but no or little surface Ig. In many cases atypical lymphocytes, immature lymphoblasts, and lymphoplasmacytoid cells have been shown also to belong to the tumor clone, as indicated by their expression of surface idiotypic markers identical to those of myeloma cells and serum M-component (6, 7). These findings indicate that B-cell tumors do not correspond to "frozen stages" of differentiation but that the same malignant clone can include cells representing a wide range of B-cell differentiation. Indeed, Preud'homme et al. (32) have reported a myeloma case expressing the idiotypic markers of the monoclonal serum protein on both B and T cells, which suggests that stem cells maturing to T and B cells probably were part of the malignant clone in this patient.

Expression of two heavy chains has also been found on the myeloma cells in a few cases of myeloma (10).

Hairy-cell leukemia

Hairy-cell leukemia is a well-recognized clinico-pathological entity, but the origin of the neoplastic cell is still under debate. Suggestions of monocytic/histiocytic origin have mainly been based on the presence of high-avidity $F_{c\gamma}$ receptors and a strong, tartrate-resistant acid phosphatase activity. However, a B-lymphocyte derivation has also been suggested, primarily on the basis of the demonstration of surface membrane Ig and Ig synthesis (33, 34). Recently, simultaneous expression of monocytic and B-lymphocytic characteristics on the same hairy cell has been observed (35). In this study, monoclonality was suggested by light-chain restriction. Hairy-cell leukemia is discussed more thoroughly in a separate chapter in this volume.

B-cell lymphomas

Many cases of CLL present with simultaneous lymph node involvement, usually as well-differentiated lymphocytic lymphomas. These lymphoma cells carry the same immunoglobulin isotype as the circulating CLL cells, with respect to both heavy- and light-chain classes, thus indicating a common clonal origin (35) (Table 1).

Almost all nodular lymphomas studied in our and other laboratories have, regardless of cytologic subtype and degree of nodularity, been of B-cell origin. They usually have a higher density of membrane-bound Ig molecules than CLL cells (36, 37). As in CLL, $\mu+/\kappa+$ is the most frequent Ig isotype expressed by nodular lymphoma cells but, in contrast to the findings in CLL, IgG is also found in some cases and IgD is much less frequently observed (Table 2). This difference in the expression of various immunoglobulin isotypes in nodular lymphomas including IgA supports the contention that these lymphomas represent a wider spectrum of B-cell differentiation than do the CLL's (38, 39, 40). Immuno-

Table 2. Ig classes in nodular lymphomas or equivalent entities.

Study	Ig+/total	μ	γ	μ + δ	μ + γ	γ + α	δ + α
Aisenberg and Long (61)	5/6	κ/λ 3/0	κ/λ 2/0	κ/λ	κ/λ	κ/λ	κ/λ
Leech et al. (36)	14/15	7/0		2/0	1/0		1/0
Stein (62)	6/6	3/1		1/1			
Christensson et al. (43)*	16/18	3/7	1/1	1/1		1/1	
Total	41/45	μ = 24/41 κ/λ = 16/8	γ = 4/41 κ/λ = 3/1	μ + δ = 6/41 κ/λ = 4/2	μ + γ = 1/41 κ/λ = 1/0	λ + α = 2/41 κ/λ = 1/1	δ + α = 1/41 κ/λ = 1/0

*Tested on frozen tissue sections.

fluorescence studies on frozen sections (Table 2) and demonstration of complement receptors in parallel sections (Figure 1) are methods which are helpful in ascertaining the monoclonality and follicle derivation of the nodular cells (41, 43)

Most *diffuse, poorly differentiated lymphocytic lymphomas* are also of B-cell origin, as indicated by their Ig content (Table 3). Many of these cases have immunologic characteristics quite similar to those of the malignant cells in nodular lymphomas, suggesting that they also have a follicular cell origin, but progress from a nodular to diffuse growth (Figure 2). Alternatively, they may originate from cells which have left the follicles (44, 45).

Not infrequently, the B-cell lymphomas also progress to leukemic stages, although the total white blood cell count may not be elevated. Immuno-fluorescent studies often lead to the detection in the circulation of a discrete monoclonal subpopulation showing the same heavy- and light-chain classes as solid tumor cells. A relatively small change in the normal κ/λ ratio may be the only sign of the occurrence of such a discrete monoclonal population. By using other lymphoma cell markers such as idiotypes, even smaller proportions of leukemic lymphoma cells may be detected (6). It is therefore probable that more patients than have hitherto been reported will be found to have leukemic spread of their lymphoma cells.

The *diffuse large-cell (histiocytic) lymphomas* appear to be an immunologi-cally heterogeneous group (46). Only in rare cases has true histiocytic origin of these tumors been established (47). Approximately 60% of these lympho-mas appear to be B-lymphocyte derived, as indicated by Ig expression (Table 4). Some of these lymphomas supervene earlier lymphoproliferative diseases such as low-grade malignant lymphomas or auto-immune diseases (46). They usually have the same immunological phenotype as found on the cells of the preceding lymphoma, thus suggesting a progressive dedifferentiation of the same cell clone.

Of the non-B, histiocytic lymphomas, approximately 10% express T-cell markers and the rest lack T- and B-cell markers (37, 48).

The histiocytic lymphoma group is heterogeneous not only with respect to immunologic characteristics but also with regard to morphology and prognosis (49). Preliminary observations seem to indicate that the B-derived lymphomas in this group have a better prognosis than the non-Bs (48, 50, 51).

The delineation between *lymphoblastic lymphomas* and *lymphoblastic* leukemias (ALL) is not clear and varies from case to case depending on the extent of involvement of peripheral blood and lymphoid tissues. The nature of T and non-T/non-B acute lymphoblastic leukemias is the subject of separate chapters in this book. B-lymphocytic leukemias (B-ALL) are rare and in children have an even poorer prognosis than the T-cell ALL (48, 51). They are usually leukemic manifestations of malignant lymphoma of the Burkitt type (52, 53, 56).

Table 3. Ig classes in diffuse poorly differentiated lymphocyte lymphomas or equivalent entities.

Study	Ig+/total	μ	γ	δ	$\mu + \delta$	$\mu + \gamma$	$\mu + \gamma + \delta$
		κ/λ	κ/λ	κ/λ	κ/λ	κ/λ	κ/λ
Aissenberg and Long (61)	12/12	5/6					
Leech et al. (36)	9/9	4	1	1	3	1/0	Light chain n.t
Preud'homme et al. (8)	8/9				3/5		
Stein (63)	14/14	1/1/3*			1/1	0/2/2*	
Christensson et al. (43)**	13/16	3/2			3/2	3/2	1/0
Total	56/60	$\mu = 28/56$ $\kappa/\lambda = 12/9$	$\gamma = 1/56$	$\delta = 1/56$	$\mu + \delta = 16/56$ $\kappa/\lambda = 6/7$	$\mu + \gamma = 9/56$ $\kappa/\lambda = 4/4$	$\mu + \gamma + \delta = 1/56$

* $\kappa^+ \lambda^+$.
** IFL on frozen sections.

Table 4. Ig classes on large-cell lymphomas (immunoblastic/histiocytic and mixed lymphoblastic/histiocytic) or equivalent entities.

Study	Ig+/total	μ κ/λ	γ κ/λ	μ+γ κ/λ	μ+γ+δ κ/λ	μ+δ κ/λ
Aisenberg and Long (61)	0/3					
Brouet et al. (64)	3/6					
Morris and Davey (65)	5/6	1/1	1/0	1/0		
Seligmann et al. (66)	5/14				1/0	
Braylan et al. (37)	11/17	6/0				One case only κ
Krüger et al. (67)	1/6					
Stein (68)	5/6	2/1/1*	1/0			
Christensson et al. (43)**	15***/22	7/1	1/1	1/0		3/0
Total	45/80	μ = 20/45 κ/λ = 16/3	γ = 4/45 κ/λ = 3/1	μ + γ = 2/45 κ/λ = 2/0	μ + γ + δ = 1/45 κ/λ = 1/0	μ + δ = 3/45 κ/λ = 3/0

* κ+λ+.
** IFL on frozen sections.
*** One case κ+λ+.

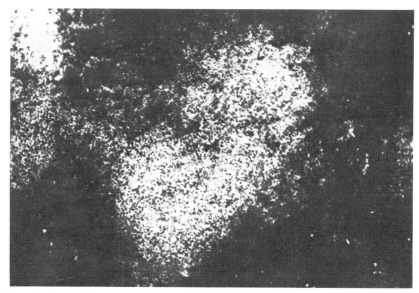

Figure 1. Immunofluorescense pattern shown by for μ chains in a frozen lymphnode section from a patient with nodular lymphoma.

In several studies (53, 56) the lymphoblastic tumors of the Burkitt type, both endemic and nonendemic, have been shown to be of B-lymphocytic origin. In most cases the cells have been shown to be monoclonally positive for surface-membrane IgM in the African type (53b, 54) as well as in the American type (52; 53a, 55). In some cases the occurrence of IgD too has been shown (8, 57). In many studies weak to moderate complement receptor activity both of C3b and C3d has been found. Mann et al. (55) have suggested an association between Burkitt lymphoma cells and normal lymphocytes of the mantle zone area of germinal centers, on morphological, immunological, and tissue distributional grounds. No definite immunological differences have been found between endemic and nonendemic Burkitt lymphomas or cases with and without proven contents of EB-virus genomes.

Non-Burkitt B-cell monoclonal proliferations have also been found in ALL, and not infrequently these cases represented a lymphoblastic transformation of typical B-lymphocytic CLL (see above) (58). Most cases studied so far have monoclonal surface IgM. A few cases of non-B/non-T cell ALL have been reported to show a cytoplasmatically detectable small amount of IgM suggesting a pre-B cell nature of this disease (59). In rare cases of ALL the simultaneous occurrence of B- and T-cell markers on the lymphoblastic cells have been found. Whether these results are due to technical errors in the assay systems or these cells represent neoplastic counterparts of prethymocytes is not clear.

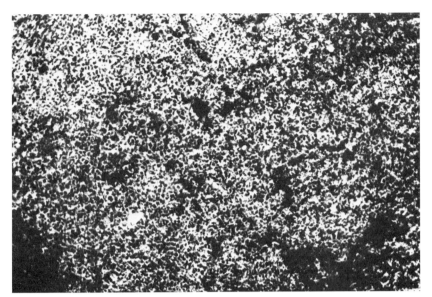

Figure 2. Immunofluorescence pattern shown by for μ chains in a frozen lymphnode section from a patient with diffuse lymphoma.

SUMMARY

Demonstration of surface membrane Ig and/or cytoplasmic Ig in various non-Hodgkin lymphomas and lymphatic leukemias is a useful marker of B-cell lymphomas/leukemias and is of interest for their identification. Recent clinical studies indicate that such an immunological classification is helpful for the prognostic evaluation of these diseases.

ACKNOWLEDGMENTS

This work was supported by the Swedish Cancer Society and the Swedish Medical Research Council. The technical assistance of M. Andersson and M. Ekman is gratefully acknowledged.

REFERENCES

1. Winchester, R.J., Fu, S.M., Hofman, T., and Kunkel, H.G.: IgG on lymphocyte surfaces: Technical problems and the significance of a third cell population. J. Immuno., 114:1210–1212, 1975.
2a. Winchester, R.J., Winfield, J.B., Siegal, F., Wennert, P., Bantwick, Z., and Kunkel, H.G.: Analysis of lymphocytes from patients with rheumatoid arthritis and systemic lupus erythematosus. Occurrence of interfering cold-reactive antilymphocyte antibodies. J. clin. Invest., 54:1082–1092, 1974.
2b. Biberfeld, G., Biberfeld, P., and Wigzell, H.: Antibodies to surface antigens of lymphocytes and lymphoblastoid cells in cold-agglutinin-positive sera from patients with Mycoplasma pneumoniae infection. Scand. J. Immunol., 5:87–95, 1976.

3. Lobo, P.I., Westervelt, F.B., and Horwitz, V.A.: Identification of two populations of immunoglobulin-bearing lymphocytes in man. J. Immunol., 114: 116–119, 1975.

4. Sternberger, L.A.: Immunocytochemistry. Prentice Hall, New Jersey, 1974.

5. Schroer, K.R., Briles, D.E., van Boxel, J.A., and Davie, J.M.: Idiotypic uniformity of cell surface immunoglobulin on chronic lymphatic lymphocytic leukemia. Evidence for monoclonal proliferation. J. exp. Med., 140:1416, 1974.

6. Mellstedt, H., Hammarström, S., and Holm, G.: Monoclonal lymphocyte population in human plasma cell myeloma. Clin. exp. Immunol., 17:371–384, 1974.

7. Biberfeld, P., Pettersson, D., and Mellstedt, H.: Ultrastructural and immunocytochemical characterization of circulating mononuclear cells in patients with myelomatosis. Acta path. microbiol. scand. A, 85:611–624, 1977.

8. Preud'homme, J.L., Brouet, J.C., Clauvel, I.P.,and Seligmann, M.: Surface IgD in immunoproliferative disorders. Scand. J. Immunol., 3:853–858, 1974.

9. Gray, H.M., Rabellino, E.M., and Pirofsky, B.: Immunoglobulins on the surface of lymphocytes IV. Distribution in hypogammaglobulinaemia, cellular immunodeficiency, and chronic lymphatic leukemia. J. clin. Invest., 50:2368–2375, 1971.

10. Seligmann, M., Preud'homme, J.L., and Brouet, J.-C.: B and T cell markers in human proliferative blood diseases and primary immunodeficiencies, with special reference to membrane bound immunoglobulins. Transplant. Rev., 16:85–113, 1973.

11. Grey, H.M., Kubo, R.T., Rabellino, E.M., Polley, M., and Ross, G.D.: Immunoglobulins and complement receptors on CLL cells. In: Shearing symposium on immunopathology, Cavtap, June 1973. Advances in Biosciences, 12:213–218, Pergamon Press, 1974.

12. Frøland, F.S., and Natvig, J.B.: Class, subclass and allelic exclusion of membrane bound Ig of human B lymphocytes. J. Exp. Med., 136:409–414, 1972.

13a. Fu, S.M., Winchester, R.J., and Kunkel, H.G.: Occurrence of surface IgM, IgD and free light chains on human lymphocytes. J. exp. Med., 139:451–456, 1974.

13b. Ross, G.D., Rabellino, E.M., Polley, M.J., and Gray, H.M.: Combined studies on complement receptor and surface immunoglobulin bearing cells and sheep erythrocyte rosette forming cells in normal and leukemic human lymphocytes. J. clin. Invest., 52:377–385, 1973.

14. Fu, S.M., Winchester, R.J., and Kunkel, H.G.: Similar idiotypic specificity for membrane IgD and IgM on human B lymphocytes. J. Immunol., 144: 250–252, 1975.

15. Kubo, R.T., Gray, H.M., and Pirofsky, B.: IgD: A major immunoglobulin on the surface of lymphocytes from patients with chronic lymphatic leukemia. J. Immunol., 112:1952–1954, 1974.

16. Preud'homme, J.L., Brouet, J.-C., and Seligmann, M.: Lymphocyte membrane markers in human lymphoproliferative diseases. In: Membrane receptors on lymphocytes. INSERM Symposium I, North-Holland, Elsevier, 1975.

17. Brouet, J.-C., and Prieur, A.-M.: Membrane markers on chronic lymphocytic leukemia cells: A B-cell leukemia with rosettes due to anti-sheep erythrocyte antibody activity of the membrane bound IgM and a T-cell leukemia with surface Ig. Clin. Immunol. Immunopathol., 2:481–487, 1974.

18. Brouet, J.-C., Flandrin, G., Sasportes, M., Preud'homme, J.L., and Seligmann, M.: Chronic lymphocytic leukemia of T-cell origin. Immunological and clinical evaluation of 11 patients. Lancet, II:890–894, 1975.

19. Preud'homme, J.L., and Seligmann, M.: Surface bound immunoglobulin as a cell marker in human lymphoproliferative diseases. Blood, 40:777–794, 1972.

20a. Salmon, S.E., and Seligmann, M.: B-cell neoplasia in man. Lancet, II:1230, 1974.

20b. Robèrt, K.-H., Bird, A.G., and Möller, E.: Mitogen induced differentiation of human CLL lymphocytes to antibody secreting cells. Scand. J. Immunol., in press.

21. Buskard, N.A., Catovsky, D., Okos, A., Goldmann, J.M., and Galton, D.A.G.: Prolymphocytic leukemia: Cell studies and treatment by lukapho-

21. resis. In: Maligne Lymphome und Monoklanale Gammapathien. Hematologie und Blut Transfusion, 18:237–253, 1976.

22. Preud'homme, J.L., and Seligmann, M.: Immunoglobulin on the surface of lymphoid cells in Waldenström's macroglobulinaemia. J. clin. Invest., 51: 701, 1972b.

23. Rudders, R.A., and Ross, R.: Partial characterization of the shift from IgG to IgA synthesis in clonal differentiation of human leukemic bone marrow derived lymphocytes. J. exp. Med., 142:549, 1975.

24. Frøland, F.S., and Natvig, J.B.: Identification of three different human lymphocyte populations by surface markers. Transplant. Rev., 16:114–162, 1973.

25. Franklin, E.C., Loewenstein, J., Wigelow, B., and Melltzer, M.: Heavy chain disease—a new disorder of serum gammaglobulins. Report of the first case. Amer. J. Med., 37:332–350, 1964.

26. Seligmann, M., Dunnon, F., Hurez, D., Mihaesco, E., and Preud'homme, J.L.: Alpha chain disease: A new immunoglobulin abnormality. Science, 162:1396–1397, 1968.

27. Seligmann, M.: Immunochemical, clinical and pathological features in alpha chain disease. Arch. Inter. Med., 135:78–82, 1975.

28. Seligmann, M., and Rambaud, J.C.: Alpha chain disease, a possible model for pathogenesis of human lymphomas. In: Immunopathology of lymphoreticular neoplasms, pp. 425–447, Plenum Press, 1978.

29. Wolfelstein-Todel, C., Mihaesco, E., and Francione, B.: Alpha chain disease protein defect: Internal deletion of human immunoglobulin A1 heavy chain. Proc. Natl. Acad. Sci. U.S.A., 71:974–978, 1974.

30. Pernis, B., Brouet, J.-C., and Seligmann, M.: IgD and IgM on the membrane of lymphoid cells in macroglobulinaemia. Evidence for identity of membrane IgD and IgM antibody activity in a case with anti-IgG receptors. Eur. J. Immunol., 4:776–778, 1974.

31. Stein, H., and Lennert, K.: In: Malignant lymphomas other than Hodgkin's disease. Lennert, K., Springer-Verlag, 1978.

32. Preud'homme, J.L. et al.: Eur. J. Immunol., 7:840, 1977.

33. Rubin, A.B., Douglas, S.D., Chessim, L.M., Glade, P.R., and Dameshek, V.: Chronically reticulo-lymphocytic leukemia. Reclassification of leukemic reticuloendotheliosis through functional characterization of circulating mononuclear cells. Amer. J. Med., 47:149–162, 1969.

34. Haak, H.L., de Manne, J.C.H., Heijmans, V., Knapp, V., and Speck, B.: Further evidence for the lymphocytic nature of leukemic reticuloendotheliosis. Brit. J. Haematol., 27:31–38, 1974.

35a. Rieber, E.P., van Heyden, H.V., Linke, R.P., Faal, J.G., Reitermüller, G., van Heyden, H.V., Valler, H.D., and Schwartz, H.: Hairy cell leukemia. Simultaneous demonstration of autochthonous surface Ig and monocytic functions of hairy cells. In: Hematology and blood transfusion vol. 20, pp. 157–163, Springer-Verlag, 1977.

35b. Braylan, R.C., Jaffe, E.S., Burbach, J.V., Frank, M.N., Johnson, R.E., and Berard, C.V.: Similarities of surface characteristics on neoplastic well differentiated lymphocytes from solid tissues and from peripheral blood. Cancer Res., 36:1619, 1976.

36. Leech, J.H., Glick, A.B., Waldron, J.A., Flexner, J.M., Horn, R.G., and Collins, R.D.: Malignant lymphomas of follicular center cell origin in man. I. Immunologic studies. J. Natl. Ca. Inst., 54:11, 1975.

37. Braylan, R.C., Jaffe, E.S., Mann, R.B., Frank, M.N., and Berard, C.V.: Surface receptors of human neoplastic lymphoreticular cells. Hematology & Blood Transfusion, 20:47–53, 1977, Springer-Verlag.

38. Lukes, R.J., Parker, J.W., Taylor, C.R., Tindle, B.H., Cramer, A.D., and Lincoln, T.L.: Immunologic approach to non-Hodgkin lymphomas and related leukemias. Analysis of the results of multiparameter studies of 425 cases. Seminars in Hematology, 15(4):322–351, 1978.

39. Lennert, K., Stein, H., and Kaiserling, E.: Cytological and functional criteria for the classification of malignant lymphomata. Brit. J. Cancer, 31, Suppl. II:29–43, 1975.

40. Shevach, E.M., Jaffe, E.S., and Green, E.: Receptors for complement and immunoglobulin on human and animal lymphoid cells. Transplant. Rev., 16:3–28, 1973.

41. Cossmann, J., Schnitzer, B., and Degan, M.J.: Immunologic surface markers in non-Hodgkin lymphomas. Amer. J. Pathol., 87:19–32, 1977.

42. Warnke, R., and Levi, R.: Immunopathology of follicular lymphomas. New Engl. J. Med., 298:481–486, 1978.

43. Christensson, B. et al. unpublished, 1979.

44. Jaffe, E.S., Shevach, E.M., Sussman, E.H., Frank, M.N., Green, E., and Berard, C.W.: Membrane receptor sites for identification of lymphoreticular cells in benign and malignant conditions. Brit. J. Cancer, 31, Suppl. II:107–120, 1975.

45. Brouet, J.C., Labaumes, S., and Seligmann, M.: Evaluation of T and B lymphocyte membrane markers in human non-Hodgkin malignant lymphomata. Brit. J. Cancer 31, Suppl., II:121–127, 1975.

46. Brouet, J.C., Preud'homme, J.L., Flandrin, G., Chelloul, N., and Seligmann, M.: Membrane markers in histiocytic lymphomas (reticulum cell sarcoma). J. Natl. Ca. Inst., 56:631–633, 1976.

47. Ralph, P., Moore, M.A.S., and Nilsson, K.: Lysosome synthesis by established human and murine histiocytic lymphoma cell lines. J. exp. Med., 143:1528–1533, 1976.

48. Belpomme, D., Lelarge, N., Mathé, G., and Davies, A.J.S.: Etiological, clinical and prognostic significance of the T/B immunological classification of primary acute lymphoid leukemias and non-Hodgkin lymphomas. In: Hematology and blood transfusion vol. 20, pp. 33–47, Springer-Verlag, 1977

49. Strauchen, J.A., Young, R.C., Devita, V.T., Anderson, T., Vantone, J.C., and Berard, C.W.: Clinical relevance of the histopathological subclassification of diffuse histiocytic lymphoma. New Engl. J. Med., 299:1382–1387, 1978.

50. Bloodmfield, C.D., Kersey, J.H., Brunning, R.D., and Gajl-Peczalska, K.J.:

Prognostic significance of lymphocyte surface markers in adult non-Hodgkin malignant lymphoma. Lancet, December 18, 1976.

51. Kersey, J., Coccia, P.F., Bloomfield, C., Nesbit, M., Mackenna, R., Brunning, R.D., Hallgren, H., and Gajl-Peczalska, J.L.: Surface markers define human lymphoid malignancies with different prognoses. In: Hematology and blood transfusion vol. 20, pp. 17–24, Springer-Verlag, 1977.

52. Flandrin, G., Brouet, J.C., Daniel, M.T., and Preud'homme, J.L.: Acute leukemia with Burkitt's tumor cells: Study of six cases with special reference to lymphocyte surface markers. Blood, 45:183–188, 1975.

53a. Gajl-Peczalska, K.J., Bloomfield, C.D., Coccia, P.F., Susin, H., Brunning, R.D., and Kersey, J.H.: B and T cell lymphomas. Analysis of blood and lymph nodes in 87 patients. Amer. J. Med., 59:674–685, 1975.

53b. Klein, E., Klein, G., Nadkarny, J.S., Nadkarny, J.J., Wigsell, H., and Clifford, P.: Surface IgM specificity of cells derived from Burkitt's lymphoma. Lancet, II:1068–1070, 1967.

54. Fialkow, P.J., Klein, E., Klein, G., Clifford, P., and Singh, S.: Immunoglobulin and glucose-6-phosphate dehydrogenase as markers of cellular origin of Burkitt lymphoma. J. exp. Med., 138:89–102, 1973.

55. Mann, R.B., Jaffe, E.S., Braylan, R.C., Nanda, K., Frank, N.M., Ziegler, J.L., and Berard, C.W.: Non-endemic Burkitt's lymphoma. A B-cell tumor related to germinal centers. New Engl. J. Med., 295:685–691, 1976.

56. Gajl-Peczalska, J.L., Bloomfield, C.D., Nesbit, M.E., and Kersey, J.H.: B-cell markers on lymphoblasts in acute lymphoblastic leukemia. Clinical and experimental immunology, 17:561–569, 1974.

57. Biberfeld, P. et al.: EBV genome positive Burkitt's lymphoma in Sweden, unpublished.

58. Brouet, J.C., Preud'homme, J.L., Seligmann, M., and Bernard, J.: Blast cells with monoclonal surface immunoglobulin in two cases of acute blast crises supervening on chronic lymphocytic leukemia. Brit. Med. J., 4:23, 1973.

59. Cooper, M.D., Kearnye, J.F., Lidyard, T.M., Grossi, E.C., and Lawton, R.A.: Studies of generation of B-cell diversity in mouse, man and chicken. Cold Spring Harbor Symposium "Quantitative Biology" no. 41, pp. 139–146, 1976.

60. Stein, H., Bruhn, H.: In: Malignant lymphomas, P. 566, Lennert, K., Springer-Verlag, 1978.

61. Aisenbrg, A.C., and Long, J.C.: Lymphocyte surface characteristics in malignant lymphoma. Amer. J. Med., 58:300–306, 1975.

62. Stein, H.: In: Malignant lymphomas, Lennert, K., p. 615, Springer-Verlag, 1978.

63. Stein, H.: In: Malignant lymphomas, p. 610. Lennert, K., Springer-Verlag, 1978.

64. Brouet, J.C., Labaume, S., and Seligmann, M.: Evaluation of T and B lymphocyte membrane markers in human non-Hodgkin malignant lymphomata. Brit. J. Cancer 31, suppl. II:121–127, 1975.

65. Morris, M.W., and Davey, F.R.: Immunologic and cytochemical properties of histiocytic and mixed histiocytic lymphocytic lymphomas. Amer. J. clin. Path., 63:403–414, 1975.

66. Seligmann, M., Brouet, J.C., and Preud'homme, J.L.: The immunological diagnosis of human leukemias and lymphomas: An overview. In: Hematology and blood transfusion vol. 20, pp. 1–15, Springer-Verlag, 1977.

67. Krüger, G., Huhlmann, C., Hellriegel, K.P., Sesterchenn, K., Samii, H.,

Fischer, R., Wustrow, F., and Gross, R.: Membranrezeptoren lymphoretiku-
läre Zellen bei hyperplastischen und neoplastischen Erkrankungen des
lymphatischer Systems. In: Maligne Lymphome und Monoklonale Gammapathien. Hematologie u. Blut Transfusion vol. 18, pp. 17–31, Lehmans, 1976.

68.   Stein, H.: In: Malignant lymphomas, p. 645, Lennert, K., Springer-Verlag,
1978.

18. LYMPHOPLASMACYTIC/LYMPHOPLASMACYTOID LYMPHOMA (LP IMMUNOCYTOMA)

(Modified Abstract)

K. LENNERT AND M. BURKERT

We apply the term malignant lymphoma, lymphoplasmacytic/lymphoplasmacytoid, or LP immunocytoma, to lymphomas whose main constituents are lymphocytes but which also have a small to moderate number of lymphocyte-derived cells capable of secreting immunoglobulin (plasma cells or plasmacytoid cells and their precursors). The ability to secrete immunoglobulin (Ig) can be suggested or proved by the following methods and features. On light microscopy, the cells have basophilic cytoplasm (with Giemsa staining of sections or, even better, imprints). On electron microscopy, they show abundant rough endoplasmic reticulum. The immunoperoxidase reaction demonstrates intracytoplasmic Ig of one light chain type. With the PAS reaction, intranuclear or intracytoplasmic globular Ig inclusions can often be recognized. Such inclusions do not occur in chronic lymphocytic leukemia of the B type (B-CLL).

LP immunocytoma can be subclassified into three subtypes that differ in cytologic composition: (a) the lymphoplasmacytic subtype, (b) the lymphoplasmacytoid subtype, and (c) the polymorphic subtype. Cases of the first subtype show not only typical lymphocytes, but also a small number of Marschalkó-type plasma cells. Proliferation centers are relatively rare. In the second subtype, there is an admixture of plasmacytoid cells. These are not always clearly distinguishable from lymphocytes. Their cytoplasm is somewhat more abundant and more basophilic than that of lymphocytes. Proliferation centers (pseudofollicular pattern) are often found in this subtype. In addition, the first and second subtypes show a few immunoblasts. Besides plasma cells and plasmacytoid cells, the third subtype shows numerous immunoblasts and often centroblasts and centrocytes; but the predominating cells are still lymphocytes. This subtype displays a diffuse growth pattern.

Chemical analysis of tumor homogenates revealed increased amounts of Ig (usually IgM, specifically IgM of one light chain type). The immunoperoxidase technique makes it possible to demonstrate monoclonal Ig in the cytoplasm of a moderate to large number of the tumor cells. This Ig is chiefly IgM, less often IgG, and rarely IgA. κ chains are more common than λ-light chains (see Table 1).

The blood serum of about one third of the patients shows an increase in

J.G. van den Tweel et al. (eds.), Malignant Lymphoproliferative Diseases, 245–247
All rights reserved.
Copyright © 1980 by Martinus Nijhoff Publishers bv, The Hague/Boston/London.

Table 1. Monoclonal intracytoplasmic immunoglobulin in the three subtypes of LP immuno-cytoma demonstrated by the immunoperoxidase technique.*

Subtype	IgM		IgG		IgA		Light chains only		Total	
	κ	λ	κ	λ	κ	λ	κ	λ	κ	λ
Lymphoplasmacytic	10	6	3	1	1	—	—	1	14	8
Lymphoplasmacytoid	31	19	2	3	1	—	8	2	42	24
Polymorphic	10	4	2	2	—	—	—	2	12	8
	51	29	7	6	2	—	8	5	68	40
Total	80		13		2		13		108	

*Study performed with M. Burkert, J. Fuchs, U. Müller-Hermelink and C.S. Papadimitriou.

the same Ig classes with a monoclonal pattern. When there is an increase in the IgM level, one may speak of Waldenström's macroglobulinemia, but this term certainly does not cover all cases of LP immunocytoma, or even all cases of monoclonal paraproteinemia. LP immunocytoma also constitutes the morphologic basis of heavy-chain diseases of the γ-and μ-chain types.

A leukemic blood picture is not uncommon in LP immunocytoma. The borderline between LP immunocytoma and B-CLL is not sharp. In such

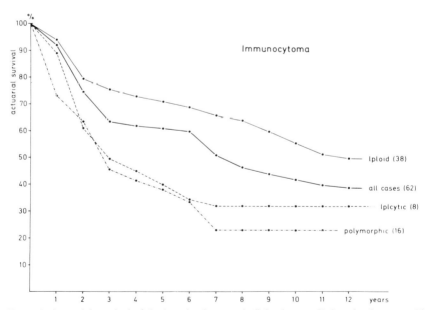

Figure 1. Actuarial survival of the lymphoplasmacytic (lplcytic, n = 8), lymphoplasmacytoid (lploid, n = 38), and polymorphic (n = 16) subtypes of LP immunocytoma and of all cases (n = 62). (Kindly provided by G. Brittinger, Essen.)

borderline cases we define a case as LP immunocytoma only when the histological picture shows a significant number of tumor cells containing intracytoplasmic Ig of one light chain type; in other words, we diagnose LP immunocytoma by means of immunomorphologic methods alone, irrespective of an increase in Ig (monoclonal) or the number of lymphocytes in the patient's blood.

LP immunocytoma may evolve into an immunoblastic lymphoma, i.e., transformation occurs from a low-grade malignant lymphoma into a high-grade one. In such cases, Ig production is less pronounced than in most cases of LP immunocytoma, but the proliferating cell alone is the same. This has been demonstrated by Seligmann and others.

The age distribution of LP immunocytoma shows a peak between 60 and 70 years for both males and females. There is a slight preponderance of males.

Data on the prognosis of LP immunocytoma are available for all three subtypes. The Kiel Lymphoma Study Group (Brittinger and co-workers, forthcoming) has shown that the lymphoplasmacytoid subtype has the best prognosis (see Figure 1.). The prognosis of the lymphoplasmacytic subtype is poorer. The worst prognosis is found in the polymorphic subtype, which is understandable, because the polymorphic subtype has many blast cells (immunoblasts and centroblasts) with a large number of mitotic figures. The number of immunoblasts is, however, hardly as high as it is in immunoblastic lymphoma; correspondingly, the prognosis is not as poor as that of immunoblastic lymphoma.

We are often criticized for separating LP immunocytoma from B-CLL. Despite the ill-defined borderline, however, we consider this distinction to be justifiable, because there are some special features in the clinical picture of LP immunocytoma. For example, there is sometimes lymphoma infiltraion of the eyes (orbit, eyeball, conjuctiva) or skin; this infiltration is often the first clinical symptom of the malignant lymphoma and rarely or never occurs in B-CLL.

For a complete list of references see:

Lennert, K., in collaboration with Stein, H., Mohri, N., Kaiserling, E., and Müller-Hermeling, H.K.: Malignant lymphomas other than Hodgkin's disease. Springer-Verlag, New York, Heidelberg and Berlin, 1978.

19. LYMPHOPROLIFERATIVE DISEASES AND MONOCLONAL GAMMOPATHY

D.Y. MASON

The term "monoclonal gammopathy" is applied to a spectrum of clinical conditions, ranging from the benign to the malignant, characterized by the presence of a monoclonal Ig paraprotein (Table 1). As will be seen from the table some of these conditions, e.g. myelomatosis, are almost invariably associated with the presence of a paraprotein, while in other conditions (e.g. non-Hodgkin's lymphoma) paraproteins are present in only a proportion of patients.

There are several objections to lumping cases together purely on the basis of whether or not we can detect monoclonal immunoglobulin in the patients's serum or urine. From the histologist's point of view it cuts across the classifications which he has painstakingly striven to establish. This is well illustrated in the case of Waldenström's macroglobulinaemia. The histological pattern of this disease may also be seen in cases in whom no IgM serum paraprotein is detectable, probably because of a block in cellular secretion. As Lennert (76) points out such cases of "macroglobulinaemia without macroglobulinaemia" are in essence identical to classical Waldenström's disease, and a term such as his category of "lymphoplasmacytoid lymphoma", which embraces both paraprotein and nonparaprotein producing forms of the disease, should be used.

Table 1. Classification of monoclonal gammopathies.

Clinical diagnosis	Associated gammopathy
Myeloma	Monoclonal Ig present in 99% of cases, IgG commonest. Approx. 50% excrete free light chains.
Waldenstrom's (primary) macroglobulinaemia	Monoclonal IgM present. Approx. 10% excrete light chains.
Primary amyloidosis	Monoclonal Ig produced by majority of patients. Light chain excretion common (usually lambda).
Non-Hodgkin's lymphoma	Approx. 7% of cases produce serum paraprotein. Usually IgM.
Benign (or secondary) monoclonal gammopathy	Found in approx. 0.2% of random sera. Frequency rises to > 10% over age of 80. Light chain excretion rare.

From the immunologist's point of view the categorization of lymphoproliferative diseases on the basis of whether or not they are associated with a detectable paraprotein is also illogical. The objection lies in the word "detectable" since our ability to find a paraprotein depends upon a number of technical factors such as the level of the paraprotein, electrophoretic mobility, Ig type, etc. Furthermore, as has been emphasized by previous contributors, monoclonal immunoglobulin is almost always present in the membrane of neoplastic B cells even if they do not secrete it. Consequently to isolate cases on the basis of detectable paraprotein production is to obscure the essential unity of B-lymphoproliferative disorders.

So is there any argument for considering the monoclonal gammopathies as a group? There is some clinical justification for this, since a number of important complications of these diseases such as renal damage, hyperviscosity syndrome and amyloidosis are directly attributable to the effects of the monoclonal Ig product. But a further argument for focussing our attention on monoclonal gammopathies is that by studying the relationship between B-cell neoplasms and the paraproteins which they produce we may learn something about normal B-cell physiology. Thus we may look upon diseases such as multiple myeloma as experiments of nature in which a single cell and its Ig product are both subject to an enormous expansion enabling us to study each of them in much greater detail than would otherwise be possible. In this way we may be able to say something about the relationship between different morphologically defined types of B cells and the Ig which they secrete.

However, the disadvantage of allowing Nature to perform our experiments is that she rarely gives us full details of how she achieves her re-

Table 2. Observation and inference in monoclonal gammopathies.

	Observation	*Inference*
1. Ig Class	Myeloma cells: IgG > IgA > IgD > IgE Kappa:lambda =2:1	Normal plasma cells: IgG > IgA > IgD > IgE Kappa:lambda =2:1
2. Tissue localization	Myeloma:Bone marrow Waldenström's:Spleen, lymph nodes, marrow.	IgG & IgA cells:Marrow IgM cells:Spleen, lymph nodes, marrow.
3. Free light chains	50% of myeloma cases	50% of normal plasma cells
4. No heavy chains	20% of myeloma cases	20% of normal plasma cells
5. IgD	IgD myeloma: Male:female =3:1 Kappa:lambda =1:9 Free light chains in 92% of cases	IgD cells: 3 times commoner in men Kappa:lambda =1:9 92% produce free light chains

markable results, and in particular we cannot assess the extent to which we are justified in extrapolating from the neoplastic to the normal B cell. This is illustrated by Table 2 which shows some of the observations which we can make about monoclonal gammopathies and the inferences which we might draw from them. Clearly some of the inferences on the right hand side of this table are justified, e.g. Line 1, whilst others are untrue (Line 2), or of doubtful validity (Lines 3 to 5).

A further objection to having nature on your scientific staff is that she does not always obtain the same result when she repeats an experiment. What, for example, are we to make of Table 3 which lists exceptions to traditional associations between clinical and immunochemical features of monoclonal gammopathies? And how are we to interpret anomalous aspects of Ig synthesis by neoplastic lymphoid cells such as the absence of heavy chain production or the synthesis of deleted heavy chains, half Ig molecules (54, 111, 115, 116), or tetramers of light chains (67). When these anomalies are common, such as the absence of heavy chain production (seen in approximately 20% of cases of myeloma) it may be fairly simple to ascertain that these features are not seen in comparable percentages of normal B-lymphoid cells. They are hence presumably associated with the neoplastic nature of the monoclone. On the other hand rare anomalies, such as heavy chain diseases, are much less readily interpreted. So that what we see when we study monoclonal paraproteins in lymphoproliferative disorders is sometimes representative of normal B-cell maturation and sometimes represents features which are either specific to neoplastic cells or associated with the immaturity of the cell. In the latter context it may be noted that there is evidence that excess light chain production is characteristic of immature B cells

Table 3. Anomalous morphological/immunochemical relationships in monoclonal gammopathies.

No. of cases	Morphological and clinical type	Paraprotein class	Authors
5	Waldenstrom's macro-globulinaemia	IgG	Tursz et al., (124)
1	Waldenstrom's macro-globulinaemia	IgG	Resegotti et al., (107)
2	Waldenstrom's macro-globulinaemia	IgA	Tursz et al., (124)
1	Waldenstrom's macro-globulinaemia	IgA	Hijmans (52)
1	Pleomorphic lympho-proliferative disorder	IgA	Child et al., (29)
1	Alpha chain disease	Gamma chain	Seligmann (113)

(47) and also that J chain synthesis (a feature of myeloma cells) is also seen in immature Ig producing cells but not in mature Ig producing cells (20). Indeed some cases of monoclonal gammopathies in which defective or blocked maturation occurs may provide closer parallels with immunodeficiency states than with normal B-lymphoid differentiation.

CELLULAR ASPECTS OF MONOCLONAL GAMMOPATHIES

There is a further objection to using monoclonal gammopathies as a basis on which to construct theories about the relationships between Ig production and cell morphology which exist in normal lymphoid tissues. This is that the neoplastic cell populations in lymphoproliferative diseases embrace a wider range of cytological types than was initially realized. This was demonstrated by Preud'homme and Seligmann in 1972 in a study of Waldenström's macroglobulinaemia where it was found that IgM of a single light chain class could be demonstrated not only in the plasmacytic cells in bone marrow but also on more than half of the peripheral blood small lymphocytes. Subsequently Mellstedt and his colleagues (84) were able to demonstrate a similar phenomenon in human multiple myeloma. This was achieved by preparing antisera against the purefied paraproteins from individual patients and then rendering these antisera specific for idiotypes on the paraprotein by extensive absorption with normal polyclonal Ig. These antisera then gave no reaction with normal peripheral lympyoid cells but stained 20% to 47% of peripheral lymphoid cells in three cases of myloma. It was demonstrated that the immunglobulin bearing the idiotype was synthesized by the peripheral blood mononuclear cells rather than absorbed from the serum. Mellstedt and his colleagues went on to show that the idiotype positive population of peripheral mononuclear cells exhibit a spectrum of ultrastructural appearances ranging from nondescript small lymphoid cells through intermediate forms to clearly plasmacytoid cells (16), and furthermore, by ^{3}H thymidine labeling (85) they were able to demonstrate that the small mononuclear compartment in myeloma has a higher proliferative rate (labeling index 11.5–14%) than does the population of mature plasmacytoid cells (labeling index 2.5–5%).

Thus the mutation which gives rise to a disease such as myloma appears to take place in a small mononuclear cell, and the plasma cells which are so prominent in a marrow aspirate represent terminal differentiation by the neoplastic clone, rather analogous to the way in which myeloid leukaemia cells may differentiate to form mature polymorphs. The parallel with myeloid leukaemia may be carried further, since in both diseases the neoplastic clones may be characterized by deficiencies of cell morphology, constituents or functions, such as nuclear anomalies or deficiencies of lysosomal proteins in myeloid leukaemia, cytoplasmic and nuclear inclusions or anomalies in Ig production and secretion in multiple myeloma.

How early in lymphoid cell maturation does the mutation which gives rise to multiple myeloma occur? It was convincingly demonstrated by Preud'-homme and his colleagues (105) that the paraprotein idiotype could be found not only on peripheral B cells in a case of myloma but also on peripheral T cells. Thus in at least some cases of myeloma the neoplastic clone may originate from the mutation of a stem cell prior to the T/B-cell dichotomy. Quite how early this cell may lie in haemopoetic/lymphoid stem cell development is unknown. There have been a number of cases reported in the literature in which multiple myeloma and acute myeloid leukaemia have been diagnosed simultaneously (Table 4) raising the possibility that a stem cell common to both lymphoid and myeloid cells may be involved. This view, which would have appeared unlikely a few years ago, now finds a precedent in reports of acute leukaemia of clearly lymphoblastoid nature arising in cases of chronic myeloid leukaemia.

These reassessments of the cellular basis of diseases such a myeloma are not of purely theoretical significance since they emphasize the difficulties of monitoring therapeutic success in myeloma by examining bone marrow aspirates. Furthermore, the ability of myeloma to spread is presumably related to the seeding potential of the small mononuclear compartment of the neoplastic clone which circulates through the peripheral blood (130).

It should be noted that Heller (50) and colleagues place a different interpretation upon idiotype positive small mononuclear cells in myeloma and have evidence that these cells acquire the paraprotein idiotype under the influence of RNA from the malignant cell clone. Such a conversion in both animal and human myeloma has been demonstrated by Heller's group using

Table 4. Simultaneous development of myeloid leukaemia and monoclonal gammopathy.

Multiple myeloma and acute myelomonocytic leukaemia	Cleary et al., (30)
Multiple myeloma and myelomonocytic leukaemia	Parker (98)
Multiple myeloma and myelomonocytic leukaemia	Taddeini and Schrader (121)
Multiple myeloma and myeloblastic leukaemia	Rosner and Grunwald (110)
Multiple myeloma and myeloid leukaemia	Videbaek (128)
Multiple myeloma and acute myeloblastic leukaemia	Tursz et al., (125)
Macroglobulinaemia and myelomomocytic leukaemia	Allen et al., (6)
Macroglobulinaemia and acute myelomonocytic leukaemia	Ligorsky et al., (77)

RNA extracted from myeloma serum or tissue (28, 44, 51). RNA from immunosuppressive plasmacytomas was also capable of inducing immuno-suppression in experimental animals. However no confirmatory evidence of these results has been forthcoming from other laboratories.

MULTIPLE MYELOMA

Diagnosis

The diagnosis of multiple myeloma is usually made without difficulty as a result of clinical, haematological, radiological and biochemical investiga-tions. Marrow aspiration usually reveals numerous plasma cells which may show morphological abnormalities such as nuclear or cytoplasmic inclusions (22, 31, 36, 120, 14, 18) Haematologists are sometimes asked to pronounce on whether bone marrow cells are reactive or neoplastic (although other investigations usually answer this question) and the phenomenon of nuclear cytoplasmic asynchrony (giving a centrally placed nucleolated nucleus with an open chromatin pattern lying in a pale blue cytoplasm) has been pro-posed as a useful cytological criterion of neoplasia (15).

Contrary to earlier reports it now appears that the cytological appearance of the myeloma cell gives no clue as to the class of paraprotein which it contains (49). Immunofluorescent staining enables this to be determined but is usually of no great diagnostic value. It does not allow one for example, to distinguish benign monoclonal gammopathies from multiple myeloma. Immunofluorescent staining may perhaps be of more practical value in the rare cases of myeloma which are nonsecretory. As will be seen in Table 5, in the majority of such cases monoclonal intracellular Ig can be demonstra-ted. Immunofluorescent staining has also been used in the investigation of the cellular basis of double paraprotelnaemia. In most cases the two para-proteins appear to be secreted by different clones although they probably arise from a common precursor (for references see van Camp et al. (127). In a few cases "double secretors" have been detected, and these may repre-sent neoplastic expansion of a "switch" B cell (127).

Although diagnosis is usually readily achieved in multiple myeloma it is worth mentioning two causes of diagnostic difficulty which are occasionally encountered. Firstly cases of early myeloma in which the clinical, radiolo-gical and laboratory abnormalities are either absent or borderline may pose diagnostic problems. Many of these patients declare themselves as frank cases of myeloma if observed over a period of a year or more. The remainder are then classified as examples of benign monoclonal gammopathy (BMG) (90, 79). It should be recognized however that the borderline between these two categories is not always sharply defined. Occasional cases are seen of

Table 5. Immunofluorescent staining of nonsecretory myeloma cells.

No. of cases	Monoclonal intracellular Ig detected	
	Results	*Authors*
1	Kappa chains detected	Fabia et al., (39)
1	IgGK detected. K staining much stronger than IgG	Arend and Adamson (7)
1	IgGK detected. Both bound and free light chain present in myeloma cells	Whicher et al., (131)
25	Monoclonal Ig detected in all cases. Imbalance in intensity of heavy and light chain staining	Preud'homme et al., (104)
1	Kappa chains detected. Nonsecretion confirmed by 14C labeling	Nilsson et al., (92)

No. of cases	Intracellular Ig not detected	
	Result	*Authors*
1	Neg. for "human Ig" ? abnormal RER and Golgi on e.m.	Gach et al., (41)
1	Neg. for G,A,M and light chains	River et al., (108)
1	Neg. for G,A,M,D,E	Indiveri et al., (59)
1	Neg. for G,A,M, kappa and lambda	Bedou et al., (10)
1	Neg. for F(ab')$_2$, G,A,M,D	Stavem et al., (119)
1	Neg. for G,A,M,D,E, and light chains	Mancilla and Davis (82)
1	Neg.	Nilsson et al., (92)

"indolent" myeloma (almost always IgG producers) reminiscent to the haematologist of "smouldering" leukaemia (93), some of which (Figure 1) subsequently progress to overt meyloma, whilst the remainder remain stable (33). Solitary myelomas, which commonly affect the vertebral column and pelvis, may remain localized for long periods (33, 87, 97).

Conversely BMG may not always present as benign a profile as its title implies (65). Lindström and Dahlström (78) in a recent study of 44 cases reported that suppression of polyclonal background immunoglobulin was frequently seen, and furthermore 40% of patients were excreting urinary light chains, although never at a concentration of greater than 50mg/100ml. The authors concluded that the distinction between myeloma and BMG is quantitative rather than qualitative.

However as mentioned above myeloma will ultimately declare itself as a progressive disease if observed over a period whereas BMG will remain stable. Since there is no evidence that delay in treating an early case of myeloma worsens the ultimate prognosis it is reasonable to await the development of symptoms before treating. Indeed in view of the mutagenic dangers of myeloma chemotherapy there is a positive reason for not institut-

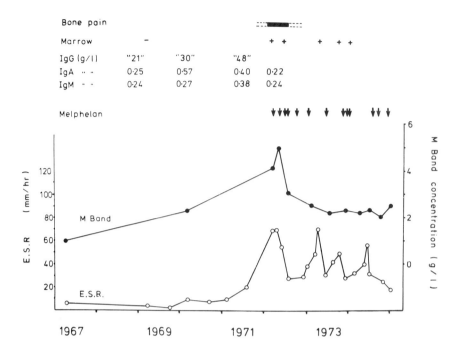

Figure 1. Details of a patient who developed overt myeloma after a period of more than four years during which asymptomatic paraproteinaemia was present.

ing treatment until symptoms develop. However, all presumed BMG or early myeloma patients require follow-up. Since the survival of patients with established myeloma is clearly related to the size of the malignant cell population (3, 37) and to whether or not renal function has been irreversibly compromised, there should be no delay in starting therapy once the typical clinical features of myeloma appear.

A second cause of diagnostic difficulty in myeloma is represented by the patient in whom bone pain is absent or minimal at presentation. Approximately one in five myeloma patients fall into this category and two-thirds of these cases present with pneumonia, renal failure or nonspecific symptoms of malaise and weight loss. Soft tissue plasmacytomas may occasionally be the presenting complaint (38, 43, 17, 96), and since the cellular morphology of these growths is frequently more primitive than that of the parent intramedullary neoplasm (99) the histologist may have difficulty in recognizing their origin. The diagnosis of multiple myeloma is usually however readily made on the basis of bone marrow examination and by electrophoretic analyses.

Clinical complications (Figure 2)

Bone pain

Bone pain, the cardinal feature of myeloma, arises from malignant plasma cells stimulating osteoclastic resorption of bone (91). However bone pain probably represents a dynamic rather than a static state in that it stems from skeletal regions in which infraction (fracture without displacement) is occurring. This was demonstrated by Charkes et al. (27) using the radio-active isotope ^{87m}Sr, which is taken up whenever reactive new bone is being formed. These workers found that painful skeletal sites were always associated with increased strontium uptake implying a recent or an impending fracture. They pointed out an obvious, though sometimes overloooked, fact that bone erosion *per se*, for example in the vault of the skull, is usually pain-less since it is not associated with infraction. It follows that any therapeutic measure which arrests or even slows the erosive process allows the site to stabilize and pain is thereby alleviated. This accounts for the rapidity with which bone pain responds to chemotherapy or radiotherapy.

Infection

Infection is an ever-present risk in myeloma patients, although awareness on the part of the physician and the patient of this hazard, and prompt insti-tution of antibiotic therapy, does much to reduce its dangers. There appears to be no reliable way of identifying patients at particular risk from infection, since it is not clearly related to the degree of suppression of background serum Ig or to the paraprotein class.

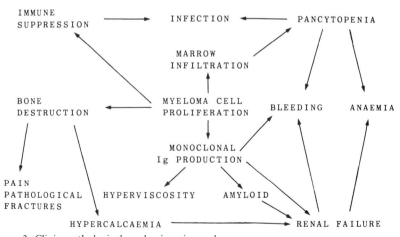

Figure 2. Clinicopathological mechanisms in myeloma.

What is the mechanism of immune suppression in myeloma? There is evidence from animal studies to suggest that a mononuclear cell population, probably of macrophages, accounts for the defect (66, 68) but these findings could be explained on the basis of an increased number of macrophages (which are normally immunosuppressive) in plasmacytoma bearing animals. In the past few years evidence has been reported that peripheral blood mononuclear cells from human myeloma patients can suppress mitogen and antigen driven B-cell activation (21, 95) but again the clinical relevance of these observations is still uncertain.

Anaemia

Anaemia is largely attributable to the effects of marrow infiltration and renal failure. However, it is important to recognize that, by a mechanism which is still quite mysterious, increased blood viscosity appears to lead to an increased plasma volume (2, 123), presumably representing a physioloical attempt to improve circulation in small vessels. This haemodilutional anaemia should be recognized in view of the dangers of overtransfusion.

Hyperviscosity

Hyperviscosity syndrome in myeloma (80) was initially recognized as a complication of IgG myeloma, but is now seen to be more frequent in IgA myeloma (102, 129) particularly when the paraprotein is secreted by the cell as a covalent 11S or higher molecular weight polymer (86, 102, 109). The major clinical manifestation is usually a haemorrhagic tendency. Invesigation of haemostatic abnormalities in myeloma patients (74), reveals what one investigator termed "a bewildering variety of abnormalities" (100), but from a clinical point of view the relevant defect in haemorrhagic myeloma patients seems to be an interference with platelet/capillary wall interactions and this is particularly likely to happen when the paraprotein is of high molecular weight.

It is worth noting that although haemorrhage is the commonest haemostatic abnormality in myeloma, patients occasionally develop thrombosis (26, 89).

Renal failure

Renal failure is the major cause of early death in myeloma patients despite recognition of the importance of adequate dehydration and correction of hypercalcaemia (42). It should be recognized however that the important prognostic indicator is the level of blood urea rather than the light chain excretion *per se*. Many patients excrete very large amounts of light chains— of the order of many grammes a day (48), without evidence of renal damage and the survival of these patients is close to that of non-light chain excreting patients. As is well known light chains damage principally renal tubules

(133), and any patient who shows evidence of nephrotic syndrome with heavy proteinuria should be suspected of having renal amyloid.

A less frequently encountered renal complication of myeloma is the development of acute renal failure (64, 19, 35, 69, 103, 112). There are several causes including hypercalcaemia, hyperuricaemia, intravascular coagulation and dehydration. The prognosis is poor (35) but prolonged survival is possible with prompt treatment.

Acute leukaemia

Acute leukaemia is now widely recognized as an occasional terminal event in multiple myeloma (110), and its incidence has been put at approximately 50 times that of the normal population (46). The malignancy is most frequently an acute myeloblastic or myelomonocytic leukaemia, although several cases of erythroleukaemia have been reported (23, 40, 88, 134). It is strongly suspected that the malignancy reflects the mutagenic effects of treatment with cytotoxic drugs. The probable course of events is that drug therapy not infrequently induces mutant clones in treated myeloma patients (34, 117), but that only an occasional clone manifests itself as a haemopoietic malignancy (57). Overt leukaemia is frequently heralded by a period of dyserythropoietic or sideroblastic anaemia (34, 63, 75).

Anaplastic lymphoid neoplasms

Anaplastic lymphoid neoplasms occasionally emerge during the management of myeloma patients (56). These cells are characterized by rapid growth and drug resistance and they appear, on the basis of immunohistological studies, to represent second mutations occurring in the myeloma cell clone (122). The ability to synthesize heavy chains may be lost by these mutant cells (94), a process known as "Bence Jones escape", although the reverse pattern may occasionally be encountered. The new cell line appears to show a greater tendency than its parent clone to grow outside the confines of the bone marrow so that the development of soft tissue plasmacytomas during treatment often heralds a rapid relapse.

Treatment

More than 20 years have elapsed since the first reports of the treatment of myeloma with cyclophosphamide and with sarcolysin (the racemic form of melphelan). Although the lives of many myeloma patients have been transformed since the introduction of these drugs, it is now apparent that remission is usually only of limited duration. The neoplastic cells in any individual patient appear to be heterogeneous with regard to drug sensitivity, so that chemotherapy at best only destroys a proportion of the malignant clone (55). Sequential studies (55) suggest that the neoplastic cells decrease in number as a result of chemotherapy in responding patients, but that they start to reaccumulate as soon as the maximal kill has been achieved (despite clinical impressions that a plateau state of variable duration is attained before relapse). The studies of Alexanian et al. (4) have shown that conventional maintenance therapy for patients who have achieved remission offers no benefit in terms of ultimate survival when compared to a nontreatment group, and indeed entails a greater risk of complications such as marrow suppression.

Once relapse occurs reinduction may be difficult. A number of regimes based upon BCNU have been proposed (8, 1, 24). Bergsagel et al. (13) recommended the use of high dose intermittent cyclophosphamide for melphelan resistant patients (Figure 3), but Kyle et al. (73) reported disappointing results with this regime.

The therapeutic limitations of simple cyclophosphamide/prednisolone or melphelan/prednisolone combinations have focussed attention on more aggressive multiple drug chemotherapy regimes (Table 6). It appears that the important factor in these drug combinations is the presence of vincristine, since it is only by the inclusion of this drug that an improvement on the conventional melphelan/prednisolone regimes can be obtained. However, although these new regimes appear to produce a higher response rate and longer remission period than conventional therapy it is doubtful if they alter the fundamental pattern of a period of remission followed by an almost inevitable relapse. It also remains to be seen whether leukocyte interferon, which was recently reported by Mellstedt et al. (83) as inducing complete remission in two cases of myeloma and a partial response in a further two patients, will find a place in the therapy of the disease.

Additional therapeutic measures in the management of myeloma should

Table 6. Recent trials of multiple drug therapy for myelomatosis.

Authors	No. of patients	Drugs	Results
Alexanian et al., (5)	462	Mel + Adr + Pred Mel + Cyc + Pred Mel + Cyc + BCNU + Pred Cyc + Adr + Pred Vin + Mel + Cyc + Pred	Vincristine regimes gave 15% higher resp. rate than all other regimes. Projected median remission time: 34 mo. (9 mo. better than previous regimes)
Case et al. (24)	72	Mel + Pred + Cyc + Vin + BCNU	Previously untreated: 87% resp. rate. Median remission: 20 mo. Previously treated: 50% resp. rate. Median remission: 22 mo.

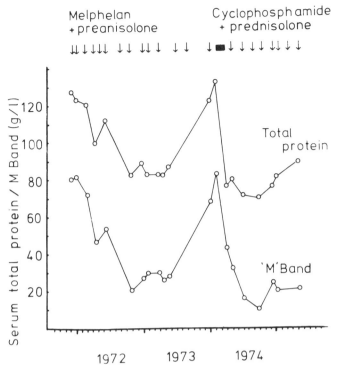

Figure 3. Details of a patient who responded to intermittent cyclophosphamide following relapse on melphelan.

not be forgotten (32). Surgery has a role to play, particularly in the management of cord compression syndromes (126). Since these patients frequently have relatively localized disease, many of them respond well and for prolonged periods to surgical decompression followed by chemotherapy. Other ancillary treatment measures include the use of radiotherapy, plasmapheresis (60, 101), anti-hypercalcaemia agents such as mithramycin (114, 118), or calcitonin (11) and the use of fluoride calcium (71). The value of the latter treatment as an adjuvant to chemotherapy appears to depend upon the use of supplemental calcium, since fluoride alone offers no benefit.

PRIMARY AMYLOIDOSIS

Although cases of primary amyloid often do not resemble myeloma clinically, the disease probably represents a very similar process of plasma cell neoplasia (61). It is now well established that the major component of primary amyloid is a protein closely homologous to the N-terminal portion of

Table 7. Clinical features of primary amyloidosis (data from (70)).

Symptoms	%	Signs	%
Fatigue	67	Hepatomegaly	45
Weight loss	55	Oedema	35
Dyspnoea	30	Purpura	17
Paraesthesiae	26	Macroglossia	12
"Hoarseness"	12	Splenomegaly	7
Syndromes		Skin lesions	4
Carpal tunnel syndrome		Nephrotic syndrome	
Cardiac failure		Peripheral neuropathy	
Orthostatic hypotension			

immunoglobulin light chains, and probably arises from the denaturation and precipitation in the tissues of circulating monoclonal light chains (usually lambda in type) (45). Patients consequently present clinically with evidence of tissue amyloid deposition (Table 7) at a much earlier stage of development of the plasma cell clone than is typically present at diagnosis in classical myeloma. However, if carefully sought, a monoclonal paraprotein will be found in the urine or serum (Table 8). In many patients the only paraprotein is found in the urine as free light chains. These may be difficult to detect, firstly because of masking by serum protein escaping via damaged glomeruli, and secondly because they frequently move further towards the anode on electrophoresis than do most paraproteins (61). Bone marrow plasma cells are not usually grossly increased in number (Table 8) but they may show cytological features suggesting neoplasia (Figure 4), as well as showing evidence of monoclonality on immunocytological staining (Figure 5).

It should be noted that monoclonal light chains may be deposited in

Table 8. Paraprotein and bone marrow findings in primary amyloid.

Authors	No. of patients	Serum and/or urine paraprotein	Marrow plasmacytosis	X-ray lesions
Barth et al., (9)	15	9	5	1
Benson et al., (12)	38	17	N.D.	N.D.
Cathcart et al., (25)	14	7	7	N.D.
Hobbs (53)	40	35	N.D.	N.D.
Isobe and Osserman (61)	26	26	26	0
Jones et al., (62)	8	3	1	0
Kyle and Bayrd (70)	132	105	0	8

N.D.: no data.

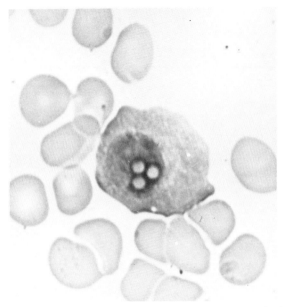

Figure 4. A plasma cell containing intranuclear inclusions from the bone marrow of a patient suffering from primary amyloidosis. Numerous such cells were present in the marrow.

tissues, causing severe tissue damage without forming recognizable amyloid. Randall and colleagues (107) have described two patients in whom multiple organs including kidney, liver, gastrointestinal tract and heart were damaged by the deposition of monoclonal light chains. Only one of these patients had overt myeloma. In both cases the light chains were kappa in type and could be demonstrated immunohistologically in the affected organs. We have seen a similar case in Oxford, and a probably related disorder has been reported by Mallick and colleagues (81) as an occasional finding amongst patients presenting at a renal clinic with "idiopathic" proteinuria.

Primary amyloid is a rare disease and experience in its treatment is necessarily limited. It has been suggested that cytotoxic therapy may be of value (62) but its benefit is restricted by the fact that irreversible tissue damage, especially of the kidneys, may be present at diagnosis. At least two patients have been reported in whom acute leukaemia developed following melphelan therapy of primary amyloidosis (72), whilst Zilko and Dawkins (132) have reported a case in whom cytotoxic therapy appeared to accelerate the development of amyloid, a finding which parallels results from experimental amyloidosis in animals.

a

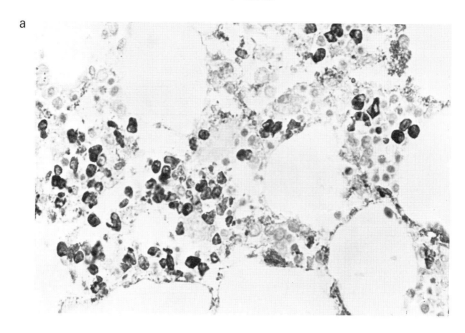

b

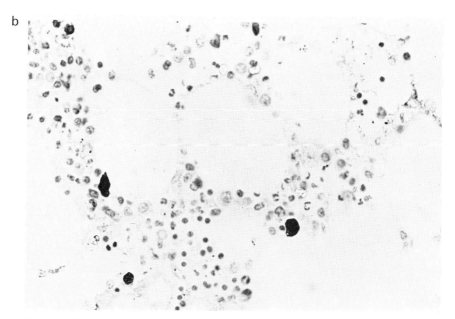

Figure 5. Bone marrow from a further case of primary amyloidosis in whom urinary lambda light chains were detected. Immunoperoxidase staining revealed an excess of lambda positive plasma cells (a) relative to kappa cells (b) providing evidence of a monoclonal population of plasma cells.

CONCLUSION

Monoclonal gammopathies are an intriguing group of diseases because of the possibility which they offer of new insight into normal lymphoid physiology and also because of their unique clinical manifestations. However the major challenge which they present is in the field of therapy. Current chemotherapy can only offer temporary remissions in diseases such as myeloma and new drug regimes are required which achieve permanent eradication of the neoplastic cell clone.

REFERENCES

1. Alberts, D.S., Durie, B.G.M., and Salmon, S.E.: Doxorubicin/B.C.N.U. chemotherapy for multiple myeloma in relapse. Lancet, 1:926, 1976.
2. Alexanian, R.: Blood volume in monoclonal gammopathy. Blood, 49:301, 1977.
3. Alexanian, R., Balcerzak, S., Bonnet, J.D., Gehan, E.A., Haut, A., Hewlett, J.S., and Monto, R.W.: Prognostic factors in multiple myeloma. Cancer, 36:1192, 1975.
4. Alexanian, R., Gehan, E., Haut, A., Saiki, J., and Weick, J.: Unmaintained remissions in multiple myeloma. Blood, 51:1005, 1978.
5. Alexanian, R., Salmon, S., Bonnet, J., Gehan, E., Haut, A., and Weick, J.: Combination therapy for multiple myeloma. Cancer, 40:2765, 1977.
6. Allen, E.L., Metz, E.N., and Balcerzak, S.P: Acute myelocytic leukaemia with macroglobulinaemia, Bence-Jones proteinaemia and hypercalcaemia. Cancer, 32:121, 1973.
7. Arend, W.P., and Adamson, J.W.: Non-secretory myeloma. Cancer, 33:721, 1974.
8. Azam, L., and Delamore, I.W.: Combination therapy for myelomatosis. Brit. Med. J., ii:560, 1979.
9. Barth, W.F., Willsron, J.T., and Waldmann, T.A.: Primary amyloidosis. Amer. J. Med., 47:259, 1969.
10. Bedou, G., Legoff, P., Besson, G., Blanguernon, P., and Garre, H.: Myelome non-excretant révélé par une compression médullaire Sem. Hop. Paris., 50: 2477. 1974.
11. Behn, A.R., and West, T.E.T.: Emergency treatment with calcitonin of hypercalcaemia associated with multiple myeloma. B.M.J., 1:755, 1977.
12. Benson, M.D., Cohen, A.S., Brandt, K.D., and Cathcart, E.S.: Neuropathy M components and amyloid. Lancet, i:10, 1975.
13. Bergsagel, D.E., Cowan, D.H., and Hasselback, R.: Plasma cell myeloma: response of melphelan resistant patients to high dose intermittent cyclophosphamide Canad. Med. Assoc. J., 107:851, 1972.
14. Bernier, G.M., Del Duca, V., Brereton, R., and Graham, R.C.: Multiple Myeloma with intramedullary masses of M-Component. Blood 46:931, 1975.
15. Bernier, G.M., and Graham, R.C.: Plasma cell asynchrony in myeloma: Correlation of light and electron microscopy. Sem. Haemat, 13:239, 1976.
16. Biberfeld, P., Mellstedt, H., and Pettersson, D.: Ultrastructural and

immunocytochemical characterisation of circulating mononuclear cells in patients with myelomatosis. Acta. Path. Microbiol. Scand. (A), 85:611, 1977.

17. Bjorkholm, M., Holm, G., Mellstedt, H., and Sjogren, A.: Extensive nodular infiltration of extra-osseous tissue in human myelomatosis. Acta. Med. Scand. 200:139, 1976.

18. Blom, J., Mansa, B., and Wiik, A.: Study of Russell bodies in human monoclonal plasma cells by means of immunofluorescence and electron microscopy. Acta. Path. Microbiol. Scand., A84:335, 1976.

19. Booth, L.J., Minielly, J.A., Smith, E.K.M.: Acute renal failure in Multiple myeloma. Canad. Med. Ass. J., 111:335, 1974.

20. Brandtzaeg, P., and Berdal, P.: J Chain in malignant human IgG immunocytes. Scand. J. Immunol. 4:404, 1975.

21. Broder, S., Humphrey, R., Durm, M., Blackman, M., Meade, B., Goldman, C., Strober, W., and Waldmann, T.: Impaired synthesis of polyclonal (non-paraprotein) immunoglobulins by circulating lymphocytes from patients with multiple myeloma. New Engl. J. Med., 293:887, 1975.

22. Brunning, R.D., and Parkin, B.A.: Intranuclear inclusions in plasma cells and lymphocytes from patients with monoclonal gammopathies. Am. J. Clin. Path., 66:10, 1976.

23. Cardamone, J.M., Kimmerle, R.I., and Marshall, E.Y.: Development of acute erythroleukaemia in B-cell immunoproliferative disorders after prolonged therapy with alkylating drugs. Am. J. Med., 57:836, 1974.

24. Case, D.C., Lee, B.J., and Clarkson, B.D.: Improved survival times in multiple myeloma treated with Melphalen, Prednisone, Cyclophosphamide, Vincristine and BCNU. M-2 protocol. Am. J. Med., 63:897, 1977.

25. Cathcart, E.S., Ritchie, R.F., Cohen, A.S., Brandt, K.: Immunoglobulin and amyloid. Amer. J. Med., 52:93, 1972.

26. Catovsky, D., Ikoku, N.B., Pitney, W.R., and Galton, D.A.G.: Thrombo-embolic complications in myelomatosis. Brit. Med. J., 3:438, 1970.

27. Charkes, N.D., Durrant, J., and Barry, W.E.: Bone pain in multiple myeloma. Studies with radioactive 87mSr. Arch. Int. Med., 130:53, 1972.

28. Chen, Y., Bhoopalam, N., Yakulis, V., and Heller, P.: Changes in lymphocyte surface immunoglobulins in myeloma and the effect of an RNA-containing plasma factor. Ann. Intern. Med., 83:625, 1975.

29. Child, J.A., Franklin, I.M., Warren, J.V., Cawley, J.C., Roberts, B.E., Burns, G.F., and Roach, T.C.: Pleomorphic B cell neoplasm with monoclonal IgG secretion. Cancer 40:2948, 1979.

30. Cleary, B., Binder, R.A., Kales, A.N., and Veltri, B.: Simultaneous presentation of acute myelomonocytic leukaemia and multiple myeloma. Cancer 41:1381, 1978.

31. Cohen, H.J., and Lefer, L.G., Intranuclear inclusions in Bence-Jones lambda plasma cell myeloma. Blood 45:131, 1975.

32. Cohen, H.J., and Rundles, R.W.: Managing the complications of multiple myeloma. Arch. Int. Med., 135:177, 1975.

33. Conklin, R., and Alexanian, R.: Clinical classification of plasma cell myeloma. Arch. Intern. Med., 135:139, 1975.

34. Dahlke, M.B., and Nowell, P.C.: Chromosomal abnormalities and dysery-thropoiesis in the preleukaemic phase of multiple myeloma. Brit. J. Haemat. 31:111, 1975.

35. Defronzo, R.A., Humphrey, R.L., Wright, J.R., and Cooke, C.R.: Acute renal failure in myeloma. Medicine 54:209, 1975.

·36. Djaldetti, M., and Lewinski, U.H.: Origin of intranuclear inclusions in myeloma cells. Scand. J. Haematol. 20:200, 1978.

37 Durie, B.G.M., and Salmon, S.E.: A clinical staging system for multiple myeloma. Cancer 36:842, 1975.

38. Edwards, G.H., and Zawadski, Z.A.: Extraosseus lesions in plasma cell myeloma. Amer. J. Med., 43:194, 1967.

39. Fabia, F., Burnichon, J., and Cornillot, P.: Essai d'interpretation physio-pathologique du myelome "non excretant". Path. Biol. 22:617, 1974.

40. Fishman, S.S., and Ritz, N.D.: Erythroleukaemia following melphalan therapy for multiple myeloma. New York State J. Med., 74:2402, 1975.

41. Gach, J., Simar, L., Salmon, J.: Multiple myeloma without M type protein-aemia. Amer. J. Med., 50:835, 1971.

42. Galton, D.A.G., and Peto, R.: Report on the First Myelomatosis Trial. Brit. J. Haem., 24:123, 1973.

43. Ghosh, M.L., and Sayeed, A.: Unusual cases of myelomatosis. Scand. J. Haem. 12:147, 1974.

44. Giacomoni, D., Yakulis, V., Wang, F., Cooke, A., Dray, S., and Heller, P.: In vitro conversion of normal mouse lymphocytes by plasmacytoma RNA to express idiotype specificities on their surface characteristic of the plasma-cytoma immunoglobulin. Cell Immunol., 11:389, 1971.

45. Glenner, G.G., Terry, W.D., and Isersky, C.: Amyloidosis, its nature and pathogenesis. Semin. Hemat., 10:6, 1973.

46. Gonzalez, F., Trujillo, J.M., and Alexanian, R.: Acute leukaemia in multiple myeloma. Ann. Intern. Med., 86:440, 1977.

47. Gordon, J., Smith, J.L.: Free immunoglobulin light chain synthesis by lympho-cytes from patients with hypogammaglobulinaemia. Clin. Exp. Immunol., 34:288, 1978.

48. Hayes, J.S., Jankey, N., Cuthbert, A.L., and Das, P.M.: Massive proteinuria in light chain disease. Arch. Intern. Med. 138:785, 1978.

49. Hayhoe, F.G.J., and Neuman, Z.: Cytology of myeloma cells. J. Clin. Path., 29:916, 1976.

50. Heller, P.: The mechanism of the immunologic deficiency in myeloma of man and mouse. Blut. 37:65, 1978.

51. Heller, P., Yakulis, V., Bhoopalam, N., Costea, N., Cabana, V., and Nathan, R.D.: Surface immunoglobulins on circulating lymphocytes in mouse and human plasmacytoma. Trans. Assoc. Amer. Phys., 85:192, 1972.

52. Hijmans, W.: Waldenström's disease with an IgA paraprotein. Acta. Med. Scand. 198:519, 1975.

53. Hobbs, J.R.: An ABC of amyloid. Proc. Roy. Soc. Med., 66:705, 1973.

54. Hobbs, J.R., Jacobs, A.: A half molecule GK plasmacytoma. Clin. Exp. Immunol. 5:199, 1969.

55. Hokanson, J.A., Brown, B.W., Thompson, J.R., Drewinko, B., and Alexanian, R.: Tumor growth patterns in multiple myeloma. Cancer 39:1077, 1977.

56. Holt, J.M., and Robb-Smith, A.H.T.: Multiple myeloma: Development of plasma cell sarcoma during apparently successful chemotherapy. J. Clin. Path., 26:649, 1973.

57. Hossfeld, D.K., Holland, J.F., Cooper, R.G., and Ellison, R.R.: Chromosome studies in acute leukaemias developing in patients with multiple myeloma. Cancer Res., 35:2808, 1975.

59. Indiveri, F., Barabino, A., Santolini, M.E., and Santolini, B.: "Non-secret-ory" multiple myeloma. Acta. Haemat. 51:302, 1974.

60. Isbister, J.P., Biggs, J.C., and Penny, R.: Experience with large volume plasmapheresis in malignant paraproteinaemia and immune disorders. Aust. N.Z.J. Med., 8:154, 1978.

61. Isobe, T., and Osserman, E.F.: Patterns of amyloidosis and their association with plasma cell dyscrazia, monoclonal immunoglobulins and Bence-Jones proteins. New. Eng. J. Med., 290:473, 1974.

62. Jones, N.F., Hilton, P.J., Tighe, J.R., and Hobbs, J.R.: Treatment of "primary" renal amyloidosis with melphalan. Lancet 3:616, 1972.

63. Khaleeli, M., Keane, W.M., and Lee, G.R.: Sideroblastic anaemia in multiple myeloma – a preleukaemic change. Blood 41:17, 1973.

64. Kjeldsberg, C.R., and Holman, B.E.: Acute renal failure in multiple myeloma. J. Urol., 105:21, 1971.

65. Kohn, J.: Benign paraproteinaemia. J. Clin. Path. 28(6):77, 1974.

66. Kolb, J-P., Arrian, S., Zolla-Pazner, D. (1977). Suppression of the humoral immune response by plasmacytomas: mediation by adherent mononuclear cells. J. Immunol. 118:702, 1977.

67. Kozuru, M., Benoki, H., Sugimoto, H., Sakai, K., and Ibayashi, H.: A case of lambda type tetramer Bence-Jones proteinaemia. Acta. Haemat., 57:359–365, 1977.

68. Krakauer, R.S., Strober, W., Waldmann, T.: Hypogammaglobulinaemia in experimental myeloma: the role of suppressor factors from mononuclear phagocytes. J. Immunol., 118:1385, 1977.

69. Krull, P., Kühn, K., Zobl, H., and Sterzel, R.B.: Akutes Nierenwersagen Bei Bence-Jones-Plasmozytom. Deutsche Med. Wsch. 98:318, 1973.

70. Kyle, R.A., and Bayrd, E.D.: Amyloidosis: Review of 236 cases. Medicine 54: 271, 1975.

71. Kyle, R.A., Jowsey, J., Kelly, P.J., and Taves, D.R.: Multiple myeloma bone disease. New. Engl. J. Med., 293:1334, 1975.

72. Kyle, R.A., Pierre, R.V., Bayrd, E.D.: Primary amyloidosis and acute leukaemia associated with melphalan therapy. Blood 44:333, 1974.

73. Kyle, R.A., Seligman, B.R., Wallace, H.J., Silver, R.T., Glidewell, O., and Holland, J.F.: Multiple myeloma resistant to Melphalen (NSC-8806) treated with Cyclophosphamide (NSC-26271), Prednisone (NSC-10023) and Chloroquine (NSC-187208). Cancer Chemother. Rep. 59:557, 1975.

74. Lackner, H.: Hemostatic abnormalities associated with dysproteinaemia. Semin. Hemat., 10:125, 1973.

75. Law, I.P., Koch, F.J., Cannon, G.B., Herbeman, R.B., and Oldham, R.K.: Acute myelomonocytic leukaemia associated with paraproteinaemia. Cancer 37:1359, 1976.

76. Lennert, K.: In: Malignant Lymphomas. Ed. K. Lennert., Springer-Verlag., p.211, 1978.

77. Ligorsky, R.D., Axelrod, A.R., Mandell, G.H., Palutke, M., and Prasad, A.S.: Acute myelomonocytic leukaemia in a patient with macroglobulinaemia and malignant lymphoma. Cancer 39:1156, 1977.

78. Lindström, F.D., and Dahlström, U.: Multiple myeloma or benign monoclonal gammopathy? A study of differential diagnostic criteria in 44 cases. Clin. Immunol. and Immunopath. 10:168, 1978.

79. Lindström, F.D., Hardy, W.B., Eberle, B.J., and Williams, R.C.: Multiple myeloma and benign monoclonal gammopathy. Differentiation by immunofluorescence of lymphocytes. Ann. Int. Med., 78:837, 1973.

80. McGrath, M.A., and Penny, R.: Paraproteinaemia—Blood hyperviscosity and clinical manifestations. J. Clin. Invest. 58:1155, 1976.

81. Mallick, N.P., Dosa, S., Acheson, E.J., Delamore, I.W., McFarlane, H., Seneviratne, C.J., and Williams, G.: Detection, significance and treatment of paraprotein in patients presenting with "Idiopathic" proteinuria without myeloma. Quart. J. Med., 45:145, 1978.
82. Mancilla, R., and Davis, G.L.: Non-secretory multiple myeloma. Am. J. Med., 63:1015, 1978.
83. Mellstedt, H., Björkholm, M., Ahre, A., Holm, G., Johnsson, B., and Strander, H.: Interferon therapy in myelomatosis. Lancet i:245, 1979.
84. Mellstedt, H., Hammarström, S., and Holm, G.: Monoclonal lymphocyte population in human plasma cell myeloma. Clin. Exp. Immunol., 17:371, 1974.
85. Mellstedt, H., Killander, D., and Pettersson N.D.: Bone marrow kinetic studies on three patients with myelomatosis. Acta. Med. Scand. 202:413, 1977.
86. Mestecky, J., Hammack, W.J., Kulhavy, R., Wright, G.P., and Tomana, M.: Properties of IgA myeloma proteins isolated from sera of patients with hyperviscosity syndrome. J. Lab. Clin. Med., 89:919, 1977.
87. Meyer, J.E., and Schulz, M.D.: "Solitary" myeloma of bone. A review of 12 cases. Cancer 34:438, 1974.
88. Meytes, D., Seligsohn, U., and Ramot, B.: Multiple myeloma with terminal erythroleukaemia. Acta. Haemat., 55:358, 1976.
89. Monta, L.E., and Ramanan, S.V.: Recurrent pulmonary embolism. A sign of multiple myeloma. JAMA 233:1192, 1975.
90. Morell, A., Maurer, W., Skvaril, F., and Barundun, S., Differentiation between benign and malignant monoclonal gammopathies by discriminant analysis on serum and bone marrow parameters. Acta. Haemat. 60:129, 1978.
91. Mundy, G.R., Raisz, L.G., Cooper, R.A., Schechter, G.P., and Salmon, S.E.: Evidence for the secretion of an osteoclast stimulating factor in myeloma. New Eng. J. Med., 291:1041, 1974.
92. Nilsson, K., Killander, D., Killander, J., and Mellstedt, H.: Short term tissue culture of two non-secretory human myelomas. Scand. J. Immunol. 5:819, 1976.
93. Nørgaard, O.: Three cases of multiple myeloma in which the preclinical asymptomatic phases persisted throughout 15–24 years. Brit. J. Cancer 25: 417, 1971.
94. Oldham, R.K., and Polmar, S.H.: Extramedullary plasmacytomas following successful radiotherapy of Hodgkin's disease. Amer. J. Med., 261:100, 1973.
95. Paglieroni, T., and Mackenzie, M.R.: Studies on the pathogenesis of an immune defect in multiple myeloma. J. Clin. Invest., 59:1120, 1977.
96. Paine, C.J., Richardson, J.V., and Eichner, E.R.: Diverse clinical expression of multiple myeloma—atypical presentations. Am. J. Med., 267:99, 1974.
97. Pankovich, A.M., and Griem, M.C.: Plasma cell myeloma. A thirty year follow up. Radiology. 104:521, 1972.
98. Parker, A.C.: A case of acute myelomonocytic leukaemia associated with myelomatosis. Scand. J. Haemat., 11:257, 1973.
99. Pasmantier, M.W., and Azar, H.A.: Extraskeletal spread in multiple myeloma. Cancer 23:167, 1969.
100. Perkins, H.A., Mackenzie, M.R., and Fudenberg, H.H.: Hemostatic defects in dysproteinaemias. Blood 35:695, 1970.
101. Powles, R., Smith, C., Kohn, J., and Hamilton Fairley, G.: Method of removing abnormal protein rapidly from patients with malignant paraproteinaemias. B.M.J. iii:664, 1971.
102. Preston, F.E., Cooke, K.B., Foster, M.E., Winfield, D.A., and Lee, D.: Myelo-

matosis and the hyperviscosity syndrome. B.J. Haemat., 38:517, 1978.

103. Preston, F.E., and Ward, A.M.: Acute renal failure in myelomatosis from intravascular coagulation. B.M.J., 1:604, 1972.

104. Preud'Homme, J-L., Hurez, D., Danon, F., Brouet, J.C., and Seligmann, M.: Intracytoplasmic and surface-bound immunoglobulins in 'nonsecretory' and Bence-Jones myeloma. Clin. Exp. Immunol., 25:428, 1976.

105. Preud'Homme, J-L., Labaume, S., and Seligmann, M.: Idiotype-bearing and antigen binding receptors produced by blood T-lymphocytes in a case of human myeloma. Eur. J. Immunol., 7:840, 1977.

106. Preud'Homme, J-L., and Seligmann, M., Immunoglobulins on the surface of lymphoid cells in Waldenström's macroglobulinaemia. J. Clin. Inv., 51:701, 1972.

107. Randall, R.E., Williamson, W.C., Mullinax, F., Tung, M.Y., and Still, W.J.S.: Manifestations of systemic light chain deposition. Am. J. Med., 60:293, 1976.

108. Resegotti, L., Palestro, G., Coda, R., Dolci, C., Poggio, E., and Leonardo, E.: Waldenström like immunocytic lymphoma with IgG serum in component. Acta. Haemat., 58:38, 1977.

109. River, G.L., Tewksbury, D.A., and Fudenberg, H.H.: "Non-secretory" multiple myeloma. Blood 40:204, 1972.

110. Roberts-Thompson, P., Mason, D.Y., and MacLennan, I.C.M.: Paraprotein polymerisation in IgA myelomatosis. B.J. Haemat., 33:117, 1976.

111. Rosner, F., and Grünwald, H.: Multiple myeloma terminating in acute leukamia. Am. J. Med., 57:927, 1974.

112. Sakurabayashi, I., Kin, K., and Tadashi, K.: Human IgA, half-molecules: Clinical and immunologic features in a patient with multiple myeloma. Blood 53:269, 1979.

113. Schubert, G.E., Veigel, J., and Lennert, K.: Structure and function of the kidney in multiple myeloma. Virchow Arch. (Path. Anat.), 355:135, 1972.

114. Seligmann, M.: Alpha chain disease. J. Clin. Path. 28 Suppl., 6:72, 1974.

115. Smith, L.E., and Powles, T.J.: Mithramycin for hypercalcaemia associated with myeloma and other malignancies. B.M.J., 1:268, 1975.

116. Speigelberg, H.L.: Human myeloma IgG half-molecules. Catabolism and biological properties. J. Clin. Invest., 56:588, 1975.

117. Spiegelberg, H.L., and Fishkin, B.G.: Human myeloma IgA half-molecules. J. Clin. Invest. 58:1259, 1976.

118. Spriggs, A.I., Holt, J.M., and Bedford, J.: Duplication of part of the long arm of chromosome 1 in marrow cells of a treated case of myelomatosis. Blood 48:595, 1976.

119. Stamp. T.C.B., Child, J.A., and Walker, P.G.: Treatment of osteolytic myelomatosis with mithramycin. Lancet i:719, 1975.

120. Stavem, P., Frøland, S.S., and Haugen, H.F.: Non-secretory myelomatosis without intracellular immunoglobulin. Scand. J. Haem., 17:89, 1976.

121. Stavem, P., Hovig, T., Frøland, S., and Skrede, S.: Immunoglobulin-containing inclusions in plasma cells in a case of IgG myeloma. Scand. J. Haematol., 13:266, 1974.

122. Taddeini, L., and Schrader, W.: Concomitant myelomonocytic leukaemia and multiple myeloma Minn Med 55:446, 1972.

123. Taylor, C.R., and Mason, D.Y.: The immunohistological detection of intracellular immunoglobulins in formalin paraffin sections from multiple myeloma and related conditions using the immunoperoxidase technique. Clin. Exp. Immunol. 18:417, 1974.

124. Tuddenham, E.G.D., and Bradley, J.: Plasma volume expansion and increased serum viscosity in myeloma and macroglobulinaemia. Clin. Exp. Immunol., 16:169, 1974.
125. Tursz, T., Brouet, J-C., Flandrin, G., Danon, F., Clauvel, J-P., and Seligmann, M.: Clinical and pathologic features of Waldenström's macroglobulinaemia and seven patients with serum monoclonal IgG and IgA. Am. J. Med., 63:499, 1977.
126. Tursz, T., Flandrin, G., Briere, J., and Seligmann, M.: Simultaneous occurrence of acute myeloblastic leukaemia and multiple myeloma without previous chemotherapy. B.M.J., 1:642, 1974.
127. Unander-Scharin, L., Waldenström, J.G., and Zettervall, O.: Surgical treatment of myelomatosis—A review of 18 cases. Acta. Med. Scand. 203:265, 1978.
128. Van Camp, B.G.K., Shuit, R.E., Hijmans, W., and Radl, J.: The cellular basis of double paraproteinaemia in man. Clin. Immunol. and Immunopath., 9:111, 1977.
129. Videbaek, A.: Unusual cases of myelomatosis Brit. Med. J., ii:326, 1971.
130. Virella, G., Preto, V., and Graca, F.: Polymerized monoclonal IgA in two patients with myelomatosis and hyperviscosity syndrome. Brit. J. Haemat., 30:479, 1975.
131. Warner, T.F.C.S., and Krueger, R.G.: Circulating lymphocytes and the spread of myeloma. Lancet 1:1174, 1978.
132. Whicher, J.T., Davies, J.D., and Greyburn, J.A.: Intact and fragmented intracellular immunoglobulin in a case of non-secretory myeloma. J. Clin. Path., 28:54, 1975.
133. Zilko, P.J., and Dawkins, L.: Amyloidosis associated with dermatomyositis and features of multiple myeloma. Am. J. Med., 59:448, 1975.
134. Zlotnik, A., and Rosenmann, E.: Renal pathologic findings associated with monoclonal gammopathies. Arch. Int. Med., 135:40, 1975.
135. Zwaan, F.E., Den Ottolander, G.J., Brederoo, P., Van Zwet, Th.L., Te Velde, J., and Willemze, R.: The morphology of dyserthropoiesis in a patient with acute erythroleukaemia associated with multiple myeloma. Scand. J. Haemat., 17:353, 1976.

20. IMMUNOBLASTIC LYMPHOMA ARISING IN ANGIOIMMUNOBLASTIC LYMPHADENOPATHY*

B.N. NATHWANI, H. RAPPAPORT, G. PANGALIS, E.M. MORAN AND H. KIM

Angioimmunoblastic lymphadenopathy (AILD) (4, 5) or immunoblastic lymphadenopathy (7) is a systemic disease clinically characterized by fever, generalized lymphadenopathy, and hepatosplenomegaly. Polyclonal hypergammaglobulinemia, and Coombs' positive hemolytic anemia are frequently present.

AILD (4, 5, 9, 12) is similar but not identical to immunoblastic lymphadenopathy (7). AILD differs from malignant lymphomas clinically by the high frequency of constitutional symptoms, generalized lymph node enlargement, hepatosplenomegaly, cutaneous manifestations, and polyclonal hypergammaglobulinemia at the time of clinical onset. Histoligically, AILD is characterized by obliteration of the architecture; small-vessel proliferation; a proliferation of small, mature lymphocytes, plasma cells, and immunoblasts which are scattered throughout the involved tissue without forming cohesive clusters or masses; and the presence of an eosinophilic intercellular material which is generally PAS-positive. Similar clinical and histologic observations have been described and reported under other designations (3, 11, 14).

Based on the study of our first group of 24 patients (4, 5), AILD was considered as a nonneoplastic disorder, a view also expressed for immunoblastic lymphadenopathy (7, 11). However, progression of both AILD (2, 10, 15) and immunoblastic lymphadenopathy (4, 7, 13) into immunoblastic lymphoma has been reported. For this reason we were particularly interested in establishing histologic criteria that would allow us to recognize the evolution of maligant lymphoma in lymph nodes exhibiting features of AILD.

Eighty-four cases of AILD with and without histologic features of IL were studied; 42 of these were interpreted as AILD, 36 as AILD plus immunoblastic lymphoma (AILD + IL), and six as AILD in an initial (diagnostic) biopsy and as AILD + IL in follow-up biopsies (8). Analysis of the histologic

* This work was supported by Grant R10 CA 18044 and 1 T32 CA 09308 awarded by the National Cancer Institute, National Institutes of Health, Department of Health, Education, and Welfare, and by Hematopathology Tutorials, Inc.

Table 1. Evolution of disease in 10 patients with AILD + IL who had a follow-up biopsy and at autopsy.

Pt.	Findings in first LN biopsy	Interval between biopsies (months)	Findings in follow-up biopsy*	Interval between last biopsy and death (months)	Autopsy
R.J.	AILD + IL clusters, islands	1	IL diffuse	1	AILD
C.O.	AILD + IL clusters**	2	IL diffuse	4	AILD + IL (LN, spleen) islands
E.L.	AILD + IL clusters, islands, clear cells	2	IL diffuse (splenectomy)	6	Not done
G.P.	AILD + IL clusters	3½	IL diffuse	1	IL (LN) diffuse
M.L.	AILD + IL clusters, clear cells	5	IL diffuse	4	IL (LN) diffuse
A.C.	AILD + IL clusters, diffuse	9½	IL diffuse (splenectomy)	½	IL (LN)
F.B.	AILD + IL clusters, islands	16	IL diffuse	2	AILD + IL (LN, BM) islands
A.Y.	AILD + IL clusters	2½	Il clusters, islands, diffuse	2	Not done
J.D.	AILD + IL clusters, diffuse	9	AILD + IL, clusters, diffuse	2	IL (LN) diffuse
L.G.	AILD + IL clusters	2½	AILD	1	IL (LN) diffuse

*Of lymph nodes, except in patients A.C., and E.L.
**A lymph node biopsy obtained 214 months earlier had shown AILD only (Table 2).
LN: lymph node; BM: bone marrow.

features in the diagnostic and follow-up biopsies in some of these patients strongly suggested that the earliest phase of malignant progression can be recognized by the presence of transformed large lymphoid cells in clusters or islands (Table 1). The clusters may be of varying sizes and may be intra-vascular or extravascular. As the disease progresses, the clusters and islands become confluent to form diffuse monomorphic areas of large lymphoid cells with or without plasmacytoid features, and when this has taken place, the malignant lymphoma is readily diagnosable. Such progression was ob-served in eight of ten patients of AILD + IL in whom a second lymph node biopsy became available in the course of the patients' illness (Table 1).

To investigate the validity of our histologic criteria for malignancy, we compared 42 patients with AILD in one or more biopsies with 36 patients diagnosed AILD + IL on the basis of the first biopsy, with respect to (a) clinical features, (b) response to therapy, (c) survival, and (d) presence and extent of malignant lymphoma at autopsy (8). We found no differences in the clinical presentation between AILD and AILD + IL. Patients with AILD, however, tended to respond better to prednisone or to chemotherapy than patients with AILD (63%) and those with AILD + IL (26%) (p = 0.01). The differences in median survival were striking. The median survival of 42 patients who had AILD only was 35 months, whereas in the 36 patients who had AILD + IL in the first biopsy the median survival was 6 months. (p = 0.0004). Malignant lymphoma was evident at autopsy in two of 10 patients (20%) in the AIL group, in contrast to 18 of 22 patients (82%) in the AILD + IL group (p = >0.005). Extranodal involvement by malignant lymphoma at autopsy was observed in only one patient (10%) with AILD, whereas it was seen in 14 patients (64%) with AILD + IL, (p = <0.025) (8).

Spontaneous clinical remission lasting longer than six months and consisting of regression of lymph node enlargement and the disappearance of clinical symptoms occurred in four patients with AILD and in three patients with AILD + IL. Of the four patients with AILD, two are alive and well 50 and 56 months, respectively, after onset of the disease. One patient died from pneunomia 45 months after onset of the disease, and at autopsy no evidence of AILD or IL was found. The fourth patient had a repeat biopsy after 60 months, revealing AILD + IL, and died 10 months therafter. Of the patients with AILD + IL, one is alive without relapse 44 months after diagnosis, and one previously reported as being alive and well 12 months after diagnosis (8) has had a relapse with involvement of the central nervous system eight months later. One patient had a relapse after nine months and died two months later.

Of 13 patients with AILD who had second lymph node biopsies after 2–214 months, the follow-up biopsies showed evidence of malignant lymphoma in six (Table 2). This tends to indicate that malignant lymphoma may develop in patients with AILD after latent periods of unpredictable duration. The four long-term spontaneous remissions in AILD would be consistent with the histologically benign appearance of the disease. The spontaneous remission in the patient with AILD + IL without relapse is not readily explained but could be attributed to either of the following possibilities: the removed tissue may have contained only focus of tumor in the host, or the total tumor cell mass outside the removed tissues may have been still small enough to be controlled by the immunological defenses of the host (8).

We were interested in correlating the functional activity of the plasma cells and that of large lymphoid cells (immunoblasts) by demonstrating cytoplasmic immunoglobulins in tissue sections by the peroxidase-antiperoxidase (PAP) method. We found in all cases tested, that the plasma cell

Table 2. Evolution of AILD to malignant lymphoma, as seen in follow-up biopsies and at autopsy.

Pt.	Findings in 1st biopsy	Interval between biopsies	Findings in 2nd biopsy	Interval between 2nd biopsy and death (months)	Autopsy
V.R.	AILD	2	AILD + IL islands, diffuse	8	IL (LN, BM, spleen, liver, kidney, lung thyroid) diffuse
H.F.	AILD	4½	Il diffuse	3	IL (LN, liver, kidney) diffuse
O.S.	AILD	5	AILD + IL islands, clear cells	14	Not done
R.J.	AILD	48	IL diffuse	3	AILD + IL (Skin) diffuse
R.L.	AILD	60	IL diffuse	10	Not done
C.O.	AILD	214	AILD + IL clusters	6	AILD + IL (LN, spleen) islands

LN: lymph node; BM: bone marrow.

population was polyclonal. In approximately half of these, scattered immunoblasts in the AILD areas showed both light chains as well as the heavy chains corresponding to those observed in the plasma cells in the same sections. In the remaining cases, only the plasma cells, and not the immunoblasts, contained immunoglobulin (Table 3) (8).

Table 3. Results of immunoperoxidase reaction in 32 patients with AILD + IL.

	Immunoglobulin chains demonstrated by monospecific antisera		
	Plasma cells	Immunoblasts in AILD areas	Immunoblasts in IL areas
Light chains (LC)	32, κ, λ	18 κ, λ 14 no LC	5 κ, λ 27 no LC
Heavy chains (HC)	18 α, γ, μ	6 α, γ, μ 7 α, γ 5 no HC	2 α, γ, μ 16 no HC
	9 α, γ	4 α, γ 1 γ 4 no HC	2 α, γ 7 no HC
	2 α, μ	2 no HC	2 no HC
	1 α	1 no HC	1 no HC
	2 no HC	2 no HC	2 no HC

The ultrastructural finding in some of these cases showed that many of the large lymphoid cells had abundant polyribosomes but no rough endoplasmic reticulum. This is in keeping with the absence of demonstrable immunoglobulin in most of the neoplastic cells by the PAP method (Table 4). Whether this indicates neoplastic dedifferentiation or lack of plasmacytic differentiation is not clear at this time. However, it is of great interest that in those cases in which clusters or islands were a prominent feature, all or most of the component cells of these clusters or islands were negative for immunoglobulins, although the scattered immunoblasts in the rest of the node contained them. This suggests a functional difference between the immunoblasts inside and outside the clusters or islands. However, in five instances in which immunoglobulin could be detected in areas of IL, it was usually in the diffuse monomorphic areas and the immunoblastic proliferation proved to be polyclonal (8).

It would have been interesting to learn in a larger series of cases whether evolution of immunoblastic lymphoma could in any way be related to changes in the serum immunoelectroporetic pattern. We were unable to establish a definite correlation between changes in serum immunoglobulin levels and the evolution of immunoblastic lymphoma. However, in seven of 14 patients with AILD + IL, in whom follow-up serum immunoglobulin determinations were available, the immunoglobulin levels decreased

Table 4. Correlation of ultrastructural findings with light microscopic and immunoperoxidase findings.

Patient	Light microscopy	Immunoperoxidase for immunoglobulin chains in large lymphoid cells	Ultrastructure
R.J.	Monomorphic IL (large lymphoid cells with plasmacytoid features)	Negative	Rare rough endoplasmic reticulum, not dilated. abundant polysomes
A.C.	Polymorphic IL (large lymphoid cells with plasmacytoid features and plasma cells)	Negative	Rare enough endoplasmic reticulum, not dilated. Abundant polysomes
G.P.	Monomorphic IL (large lymphoid cells with plasmacytoid features)	Positive for κ, λ, α, γ	Occasional rough endoplasmic reticulum, rarely dilated with immunoglobulin. Abundant polysomes

Table 5. Follow-up serum immunoglobulin (Ig) levels in 14 patients with AILD + IL.

Initial Ig	No. of patients	Follow-up Ig	No. of patients
Polyclonal hypergammaglobulinemia	11	Essentially no change	3*
		Increase of polyclonal hypergammaglobulinemia	2
		Decrease of Ig to normal	1
		Hypogammaglobulinemia	5
Normal	3	Normal Ig	2
		Hypogammaglobulinemia	1

*In one patient, IgG decreased from 3980 mg% to 2420 MG%. IgA remained about the same (610 vs, 565 mg%), and IgM increased from 350 mg% to 740 mg%.

during the course of the disease, and in six patients, hypogammaglobulinemia developed (Table 5). This could suggest that as the functioning plasma cells and large lymphoid cells of AILD are replaced by a neoplastic immunoblastic population, the capacity for forming immunoglobulin diminishes and hypogammaglobulinemia may ensue. In two patients, the serum immunoglobulin levels increased, suggesting an increase in the immunoglobulin-producing cell mass (8).

REFERENCES

1. Fisher, R.I., Jaffe, E.S., Braylan, R.C., Andersen, J.C., and Tan, H.K.: Immunoblastic lymphadenopathy. Evolution into a malignant lymphoma with plasmacytoid features. Am. J. Med., 61:553–559, 1976.
2. Flandrin, G.: Adénopathies angio-immunoblastiques avec anémie auto-immune et hyperimmunoglobulinémie polyclonale. Nouv. Presse Med., 5:1521–1524, 1976.
3. Flandrin, G., Daniel, M.T., El Yafi, G., and Chelloul, N.: Sarcomatoses ganglionnaires diffuses a différenciation plasmocytaire avec anémie hémolytique auto-immune. Acutual. Hematol. (Paris), 6:25–41, 1972.
4. Frizzera, G., Moran, E.M., and Rappaport, H.: Angio-immunoblastic lymphadenopathy with dysproteinaemia. Lancet, i:1070–1073, 1974.
5. Frizzera, G., Moran, E.M., and Rappaport, H.: Angio-immunoblastic lymphadenopathy. Diagnosis and clinical course. Am. J. Med., 59:803–818, 1975.
6. Howarth, C.B., and Bird, C.C.: Immunoblastic sarcoma arising in child with immunoblastic lymphadenopathy. Lancet, ii:747–748, 1976.
7. Lukes, R.J., and Tindle, B.H.: Immunoblastic lymphadenopathy. A hyperimmune entity resembling Hodgkin's disease. N. Engl. J. Med., 292:2–8, 1975.
8. Nathwani, B.N., Rappaport, H., Moran, E.M., Pangalis, G.A., and Kim, H.: Malignant lymphoma arising in angioimmunoblastic lymphadenopathy. Cancer, 41:578–606, 1978.
9. Pangalis, G.A., Moran, E.M., and Rappaport, H.: Blood and bone marrow find-

ings in angioimmunoblastic lymphadenopathy. Blood, 51:71–83, 1978.

10. Pruzanski, W., Sutton, D.M.C., and Pantalony, D.: Angioimmunoblastic lymphadenopathy: An immunochemical study. Clin. Immunol. Immunopathol., 6:62–76, 1976.

11. Radaszkiewicz, T., and Lennert, K.: lymphogranulomatosis X. Klinisches Bild, Therapie und Prognose. Dtsch. Med. Wochenschr., 100:1157–1163, 1975.

12. Rappaport, H., and Moran, E.M.: Angio-immunoblastic (immunoblastic) lymphadenopathy. N. Eng. J. Med., 292:42–43, 1975.

13. Toth, J., and Garam, T.: Immunoblastic lymphadenopathy proceeding to sarcoma. Lancet, i:102, 1977.

14. Westerhausen, M., and Oehlert, W.: Chronisches pluripotentielles immunoproliferatives Syndrom. Dtsch. Med. Wochenschr., 97:1407–1413, 1972.

15. Yataganas, X., Papdimitriou, C., Pangalis, C., Loukopoulos, D., Fessas, Ph., and Papacharalampous, N.: Angio-immunoblastic lymphadenopathy terminating as Hodgkin's disease. Cancer, 39:2183–2189, 1977.

21. INTERRELATIONS OF B-CELL NEOPLASMS

C. R. TAYLOR

INTRODUCTION

In the accompanying paper "Changing Concepts in the Classification of Lymphoma" (this volume) it was argued that pathologists, in attempting to identify and classify lymphomas, continue to follow the basic precepts of Mallory and Willis, that "there occur tumours corresponding to almost all kinds of normal tissues; ... clearly our classification of tumours will run parallel with our classification of normal tissues" (35).

It follows that our concepts of the interrelations of different histological forms of lymphoma depend upon our concepts of the nature and interrelations of the normal cells from which the lymphomas are believed to be derived. Thus four common neoplastic processes, namely chronic lymphocytic leukemia (and small lymphocytic lymphoma "well differentiated" as the tissue manifestation), follicular center cell lymphoma, immunoblastic sarcoma (previously designated reticulum cell sarcoma or histiocytic lymphoma) and multiple myeloma/plasmacytoma, that clearly are separable in terms of morphology and behavior, were believed to be of separate lineage on the basis of their supposed derivation from four distinct cell types, the circulating small lymphocyte, the follicular center cell, the immunoblast and the plasma cell.

The immunological approaches outlined elsewhere in this monograph, have profoundly influenced current thinking regarding the interrelations of these four cell types, leading naturally to a radical revision of concepts of the interrelations of the corresponding neoplasms.

In essence the whole problem stands or falls with one question, "Is there any justification for believing that B-cell CLL, follicular center cell lymphoma, B-cell immunoblastic sarcoma and multiple myeloma are derived from our separate cells of origin?" The evidence of basic immunology suggests that there is not, for the progenitor cells of these neoplasms appear to be of common lineage.

IMPLICATIONS OF AN IMMUNE-BASED CLASSIFICATION

If B-cell CLL (and malignant lymphoma lymphocytic well differentiated), follicular center cell lymphomas, B-immunoblastic sarcoma and multiple

J.G. van den Tweel et al. (eds.), Malignant Lymphoproliferative Diseases, 281–293
All rights reserved.
Copyright © 1980 by Martinus Nijhoff Publishers bv, The Hague/Boston/London.

myeloma are all in fact manifestations of neoplasia of a single cell family, how is it that they are morphologically so diverse and so different in behavior? The beginning of a rational explanation may be found by reference to the principles of cellular immunology. This does not involve complete abandonment of traditional histologic criteria, but it does require us to view some of the traditional histological approaches in a somewhat different light.

It has been postulated that neoplastic lymphocytes may mimic the morphology and behavior of the normal lymphocyte population from which they are derived. The results of the immunologic studies described in this volume are best considered in conjunction with four principal facets of normal lymphocyte behavior and function that may be expressed, to a greater or lesser degree, by neoplastic lymphocytes:

(1) The functional separation of lymphocytes into B cells and T cells;
(2) The morphological and behavioral changes occurring in lymphocyte transformation;
(3) Lymphocyte circulation;
(4) Lymphocyte homing.

The functional division into T cells and B cells: translation into morphology

The division of malignant lymphomas into B- or T-cell functional subtypes was proposed in the initial classification of Lukes and Collins (16). Subsequent application of surface marker techniques to the study of lymphoproliferative disease in man has confirmed the essence of this proposal, and has contributed to a clearer clinical and morphologic definition of B- and T-cell lymphocytic neoplasms (11, 14, 17, 18, 26).

Normal B and T lymphocytes cannot be distinguished reliably by morphological criteria, but only by surface marker methods. It might be expected that the corresponding neoplastic cells of B- or T-cell type might also be indistinguishable by morphology alone. However, in examining neoplastic cells by light microscopy, one assesses and compares cell populations rather than individual cells. On this basis there appear to be some valid distinctions between certain B and T cell neoplasms.

The distinguishing morphological features of the B lymphocyte in the follicular center phase of its life cycle were the first to be clearly recognized (12, 13, 15), and the morphologic recognition of follicular center cell lymphomas in fact preceded more comprehensive B and T-cell subclassifications of lymphoma. Two principal morphologic forms of follicular center cells were recognized. They were termed germinocytes and germinoblasts (later amended to centrocytes and centroblasts) by Lennert and colleagues (13, 14), or cleaved and noncleaved cells by Lukes and Collins (15, 16). These terms may be regarded as equivalent for the cell types they represent, but not for the corresponding lymphomas, since the lymphomas are defined on the basis of differing cellular composition in the two classification schemes (see Table 1 in "Changing Concepts in the Classification of Lymphoma" in this volume).

Several other B and T cell lymphomas have since been distinguished by surface marker techniques, but are more difficult to identify by morphology alone. Distinctive morphological features (convoluted cell type) were ascribed to an aggressive lymphoma/leukaemia particularly prevalent in young males and presenting as a mediastianal mass, as lymphadenopathy, or as acute lymphocytic leukaemia (1). The characteristic convoluted nuclear morphology has been observed in a varying proportion of cells, with varying degrees of difficulty by different observers, according to the precise criteria employed (21). Cases of this pathological entity are now accepted, on the basis of surface marker studies, as being of T-lymphocytic origin (11, 17, 18).

Tumors composed of neoplastic plasma cells, or of cells showing evidence of "plasmacytoid" differentiation can be recognized with some confidence, as belonging to the B-cell series. Lymphocytic plasmacytic lymphoma or lymphoplasmacytoid lymphoma (immunocytoma), being in part the morphologic expression of Waldenström's disease, is an example of such a lymphoma. Cases show B-cell surface markers and contain or secrete monoclonal cytoplasmic immunoglobulin, mostly of IgM class. Multiple myeloma, though a neoplasm of plasma cells, and thus closely related to other B lymphomas in a developmental sense, has, by tradition, been excluded from most lymphoma classifications, even those which purport to be based on immunologic principles. Clinical and behavioral differences notwithstanding, myeloma clearly should be considered in relation to the other lymphocyte-derived neoplasms, for the plasma cell is nothing more than a highly specialized B lymphocyte. Similarly, a place should be found for plasmacytoma, representing a plasma cell neoplasm occurring in an extramedullary situation.

Finally, with regard to B-cell lymphoma/T-cell lymphoma and their distinction by morphology, there is growing evidence that immunoblastic sarcoma is divisible into B- and T-cell subtypes. This condition, that previously passed under the terms reticulum cell sarcoma (24) or malignant lymphoma histiocytic (23), appears to represent the neoplastic analogue of the transformed lymphocyte (see below). Surface marker and immunoperoxidase studies have revealed a B- and T-cell subdivision of tumors of this basic morphologic type, and have led to the recognition of several morphological criteria for distinguishing B-immunoblastic sarcoma from T-immunoblastic sarcoma in most cases (18, 25, 30, 31). In making this distinction the finding of "plasmacytoid" features in the neoplastic cells is the strongest morphologic indicator of a B-cell origin.

The morphological changes associated with lymphocyte transformation

Formerly the small lymphocyte was regarded as a quiescent end stage cell. Its potential for radical morphological and functional changes following antigenic stimulation was revealed in the process of lymphocyte transformation, and the small B lymphocyte was recognized as the precursor of the plasma cell series (review (22). In fact, following specific antigenic stimulation, B lymphocytes bearing immunoglobulin receptors undergo metamorphosis to large transformed lymphocytes (or immunoblasts) (6) prior to maturation to the plasma cell (Figure 1). These large transformed lymphocytes (immunoblasts) have no morphological resemblance to the lymphocytes from which they are derived. Prior to the advent of cellular immunology, these large primitive-appearing cells (immunoblasts) were considered to constitute a class entirely separate from lymphocytes and were regarded as variants of reticulum cells or histiocytes. Thus the malignant counterparts of these cells formerly were designated as either reticulum cell sarcoma or

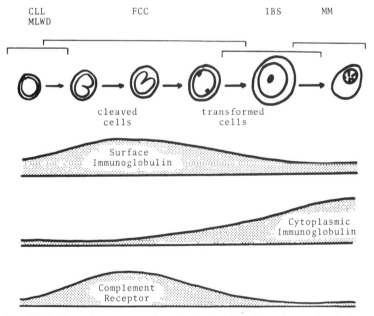

Figure 1. Simplified schematic representation of principal B-cell lymphomas in relation to the process of B-lymphocyte transformation (including the follicular center stage) and maturation to the plasma cell. Variations in the expression of surface immunoglobulin, cytoplasmic immunoglobulin and complement receptor are indicated by the shaded areas. The neoplastic cells mimic the morphology and behavior of their normal counterparts (from Taylor (29).

malignant lymphoma histiocytic (28, 30, 32). However, using immunological marker methods, these cells may now be recognized as transformed B or T lymphocytes (27, 14, 17, 18, 26, 11). The corresponding neoplasms are thus properly termed immunoblastic sarcomas, and further can be subdivided into B or T-cell subtypes as described above.

The different morphological types of lymphoma can be related to this transformation-maturation process according to the concept that neoplastic lymphocytes mimic the morphology and behavior of their corresponding normal counterparts (this is illustrated for the B-cell series in Figure 1). Thus small lymphocytic lymphoma, follicular center cell lymphoma, immunoblastic sarcoma, and plasmacytoma/myeloma can now be seen to be various expressions of neoplasms of a single cell type, the B lymphocyte, rather than four entirely distinct neoplasms as implied by earlier classification schemes. This is not to imply that morphological distinctions between these neoplasms are valueless, for there are real differences in clinical behavior which influence the prognosis and the choice of therapy. However, it may ultimately be of more value to both pathologist and clinician to recognize the essential common origin of these four neoplasms, realizing that intermediate forms may occur, rather than to continue to consider these diseases to be entirely separate processes. In many respects this concept returns to the "fluid lymphoma" school of Willis and others:

I join Warthin, Ginsburg, Herbut et al., and others, who regard all lymphoid tumours as related variants of one disease.... The names used for the principal variants have descriptive and clinical value but do not denote distinct pathological entities.

While many tumours fall into one or another (of these main diagnostic groups) they show all possible combinations and transitions. These will cause us perplexity only if we allow the names of our (four) main subgroups to assume the status of distinct species (35).

The radical differences in histological appearance between the four B-cell tumors listed above may then be explained on the basis of a predominance of one or another of the different morphological variants of the B lymphocyte. This concept is illustrated in Figure 2.

A similar scheme to that proposed above may be prepared for the T-cell lymphomas, taking account of the transformation of the small T lymphocyte to the T immunoblast. However, the product of T lymphocyte transformation, namely the sensitized effector T cell, is not distinguishable on morphologic grounds from the small T cell prior to transformation. In addition, a further complication in defining the various stages of T-cell transformation is the lack of a good immunological or immunohistological marker in the

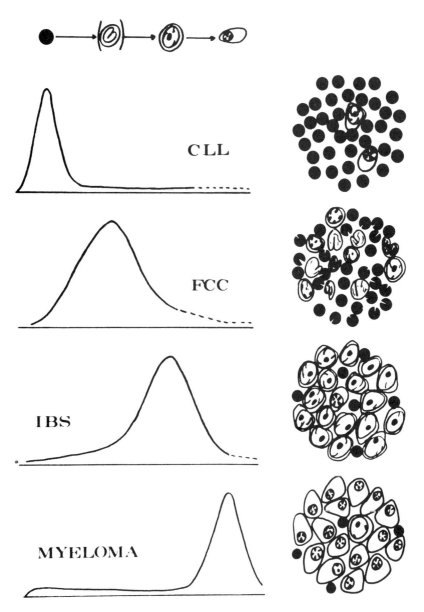

Figure 2. Interrelations of B-cell neoplasms. Schematic depicts four morphologically diverse B-cell neoplasms as composed of the same three basic morphologic forms of the B cell, namely the small lymphocyte, the immunoblast and the plasma cell, illustrated at the top of the figure as morphologic phases in B cell transformation/maturation (Figure 1). The different histologic pictures are produced simply by changes in the proportions of the different forms of the B cell within the neoplastic clone. FCC lymphoma forms a partial exception in that special variants of the B cell (the follicular center cells), representing intermediate stages of B-cell transformation in the follicle, are also present. CLL = chronic lymphocytic leukaemia/small lymphocytic lymphoma; FCC = follicular center cell lymphoma; IBS = immunoblastic sarcoma (B-cell type).

T-cell series, corresponding to surface or cytoplasmic immunoglobulin in the B-cell series.

Monoclonality and monomorphism

Neoplasms are conventionally regarded as monoclonal proliferations. The evidence of immunologic studies supports this contention for the vast majority (if not all) of the lymphomas. Neoplastic (monoclonal) populations have traditionally been regarded as having a uniform morphologic aspect; this monomorphous appearance serves as one of the keystones of histological diagnosis of neoplasia within the lymphoid system. With reference to lymphomas, and possibly to other neoplasms, these last assumptions represent a false strain of logic.

For example, in multiple myeloma, a neoplasm of "plasma cells", it has generally been assumed that the neoplasm proliferates by division of the characteristic malignant cells, i.e. malignant plasma cell begets malignant plasma cell. Yet normal plasma cells do not proliferate to give other normal plasma cells; plasma cells are derived from small lymphocytes by the process of B-lymphocyte transformation. It thus seems more probable that neoplastic plasma cells are derived from neoplastic small lymphocytes by some parody of the normal process of transformation, in strict analogy to the origin of normal plasma cells. If this is so in myeloma, then the neoplastic clone is by definition not monomorphous, for it must include neoplastic small lymphocytes, neoplastic immunoblasts, and forms intermediate in morphology, as well as the neoplastic plasma cells that characterize the process morphologically. Attention to immunologic studies reveals that this is indeed the case and that in multiple myeloma, circulating small lymphocytes can be identified and shown with certainty to be part of the neoplastic clone by the use of anti-idiotype sera (19, 20), and immunoblasts and a range of forms intermediate between immunoblasts and plasma cells can be identified by immunohistologic methods (31).

Similarly, a wide range of morphologic forms within a single neoplastic clone can be identified by a combination of surface markers and immunohistologic methods in lymphocytic plasmacytic lymphoma, in lymphocytic lymphoma (well differentiated), in follicular center cell lymphoma, and in B-cell immunoblastic sarcoma. In each of these tumors almost the whole range of B-cell types appears to be represented (see "Immunoperoxidase Techniques in Lymphoma Research", Taylor, in this volume.) It can be seen that the histological classification of these neoplasms is based upon the apparent "monomorphism" of the predominating form of the neoplastic cell, and that minor populations of the neoplastic clone with different morphologic and behavioral features may exist, but are not usually recognized by the pathologist as part of the neoplastic process. This is illustrated diagrammatically in Figure 2.

The implications of the views illustrated in Figures 1 and 2 upon our understanding of the interrelations of B-cell lymphomas and upon the nature of composite lymphomas are therefore profound. With regard to composite umors, neoplasms formed of admixtures of CLL (lymphocytic lymphoma), follicular center cell lymphoma (including all of the histologic subtypes), immunoblastic sarcoma and myeloma/plasmacytoma, can no longer be regarded as being composed of two or more separate neoplastic processes, each of distinct cellular origin; rather these tumors should be regarded as simultaneous diverse expressions of a single neoplastic cell line (the B lymphocyte). In this respect it may be of more value to the clinician to know that he is dealing with different morphologic and behavioral expressions of a single neoplasm than with two or more completely separate malignant processes.

Lymphocyte circulation

The work of Gowans and Knight (9) demonstrated that small lymphocytes circulate extensively throughout the blood, lymph and peripheral lymphoid organs. The process of lymphocyte circulation appears to constitute an essential part of the function of the lymphocyte in the immune system (22). In the "resting" nonantigenically stimulated host the majority of the circulating lymphocytes have the morphological appearance of small lymphocytes. However, following antigenic stimulation, increased numbers of partially transformed cells enter the efferent lymph and hence the peripheral blood (10) and serve to disseminate the immune response to all the lymphoid tissues of the body.

Again, following the hypothesis that neoplastic lymphocytes mimic the behavior of their normal counterparts, it is possible to relate the clinico-pathological course of various lymphocytic neoplasms to the behavior of the corresponding normal lymphocyte types. For example, lymphocytic neoplasms composed primarily of small lymphocytes frequently show a large or even predominating circulating cell component and appear as chronic lymphocytic leukaemia. In other cases, a noncirculating cell component predominates and the disease manifests as lymphocytic lymphoma well differentiated, though in many cases examination of peripheral blood by surface marker methods reveals that part of the neoplastic clone is in fact circulating. In this respect, CLL and lymphocytic lymphoma may be regarded as two ends of a spectrum of disease with many intermediate expressions (2) depending upon the proportion of the neoplastic cells in the circulating phase.

A similar situation appears to exist in relation to acute lymphoblastic leukaemia (ALL) of childhood. Combined immunologic and morphologic studies reveal a continuous spectrum of disease from the overt leukaemic to the frankly lymphomatous (4, 34). Immunological studies show that the leukaemic forms are mostly nonmarking (null cell), while the lymphomas most often show B (small noncleaved, Burkitt-like) or T (convoluted lymphoblastic) cell markers. The position of the ALL cell (lymphoblast) in the transformation sequence shown in Figure 1 is unclear. It appears to represent an intermediate phase in the transformation process, either a regression to the early stages of lymphogenesis in the foetus or possibly simply the morphologic expression of a rapidly cycling cell (short cell cycle with rapid proliferation) with short G_1 and G_2, and with mitosis following almost immediately upon completion of S phase. Some would use the term "lymphoblast" to include not only null (nonmarking) cell ALL, but also convoluted leukaemia/lymphoma and the morphologically similar Burkitt (or Burkitt-like) lymphoma that less frequently shows leukaemic manifestations (see "Changing Concepts in the Classification of Lymphoma", Taylor, in this volume).

In follicular center cell lymphoma the great majority of the neoplastic cells are confined to the tissues. Nevertheless, examination of peripheral blood, using surface marker methods, has revealed that circulating lymphoma cells are present in a proportion of cases (7, 8); the circulating cells carry the same monoclonal immunoglobulin markers as shown by the tissue lymphoma cells. In some of these cases the circulating cell component is recognizable by morphological criteria (cleaved cells); in others not so.

In immunoblastic sarcoma and plasmacytoma/myeloma the predominant neoplastic cells, resembling the immunoblast or plasma cell respectively, are rarely detected in the circulation in a morphologically recognizable form. However, studied of idiotypic immunoglobulin markers in multiple myeloma (19, 20) have revealed that some cells of the neoplastic clone do in fact circulate, though these are not recognizable by morphologic criteria as they are cytologically indistinguishable from normal small lymphocytes (see above).

Thus with reference to certain B-cell lymphomas the overall disease presentation, as lymphoma or leukaemia, appears to be governed by the degree to which the neoplastic lymphocytes reproduce the behavior of their normal counterparts (circulation, homing, etc). However, as illustrated in Figure 2, not all of the neoplastic cells necessarily display the same morphologic and behavioral characteristics, and in many cases (e.g. myeloma and follicular center cell lymphoma) subpopulations of the neoplastic clone may manifest morphologic and behavioral attributes at variance with the predominant cell type upon which classification is based (30, 32).

Again, less evidence is available with reference to T-cell lymphomas, but in general small lymphocytes may manifest primarily as leukaemia, large immunoblastic neoplasms manifest primarily as lymphoma, and neoplasms of cells of intermediate type may present anywhere along the spectrum of lymphoma to leukaemia or may show mixed manifestations. These patterns of behavior correlate with those anticipated by analogy with the corresponding normal cell types.

Lymphocyte homing

Studies of lymphocyte depleted animals involving thymectomy, bursectomy, and a variety of lymphocyte reconstitution experiments, reveal not only that lymphocytes circulate, but also that B and T lymphocytes preferentially "home" to certain anatomical regions or zones within the peripheral lymphoid tissue (22). Thus within the lymph node, B lymphocytes particularly localize in follicular center cell areas (cortex), and T lymphocytes localize within the deep cortex (paracortex). Within the spleen the corresponding areas are the B-cell follicle and the periarteriolar lymphocyte sheath (T zone) (22). In addition, T lymphocytes show a propensity to localize within the superficial dermis.

The pattern of tissue involvement by B- or T-cell lymphocytic neoplasms may in many cases be more easily understood with reference to these normal patterns of B- and T-lymphocyte circulation and homing. Thus lymphomas of follicular center cells not surprisingly, form follicles, and the loss of obvious follicle formation, as occurs in diffuse follicular center cell lymphomas, might then be interpreted as giving evidence of some loss of functional differentiation. T-cell lymphocytic neoplasms appear particularly to involve the paracortical areas of the lymph node (T-zone lymphoma, Lennert) (14, 26), or when composed of small T lymphocytes with a prominent circulating component, often seem also to involve the skin (Sézary syndrome, T-cell CLL) (3).

CONCLUSIONS

Lymphocytic neoplasms may best be understood by reference to the behavior of the corresponding normal lymphocyte (30, 32). This is not a novel idea, and in fact represents nothing more than the application to lymphocytic neoplasms of principles applied to neoplasia in general (35).

Chronic lymphocytic lymphoma, follicular center cell lymphomas, immunoblastic sarcoma and myeloma are neoplastic derivatives of the B lymphocyte. Their diverse morphologic, immunologic and behavioral aspects are not reflections of different cellular origins, but rather are expressions of variations in morphology and behavior that occur in the normal B lymphocyte during development and maturation. "There is only one B-cell lymphoma—but there are many variations on the theme" (30).

This is nothing new for we return to Custer (5): "Malignant lymphoma appears to be a single neoplastic process having a multiplicity of histological patterns. The pattern may be a static one; . . . frequently it is a changing one, and two or more patterns may exist in the same patient, even in the same tumor mass."

Recognition of the morphologic diversity within the malignant lymphomas, even in those that superficially appear quite monomorphous, should allow us to make a more reasonable interpretation of the histologic findings in lymphoma. The finding of cases that do not fit exactly with the rigid morphologic framework of existing classification schemes should evoke no surprise, for all constitute a spectrum of disease, and the morphologic divisions are but arbitrary divisions of convenience.

In remains for us to study critically those features that appear to be direct predictors of the behavior of the neoplasm—for example, the number of transformed cells (immunoblasts and lymphoblasts) that serve as the most direct indicators of the bahavior of the neoplastic population. Thus far such direct parameters of the behavior of neoplastic cell populations have largely been lost in the complexities of morphologic classification, though they in fact form part of the basis for such classification schemes. It may now be possible to examine the clinicopathologic correlation of some of these parameters more directly. Knowing the morphology of a lymphocytic neoplasm, it is becoming possible to predict the probable pattern of nodal involvement, whether or not it is like to circulate (leukaemia), whether or not it is a rapidly proliferating tumour (the proportion of transformed lymphocytes), and whether it is of B- or T-cell subtype.

SUMMARY

In spite of their diverse morphologic and behavioral characteristics the different lymphocytic leukaemias and malignant lymphomas are composed of neoplastic derivatives of a single cell type—the lymphocyte. Within the B-lymphocyte series differences in cytologic, histologic and behavioral patterns may be accounted for by variation in the proportion of neoplastic lymphocytes in different phases of the lymphocyte transformation cycle or maturation process. That is, there is only one lymphocytic (B cell) neoplasm (leukaemia/lymphoma), but there are many variations upon the theme. Implicit in this approach is an acceptance of the fact that the different morphologic expressions of lymphoma are not indicative of an entirely separate cellular origin, but rather represent arbitrary divisions in a continuous spectrum of disease, with intermediate forms between the leukaemias and the lymphomas and between the different lymphomas themselves. Many of these concepts are not new; some have an ancient lineage. These are reviewed briefly.

REFERENCES

1. Barcos, M.P., and Lukes, R.J.: Malignant lymphoma of convoluted lymphocytes: A new entity of possible T-cell type. In: Conflicts in childhood cancer:

an evaluation of current management, pp. 147–178, Sinks, L.F., Godden, J.O., (eds.), Liss, New York, 1975.

2. Braylan, R.C., Jaffe, E.S., Burbach, J.W., Frank, M.M., Johnson, R.E., and Berard, C.W.: Similarities of surface characteristics of neoplastic well-differentiated lymphocytes from solid tissues and from peripheral blood. Cancer Res., 36:1619–1625, 1976.

3. Brouet, J.-C., Flandrin, G., Sasportes, M., Preud'homme, J.-L., and Seligmann, M.: Chronic lymphocytic leukaemia of T-cell origin. Immunological and clinical evaluation in eleven patients. Lancet, 2:890–893, 1975.

4. Coccia, P.F., Kersey, J.H., Kazamiera, J., Gajl-Peczalska, K.J., Krivit, W., and Nesbit, M.E.: Prognostic significance of surface marker analysis in childhood non-Hodgkin's lymphoproliferative malignancies. Am. J. Hematol, 1:405–417, 1976.

5. Custer, R.P.: Borderlands dim in malignant disease of the blood forming organs. Radiology, 61:764–770, 1953.

6. Dameschek, W.: "Immunoblasts" and "immunocytes"—an attempt at a functional nomenclature. Blood, 21:243–245, 1963.

7. Gajl-Peczalska, K.J., Bloomfield, C.D., Coccia, P.F., Sosin, H., Brunning, R.D., and Kersey, J.G.: B and T cell lymphomas. Analysis of blood and lymph nodes in 87 patients. Am. J. Med., 59:674–685, 1975.

8. Garrett, J.V., Newton, R.K., and Scarffe, J.H.: Letter: Abnormal blood lymphocytes in non-Hodgkin's lymphoma. Lancet, 1:542, 1977.

9. Gowans, J.L., and Knight, E.J.: The route of re-circulation of lymphocytes in the rat. Proc. R. Soc. London Ser. B, 159:257–282, 1964.

10. Hall, J.G., Morris, B., Moreno, G., and Bessis, M.: The ultrastructure and function of the cells in lymph following antigenic stimulation. J. Exp. Med., 125:91–110, 1967.

11. Jaffe, E.S., Braylan, R.C., Nanba, K., Frank, M.M., and Berard, C.W.: Functional markers: a new perspective on malignant lymphomas. Cancer Treat Rep., 61:1001–1007, 1977.

12. Kojima, M., Imai, Y., and Nori, N.: A concept of follicular lymphoma. A proposal for the existence of a neoplasm originating from the germinal center. Gann Mongr. Cancer Res., 15:195–207, 1973.

13. Lennert, K.: Follicular lymphoma. Gann Monogr. Cancer Res., 15:217–231, 1973.

14. Lennert, K.: Morphology and classification of malignant lymphomas and so-called reticuloses. Acta Neuropathol Suppl, 6:1–16, 1975.

15. Lukes, R.J., and Collins, R.D.: New observations on follicular lymphoma. Gann Monogr. Cancer Res., 15:209–215, 1973.

16. Lukes, R.J., and Collins, R.D.: New approaches to the classification of the lymphomata. Br. J. Cancer 31, Suppl., 2:1–28, 1975.

17. Lukes, R.J., Taylor, C.R., Parker, J.W., Lincoln, T.L., Pattengale, P.K., and Tindle, B.H.: A morphologic and immunologic surface marker study of 299 cases of non-Hodgkin's lymphomas and related leukemias. Am. J. Pathol., 90:461–486, 1978.

18. Lukes, R.J., Parker, J.W., Taylor, C.R., Tindle, B.H., Cramer, A.D., and Lincoln, T.L.: Immunologic approach to non-Hodgkin's lymphoma and related leukemias. An analysis of the results of multiparameter studies of 425 cases. Semin. Hematol., 15:322–351, 1978.

19. Mellstedt, H., Hammarstrom, S., and Holm, G.: Monoclonal lymphocyte population in human plasma myeloma. Clin. Exp. Immunol., 17:371–384, 1974.

20. Mellstedt, H., Pettersson, D., and Holm, G.: Monoclonal B-lymphocytes in peripheral blood of patients with plasma cell myeloma. Relation to activity of the disease. Scand. J. Haematol., 16:112–120, 1976.
21. Nathwani, B.N., Kim, H., and Rappaport, H.: Malignant lymphoma, lymphoblastic. Cancer, 38:964–983, 1976.
22. Nossal, G.J.V., and Ada, G.L.: Antigens, Lymphoid Cells and the Immune Response. London: Academic Press, 1971.
23. Rappaport, H., Winter, W.J., and Hicks, E.B.: Follicular lymphoma: A reevaluation of its position in the scheme of malignant lymphoma, based on a survey of 253 cases. Cancer, 9:792–821, 1956.
24. Robb-Smith, A.H.T.: The classification and natural history of the lymphadenopathies. Treatment of cancer and allied diseases vol. 9 (2nd ed), Pack, G.T., Ariel, I.M., (eds), Hoeberg, New York, 1964.
25. Robb-Smith, A.H.T., and Taylor, C.R.: An approach to lymph node diagnosis. Harvey Miller Publishers, London, in press.
26. Stein, H.: Classification of non-Hodgkin's lymphomas on the basis of morphological and immunological features shared by normal and neoplastic lymphatic cells. Immun. Infekt., 4:52–69, 1976.
27. Taylor, C.R.: The nature of Reed-Sternberg cells and other malignant cells. Lancet, 2:802–807, 1974.
28. Taylor, C.R.: An immunohistological study of follicular lymphoma, reticulum cell sarcoma and Hodgkin's disease. Eur. J. Cancer, 12:61–75, 1976.
29. Taylor, C.R.: Hodgkin's disease and the lymphomas, vol. 1. Annual research review 1976, Horrobin, D.F., (ed.), Eden Press, Montreal, 1977.
30. Taylor, C.R.: Hodgkin's disease and the lymphomas, vol. 2. Annual research review 1977, Horrobin, D.F., (ed.), Eden Press, Montreal, and Churchill Longman Livingston, Edinburgh/London, 1978.
31. Taylor, C.R.: Immunocytochemical methods in the study of lymphoma and related conditions. J. Histochem. Cytochem., 26:495–512, 1978.
32. Taylor, C.R.: Classification of lymphomas: "new thinking" on old thoughts. Arch. Pathol. Lab. Med., 102:549–554, 1978.
33. Taylor, C.R., Parker, J.W., Pattengale, P.K., and Lukes, R.J.: Malignant lymphomas: an exercise in immunopathology. Proc. XII International Cancer Conference. Pergamon Press, Oxford, in press.
34. Williams, A.N., Taylor, C.R., Higgins, A.R., Quinn, J.J., Schneider, B.K., Swanson, V., Parker, J.W., Pattengale, P.K., Chandor, S.B., Powars, P., Lincoln, T.L., Tindle, B.H., and Lukes, R.J.: Childhood leukemia and lymphoma. I. Correlation of morphology and immunological studies. Cancer, 42:171–181, 1978.
35. Willis, R.A.: Pathology of Tumours. Butterworths, London, 1948.

22. CLINICAL MANIFESTATIONS, STAGING, AND MANAGEMENT OF THE NON-HODGKIN'S LYMPHOMAS: AN OVERVIEW

S. A. ROSENBERG

INTRODUCTION

The management of patients with malignant lymphomas has undergone considerable change during the past ten years. As a result of advances in diagnostic and therapeutic methods, treatment results have dramatically improved for patients with Hodgkin's disease (1, 2). The situation is not the same for patients with lymphomas other than Hodgkin's disease, the so-called non-Hodgkin's lymphomas (3).

Problems in this field are reflected by the continued proposals of new histopathologic classifications and nomenclature (4, 5, 6, 7). In part, this is due to new knowledge and concepts of the function of the lymphoid system. However, the search for new classifications and clinico-pathologic correlations is also motivated by the frustrations of managing these patients. The non-Hodgkin's lymphomas are a diverse group of diseases varying from very aggressive and rapidly fatal to some of the most indolent and well-tolerated malignancies of man.

Children with lymphomas must be considered separately because they present quite different clinico-pathologic problems and require different management programs than for adults (8).

Recommendations for management of the patients with non-Hodgkin's lymphomas are made more difficult not only by changing nomenclature but also by problems in defining histologic subgroups, variable diagnostic criteria of investigators reporting treatment results, reporting of benefit of treatment results in terms of remissions rather than survival changes, and the general lack of well-controlled clinical trials in this field of study.

Yet these diseases are relatively common, and physicians must select management methods based upon currently available evidence and experience.

CLASSIFICATION RECOMMENDATIONS

The Rappaport classification is still the most useful system for the clinician at this time. The Rappaport, and other classifications, can be utilized to combine several easily identifiable sugroups into those of good prognoses and those with poor prognoses.

The diffuse histiocytic subgroup of Rappaport is undoubtedly a heterogenous group. The new classifications and proposals attempt to separate patients into meaningful clinical categories within the larger subgroup of diffuse histiocytic. An interesting concept and subgroup are those within this Rappaport group, indentified by Lukes and Collins as immunoblastic sarcomas of both B- and T-cell types. A recent study from the National Cancer Institute suggests that a modification of the Lukes and Collins classification can separate prognostic subgroups with the Rappaport diffuse histiocytic group (8b) However, these interesting studies, concepts, and terminology cannot yet be translated into management decisions for patients with diffuse histiocytic lymphoma.

MANAGEMENT CONSIDERATIONS OTHER THAN PATHOLOGIC GROUP

There are very important variables and considerations which must be used in arriving at management decisions other than the histologic subtype. These are:

1) the extent of the disease, or stage of the patient (9);
2) the site, or sites, of involvement;
3) the size or mass of the tumor in various sites;
4) the symptoms of the patient, both local and systemic;
5) the threat of serious problems, i.e. ureteral obstruction, airway compromise, meningeal involvement;
6) bone marrow function;
7) the age of the patient;
8) the variable of time, or the "tempo" of the patient's tumor progression.

Also to be considered in selecting a treatment program are the experience and facilities available to the physician and whether or not the patient, with informed consent, is willing to participate in a clinical trial.

DIAGNOSTIC STUDIES

Management decisions for patients with lymphomas should not be made until the extent of the disease is determined, within the limitations of our currently available methods.

It is axiomatic that all patients should have a careful history and physical examination. In addition to routine blood counts and screening chemistries, the bone marrow should be evaluated for involvement by an adequate biopsy, usually of the posterior iliac crest. Paradoxically, bone marrow involvement will be found frequently in patients in the lymphocytic group, who have good prognoses, and infrequently in the histiocytic group. One adequate needle biopsy, with the Jamshidi needle, is usually sufficient. Additional biopsies will improve the yield (10) and should be obtained if the initial biopsy is inadequate or scanty or, in a patient in the lymphocytic group, if the demonstration of bone marrow involvement would change the management recommendation.

The lower extremity lymphogram is important to obtain in all patients in whom there is no specific contraindication (i.e. serious cardiopulmonary disease). The opacified retroperitoneal lymph nodes, whether normal or abnormal, can be valuable indicators of the tempo of the disease and can indicate progression or regression during and after the completion of treatment programs. There may be abnormal abdominal lymph nodes, especially in the mesentery, which are not seen on the lymphogram. These may be better demonstrated by computerized axial tomography or laparotomy, but the ease of making sequential comparative examinations after lymphography by subsequent plain abdominal roentgengram makes the lymphogram an indicated and valuable procedure.

The use of diagnostic laparotomy should be much more restricted for patients with non-Hodgkin's lymphomas than for those with Hodgkin's disease. It is recommended primarily for the patient under 50 years of age with favorable lymphoma, who after bone marrow biopsy and lymphography, is found to have clinical stage I or II disease (according to the Ann Arbor classification). Its primary purpose is to demonstrate stage III or IV disease, situations in which radiation therapy is not recommended, whereas it is for those with localized disease. Exploratory laparotomy is not usually indicated for patients with unfavorable lymphomas. The yield in finding occult disease is low, especially in those under age 40 (11). A significant number of patients in the poorer prognostic group will have their disease discovered at laparotomy and a second procedure is usually not indicated to clarify the extent of intra-abdominal disease.

Isotope scans to evaluate the bones, liver and spleen, or gallium scans have limited usefulness in this group of diseases. They should not be considered diagnostic, and other radiologic or biopsy methods should be used to establish sites of involvement which would change the management recommendation.

MANAGEMENT RECOMMENDATIONS

Favorable prognostic group

Patients with favorable type lymphomas of stage I and II extent are uncommon. However, approximately 10 percent of patients will have localized disease even after extensive diagnostic evaluation, including laparotomy. Radiation therapy to the involved sites is indicated. These are very radiosensitive tumors and local control of the disease may be possible for many years. No controlled trial clarifies the extent of irradiation which should be used (3). Cures should not be concluded for these patients, even if disease recurrence is not seen for five to ten years. The disease may be so indolent and well tolerated that clinical recurrence may not be evident for many years.

Patients with favorable lymphomas of stage III and IV extent are probably not curable by any known therapy program. This has been true despite the observation that these patients are highly responsive to a variety of treatment programs, including combination chemotherapy, radiation therapy, or both. Despite documented complete remission, the disease usually recurs at a rate of about 10–15 percent per year for a period of ten years or longer after treatment completion (12). The only exception to this observation has been a small group of patients with nodular mixed lymphoma treated at the National Cancer Institute (NCI), with the C-MOPP (cyclophosphamide, vincristine, procarbazine, and prednisone) program (13). This group has reported a low risk of recurrence after complete remission. These results have not yet been confirmed by others.

It is therefore recommended that a palliative treatment approach should be adopted for patients with favorable lymphomas of stage III and IV extent. In some patients, no initial treatment is required if they are asymptomatic, and the size or location of the lymphadenopathy poses no major threat (14). Much can be learned in these patients, who are usually over age of 50, by observing their status and lymph node size over a period of months before recommending a treatment program. Some will be stable over many months, even years, and treatment can be delayed. For a few, especially the elderly, it may never be required. Some will have spontaneous regressions, usually with subsequent recurrences. For other patients, within the first year and, in time, for most patients, the lymph nodes will gradually enlarge. If the rate of growth is rapid, i.e. over a few months, and if systemic symptoms are noted, combination chemotherapy with a regimen employing cyclophosphamide, vincristine, and prednisone is advised. The so-called CVP regimen of the NCI is a good one (15). The drugs are usually given in cycles until thorough examination shows that a complete remission is obtained, and then discontinued. If the disease progresses slowly over a period of many months, or the patient is anxious because of the appearance of the lymphadenopathy, continuous or intermittent oral single agent alkylating agent therapy can be satisfactory. Chlorambucil is a well-tolerated drug for this purpose. A dose of 6–12 mg/day is usually given until good disease regression is noted. A daily dose may then be reduced, or given bimonthly at 20–40 mg per dose, monitoring peripheral blood counts, or may be discontinued.

Local irradiation for major bulky sites of disease should always be considered in the palliative program for these patients, especially for ureteral obstruction, lower extremity edema, mediastinal masses, chylous effusions with paravertebral masses and cosmetic problems.

Low dose whole body irradiation (16, 17) is an acceptable alternative to systemic chemotherapy for patients with stage III and IV disease provided they have not been treated extensively with prior chemotherapy, platelet counts are adequate, and radiotherapists experienced with the technique are available.

A challenging problem is the occasional younger patient, in the 20 to 40 year-old range, who has stage III or IV favorable lymphoma. Despite the relatively good prognosis, the patient's life will probably be shortened by the disease. It is tempting and understandable for physicians to recommend aggressive treatment for younger patients with these very responsive lymphomas. Complete remissions are often obtained. Yet, no survival benefit is available to support this approach. The physician and patient should acknowledge this fact before proceeding.

Unfavorable lymphomas

Despite the overall poorer prognoses of this group of patients, the clinical problems and responses to therapy are quite variable. Paradoxically, prolonged disease-free survival is more often possible and demonstrable for this group of patients than for the "favorable" group, despite their poorer natural history. An active treatment program is always indicated, no matter how limited the disease, how asymptomatic the patient, or, at the other extreme, how widespread the tumor or how critically ill the patient.

A high proportion of patients with stage I and I_E disease, diffuse histiocytic lymphoma, limited to a single lymph node region, or an isolated extranodal site, may be cured of their disease by surgery and/or radiotherapy. In some patients who present with gastrointestinal tumor, surgery has been required to establish the diagnosis. Radical surgical procedures and lymph node dissections should not be performed, but radiation therapy in adequate doses should be used to control the primary tumor and regional lymph node areas. If careful staging methods are employed, patients with stage I and I_E disease can be cured in approximately 75 percent of the cases (18).

Patients with stage II and II_E disease are more difficult to manage. Despite careful evaluation and staging, only 25–40 percent are permanently controlled by surgery and/or radiation therapy. It is recommended that combined modality programs be used for these patients in a sequence which is best individualized to a particular clinical setting and problem. Surgery may be necessary to establish the diagnosis, and radiotherapy may be very effective in reducing large tumor masses. However, combination chemotherapy, such as the C-MOPP regimen of the NCI (13), or the CHOP (cyclophosphamide, Adriamycin, vincristine, and prednisone) regimen of the Southwest Oncology Group (19) should improve the cure rates of these patients. Clinical trials have not yet established this point however.

Patients with stage III and IV unfavorable lymphomas should all receive combination chemotherapy. Despite widespread disease and an unfavorable nature history, a prolonged disease-free survival and probable cure is possible in a significant proportion of these patients (13). Those with disease limited to lymph nodes, or stage III, extent, have the best chemotherapy results and more than 50 percent can be cured with the chemotherapy programs. Those with stage IV disease, especially with bone marrow involvement, do not fare as well; probably less than 25 percent being controlled for long periods. The role of radiation therapy in these patients with stages III and IV disease is not established.

It may be that within the diverse group of patients with unfavorable lymphomas, as grouped in this discussion, there are different clinical entities which should have different treatment approaches and prognoses. There is some evidence that the newer classifications and immunologic-morphologic techniques can help identify these subgroups (8b, 20, 21). However, we must await more information before patients can be selected within this poorer prognostic category for different management programs.

Lymphoblastic lymphomas

An important clinico-pathologic entity has been recognized by Lukes and others which had been previously included in the diffuse lymphomas, poorly differentiated lymphocytic type of Rappaport (22, 23).

These patients are rare but have distinctive clinical features. The disease occurs in younger individuals, often presenting with large mediastinal masses. The disease merges clinically and morphologically with acute lymphoblastic leukemia of poor prognosis. Despite initial drug and radiosensitivity, recurrent and subsequent involvement of the bone marrow and meninges is common, with a rapidly fatal course.

Systemic chemotherapy programs of the types used for unfavorable childhood acute leukemia (24, 25), or adult lymphoblastic leukemia, are indicated no matter how localized the lymphoblastic lymphoma appears to be. Central nervous system prophylaxis employing intrathecal methotrexate and cranial irradiation, or a comparable program, is required to prevent meningeal relapse. The St. Judes' program for unfavorable childhood acute leukemia (24) is an acceptable one, although there is inadequate data to compare different treatment regimes at this time.

REFERENCES

1. Kaplan, H.S.: Hodgkin's disease. Harvard University Press, Cambridge, Mass., 1972.
2. DeVita, V.T., Jr., Lewis, B.J., and Rozencweig, M., et al.: The chemotherapy of Hodgkin's disease: past experiences and future directions. Cancer, 42:979–990, 1978.
3. Glatstein, E., Donaldson, S.S., and Rosenberg, S.A., et al.: Combined modality therapy in malignant lymphomas. Cancer Treat. Rep., 61:1199–1208, 1977.
4. Lukes, R.J., and Collins, R.D.: Lukes-Collins classification and its significance. Cancer Treat. Rep., 61:971–979, 1977.
5. Lennert, K., Mohri, N., and Stein, H., et al.: The histopathology of malignant lymphoma. Br. J. Haematol., 31 (suppl.):193–203, 1975.
6. Dorfman, R.F.: Pathology of the non-Hodgkin's lymphomas: new classifications. Cancer Treat. Rep., 61:945–951, 1977.
7. Bennett, M.H., Farrer-Brown, G., and Henry, K., et al.: Classification of non-Hodgkin's lymphomas. Lancet, 2:405–406, 1974.
8a. Murphy, S.B.: Current concepts in cancer: Childhood non-Hodgkin's lymphoma. N. Engl. J. Med., 299:1446–1448, 1978.
8b. Strauchen, J.A., Young, R.C., and DeVita, V.T., et al.: Clinical relevance of the histopathological subclassification of diffuse histiocytic lymphoma. N. Engl. J. Med., 299:1382–1387, 1978.
9. Carbone, P.P., Kaplan, H.S., and Musshoff, K., et al.: Report of the committee of Hodgkin's disease staging classification. Cancer Res., 31:1860–1861, 1971.
10. Brunning, R.D., Bloomfield, C.D., and McKenna, R.W., et al.: Bilateral trephine bone marrow biopsies in lymphoma and other neoplastic diseases. Ann. Intern. Med., 82:365–366, 1975.
11. Goffinet, D.R., Warnke, R., and Dunnick, N.R., et al.: Clinical and surgical (laparotomy) evaluation of patients with non-Hodgkin's lymphomas. Cancer Treat. Rep., 61:981–992, 1977.
12. Portlock, C.S., Rosenberg, S.A., and Glatstein, E., et al.: Treatment of advanced non-Hodgkin's lymphomas with favorable histologies: preliminary results of a prospective trial. Blood, 47:747–756, 1976.
13. Anderson, T., Bender, R.A., and Fisher, R.I., et al.: Combination chemotherapy in non-Hodgkin's lymphoma: results of long-term followup. Cancer Treat. Rep., 61:1057–1066, 1977.
14. Portlock, C.S., and Rosenberg, S.A.: Chemotherapy of the non-Hodgkin's lymphomas: the Stanford experience. Cancer Treat. Rep., 61:1049–1055, 1977.
15. Bagley, C.M., Jr., DeVita, V.T., and Berard, C.W., et al.: Advanced lymphosarcoma: intensive cyclical combination chemotherapy with cyclophosphamide, vincristine, and prednisone. Ann. Intern. Med., 76:227–234, 1972.
16. Chaffey, J.T., Hellman, S., and Rosenthal, D.S., et al.: Total-body irradiation

in the treatment of lymphocytic lymphoma. Cancer Treat. Rep., 61:1149–1152, 1977.

17. Young, R.C., Johnson, R.E., and Canellos, G.P., et al.: Advanced lymphocytic lymphoma: randomized comparisons of chemotherapy and radiotherapy, alone or in combination. Cancer Treat. Rep., 61:1153–1159, 1977.

18. Bush, R.S., Gospodarowicz, M., and Sturgeon, J., et al.: Radiation therapy of localized non-Hodgkin's lymphoma. Cancer Treat. Rep., 61:1129–1136, 1977.

19. McKelvey, E.M., Gottlieb, J.A., and Wilson, H.E., et al.: Hydroxyldaunomycin (adriamycin) combination chemotherapy in malignant lymphoma. Cancer, 38:1484–1493, 1976.

20. Bloomfield, C.D., Kersey, J.H., and Brunning, R.D., et al.: Prognostic significance of lymphocyte surface markers in adult non-Hodgkin's malignant lymphoma. Lancet, 2:1330–1333, 1976.

21. Lukes, R.J., Taylor, C.R., and Chir B., et al.: A morphologic and immunologic surface marker study of 299 cases of non-Hodgkin lymphomas and related leukemias. Am. J. Pathol., 90:461–486, 1978.

22. Nathwani, B.N., Kim, H., and Rappaport, H.: Malignant lymphoma, lymphoblastic. Cancer, 38:964–983, 1976.

23. Barcos, M.P., and Lukes, R.J.: Malignant lymphoma of convoluted lymphocytes: a new entity of possible T-cell type. In: Conflicts in childhood cancer: an evaluation of current management, pp. 147–178, Sinks L.F., and Godden, J.O. (eds), Alan R. Liss, Inc., New York, Prog. Clin. Biol. Res., vol. 4, 1975.

24. Murphy, S.B.: Management of childhood non-Hodgkin's disease. Cancer Treat. Rep., 61:1161–1173, 1977.

25. Weinstein, H.J., Vance, Z.B., and Jaffe, N., et al.: Improved prognosis for patients with mediastinal lymphoblastic lymphoma. Blood, 53:687–694, 1979.

T-CELL LYMPHOMAS

23. THE T-CELL-DERIVED NEOPLASMS: AN OVERVIEW

J.G. VAN DEN TWEEL

It is known from several studies that approximately 10–20% of the non-Hodgkin lymphomas are T cell-derived neoplasms. Initially, this was shown by immunological methods such as spontaneous rosette formation with sheep red blood cells or specific antibodies against human T-lymphocyte subsets, but since methods became available to study the morphological features of these cells, it has become evident that at least a proportion of these tumors have characteristic cytological and cytochemical features.

In this chapter I shall discuss the morphological, clinical, and immunological aspects of the various T-cell neoplasms and the criteria for the differential diagnosis.

LYMPHOMA/LEUKEMIA OF SMALL T CELLS

Definition

This term refers to an abnormal proliferation of small lymphocytes among which the neoplastic cells carry T-cell markers. The disease can start either as leukemia or as lymphoma, but both entities can be present at the time of presentation.

Incidence

Chronic lymphocytic leukemia and lymphoma of small T lymphocytes are considered to be rare disorders. Two percent of all CLLs are estimated to be of T-cell origin.

There seems to be no age or sex preference associated with this disease. The age of onset for the T-cell CLL group ranges from 25 to 80 years. There are too few data available to provide any indication of racial prevalence for this particular disorder. It is interesting, however, that several reports come from laboratories in Japan, where CLL is a relatively rare disease.

J.G. van den Tweel et al. (eds.), Malignant Lymphoproliferative Diseases, 305–314
All rights reserved.
Copyright © 1980 by Martinus Nijhoff Publishers bv, The Hague/Boston/London.

Clinical features

Table 1 gives the clinical features of patients presenting with T-cell CLL and small T-cell lymphoma. These data suggest that the two neoplasms might differ in some of their clinical features, but the number of patients studied is still too small to permit any firm conclusions.

Morphological features

The findings in the literature show that T-cell CLL cases can display a variety of morphological features ranging from proliferation of large lymphocytes with irregular and bizarre nuclei to cells with the characteristics of prolymphocytes and well-differentiated small lymphocytes. The irregular nuclear morphology is an important feature (Figure 1). Some lymphocytes contain numerous azurophilic granules (1). Cytochemistry shows focal reactivity of acid phosphatase, acid nonspecific esterase, and β-glucuronidase. In lymph nodes there is often an increased number of epitheloid venules.

Immunological studies

The neoplastic leukemic and lymphoma cells show E-rosette formation at 4°C, lack SIg, IgG-Fc, and EAC receptors (B-cell markers), and show a variable positive response to different anti-T-cell antisera (1). Some studies indicate that, at least in some cases of T-CLL, the malignant cells are derived from T-suppressor cells (2). The possibility of the existence of a T-helper type CLL is discussed in chapter 24 in this volume.

Table 1. Some clinical features of patients with T-cell CLL or small T-cell lymphoma.

	T-CLL (11 patients)*	Small T cell lymphoma (5 patients)**
Sex ratio (male:female)	6:5	1:4
Age range (years)	25–78	68–80
Splenomegaly	10/11	5/5
Hepatomegaly	4/11	3/5
Peripheral node enlargement	1/11	5/5
Skin involvement	4/11	0/5
Marrow involvement	11/11	4/4

* Brouet et al., (1)
** Data from the Department of Pathology, University of Southern California Medical School Los Angeles.

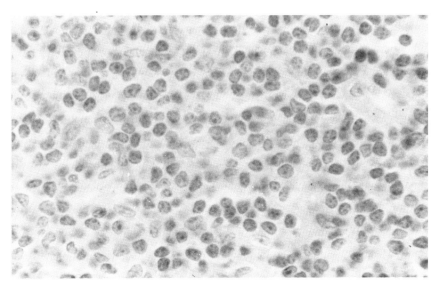

Figure 1. T-CLL. Diffuse infiltration of the lymph node by slightly irregular small T lymphocytes (H-E × 360).

Differential diagnosis

Leukemia/lymphoma of small T cells must be differentiated from small
B-cell neoplasms and from small cleaved (centrocytic) FCC lymphomas.
The morphological criteria, together with immunologic markers, should
facilitate differentiation between these disorders if the clinical picture has
not already done so.

SÉZARY'S SYDROME AND MYCOSIS FUNGOIDES

Definition

Although Sézary's syndrome and mycosis fungoides are both cutaneous
T-cell neoplasms and although the tumor cells have many features in common, there is still controversy as to the relationship between the two processes. Some authors consider these diseases to be unrelated, whereas others
consider both disorders as variants of one disease.

Incidence

The incidence of Sézary's syndrome and mycosis fungoides is very low;
according to studies done in Denmark and Sweden, it appears to be less

than 1:500,000. The age range given in different reports differs; some patients between 15 and 19 years have been described by Brehmer, but most of the patients are between 40 and 85 years old. The incidence seems to be lower in Negroes. Family incidence of mycosis fungoides is extremely rare; one case of occurrence in both a mother and daughter has been described.

Clinical features

The clinical features of Sézary's syndrome and mycosis fungoides differ. Mycosis fungoides is primarily a skin disorder, sometimes with subsequent organ involvement, whereas Sézary's syndrome is characterized by skin involvement and a leukemic blood picture. The skin involvement in mycosis fungoides has three stages: a premycotic stage, a plaque stage, and a tumor stage, but in Sézary's syndrome there is a characteristic erythroderma with edema, especially conspicuous in the face, which is accompanied by pigmentation and fissures of palms and soles. Lymphadenopathy occurs in all patients with Sézary's syndrome and is secondary to the skin lesions. Both diseases are ultimately lethal, although most patients survive for several years.

Morphological features

The diagnosis Sézary's syndrome may be indicated by the finding of "cerebriform" cells in the peripheral blood smear. Cerebriform cells are small- or medium-sized lymphocytes with coarse deep irregular foldings of the nuclear membrane. The chromatin is condensed, like that of a small lymphocyte. Cytoplasm is moderate in amount and stains lightly. In PAS-stained sections a necklace of positive granules may be seen around the nucleus. This is a typical, but not invariable, feature.

Mycosis fungoides is usually diagnosed in a skin biopsy specimen, which shows sub-epidermal infiltrates of polymorphous lymphoid cells, including some with cerebriform nuceli. Larger and more bizarre lymphocytes are also present and some, with prominent nucleoli, bear a superficial resemblance to Reed-Sternberg cell variants. Typically intra-epidermal lymphoid aggregates are present (Davier-Pautier abscesses). Typical infiltrates are found in lymph nodes (4).

Immunologic features

Sézary cells typically form E rosettes and show specific reactivity with anti-T-cell sera. Specific T-cell functions have been demonstrated in Sézary cell populations (helper cell effect) by Broder et al. (5). The cells usually express receptors for IgM.

Differential diagnosis

The differential diagnosis with respect to B-cell CLL and small cleaved FCC with circulating cells is based on morphologic and immunologic criteria. Differentiation from T-cell CLL, which may also involve the skin, is made primarily on morphological grounds.

T-ZONE LYMPHOMA

Definition

This neoplasm is defined as a lymphoma associated with neoplastic proliferation of small and large T lymphocytes in the paracortex with relative sparing of the follicular centers. Usually there is also an admixture of plasma cells.

Incidence

This type of lymphoma probably accounts for somewhat more than 1% of all non-Hodgkin's lymphomas. There seems to be no predilection for either sex. The patients range in age from 18 to 23 years (6).

Clinical features

General manifestations, lymphadenopathy and hepato- and splenomegaly are rather frequent features. Some patients present with tonsillar infiltrates and involvement of the lungs, pleura and bone marrow. The prognosis is poor; most patients die within 18 months after diagnosis.

Morphological features

The most important histological feature is the selective neoplastic involvement of the thymus-dependent areas with relative sparing of the follicles (Figure 2). There is an increase in the number of venules in the interfollicular tissue. The proliferating cells include T lymphocytes, T immunoblasts (transformed T cells), and plasma cells. Acid phosphatase is strongly positive.

Immunological studies

The tumor cells form E rosettes.

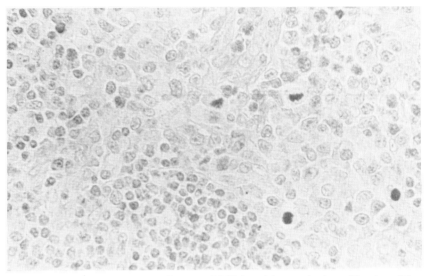

Figure 2. T-zone lymphoma. Rest of a normal follicle and the neoplastic proliferation of blast cells, polymorphic lymphocytes, plasma cells and eosinophilic granulocytes (× 480, courtesy, Prof. Lennert).

Differential diagnosis

Immunoblastic lymphadenopathy and Hodgkin's disease must be excluded. If there are many immunoblasts present, the disease has to be differentiated from T-cell immunoblastic sarcoma.

CONVOLUTED CELL LYMPHOMA (MALIGNANT LYMPHOMA LYMPHOBLASTIC, CONVOLUTED TYPE)

Definition

This term refers to a highly aggressive T-cell neoplasm, often associated with a mediastinal tumor and acute lymphocytic (lymphoblastic) leukemia, in which the nuclei usually have a characteristic convoluted morphology (7).

Incidence

Convoluted cell lymphoma accounts for approximately 40% of all T-cell lymphomas and 4–6% of all non-Hodgkin's lymphomas (6). The tumor has a relatively high incidence in older children and young adults, although it can occur at any age. In the younger age group there is male:female ratio of approximately 5:1 as against 1.6:1 in the adult group. To date, most patients with this disease have been Caucasian.

Clinical features

The patients usually present with painless asymptomatic lymph node enlargement or symtoms directly attributable to compression of the trachea or esophagus by a mediastinal tumor or pleural effusion. The reported incidence of a mediastinal mass in comparable studies ranges from 50% (9) to approximately 80% (7). A high percentage of the patients present with or develop leukemia (T-cell ALL); in the study done by Barcos and Lukes the total was 20 out of 27 and in the study by Nathwani 23 out of 30. The inferred prognosis is very poor, the majority of patients dying within a year after diagnosis.

Morphological features

Convoluted cells have dispersed fine chromatin, small nucleoli, and a nucleus with multiple fine indentations giving an overall convoluted appearance, seen best electron microscopically or in thin sections. The cytoplasm is scanty and slightly basophilic. Only a proportion of the neoplastic cells of any given patient show this morphology, but Barcos and Lukes consider it a valuable diagnostic feature when present (Figure 3). Focal acid phosphatase staining also has diagnostic value.

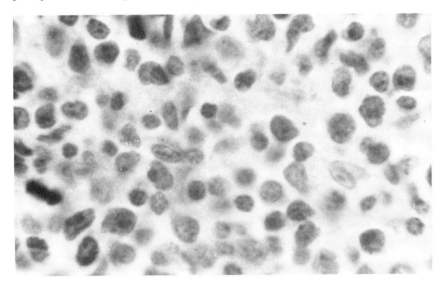

Figure 3. Convoluted lymphoma: numerous large blast cells with convoluted nuclear contours.

There is still some disagreement as to whether all cases belonging to this clinical group show a mediastinal mass or diagnostic nuclear convolutions.

Immunological studies

Of 29 cases studied by Dr. Lukes' group, only eight showed E-rosette formation by more than 50% of the neoplastic cells. In 14 cases less than 20% of the neoplastic cells formed rosettes, and in occasional cases rosette-forming cells were not identifiable, even though the morphological and clinical features were identical to those in other cases belonging to the group. Monoclonal surface immunoglobulin was not seen in any of the cases. C_3 receptor was detected in more than 30% of cells in five cases.

Stein and colleagues noted that in many respects the neoplastic cells resembled those of fetal thymocytes at 10 to 15 weeks of gestation, particularly in the presence of a complement receptor on E-rosetting cells (see chapter 2 in this volume).

Differential diagnosis

The differential diagnosis concerns other diffuse lymphomas in which some degree of nuclear irregularity may be found (e.g., follicular center cell tumors and Sézary's syndrome). The primitive appearance of the nucleus is the best guide in borderline cases, and is essential for the diagnosis. If convolutions are difficult to find or absent, the differential diagnosis concerns ALL tissue involvement and Burkitt's lymphoma with or without leukemic manifestations.

It should be underlined that convoluted lymphoma must be regarded as lymphoma-leukemia, because both manifestations of the neoplasm usually occur in the course of the disease and either one may occur as the presenting feature.

T-CELL IMMUNOBLASTIC SARCOMA

Definition

The diagnosis immunoblastic sarcoma (IBS) corresponds roughly with reticulum cell sarcoma and malignant lymphoma histiocytic in earlier classifications. The division into T- and B-cell subtypes (T-IBS, B-IBS) was initially made on theoretical grounds in order to gain correspondence with the two known lymphocyte subclasses. This separation has proved to be justified because surface marker studies have revealed morphological and clinical differences between T-IBS and B-IBS.

Incidence

The IBS group accounts for approximately 8% of the non-Hodgkin's lymphomas in American studies, half of them being of the T-cell type, the other half the B-cell type.

In the Kiel Lymph Node Registry, 15.4% were classified as malignant lymphoma, immunoblastic. The disease occurs in all races.

Morphological features

The histological features of T-cell immunoblastic sarcoma are perhaps less well defined than those of the corresponding B-cell tumor, partly because proof of T-cell origin is often difficult to obtain because fresh cell suspensions are required for surface marker studies. Even when such suspensions are available, cytocentrifuge E-rosette preparations must be examined to determine whether definite rosettes are formed by the neoplastic immunoblasts.

T-cell immunoblastic sarcoma characteristically involves the node diffusely, with an initial preferential involvement of T-cell zones and some sparing of residual follicles in the early stages (this stage might be the T-zone lymphoma described by Lennert). The malignant immunoblasts are generally smaller than those seen in B-cell immunoblastic sarcoma, and the nucleoli are less conspicuous (e.g., single large centrally positioned nucleoli, common in B-cell IBS, are less often a feature of T-cell IBS).

Furthermore, the chromatin is more widely dispersed and the nuclear outline is often irregular. In addition, there is much less cytoplasmic basophilia in T-cell immunoblastic sarcoma and plasmacytoid immunoblasts are not present, though mature plasma cells may occur scattered throughout the tumor or at the margins of tumor invasion.

Immunologic studies

By definition, recognizable neoplastic cells spontaneously form rosettes with sheep red blood cells, thus providing evidence of a T-cell lineage. The percentage of tumor cells forming rosettes is however variable, ranging from 10 to 80. The percentage of SIg cells in suspensions of nodes affected by T-IBS is usually reduced, but occasionally elevated "polyclonal" patterns are seen, possibly as an indication of adsorption of immunoglobulin to the tumor cells.

Differential diagnosis

The features of value for the distinction between T-IBS and B-IBS have been given in the description of T-IBS morphology. The differentiation from large noncleaved or large cleaved FCC can usually be made by the finding of deeply cleft cells in the follicle center tumors, whereas in T-IBS nuclear folding is finer and multiple unfoldings are present. The presence of histiocytes in T-IBS often provides a clue to the correct diagnosis.

Clinical studies in this field are in an early stage, but preliminary results suggest that T-IBS is more responsive to therapy and generally behaves less aggressively than is the case for B-IBS.

REFERENCES

1. Brouet, J.C., Flandrin, G., Sasportes, M., Preud'Homme, J.L., and Seligmann, M.: Chronic lymphocytic leukemia of T cell origin. Immunological and clinical evaluation is eleven patients. Lancet, II:890, 1975.
2. Uchigama, T., Sagawa, K., Takatsuki, K., and Uchino, H.: Effect of adult T-cell leukemia cells on pokeweed mitogen induced normal B-cell differentiation. Clinical Immunol. Immunopath., 10:24, 1978.
3. Zucker-Franklin, D.: Properties of the Sézary lymphoid cell. An ultrastructural analysis. Mayo Clin. Proc., 49:567, 1974.
4. Scheffer, E., and Meijer, C.J.L.M.: Early involvement of lymph node in mycosis fungoides. This volume, chapter 29.
5. Broder, S., Edelson, R.L., Lutzner, M.A., Nelson, D.L., MacDermott, R.P., Durm, M.E., Goldman, C.K., Meade, B.D., and Waldmann, T.A.: The Sézary syndrome. A malignant proliferation of T helper cells. J. clin. Invest., 58:1297–1306, 1976.
6. Lennert, K.: Malignant lymphomas. Springer Verlag, p. 196, 1978.
7. Barcos, M.P., and Lukes, R.J.: Malignant lymphoma of convoluted lymphocytes. A new entity of possible T cell type. Conflicts in childhood cancer vol. 4, p. 147.
8. Lukes, R.J., Parker, J.W., Taylor, C.R., and Tindle, B.H., Cramer, A.D., and Lincoln, T.: Immunologic approaches to non-Hodgkin lymphomas and related leukemias. Analysis of the results of multiparameter studies of 425 cases. Sem. in Hematology 15:3200, 1978.
9. Nathwani, B.N., Kim, H., and Rappaport, H.: Malignant lymphoma, lymphoblastic. Cancer, 38:964, 1976.

24. T-CELL NEOPLASIA IN THE PERSPECTIVE OF NORMAL T-CELL DIFFERENTIATION

H. STEIN, G. TOLKSDORF AND K. LENNERT

INTRODUCTION

Until it is possible to classify malignant lymphomas according to their etiology, the best way to do so is unquestionably, according to cell origin. It does not appear to be reasonable or practical to distinguish as many types of T-cell neoplasm as there are normal T-cell subsets (up to 20 have been distinguished in mice). However, since we do not know in advance just what is reasonable, in other words, which types of T-cell neoplasia differ in clinical and therapeutic behavior, the subtyping of neoplasms as far as possible is imperative. After experience with these subtypes has been collected, it will not be difficult to combine some or many of them into groups of tumors that show similar clinical and therapeutic behavior.

In the following, we present a concept for the classification of T-cell neoplasms that is based on our knowledge of normal T-cell differentiation, and therefore starts with a description of the cells and events occurring in normal T-cell maturation and differentation.

MATURATION AND DIFFERENTIATION OF THE T-CELL SERIES IN RELATION TO IMMUNOLOGIC, MORPHOLOGIC, AND ENZYME-CYTOCHEMICAL PROPERTIES

According to the findings of Gatien et al. (10), the first T cells are recognizable in the fetal thymus during the 10th gestational week. Up to 85% of these cells express complement (C3) receptors (Figure 1); the other 15% are devoid of C3 receptors. The cells of this gestational age also lack receptors for sheep erythrocytes (E) (Figure 1). With increasing fetal age, however, receptors for sheep E are demonstrable and the number of cells bearing C3 receptors declines. At birth, the thymus is completely devoid of C3 receptor-bearing cells. We were able to confirm these findings. Furthermore, the C3 receptor-positive and sheep E receptor-negative cells obviously mature into the C3 receptor-negative and sheep E receptor-positive cells via an intermediate cell type that expresses both C3 and sheep E

J.G. van den Tweel et al. (eds.), Malignant Lymphoproliferative Diseases, 315–329
All rights reserved.
Copyright © 1980 by Martinus Nijhoff Publishers bv, The Hague/Boston/London.

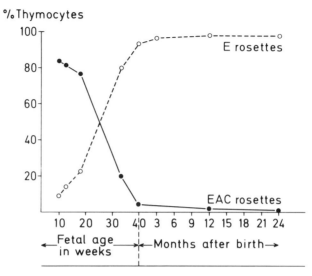

Figure 1. Expression receptors for C3 (EAC rosettes) and sheep erythrocytes (E rosettes) by fetal and postnatal thymocytes in relation to age (modified from Gatien et al. (10)).

receptors simultaneously (20). We observed the highest percentage of sheep E and C3 receptor-positive cells in the 12th week of gestation. The percentage then decreases with increasing fetal age. Starting at about the 15th gestational week, an increasing number of cells that are capable of binding sheep E not only at 4°C but also at 37°C are demonstrable; at birth, all thymocytes are capable of binding sheep E at 37°C.

On the basis of these data, we distinguish three maturation forms of thymocytes (see Table 1):

1) *Prethymocytes,* which usually express C3 receptors and invariably lack

Table 1. Immunologic features of cells of the T-cell axis.

	HTLA	$E_s 37°$	$E_s 4°$	C3R	IgM-FcR	IgG-FcR	Ia-like
Prethymocytes	+	−	−	+++	?	−	−
Prothymocytes	++	+/−	+	++	?	−	−
Mature thymocytes	+++	+	+	−	?	−	−
Helper T cells	+	−	+	−	+	−	−*
Suppressor T cells	+	−	+	−	−	+	−*
Others	+	−	+	?	?	?	?*

HTLA = human T-lymphocyte antigen; $E_s 37°$ = sheep erytrhocyte rosettes stable at 37°0; $E_s 4°$ = sheep erythrocyte rosettes stable at 4°C.; C3R = receptor for C3; IgM-FcR = IgM-Fc receptor; IgG-FcR = IgG-Fc receptor; Ia-like = Ia-like antigen.

receptors for sheep E. They are also devoid of IgG-Fc receptors and Ia-like antigen.

2) *Prothymocytes*, which are characterized by the simultaneous presence of C3 and sheep E receptors.

3) *Mature thymocytes*, which are invariably devoid of C3 receptors but have sheep E receptors that are capable of binding at 37°C.

These three types of thymocyte have to be distinguished from T cells that have emigrated from the thymus and circulate in the blood or have settled in T-dependent regions of peripheral lymphoid tissue. These peripheral T cells (see lower part of Table 1) differ from thymocytes in that they have sheep E receptors capable of binding only at 4°C.

It has been shown that the population of human peripheral T cells includes two subpopulations that are identifiable by surface receptors capable of binding either the Fc portion of IgM (17) or the Fc portion of IgG (9, 26). The T-cell fraction with IgM receptors was found to include the T cells that act as helpers in the differentiation of B lymphocytes into plasma cells in response to pokeweed mitogen stimulation. In contrast, the T-cell fraction with IgG receptors included the cells with suppressor activity (19). As far as we know, other functional forms of T cells are not identifiable in man by special properties at the single-cell level.

Table 2 shows the morphologic and enzyme-cytochemical features of the T-cell populations distinguished above. Some prethymocytes, many prothymocytes, and a few mature thymocytes have convoluted nuclei and are thus very similar in morphology to lymphoblastic lymphoma cells. All thymocytic forms are devoid of azurophil granules. An important and highly characteristic feature of thymocytes, particularly the immature forms, is their strong focal acid phosphatase reactivity (20). All three types of thymocytes are negative for acid nonspecific esterase, the only exception being a small proportion made up of medium-sized mature thymocytes

Table 2. Morphologic and enzyme cytochemical features of cells of the T-cell axis.

	Convoluted nuclei	Azurophil granules	TDT	Acid phosphatase	Acid nonspecific esterase
Prethymocytes	+	−	+	+ + +	−
Prothymocytes	+	−	+	+ + + +	−
Mature thymocytes	−/+	−	+	+ +	−
Helper T cells	−	−	−	+	+
Suppressor T cells	−	+	−	+	−
Others	?	?	?	?	?

TDT = terminal deoxynucleotidyl transferase.

showing a dotlike acid nonspecific esterase reaction product. The enzyme terminal deoxynucleotidyl transferase (Tdt) is present in all maturation forms of thymocyte, whereas it is not detectable in peripheral T cells (8).

Peripheral T cells (see lower part of Table 2) cannot be subtyped by their morphology and acid phosphatase reactivity alone. So far, only two nonimmunologic properties are known to be of help in separating the helper T-cell fraction from the suppressor T-cell fraction. The IgM-Fc receptor-positive T-cell fraction that shows helper cell activity is identifiable by enzyme cytochemistry: these cells have one or two solitary dots of acid nonspecific esterase activity (11). All other T-cell subsets have proved to be acid nonspecific esterase negative. IgG-Fc receptor-positive T cells, i.e., the T-cell fraction that displays suppressor activity (18), often contain azurophil granules (11).

It is well known that T cells can undergo antigen- or mitogen-induced blast transformation. The large blast cells are usually called immunoblasts. The blast reaction apparently serves the multiplication of T cells. On the basis of the following findings, we presume that each T-cell subset has its own "immunoblast": (a) Concanavalin A (Con A)-induced blasts are predominantly acid nonspecific esterase positive, whereas phytohemagglutinin (PHA)-induced blasts are negative (13, 24). (b) There are clear differences in the SDS-electrophoretic pattern of surface glycoproteins between Con A blasts, PHA blasts, and blasts of a mixed lymphocyte culture (1).

Table 3 summarizes our concept of the maturation and differentiation of the cells of the T-cell lineage. Prethymocytes mature via prothmocytes into mature thymocytes. Emigrated thymocytes differentiate into specialized T cells, such as helper T cells, suppressor T cells and cytotoxic T cells. Each specialized T-cell subset appears to multiply via its own immunoblasts, which shares the basic properties of the cell from which it is derived.

Table 3. Maturation and differentiation of cells of the T-cell axis and their predominant cytologic appearance.

Maturation and differentiation forms	Cytology
Prethymocytes	Lymphoblastic
↓	
Prothymocytes	Predominantly lymphoblastic
↓	
Mature thymocytes	Lymphoblastic/ Lymphocytic
↓	
Suppressor T cells Helper T cells Other T subsets	Lymphocytic
↕ ↕ ↕	
Immunoblasts Immunoblasts Immunoblasts	Immunoblastic

The right side of Table 3 shows the basic cytologic appearance of each T-cell type. A majority of the prethmocytes and prothymocytes and a minority of the mature thymocytes are lympho*blastic* in morphology. Some prothymocytes, many mature thymocytes, and all peripheral blood T cells and resting T cells in lymphoid tissue have a lympho*cytic* appearance. T immunoblasts are large cells with a large pale nucleus containing one or two prominent nucleoli; their cytoplasm varies in amount and is basophilic. T immunoblasts are usually indistinguishable from B immunoblasts.

CLASSIFICATION OF T-CELL LYMPHOMAS IN RELATION TO CELL ORIGIN

The concept for the classification of T-cell lymphomas presented here (cf. Table 4) distinguishes three main morphologic groups corresponding with the three main cytologic types of T cells mentioned above. Within each of the three morphologic groups, entities are defined according to the maturation and differentiation forms of the T-cell axis described above.

Lymphoblastic lymphomas and leukemias of the T type

We apply the terms lymphoblastic lymphoma and lymphoblastic leukemia to lymphoid neoplasms in which medium-sized cells with a large nucleus and relatively homogeneously distributed nuclear chromatin are the main proliferating cells. In all subtypes of lymphoblastic lymphoma or leukemia, with the exception of the Burkitt type, the nucleoli are usually small and not

Table 4. Classification of non-Hodgkin's lymphoma of the T type based on cytology and immunology.

1. Lymphoblastic lymphomas of the T type
    Thymocytic type
        Prethymocytic subtype
        Prothymocytic subtype
        Mature thymocytic subtype
        Peripheral T-cell type
        Helper T-cell subtype
        Suppressor T-cell subtype
        Others
2. Lymphocytic lymphomas of the T type
    Chronic lymphocytic leukemia of the T type
    Prolymphocytic leukemia of the T type
    Mycosis fungoides and Sézary's syndrome
    T-zone lymphoma
3. Immunoblastic lymphomas of the T type
    Helper T-cell subtype
    Others

prominent; the cytoplasm is sparse and moderately basophilic in most instances. It should be mentioned, however, that lymphoid neoplasms with this morphology do not have the same cellular origin. They include pre-B-lymphoblastic, null-type lymphoblastic as well as T-lymphoblastic neoplasms. The pre-B-cell type and the null-cell type are usually, if not always, leukemic. The null-cell type is probably derived from stem cells. With the exception of the controversial marker "convoluted nuclei", there are no known morphologic criteria for classifying lymphoblastic lymphomas and leukemias—other than the Burkitt type—by their cellular origin. On the other hand, it is easy to classify these neoplasms reliably with the help of immunologic and enzyme cytochemical markers.

So far, we have collected 24 cases of lymphobalstic neoplasia of the T type that were diagnosed on the basis of immunologic and enzyme cytochemical methods (21). Since it is not possible to present the individual

Cytology	Immunology/Enzyme cytochemistry					
		Thy type			Periph. T type	
		Prethy	Prothy	M.Thy	T_H	T_S
	S-Ig	−	−	−	−	−
	Ia-like antigen	−	−	−	−	−
	C3b receptor	++/−	+	−	−	−
	C3d receptor	++/−	+	−	−	−
	Mouse-E rosettes	−	−	−	−	−
	Sheep-E rosettes stable at 37°C	−	+/−	+	−	−
	stable at 4°C	−	+	+	+	+
	HTLA	+	+	++	+	+
	Tdt	+	+	+	−	−
	Acid phosphatase	++	+++	++	+	+
	Acid esterase	−	−	−	+	−
	Convoluted nuclei	+	++	?	+	−

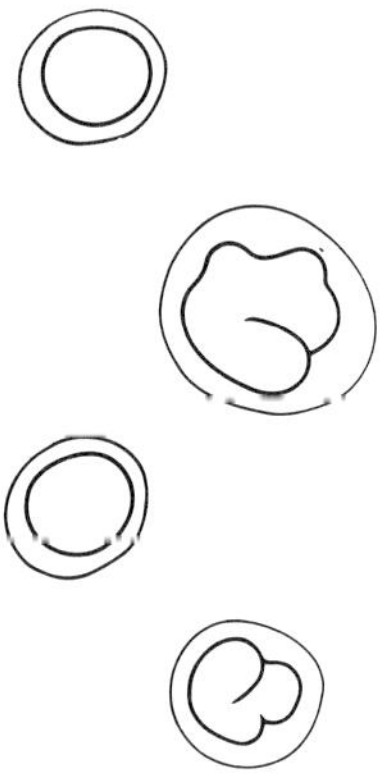

Figure 2. Cytologic, immunologic, and enzyme cytochemical features of T-lymphoblastic lymphoma with or without convoluted nuclei. Thy type = thymocytic type; Periph. T type = peripheral T-cell type; Prethy = prethymocytic subtype; Prothy = prothymocytic subtype; M. Thy = mature thymocytic subtype; T_H = helper T-cell subtype; T_S = suppressor T-cell subtype; S-Ig = surface immunoglobulin; E = erythrocyte; HTLA = human T-lymphocyte antigen; Tdt = terminal deoxynucleotidyl transferase.

results of our analyses here, the four main types of pattern we observed are shown in Figure 2. The *first* pattern is characterized by the presence, or sometimes, the lack of C3 receptors, the consistent lack of sheep E receptors, the presence of strong focal acid phosphatase activity, and the absence of acid nonspecific esterase activity. This pattern corresponds to that of pre-thymocytes. Thus, we call the neoplasms with such a pattern lymphoblastic lymphoma of the prethymocytic subtype. The *second* pattern is characterized by the simultaneous presence of C3 and sheep E receptors and the presence of acid phosphatase activity, but usually the absence of acid nonspecific esterase activity. This pattern is identical to that of prothymocytes. Thus, we call the neoplasm lymphoblastic lymphoma of the prothymocytic sub-type. The *third* pattern is characterized by the complete absence of C3 receptors, the presence of sheep E receptors capable of binding at 37°C, the presence of acid phosphatase activity, and the absence of acid non-specific esterase activity. This pattern corresponds to that of mature thy-mocytes, which led to the term lymphoblastic lymphoma of the mature thymocytic subtype. The *fourth* pattern we observed is characterized by the lack of C3 receptors, the presence of sheep E receptors capable of bind-ing only at 4°C, and the presence of both acid phosphatase and acid non-specific esterase activity. This pattern is the same as that of a majority of the peripheral-blood T cells. Thus, we proposed the term lymphoblastic lymphoma of the peripheral T-cell type. The strong focal acid nonspecific esterase reactivity of the tumor cells suggest that they are related to the helper T-cell fraction.

The literature contains a report (4) on one case of lymphoblastic lympho-ma of the T type whose cells acted as suppressor cells in the pokeweed mitogen-stimulated B-cell system. Unfortunately, no information was given concerning the surface and enzyme markers in that case.

Cytologic studies have revealed a more or less distinct pattern of con-voluted nuclei in the prethymocytic and prothymocytic subtypes. The one

Table 5. Incidence of the subtypes of T-lymphoblastic lymphoma in the series of various authors.

Lymphoblastic lymphoma, including ALL	Jaffe et al. (12) (n = 5)	Thiel et al. (22) (n = 16)	Kung et al. (14) (n = 9)	Stein et al.	
				1st series 1976 (n = 8)	2nd series 1979 (n = 24)
Prethymocytic subtype	2	7	0	2	6
Prothymocytic subtype	2	2	9	6	16
Mature thymocytic subtype	1	2	0	0	1
Peripheral T-cell subtype	0	5	0	0	1

case of the mature thymocytic subtype in our series was nonconvoluted, and the one case of the peripheral T-cell type was hyperconvoluted, the nuclei showing some resemblance to those of Sézary cells. On the whole, convoluted nuclei appear to be a reliable marker of T-lymphoblastic neoplasms. This morphologic marker cannot be used in all cases, however, because it is not always clearly present.

Table 5 gives data on the frequency of T-lymphoblastic lymphoma and leukemia in our own series and those of other investigators. To get an idea of the relative frequency of the subtypes, we subclassified the cases of the other authors according to our concept. The data vary from author to author. The cases in the series investigated by Thiel et al. (22) appear to be selected. According to the findings of Kung et al. (14) and our own, the prothymocytic subtype is by far the most common subtype. All other subtypes are comparatively rare. They can apparently be arranged in the following order of frequency: prethymocytic subtype, peripheral T-cell subtype, and mature thymocytic subtype.

In our series, females predominated among the patients with the prethymocytic subtype. This trend was recently confirmed by Thiel et al. (23), who found eight women among 13 patients with lymphoblastic lymphoma of the prethymocytic subtype. For all other subtypes, males predominated.

The prothymocytic subtype is associated with a mediastinal mass in up to 90% of the cases. Another frequent finding is a pleural effusion containing neoplastic cells.

The data available at present do not allow clear-cut conclusions about differences in patho-anatomic and clinical behavior among the various types. The number of cases investigated immunologically and clinically is still too small, and there has not yet been enough time for a follow-up analysis.

Lymphocytic lymphomas and leukemias of the T type

The next main morphologic group of T-cell neoplasms is made up of lymphocytic lymphomas and leukemias, including chronic lymphocytic leukemia of the T type (T-CLL), prolymphocytic leukemia of the T type (T-PLL), Sézary's syndrome, mycosis fungoides, and T-zone lymphoma.

T-CLL

As shown in Figure 3, the cells of T-CLL lack B markers and show the characteristics of peripheral T cells, namely, sheep E receptors that bind only at 4°C and the absence of Tdt.

The available data suggest that there are at least two types of T-CLL, namely, T-CLL of helper T cells and T-CLL of suppressor T cells. The existence of T-CLL of suppressor T cells has already been proved. Uchi-

Cytology	Immunology/Enzyme cytochemistry		
		Helper type	Suppressor type
	S - Ig	−	−
	C3b receptor	−	−
	C3d receptor	−	−
	IgM - Fc receptor	+	−
	IgG - Fc receptor	−	+
Helper subtype	Mouse - E rosettes	−	−
	Sheep - E rosettes stable at 37°C	−	−
	stable only at 4°C	+	+
	HTLA	+	+
	Tdt	−	−
	Acid phosphatase	+	+
	Acid esterase	+	−
	Azurophil granules	−	+/−
Suppressor subtype			

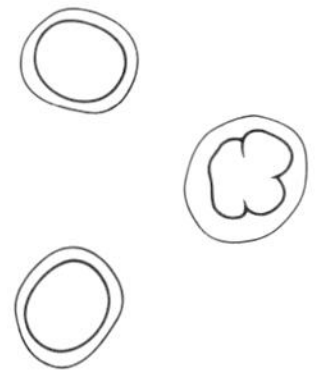

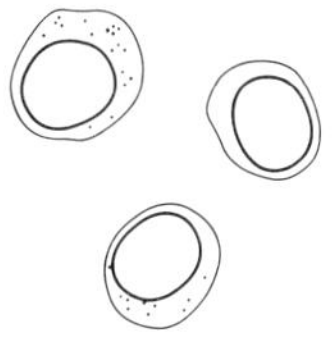

Figure 3. Cytologic, immunologic, and enzyme cytochemical features of chronic lymphocytic leukemia of the T type. Abbreviations as in Figure 2.

yama et al. (25) recently showed by cocultivation of leukemic cells and B cells in the presence of pokeweed mitogen that the cells from three out of six cases of T-CLL had a marked suppressive effect on B-cell differentiation into plasma cells. Unfortunately, these investigators did not report on the cytology or enzyme cytochemistry in their cases of suppressor T-type CLL.

On the basis of present knowledge and our own data (see below), we think that there might also be a helper T-cell type of CLL. This type would usually be IgM-Fc receptor positive and IgG-Fc receptor negative, show dotlike acid nonspecific esterase activity, lack azurophil granules, and have a propensity to involve the skin. The cells of suppressor T-type CLL are probably IgM-Fc receptor negative, IgG-Fc receptor positive, and acid nonspecific esterase negative, and contain azurophil granules in many instances (Figure 4).

In the last two years we have investigated five cases of T-CLL. The cells from four of these patients exhibited a focal or dotlike acid nonspecific esterase reaction product (Figure 4a) and lacked IgG-Fc receptors, as do the cells of the normal T-cell subpopulation that act as helpers. The leukemic cells of the fifth patient had markedly abundant cytoplasm which contained azurophil granules in 20–30% of the cells but did not show any acid nonspecific esterase activity (Figure 4b and c). On the basis of these findings, we presumed that this case was derived from suppressor T cells.

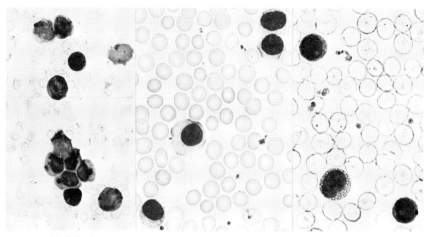

Figure 4. (a) Cells from a case of chronic lymphocytic leukemia of the T type (T-CLL) rosetted with sheep erythrocytes and stained for acid nonspecific esterase. The neoplastic T cells show a dotlike esterase reaction product, as do normal helper T cells. Cytocentrifuge slide. × 800. (b) Cells from another case of T-CLL with Pappenheim staining. Note the abundant cytoplasm and the presence of azurophil granules in the cytoplasm. Blood smear. × 800. (c) Cells from the same case as (b) stained for acid nonspecific esterase. The leukemic cells are negative. The enzyme-positive cell in the lower right corner is a residual nonneoplastic helper T cell. Blood smear. × 560.

T-PLL

This T-type leukemia is rare. Since we have not yet performed our own analyses of T-PLL, the reader is referred to the literature (6, 7).

Sézary's syndrome and mycosis fungoides

The neoplastic cells of Sézary's syndrome, mycosis fungoides, and T-CLL share the basic characteristics of peripheral T cells mentioned above and shown in Figure 5. The main differences between T-CLL on the one hand and Sézary's syndrome and mycosis fungoides on the other are the presence of so-called Sézary and mycosis cells in the latter two neoplasias and the epidermotropism of these cells.

The neoplastic cells of Sézary's syndrome (5) and mycosis fungoides usually express receptors for IgM. Functional studies have produced the most interesting results. Broder et al. (3) showed that cells from five out of seven patients with Sézary's syndrome were able to help B cells mature into plasma cells. Recently, Ballieux et al. (2) reported that in a patient with Sézary's syndrome the neoplastic T cells lacking demonstrable IgM-Fc receptors were capable of helping B cells transform into antibody-secreting cells. This observation suggests that the relationship between helper T-cell function and the expression of IgM-Fc receptors is not an absolute one.

Cytology	Immunology/Enzyme cytochemistry	
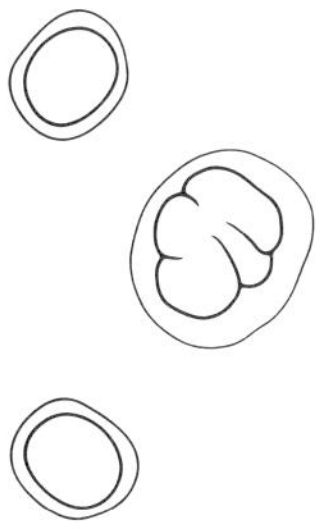	S-Ig	—
	Ia-like antigen	—
	C3 receptor	—
	IgM-Fc receptor	+
	IgG-Fc receptor	—
	Mouse-E rosettes	—
	Sheep-E rosettes	
	stable at 37°C	—
	stable at 4°C	+
	HTLA	+
	Tdt	—
	Acid phosphatase	+
	Acid esterase	+
	Helper cell activity	+

Figure 5. Cytologic, immunologic, and enzyme cytochemical features of mycosis fungoides and Sézary's syndrome. Abbreviations as in Figure 2.

Suppressor activity was not observed in any of the published cases. This is consistent with the invariable absence of azurophil granules and presence of acid nonspecific esterase activity in neoplastic cells in the four cases of Sézary's syndrome and the one case of mycosis fungoides we have analyzed. Since the neoplastic cells of mycosis fungoides exhibit exactly the same immunologic and enzyme cytochemical features as do the cells of Sézary's syndrome, these two lezions appear to be closely related. The dermotropism of the neoplastic cells of both neoplasias also suggests that affinity to the skin is a common property of helper T cells in a special stage of maturation or functional differentiation.

T-zone lymphoma

The fourth type of T-lymphocytic lymphoma is T-zone lymphoma (15, 16). So far, we have investigated only three cases with immunologic methods. In all three we found a mixture of B and T cells in the tumor tissue. The B cells showed a polytypic surface immunoglobulin pattern and both complement receptor subtypes, which are characteristic of germinal center cells. The T cells were identifiable by their capacity to bind sheep E at 4°C. Morphologic comparison of the neoplastic cells in lymph-node sections with rosetted cells in suspension revealed that the sheep E-binding cell population was the neoplastic one. We have no data on the T-cell subset involved in this disease. From an immunologic standpoint, all we can say is that T-zone lymphoma appears to be a neoplasm of peripheral T cells.

Immunoblastic lymphoma of the T type

The third main group of T-cell neoplasms comprises immunoblastic lymphoma or the large-cell type of lymphoma. Reports on the incidence of T-type tumors among the immunoblastic or large-cell lymphomas are contradictory, probably because of differences in the morphologic definition of this type of neoplasia. In our experience T-immunoblastic lymphoma is rare. Our series of 19 immunologically characterized cases of immunoblastic lymphoma includes only one with T-cell properties. Figure 6 shows the cytology of this case and the ability of the tumor cells to bind sheep E. Half of the tumor cells displayed a dotlike acid nonspecific esterase reaction product, suggesting that the cells were related to the helper T-cell lineage. We assume that other types of T-immunoblastic lymphoma related to the various T-cell subsets will be detected in the future.

CONCLUDING REMARKS

The concept for the classification of T-cell lymphomas and leukemias presented here may be somewhat idealized, since there are cases with marker constellations that do not fit into this concept. We shall end this presentation with a description of a case of CLL in which the cells expres-

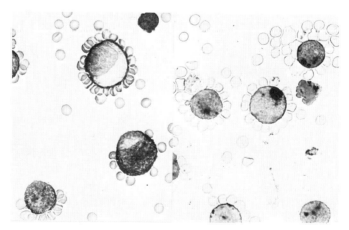

Figure 6a and b. Suspended cells from a case of T-immunoblastic lymphoma rosetted with sheep erythrocytes and stained with Pappenheim (a) or for acid nonspecific esterase (b) × 560.

Table 6. Immunologic and enzyme cytochemical features of an unusual case of chronic lymphocytic leukemia

Property	%
SIg (μ, δ, κ)	35
Mouse E rosettes	60
Ia-like antigen	63
Polyacrylic acid beads	97
EAC 3b	18
EAC 3d	91
IgG-EA	72
Sheep E rosettes at 37°C	0
Sheep E rosettes at 4°C	85
Sheep E rosettes in the presence of anti-κ or anti-λ	70
Trypsinized sheep E rosettes	0
Acid nonspecific esterase (dot-like reaction product)	70

sed a quite unusual array of immunologic and enzyme cytochemical features (Table 6).

The leukemic cells displayed readily detectable amounts of IgM and IgD on their surface. The light chains were restricted to κ. The cells also had receptors for mouse E, expressed Ia-like antigen, and bound polyacrylic acid beads. Thus, these leukemic CLL cells exhibited four different markers specific to or characteristic of B cells. Moreover, the leukemic cells bore receptors for C3d and for the Fc portion of IgG, as do cells from most patients with CLL of the B type.

Two independent T-cell markers were detectable in the leukemic cells, namely, sheep E receptors and dotlike acid nonspecific esterase activity. The sheep E rosettes were stable only at 4°C. Sheep E rosette formation was not affected by anti-immunoglobulin sera, but was completely inhibited by pretreatment of the sheep E with trypsin or pretreatment of the leukemic cells with an anti-T-cell serum. This indicates that the sheep E were bound by a surface structure having the same properties as the usual sheep E receptor of normal T cells.

It is clear that the features of this case of CLL do not fit into any of the known categories of T or B cells. There are at least two possible interpretations:

1) This leukemia might have arisen from a small population of normal cells that usually express these features or develop this marker constellation in response to appropriate stimuli.

2) The expression of almost all known markers is a manifestation of the disordered differentiation of the malignant cells.

REFERENCES

1. Andersson, L.C., and Gahmberg, C.G.: Membrane glycoprotein pattern of normal and malignant human leukocytes. In: Function and structure of the immune system. Advances in experimental medicine and biology, vol. 114, pp. 623–628, Müller-Ruchholts, W., and Müller-Hermelink, H.K., Plenum Press, New York and London, 1979.

2. Ballieux, R.E., Heijnen, C.J., UytdeHaag, F., and Zegers, B.J.M.: Regulation of B cell activity in man: Role of T cells. In: Activation of antibody synthesis in human B lymphocytes. Immunol. Rev., in press.

3. Broder, S., Lawrence, E., Durm, M., Goldman, C., Muul, L., and Waldmann, T.A.: Further characterization of neoplastic helper T cells from patients with the Sézary syndrome. In: Regulatory mechanisms in lymphocyte activation, pp. 689–691, Lucas, D.O., Academic Press, New York, 1977.

4. Broder, S., Poplack, D., Whang-Peng, J., Durm, M., Goldman, C., Muul, L., and Waldmann, T.A.: Characterization of a suppressor-cell leukemia. Evidence for the requirement of an interaction of two T cells in the development of human suppressor effector cells. New Engl. J. Med., 298:66–72, 1978.

5. Brouet, J.C.: T-cell neoplasia. Presented at the IV. C.N.R.S. International Colloquium on Lymphoid Neoplasias, and 1977 Plenary Session of the E.O.R.T.C., Paris, June 1977.

6. Brouet, J.C., Flandrin, G., Sasportes, M., Preud'Homme, J.-L., and Seligmann, M.: Chronic lymphocytic leukaemia of T-cell origin. Immunological and clinical evaluation in eleven patients Lancet, II: 890–894, 1975.

7. Catovsky, D., Pettit, J.E., Galton, D.A.G., Spiers, A.S.D., and Harrison, C.V.: Leukaemic reticuloendotheliosis ("hairy" cell leukaemia): A distinct clinico-pathological entity. Brit. J. Haemat., 26:9–27, 1974.

8. Chang, L.M.S.: Development of terminal deoxynucleotidyl transferase activity in embryonic calf thymus gland. Biochem. biophys. Res. Commun., 44:124–131, 1971.

9. Ferrarini, M., Moretta, L., Abrile, R., and Durante, M.I.: Receptors for IgG molecules on human lymphocytes forming spontaneous rosettes with sheep red cells. Eur. J. Immunol., 5:70–72, 1975.

10. Gatien, J.G., Schneeberger, E.E., and Merler, E.. Analysis of human thymocyte subpopulations using discontinuous gradients of albumin: Precursor lymphocytes in human thymus. Eur. J. Immunol., 5:312–317, 1975.

11. Grossi, C.E., Webb, S.R., Zicca, A., Lydyard, P.M., Moretta, L., Mingari, M.C., and Cooper, M.D.: Morphological and histochemical analyses of two human T-cell subpopulations bearing receptors for IgM or IgG. J. exp. Med., 147:1405–1417, 1978.

12. Jaffe, E.S., Braylan, R.C., Frank, M.M., Green, I., and Berard, C.W.: Heterogeneity of immunologic markers and surface morphology in childhood lymphoblastic lymphoma. Blood, 48:213–222, 1976.

13. Knowles, D.M., II, Hoffman, T., Ferrarini, M., and Kunkel, H.G.: The demonstration of acid α-naphthyl acetate esterase activity in human lymphocytes: Usefulness as a T-cell marker. Cell. Immunol., 35:112–123, 1978.

14. Kung, P.C., Long, J.C., Ratliff, R.L., Harrison, T.A., and Baltimore, D.: Terminal deoxynucleotidyl transferase in the diagnosis of leukemia and malignant lymphoma. Amer. J. Med., 64:788–794, 1978.

15. Lennert, K.: Klassifikation und Morphologie der Non-Hodgkin-Lymphome.

In: Maligne Lymphome und monoklonale Gammopathien. Hämatologie und Bluttransfusion, vol. 18, pp. 145–166, Löffler, H., (ed.), Lehmanns, München, 1976.

16. Lennert, K., Mohri, N., Stein, H., and Kaiserling, E.: The histopathology of malignant lymphoma. Brit. J. Haemat., 31: (Suppl.), 193–203, 1975.

17. Moretta, L., Ferrarini, M., Durante, M.L., and Mingari, M.C.: Expression of a receptor for IgM by human T cells in vitro. Eur. J. Immunol., 5:565–569, 1975.

18. Moretta, L., Mingari, M.C., Moretta, A., and Cooper, M.D.: Human T lymphocyte subpopulations: Studies of the mechanism by which T cells bearing Fc receptors for IgG suppress T-dependent B cell differentiation induced by pokeweed mitogen. J. Immunol, 122:984–990, 1979.

19. Moretta, L., Webb, S.R., Grossi, C.E., Lydyard, P.M., and Cooper, M.D.: Functional analysis of two human T-cell subpopulations: Help and suppression of B-cell responses by T cells bearing receptors for IgM or IgG. J. exp. Med., 146:184–200, 1977.

20. Stein, H., and Müller-Hermelink, H.K.: Simultaneous presence of receptors for complement and sheep red blood cells on human fetal thymocytes. Brit. J. Haemat., 36:227–233, 1977.

21. Stein, H., Petersen, N., Gaedicke, G., Lennert, K., and Landbeck, G.: Lymphoblastic lymphoma of convoluted or acid phosphatase type – a tumor of T precursor cells. Int. J. Cancer, 17:292–295, 1976.

22. Thiel, E., Dörmer, P., Rodt, H., Huhn, D., Bauchinger, M., Kley, H.P., and Thierfelder, S.: Quantitation of T-antigenic sites and Ig-determinants on leukemic cells by microphotometric immunoradiography. Proof of the clonal origin of thymus-derived lymphocytic leukemias. In: Immunological diagnosis of leukemias and lymphomas. Haematology and Blood Transfusion, vol. 20, pp. 131–144, Thierfelder, S., Rodt, H., and Thiel, E. (eds), Springer, Berlin, Heidelberg and New York, 1977.

23. Thiel, E., Rodt, H., Netzel, B., Huhn, D., Wündisch, G.F., Haas, R.J., Bender-Götze, C., and Thierfelder, S.: T-Zell-Antigen positive, E-Rosetten negative akute Lymphoblastenleukämie. Blut, 36:363–369, 1978.

24. Tötterman, T.H., Ranki, A., and Häyry, P.: Expression of the acid α-naphthyl acetate esterase marker by activated and secondary T lymphocytes in man. Scand. J. Immunol., 6:305–310, 1977.

25. Uchiyama, T., Sagawa, K., Takatsuki, K., and Uchino, H.: Effect of adult T-cell leukemia cells on pokeweed mitogen-induced normal B-cell differentiation. Clin. Immunol. Immunopath., 10:24–34, 1978.

26. Yoshida, T.O., and Andersson, B.: Evidence for a receptor recognizing antigen complexed immunoglobulin on the surface of activated mouse thymus lymphocytes. Scand. J. Immunol., 1:401–408, 1972.

25. CLINICAL MANIFESTATIONS OF T-CELL LYMPHOMAS

A.M. LEVINE

CUTANEOUS T-CELL LYMPHOMAS

The cutaneous T-cell lymphomas include Mycosis fungoides and Sézary syndrome. Although these diseases have been considered separate entities in the past, current evidence would suggest that they represent instead, a spectrum of the same disease. The evidence for this concept is as follows. First, in each variant, the malignant cell appears identical in all respects. Thus, the morphology on light microscopy and electron microscopy is similar, with characteristic deep nuclear convolutions, causing the so-called "cerebriform" nuclear appearance. Second, the histologic appearance of involved skin in Sézary syndrome and Mycosis fungoides is similar. Third, a clinical relationship between these two variants is known to exist, with well-documented cases of Sézary syndrome proceeding to develop classic changes of Mycosis fungoides, and vice versa. Last, and most recent, it is now known that both diseases are neoplasms of "T" lymphocytes. In selected well-studied cases, the malignant T lymphocyte has been identified as a helper T cell in function, which may explain the hyperglobulinemia (IgA primarily) which has been noted clinically. Although the malignancies appear pathophysiologically similar, the morphologic expression on the skin varies from patient to patient, leading some investigators to speculate that these variations may reflect differing host responses to the malignant cell, rather than separate disease entities.

Mycosis fungoides usually begins as a nonspecific psoriaform eruption on the skin. Although the psoriaform lesions may be present for many years, it may be impossible to make the histologic diagnosis of Mycosis fungoides at this stage. In its first histologically recognizable form, Mycosis fungoides is seen as plaques on the skin. These plaques may be quite pruritic, and may involve any dermatologic area. After the plaque stage, the disease progresses, with development of tumors and ulcers on the skin. It is estimated that approximately five years elapse between the time that the diagnosis can first be made to the time that generalized tumors appear. After the typical tumor stage, the disease disseminates, with involvement first of lymph nodes, then of spleen, liver, and potentially, any parenchymal organ. Sur-

J.G. van den Tweel et al. (eds.), Malignant Lymphoproliferative Diseases, 331–339
Copyright © 1980 by Martinus Nijhoff Publishers bv, The Hague/Boston/London.

vival at this stage is quite short, with median survivals in the range of one to two years.

Sézary syndrome, in similar manner, may be present for many years in a relatively benign manner, confined for the most part to the skin. The patient with Sézary syndrome typically develops an edematous, erythematous, intensely pruritic eruption, usually involving the entire skin surface. The clinical picture resembles that which is seen in a severe sunburn. After many years of disease limited to the skin, the patient with Sézary syndrome, similar to Mycosis fungoides, usually develops dissemination of disease, with involvement of lymph nodes, liver, spleen, bone marrow, and other organs.

Peripheral blood involvement in these diseases has been a matter of interest within the past several years. The typical malignant cell may be seen circulating in the peripheral blood at diagnosis in the vast majority of patients with Sézary syndrome. In contrast, older reports in the literature indicate that this is a much rarer event in the patient with Mycosis fungoides, occurring in only 20 to 30% of patients. Using more advanced technical methodology, however, recent investigations have demonstrated the presence of these cells in the peripheral blood of approximately 50 to 70% of Mycosis fungoides patients. The occurrence of peripheral blood involvement in the absence of marrow involvement has led to much speculation regarding the primary site of Sézary cell production. Based upon kinetic data, recent investigations have indicated that the malignant cell is not primarily produced either in the skin or in the peripheral blood, but rather, in another, as yet undefined site. Shackeny and his coworkers have suggested that this site might be the lymph nodes.

Beacuse the cutaneous T-cell lymphomas are relatively rare diseases, a large body of information does not yet exist regarding the usual staging or extent of disease at diagnosis in the majority of patients. Since lymph node involvement is known to be associated with poorer prognosis and short survival, the results of lymphangiography in a large number of patients would be of interest. A recent study from Stanford University, involving 97 patients, indicated that lymphangiography did not contribute significantly compared to physical examination for palpable lymphadenopathy. An additional problem in this regard is the fact that palpable lymphadenopathy remains a sign of poor prognosis even when the enlarged lymph nodes are found, on biopsy, not to be involved with Mycosis fungoides, but rather, with dermatopathic lymphadenitis. Because of this finding, some investigators have suggested that dermatopathic lymphadenitis may represent the earliest stage of lymph node involvement in the patient with Mycosis fungoides.

Aside from palpable lymphadenopathy, other indicators of poor prognosis in these diseases include older age at diagnosis (greater than 50 years), greater extent of disease on the skin (tumors or ulcers), and the lack of attainment of complete remission after a given therapeutic modality has been employed.

Many modalities of therapy have been shown to be effective in the management of the patient with cutaneous T-cell lymphoma. In general, however, early stages of disease respond quite well to most modalities, whereas late stage disease remains far more resistant. The application of chemotherapeutic agents to the skin has been used for many years, and appears quite effective in the management of early plaque or erythrodermatous disease. The agent most widely used is nitrogen mustard, which is dissolved in tap water (10 mgm vial with 50 cc of water), and applied with a sponge or hand to all body surface areas except the axilla, perineum, scalp and eyelids. This application is repeated daily until good control is achieved, and is then repeated weekly in an attempt to maintain the remission. Approximately 50 to 75% of patients with early stage disease will respond completely, with continued good control lasting an average of two to three years. The most frequently encountered problem with topical nitrogen mustard is the development of hypersensitivity reactions to the drug, which occur in as many as two-thirds of patients during the course of therapy. Recent investigations have reported an equal efficacy to the use of topical BCNU in these patients; additionally, BCNU does not appear to cross-react with nitrogen mustard. Argyropoulos et al. have recently reported on the preliminary evaluation of fifteen different chemotherapeutic agents applied topically to patients with cutaneous T-cell lymphomas, using a patch test technique. Many of these agents appear promising, including cytosine arabinoside, dianhydrogalacticol, and others.

Photochemotherapy has also been used with success in patients with cutaneous T-cell lymphomas. It has long been known that sunlight exerts a beneficial effect on early stages of disease. Long wave ultra-violet (UV) light (UV-A: 320–400 nm "black light") offers an advantage over conventional ultraviolet rays, since approximately 60% of UV-A reaches the dermis, with less than 1% delivered to the subcutaneous tissues. Photosensitizing agents, for example, Methoxsalen, are activated by UV-A, and bind covalently and reversibly to the pyrimidine bases in DNA, causing decreased DNA synthesis and cell division. The photosensitizing agents are given orally two hours prior to UV-A exposure. Treatments are given initially two or three times per week, and are then decreased in frequency as lesions are controlled. Although the results appear encouraging, this modality has been used only a relatively short time. Of 12 patients reported by Roenigk et al., eight remain in complete remission at three years, while three have developed progressive disease. No significant systemic toxicity has yet been reported, although experience with this modality is quite limited.

Radiotherapy has been used extensively in the treatment of these diseases, and newer techniques appear quite exciting in the long-term management of some patients. Traditional orthovoltage radiation has been used for many years, and, when given to localized lesions, can produce permanent control in most patients. The disadvantage of orthovoltage radiation, however, is the risk of bone marrow depression, since 75% of the energy is delivered to a depth greater than one centimeter from the skin surface. Additionally, only small fields may be treated, as total body irradiation with this modality is tedious and inaccurate. Because of these disadvantages, recent investigators have explored the use of electron beam radiotherapy in the patient with cutaneous T-cell lymphoma. The maximum range of the electron is approximately one centimeter, with less than 5% of the radiation delivered below two centimeters from the skin surface. The radiation dosage may be delivered in a uniform manner, making treatment of the entire skin surface possible. Using high dose electron beam therapy (3,000 to 4,000 rads). Hoppe and his coworkers at Stanford University were able to produce a complete remission in 91% of 92 patients with limited and generalized plaque disease. Approximately 40% of these patients remain alive, without relapse, and without evidence of disease at nine years. It is possible that these patients have been cured. Ninety-six percent of the total group remain alive at nine years. These investigators were able to demonstrate that high dose electron beam therapy was significantly superior to lower doses (less than 3,000 rads). Although early stage disease was treated very effectively, patients with tumors on the skin, or dermatopathic lymphadenitis, lived an average of three years, with only a few patients remaining disease-free, although 72% attained a complete remission. The median survival of patients with pathologically involved lymph nodes or other visceral organs was only 1.7 years. Similar results have recently been reported from other centers.

Antithymocyte globulin has been used in a limited number of patients with cutaneous T-cell lymphomas, and has been shown to be transiently effective in some, although systemic toxicity (fever, nausea, vomiting) does occur. This modality will undoubtedly be investigated further.

Single agent chemotherapy has been used for the treatment of patients with advanced disease. Although selected agents have produced objective responses, for the most part these responses have been of short term duration. A recent study from the Southwest Oncology Group reports more promising results using combination chemotherapy. Twenty-four patients were treated with either CHOP (adriamycin, cyclophosphamide, vincristine and prednisone), HOP (adriamycin, vincristine and prednisone), or COP-Bleo (cyclophosphamide, vincristine, prednisone and bleomycin). The objective response rate was 95%, with complete remission rate of 29% for the group. The median survival for all patients was 95 weeks, and was similar in all three groups. COP-Bleo appeared best tolerated, with less hematologic toxicity and longer duration of complete and partial remission.

Recently, the use of electron beam radiotherapy together with combination chemotherapy has been described in the management of patients with advanced disease. Using high dose (3,000 rads) whole-body electron therapy with six cycles of MOPP (nitrogen mustard, vincristine, procarbazine and prednisone), Griem et al. have demonstrated 70% three year disease-free survival in nine patients. The use of such combined modes of therapy will certainly be investigated further.

CONVOLUTED LYMPHOCYTIC (LYMPHOBLASTIC) LYMPHOMA

Convoluted lymphocytic lymphoma was first described by Barcos and Lukes in 1975. These investigators noted a particular type of lymphoma, occurring primarily in older children or adolescents, which presented quite characteristically with the onset of a mediastinal mass. The disease was noted to progress rapidly in the majority of cases, to involve the bone marrow and peripheral blood. The malignant cells, which were noted to have striking nuclear convolutions, had a very primitive appearance. Retrospectively, these cells were, for the most part, considered to be lymphoblasts by prior investigators, and the disease was considered to be equivalent to acute lymphocytic leukemia of childhood. When surface marker studies were performed on malignant cells from these patients, it was found that they did not mark as the characteristic "null" (non-B/non-T) cells of acute lymphocytic leukemia (ALL), but rather, these cells marked as "T" cells. Convoluted lymphocytic lymphoma was clearly confused with ALL in the past, and explains the subgroup of patients with acute lymphocytic leukemia, somewhat older than the usual patient, who presented with a mediastinal mass, high white count, and had a course of disease which was far more aggressive than the typical case of ALL.

The same entity has now been described in the adult population. The disease is quite characteristic in its onset, course, and natural history. Males are affected more frequently than females. Any age group may be affected, although the peak incidence of disease seems to occur in young adults. The most common mode of presentation is that of a mediastinal mass, which is usually accompanied by symptoms and signs of compression of vital intrathoracic structures. Dyspnea, dysphagia, superior vena caval syndrome, pericarditis and congestive heart failure are common modes of presentation. Frequently, these symptoms are of an emergent nature, requiring immediate diagnosis and management. Biopsy of involved mediastinal tissue will reveal the typical morphologic appearance of convoluted lymphocytic lymphoma. In the classification schema of Rappaport, this tumor would have been considered part of the spectrum of poorly differentiated lymphocytic lymphoma, diffuse, and its inclusion in this group must certainly be responsible for some of the prior reports of poor prognosis in that heterogeneous group of lymphoma. With the newer concepts of this disease, Rappaport and Nathwani have termed the disorder "lymphoblastic lymphoma".

Between 50 and 75% of patients with convoluted lymphocytic lymphoma present with a mediastinal mass. From the mediastinum, the disease progresses predictably to involve the bone marrow, occurring, again, in approximately 75% of patients. Most patients with bone marrow involvement will demonstrate tumor cells circulating in the peripheral blood. Approximately half of the patients with bone marrow involvement progress to develop disease in the central nervous system, usually presenting as a meningitic picture. The disease is a very aggressive one, with a median survival of approximately one year, in spite of multiagent chemotherapy.

When treated with a variety of chemotherapeutic agents, most patients will respond dramatically. However, in spite of rapid disappearance of disease, the tumor characteristically relapses with equal rapidity, either in the peripheral nodal regions, the bone marrow, or the central nervous system. Chemotherapeutic agents which are usually not employed in non-Hodgkin's lymphoma, such as cytosine arabinoside, and L-asparaginase, have been shown to be quite effective in convoluted lymphocytic lymphoma. Based upon the knowledge that this disease will predictably relapse, in spite of aggressive chemotherapy, and that the disease often relapses in the central nervous system, newer therapeutic techniques have been devised which attempt to treat the central nervous system prophylactically, as in acute lymphocytic leukemia. Additionally, aggressive, multiagent regimens, similar to those used in childhood lymphoma, are being used with initial excellent response. A modification of the LSA-2/L-2 regimen, devised by Wollner, and consisting of the cyclic administration of eleven different chemotherapeutic agents, given over a three-year period of time, appears to be quite effective in the management of this disease. However, these newer treatment modalities have only recently been instituted, and further study will be required before firm recommendations can be made.

IMMUNOBLASTIC SARCOMA OF T CELLS

Immunoblastic sarcoma was described by Lukes and Collins in 1974. This represents a lymphoma of transformed lymphocytes, which was though to occur in the setting of genetic predisposition, abnormal immune status, and chronic antigenic stimulation. Although originally thought to be exclusively of B-cell origin, T-cell immunoblastic sarcoma has now been recognized. Eighteen patients with immunoblastic sarcoma of T-cell origin have recently been studied by Levine et al. A two to one female predominance was found. The median age of these patients was 47 years. The majority of patients (16) originally presented because of lymphadenopathy.

Three patients had histories of immune disease, two patients had prior histories of carcinoma (vulvar and ovarian), and one patient had a two-year history of poorly differentiated lymphocytic lymphoma, diffuse, prior to transforming to immunoblastic-sarcoma. Systemic symptoms, consisting of fever, night sweats and weight loss, were present in eleven of the patients (61%). The majority (90%) had widely disseminated disease at diagnosis, with bone marrow involvement in 50%, and hepatic involvement in 60%. Half of the patients had disease in the mediastinum and/or hilum. Lymphocytopenia (absolute lymphocyte count less than 1,000/dl) was present in 40%, and when present, was an indicator of shorter survival. It was of interest that seven patients (47%) demonstrated diffuse, polyclonal hypergammaglobulinemia on serum protein electrophoresis, since one might speculate that the tumor in these patients may have had helper T-cell function. In this regard, a patient recently reported by Lawrence et al., who had Sézary syndrome, was found to have malignant cells with helper T-cell function. The patient evolved to develop an immunoblastic sarcoma of T-cell origin. At the time of transformation, the malignant T cells were found to retain their helper cell function.

In spite of multiagent chemotherapy (BACOP, CHOP-Bleo, or COPP: bleomycin, adriamycin, cyclophosphamide, vincristine, prednisone and/or procarbazine), the median survival of these 18 patients was only 26 months. Disseminated disease (Stage III or IV), and presence of lymphocytopenia were found to be independent factors in predicting shorter survival. The optimal therapeutic modalities for these patients have yet to be defined.

CHRONIC LYMPHOCYTIC LEUKEMIA OF T-CELL ORIGIN

Chronic lymphocytic leukemia (CLL) is almost exclusively a disease of B-cell origin. However, approximately 40 cases of T-cell CLL have now been described in the literature. Morphologically, T-cell CLL appears heterogeneous, with some cases demonstrating a prolymphocytic appearance, and others demonstrating dense azurophilic granules in the cytoplasm.

Clinical differences exist between the T-cell and B-cell variants of this disease. As opposed to the male predominance seen in B-cell CLL, females appear to be affected with equal frequency in the T-cell variant. Although the median age is similar for both types, a greater range in age has been shown for the T-cell variant, with several reported cases in the second and third decades of life. The incidence of splenomegaly appears greater in patients with T-cell CLL, with only 20% of patients lacking this finding, and many patients reported to have splenomegaly of massive proportions. The skin appears to be involved, again, with greater frequency in the T-cell variety, reported in approximately 50% of patients. Skin disease may consist of generalized erythroderma, localized erythroderma, or single or multiple cutaneous nodules. The lesions have been reported to be intensely pruritic. Further, whereas approximately 50% of patients with B-cell CLL are found to have hypogammaglobulinemia on serum protein electrophoresis, the majority of patients with T-cell variant appear to have normal immunoglobulin levels, or diffuse polyclonal hypergammaglobulinemia.

The natural history and optimal therapy for patients with T-cell CLL has yet to be ascertained. From the few reports in the literature, however, the survival of these patients appears to be shorter than the seven to nine year median survival described for the B-cell variety. Further reports concerning these patients are awaited with great interest.

REFERENCES

1. Argyropoulos, C.L., Lamberg, S.I., and Clendenning, W.E., et al.: Preliminary evaluation of 15 chemotherapeutic agents applied topically in the treatment of mycosis fungoides. Cancer Treat. Rep., 63:619–622, 1979.
2. Brouet, J.C., Flandrin, G., and Sasportes, M. et al.: Chronic lymphocytic leukemia of T cell origin. Lancet, 890–893, November 8, 1975.
3. Castellino, R.A., Hoppe, R.T., and Blank, N. et al.: Experience with lymphography in patients with mycosis fungoides. Cancer Treat. Rep., 63:581–586, 1979.
4. Catovsky, D., and Galetto, J. et al.: Prolymphocytic leukemia of B and T cell type. Lancet:232–234, August 4, 1973.
5. Edeslon, R.L., Raafat, J., and Berger, C.L. et al.: Antithymocyte globulin in the management of cutaneous T cell lymphoma. Cancer Treat. Rep., 63:675–680, 1979.
6. Greim, M.L., Tokars, R.P., and Petras, V. et al.: Combined therapy for patients with mycosis fungoides. Cancer Treat. Rep., 63:655–658, 1979.
7. Grozea, P.N., Jones, S.E., and McKelvey, E.M. et al.: Combination chemotherapy for mycosis fungoides. A Southwest Oncology Group Study. Cancer Treat. Rep., 63:647–654, 1979.
8. Hoppe, R.T., Cox, R.S., and Fuks, Z. et al.: Electron-beam therapy for mycosis fungoides: The Stanford University Experience. Cancer Treat. Rep., 63:691–700, 1979.
9. Lawrence, E.C., Broder, S., and Jaffe, E.S. et al.: Evolution of a lymphoma with helper T cell characteristics in Sézary syndrome. Blood, 52:481–492, 1978.
10. Levine, A.M., Taylor, C.R., Koehler, S., et al.: Immunoblastic sarcoma of T versus B cell origin. I. Clinical features. Submitted for publication.
11. Lichtenstein, A., Levine, A.M., and Lukes R.J., et al.: Immunoblastic sarcoma: A clinical description. Cancer, 43:343–352, 1979.
12. Lutzner, M., Edelson, R., and Schein, P., et al.: Cutaneous T cell lymphoma: the Sézary syndrome, mycosis fungoides, and related disorders. Annals. Int. Med., 83:534, 1972.
13. Nathwani, B.N., Kim, H., and Rappaport, H.: Malignant lymphoma, lymphoblastic. Cancer, 38:964–983, 1976.
14. Roenigk, H.H., Jr.: Photochemotherapy for mycosis fungoides: Long-term follow-up study. Cancer Treat. Rep., 63:669–674, 1979.

15. Rosen, P.J., Feinstein, D.I., and Pattengale, P.K., et al.: Convoluted lympho-cytic lymphoma in adults: A clinicopathologic entity. Annals. Int. Med., 89:319–324, 1978.
16. Schackney, S., Edelson, R., and Bunn, P.: The kinetics of Sézary cell production. Cancer Treat. Rep., 63:659–662, 1979.
17. Uchiyama, T., and Yodoi, J., et al.: Adult T cell leukemia: Clinical and hemato-logic features of 16 cases. Blood, 50:481–492, 1977.
18. Wollner, B., Burchenal, J.H., and Lieberman, P.M., et al.: Non-Hodgkin's lymphoma in children: A comparative study of two modalities of therapy. Cancer, 37:123–134, 1976.

26. CUTANEOUS T-CELL LYMPHOMA: MORPHOLOGICAL AND IMMUNOLOGICAL ASPECTS

C.J.L.M. MEIJER, E.M. VAN DER LOO, W.A. VAN VLOTEN, C.J. CORNELISSE AND E. SCHEFFER

The term cutaneous T-cell lymphoma (CTCL) has been proposed by Lutzner et al. (1) for lymphoproliferative diseases sharing the following characteristics:

1) the disease is primarily confined to the skin and secondarily involves other organs;

2) the neoplastic cell is a morphologically characteristic lymphoid cell of thymus-derived nature; it involves preferentially T-cell-dependent areas of lymphoid tissues;

3) the neoplastic cells infiltrate into the epidermis.

At least three diseases meet these criteria and have a malignant course: mycosis fungoides, Sézary's syndrome and the pagetoid reticulosis of Woringer-Kolopp (2). Clinical details of these diseases are described by W.A. van Vloten in chapter 27 in this volume.

Lymphomatoid papulosis (3) has not been placed in this group of diseases, although the histological infiltrate has a malignant appearance and the infiltrate cells are T cells (1). However, the clinical course is usually benign and not that of a lymphoma. Only in a few cases progression to a lymphoma has been noticed (4, 5). Maybe this disease can be regarded as "occupying the no-man's-land between a disordered immunologic state and malignancy" (5).

Although Edelson (44) has recently amplified the concept of CTCL by omitting as criterion the distinctive morphology and epidermotropism of the neoplastic T cells, we will focus on the above-mentioned diseases.

HISTOPATHOLOGICAL ASPECTS OF CUTANEOUS T-CELL LYMPHOMA

In the classical Alibert form, three clinical stages of mycosis fungoides can be distinguished. (a) the premycotic or eczematous stage, (b) the plaque or

J.G. van den Tweel et al. (eds.), *Malignant Lymphoproliferative Diseases, 341–353*
All rights reserved.
Copyright © *1980 by Martinus Nijhoff Publishers bv, The Hague/Boston/London.*

infiltration stage, and (c) the tumor stage. The plaque stage has a characteristic histological picture, whereas that of the premycotic stage of MF is often nonspecific (1). In the plaque stage a bandlike pleomorphic dermal infiltrate is found. This infiltrate contains atypical lymphoid cells which may vary considerably in diameter. Because of their lobulated, indented, or cerebriform nuclei, they are called atypical or cerebriform mononuclear cells (6) (CMC). The larger ones which also have a hyperchromatic nucleus are the so-called "mycosis cells". The CMC show a striking tendency to infiltrate the epidermis and epithelia of adnexa and can form aggregates in acantholytic spaces of the epidermis, i.e. Pautrier abscesses.

Due to the presence of histiocytes, lymphocytes, plasma cells and eosinophils in variable numbers, the infiltrate has often a rather pleomorphic appearance. Mitotic figures are scarce.

In the tumor stage the infiltrate is found in the deeper layers of the dermis and acquires a monomorphic appearance due to the predominance of tumor cells.

Sézary's syndrome (7, 8) is manifested as a generalized exfoliative erythroderma with lymphadenopathy, hyperkeratosis of palms and soles, and atypical or cerebriform mononuclear cells (Sézary cells) in the peripheral blood. Many authors (1) consider Sézary's syndrome to be a leukemic variant of mycosis fungoides. Histologically the skin infiltrate of Sézary's

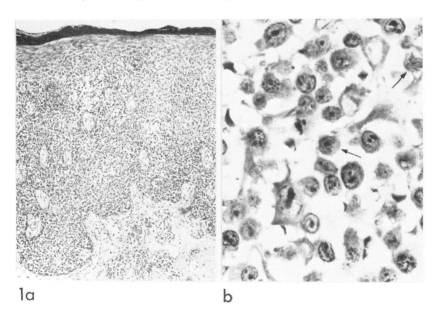

1a   b

Figure 1. Skin biopsy from a patient with generalized Woringer-Kolopp's disease.
a: Predominantly intra-epidermal localization of the infiltrate × 34.
b: Detail of the infiltrate; arrows indicate CMC × 535.

syndrome resembles that of mycosis fungoides, but the relative number of CMC in the infiltrate of the former is often higher.

Woringer-Kolopp's disease (2, 9, 10, 11) is a very rare malignant lymphoma of the skin, histologically characterized by the presence of large numbers of tumor cells confined almost entirely to the epidermis (Figure 1). Because morphologically these tumor cells are cerebriform mononuclear cells (10), it has been suggested that this disease is an epidermotropic variant of mycosis fungoides (2, 10). Two clinical forms have been described: a localized form with a slow evolution and a good prognosis (9, 11) and a generalized form with rapid progression and a fatal outcome (10).

In the following we shall discuss recent developments in the research on cutaneous T-cell lymphomas concerning: (a) the role of the Langerhans cells, (b) the nature of the cerebriform mononuclear cells, and (c) the early diagnosis of MF involvement of skin and lymphnodes.

The role of the Langerhans cell

The role of the Langerhans cells in MF has recently received much attention, because these cells were found to be capable of picking up several contact sensitizing antigens (12) and other antigens including tick-bite antigen (13), antigen-antibody complexes (14), and viral antigens (15). Ultrastructurally, Langerhans cells (16) have a nucleus with an irregular shape and a thin layer of chromatin along the nuclear membrane. The cytoplasm is electron-lucent and contains varying numbers of cell organelles, a few lysosomes, and a well-developed Golgi area with numerous vesicles, mitochondria, and short profiles of rough and smooth endoplasmatic reticulum. In man the most important characteristic feature is the presence of rodlike structures in the cytoplasm, called the Langerhans or Birbeck granules.

Besides these granules, Langerhans cells show ultrastructural features giving them a close resemblance to "indeterminate" cells in the skin (16, 17), veiled cells in the lymphatics (18) and interdigitating reticulum cells (18, 19, 20) (IDC) in the thymus-dependent areas of the lymph nodes. Langerhans cells possess Fc and C_3 receptors (21) and express Ia-like antigens (22). They have adenosin-tri-phosphatase and alpha naphtyl acetate esterase activity (16, 18). These membrane characteristics are shared by at least a proportion of the veiled cells and a number of the interdigitating reticulum cells (18). Moreover, Birbeck granules may be found in a number of veiled cells and interdigitating reticulum cells (18, 20). All these findings have led to the hypothesis (18) that Langerhans cells can travel as veiled cells through the lymphatics to the paracortical areas of the lymph node. Although they belong to the mononuclear phagocyte series (21), the main function of these cells appears not to be phagocytosis but the presentation of antigens to lymphocytes (12, 21) thus giving rise to a T-cell response.

Not only the observed close contact between Langerhans cells and related cells on the one hand and CMC on the other hand (23, 24), but also the presence of Langerhans cells in Pautrier abscesses (23) suggest an interaction between Langerhans cells and CMC. Moreover, Pautrier abscesslike structures are never found in gut epithelia; Langerhans cells are not present in these epithelia. Tan et al. (25) have suggested that MF might be a disease of antigen persistence. In this respect it is of interest that in mycosis fungoides and Sézary's syndrome we were recently able to demonstrate viruslike particles with the ultrastructural characteristics of C-type viruses and the biochemical characteristics of retraviruses exclusively in the Langerhans cell series (Figure 2) (26).

Nature of the cerebriform mononuclear cell

Electron microscopically, the CMC is characterized by a deeply indented cerebriform nucleus with heterochromatin localized along the nuclear

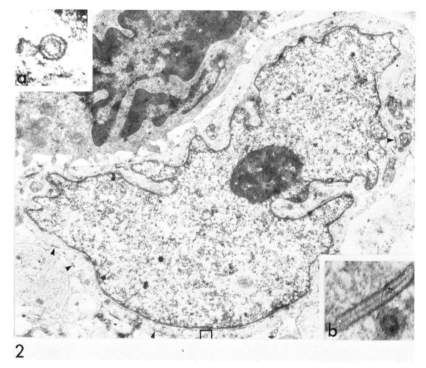

Figure 2. Viruslike particle containing Langerhans cell (× ca. 13,500) in close contact with CMC, localized in the dermis of a patient with MF. Arrowheads indicate Birbeck granules.
Inset *a:* C type viruslike particles (× ca. 68,000).
Inset *b:* Birbeck granule (× ca. 9,010).

membrane, and scanty cytoplasm poor in organelles (27, 28, 29). Recently several investigators (30, 31, 32) have shown that the atypical or cerebriform mononuclear cells in mycosis fungoides and Sézary's syndrome are Tlymphocytes.

The evidence put forward includes:

1) CMC form rosettes with uncoated sheep erythrocytes, are killed by specific anti-T-cell sera (30) and lack surface membrane immunoglobulin (30, 32).

2) CMC behave like T lymphocytes (24) in that they home specifically in thymus dependent areas of lymph nodes and spleen and are often found in close contact with IDC.

Recently, a helper T-cell function was claimed for these cells (33) on the grounds that Sézary cells were able to help PWM-stimulated lymphocytes to synthesize immunoglobulins in vitro. Furthermore Worman et al. (34) have shown that these cells form rosettes with ox erythrocytes coated with rabbit IgM antibodies, thus indicating the presence of an Fc μ receptor known to be present on helper T cells.

CMC are not specific for cutaneous T-cell lymphomas; they are also found in nonlymphomatous dermatoses (35) in the synovium and synovial fluid of patients with rheumatoid arthritis, in normal spleen and lymph nodes, in human cord blood, and in the blood of healthy donors (6). Moreover, they have been observed in cultures of PHA- or PWM-stimulated blood lymphocytes (36). These CMC are T cells since they invariably form rosettes with sheep red blood cells, lack surface membrane Ig, and are unable to form rosettes with mouse complement-coated or IgG coated erythrocytes (6). Recently we showed the presence of an Fc μ receptor on the CMC in the blood of healthy donors. All these marker studies indicate that in reactive processes the CMC are a morphologically distinct subpopulation of T cells, possibly with a helper T-cell function. CMC are not restricted to the human species; we have observed them in lymph nodes of guinea pigs, mice and rabbits after antigenic stimulation and were able to demonstrate T-cell membrane characteristics on these cells in guinea pigs and mice.

It is conceivable that the typical "mycosis" and "Sézary" cells in CTCL are variants of the CMC in reactive processes. Some characteristics of CMC in reactive processes, mycosis cells and Sézary cells are summarized in Table 1. The most important differences between the CMC in reactive processes and the CMC characteristic for cutaneous T-cell lymphomas are found in the size, the DNA content, and the degree of nuclear indentation as expressed by the nuclear contour index (see below). These differences have led to practical applications for the diagnosis of early MF lesions in skin and lymph nodes.

Table 1. Properties of CMC in reactive processes, mycosis fungoides and Sézary's syndrome.

	Reactive processes	*Mycosis cells*	*Sézary cells*
Size	Medium to large lymphocytes	> than large lymphocytes	Large lymphocytes or >
Localization in lymphatic tissue	Preferentially in thymus dependent areas	Preferentially in thymus dependent areas	Preferentially in thymus dependent areas
E rosettes	+	+/−	+/−
Fcγ	−	−	−
Fcμ	+	?	+
sIg	−	−	−
DNA content	Diploid or tetraploid	Hypertetraploid and aneuploid	Hypertetraploid and aneuploid
Degree of nuclear indentation (expressed in NCI)	6.5–11.5	6.55–20.6	6.5–24.2

*NCI = nuclear contour index.
A CMC is mathematically defined by an NCI > 6.5.

Early diagnosis of MF skin lesions

DNA cytophotometry. Histologically, the early diagnosis of mycosis fungoides in the premycotic and early plaque stages may be difficult (37). The abnormal DNA content of CMC in mycosis fungoides has been used as criterion to differentiate early MF skin lesions from benign skin disorders (38). The results are described by W.A. van Vloten in chapter 27 of this volume.

Computer-assisted morphometry. An other practical application (39) was based upon the fact that the number of the CMC present in skin infiltrates and the degree of nuclear indentation of these CMC were greater in cutaneous T-cell lymphomas than in reactive processes. To express the degree of nuclear indentation (Figure 3), a size-independent shape parameter was used, i.e. the nuclear contour index (40) which is derived from the contour perimeter and area as follows:

$$\text{contour index} = \frac{\text{perimeter}}{\sqrt{\text{area}}}.$$

This parameter takes the minimum value of 3.54 for a circular contour.

Measurements were done on the EM photographs of skin infiltrates with a semiautomated morphometry system consisting of a graphic tablet interfaced to a PDP 11/10 minicomputer. The nuclear contour index (NCI) of at least 75 randomly chosen lymphoid cells was measured. Mononuclear phagocytes were distinguished from lymphoid cells by the presence of an

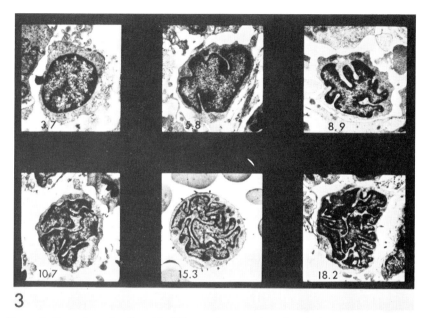

Figure 3. Examples of cells with different degrees of nuclear indentation, expressed as nuclear contour index.

organelle-rich cytoplasm with numerous azurophilic granules and lyso-somes. Typical examples of nuclear contour index histograms of a patient with cutaneous T-cell lymphoma and a patient with a chronic eczema are

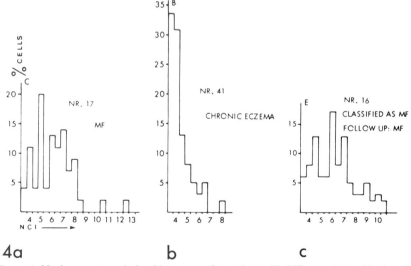

Figure 4. Nuclear contour index histogram of a patient with MF; a patient with chronic eczema, and a patient with suspected MF. This last patient was correctly classified in the malignant group 18 months before a definite histological diagnosis could be made.

given in Figure 4. These histograms showed the following characteristics:

1) Cutaneous T-cell lymphomas have more CMC (defined as cells with an NCI above 6.5), than those in reactive processes.
2) The degree of nuclear indentation (expressed as the NCI value) is higher in cutaneous T-cell lymphomas than in reactive processes.
3) Cells with an NCI larger than 11.5 were never found in reactive processes.

The lymphoid cells in skin infiltrates from 12 patients with cutaneous T-cell lymphoma and 10 patients with chronic benign skin lesions were measured.

A nonlinear discriminant analysis program (Alloc 3) developed by Habbema and Hermans (41) at the Department of Medical Statistics of the University of Leiden was used to evaluate the statistical differences between the nuclear contour index histograms of benign and malignant cases. This program selected the 25th and 70th percentile of the nuclear contour index histogram as the best discriminating parameters for assigning a patient to the malignant or benign group.*

The classifications together with the computed probability (posterior probability) of this group, are shown in Figure 5. It appears that all of these cases were classified correctly with a probability greater than 95%. Only one case with atopic dermatitis was classified as benign with a probablity of 85%. The same classification rule was applied to a group of 10 skin lesions suspected of cutaneous T-cell lymphomas but in which the histological

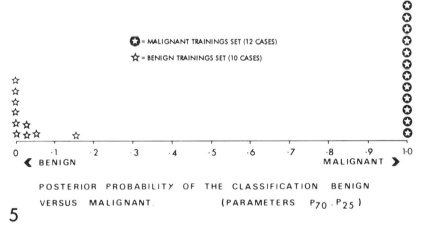

5

Figure 5. Probability of classification of the malignant (cutaneous T-cell lymphoma) and a benign (chronic skin lesions) training set.

* The 25th percentile of the nuclear contour index distribution is the nuclear contour index value reached by 25% of the lymphoid cells.

diagnosis was not conclusive. Two of these patients (K.O., V.E.) showed a clinical picture compatible with parapsoriasis en plaque. The classification results are shown in Table 2. None of the patients classified as benign developed MF in the follow-up period. Of the 7 patients classified as malignant, 5 developed mycosis fungoides and one was found to have lymphomatoid papulosis; one patient has rheumatoid arthritis combined with a dermatitis, which has been present for three years and clinically is still suspected of mycosis fungoides. In general, there is good correlation between these results and the classification based on abnormal DNA values (Table 2).

Early diagnosis of mycosis fungoides in lymph nodes

Early diagnosis of mycosis fungoides in lymph nodes is important because lymph-node involvement in mycosis fungoides has a poor prognosis and often is associated with a visceral localization of the disease (42). Hence, localization of mycosis fungoides in lymph nodes affects the choice of therapy. All differences between the CMC in mycosis fungoides and those in reactive processes, as shown in Table 1, have therefore been evaluated for their importance in diagnosing of early MF involvement. The observation of differences in size between CMC in mycosis fungoides and those in reactive processes (see Table 1), has led to new histologic criteria for the diagnosis of early MF involvement of lymph nodes (43). For details see chapter 29.

Using DNA cytophotometry on imprints of lymph nodes from mycosis fungoides patients, van Vloten et al. demonstrated cells with abnormal

Table 2. Classification of suspected cases of cutaneous T-cell lymphoma according to NCI values and DNA content of lymphoid cells in the skin.

Pat	Probability of classification in the malignant group	DNA	Diagnosis in follow-up (1–3 years)
LA	100	A	MF
RU	100	N	Dermatitis with RA MF still suspect
VI	65	A	MF
BE	100	A	Lymphomatoid papulosis
KO	97.6	A	MF
ZU	100	A	MF
VE	100	N	MF
ZW	0	N	Lymphomatoid reaction
ST	0.5	N	Chronic eczema
WE	0	N	Pseudo lymphoma

A = abnormal   N = normal.
The DNA content is considered to be abnormal when hypertetraploid and aneuploid cells are present.

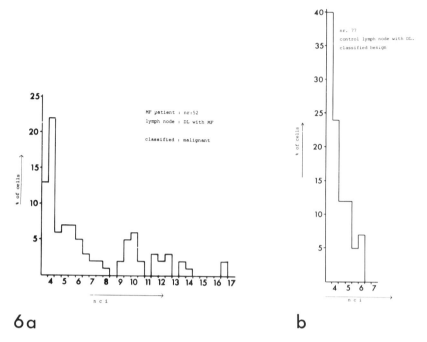

6a   b

Figure 6. Nuclear contour index histograms of lymph-node cell suspensions.
a: Dermatopathic lymph node (DL) with MF involvement.
b: Control DL lymph node.

DNA content in lymph nodes showing involvement (for details see chapter 27).

Recently we performed computer assisted morphometry on EM preparations of cell suspensions deriving from lymph nodes of patients with mycosis fungoides (Figure 6) The training set consisted of 8 lymph nodes showing dermatopathic lymphadenopathy with MF involvement and 8 lymph nodes showing dermatopathic lymphadenopathy obtained from patients with an unrelated disease. Discriminant analysis selected the mean nuclear contour index and standard deviation of the randomly measured lymphoid cells as the best discriminating parameter.

All lymph nodes from the training set (8 malignant, 8 benign) were correctly classified with a probability greater than 95%. When this classification rule was used on 10 lymph nodes in which MF involvement was suspected, 6 were classified as benign and 4 as malignant (Table 3). Only in two patients (P.K. and T.O.) there was disparity between the histological classification and the classification based on computer assisted morphometry. However, in this group of patients DNA cytophotometry too gave differences between the histological classification and the classification based on cells with abnormal DNA content (Table 3).

Table 3. Classification of lymph nodes suspected of mycosis fungoides involvement, according to NCI values and DNA content.

Pat	Sex	Probability of classification in the malignant group	DNA	Diagnosis
AI	M	95.5	N*	DL with MF
HA	M	0.3	N	DL
PK	F	0.5	A	DL with MF
MO	M	0	A	DL
WE	M	0.5	N	DL
TO	M	100	N	DL
JO	M	10.3	N	DL
LA	M	100	A	DL with MF
KL	M	100	N	DL with MF
RE	F	0.6	N	DL

DL = dermatopathic lymphadenopathy.
*A = abnormal N = normal.
The DNA content is considered to be abnormal when hypertetraploid and aneuploid cells are present.

In conclusion it may be said that DNA cytophotometry and computer assisted morphometry on lymphoid cells can give additional objective information for the early diagnosis of MF lesions in skin and lymph nodes.

REFERENCES

1. Lutzner, M.A., Edelson, R., Schein, P., Green, I., Kirkpatrick, C., and Achmed, A.: Cutaneous T cell lymphomas: The Sézary syndrome, mycosis fungoides and related Disorders. Ann. Int. Med., 83:534–552, 1975.
2. Woringer, M.M.F., and Kolopp, P.: Lesion erythématosquameuze polycyclique de l'avant-bras evoluant depuis 6 ans chez un garconnet de 13 ans. Histologiquement infiltrat intra-epidermique d'apparence tumorale. Ann. Dermat., 10:945–958. 1939–1940.
3. Macaulay, W.L. Lymphomatoid papulosis. A continuing, selfhealing eruption, clinically benign, histologically malignant. Arch. Dermatol., 97:23–30, 1968.
4. Fine, R.M., Meltzer, H.D., and Rudner, E.J.: Lymphomatoid papulosis eventuating mycosis fungoides. South Med. J., 67:1492–1497, 1974.
5. Wilson Jones, E.: Question. Am. J. Dermatopathology, 1:91–92, 1979.
6. Meijer, C.J.L.M., van Leeuwen, A.W.F.M., van der Loo, E.M., van de Putte, L.B.A. and van Vloten, W.A.: Cerebriform (Sézary like) mononuclear cells in healthy individuals: a morphologically distinct population of T cells. Virchows Arch. B Cell Path., 25:95–104, 1977.
7. Hamminga, A.L., Hartgrink-Groeneveld, C.A., and van Vloten, W.A.: Sézary's syndrome: a clinical evaluation of eight patients. Brit. J. Derm., 100:291–296, 1979.
8. Sezary, A., and Bouvrain, Y.: Erythrodermie avec presence de cellules monstrueuses dans derme et dans sang circulant. Bull. Soc. Fr. Dermatol. Syphiligr., 45:254–260, 1938.
9. Braun-Falco, O., Marghescu, S., and Wolff, U.H.: Pagetoide-reticulose Morbus Woringer-Kolopp. Der Hautarzt, 24:11–21, 1973.

10. Degreef, H., Holvoet, C., van Vloten, W.A., Desmet, V., and de Wolff-Peeters, C: Woringer-Kolopp Disease. An epidermotropic variant of mycosis fungoides. Cancer, 38:2154–2165, 1976.
11. Lever, W.F.: Localized Mycosis Fungoides with prominent epidermotropism: Woringer-Kolopp Disease. Arch. Dermatol., 133:1254–1256, 1977.
12. Silberberg-Sinakin, I., Thorbecke, G.J., Baer, R.L., Rosenthal, S.A., and Berezowsky, V.: Antigen-bearing Langerhans cells in skin, dermal lymphatics and in lymph nodes. Cell Immunol., 25:137–143, 1976.
13. Allen, J.R., Khalil, H.M., and Wikel, S.K.: Langerhans cells trap tick salivary gland antigens in tick-resistant guinea pigs. J. Immunology, 122:563–565, 1979.
14. Silberberg-Sinakin, I., Fedorko, M.E., Baer, R.L., Rosenthal, S.A., Berezowsky, V.E., and Thorbecke, G.J.:Langerhans cells, target cells in immune complex reactions. Cellular Immunology, 32:400, 1977.
15. Nagao, S., Inaba, S., and Iijima, S.: Langerhans cells at the site of vaccinia virus inoculation. Arch. Derm. Res., 256:23–31, 1976.
16. Wolff, K.: The Langerhans cell. In: Current problems of dermatology, vol. 4, pp. 79–145, Mali, J.W.H., (ed.), Karger, Basel, 1972.
17. Rowden, G., Philips, T.M., and Lewis, M.G.: Ia antigens on indeterminate cells of the epidermis: Immunoelectronmicroscopic studies of surface antigens. Brit. J. of Derm., 100:531–541, 1979.
18. Drexhage, H.A., Lens, J.W., Coetanoo, J., Kamperdijk, E.W.A., Mullink, R., and Balfour, B.M.: Structure and functional behaviour of veiled cells, resembling Langerhans cells, present in lymph draining from normal skin and skin after the application of the contact sensitizing agent dinitrofluorobenzene. Third Leiden Conference on Mononuclear Phagocytes. Functional aspects, van Furth R., (ed.), Martinus Nijhoff Medical Division 1979, in press.
19. Kaiserling, E., und Lennert, K.: Die interdigitierende Reticulum zelle im Menschliechen Lymphknoten. Eine spezifische Zelle der Thymusabhangigen Region. Virchows Arch. B. Cell. Path., 16:51–61, 1974.
20. Kamperdijk, E.W.A., Raaymakers, E.M., de Leeuw, J.H.S., and Hoefsmit, E.Ch.M.: Lymphnode macrophages and reticulum cells in the immune respons. I. The primary respons to paratyphoid vaccine. Cell and Tissue Research, 192:1–10, 1978.
21. Stingl, G., Dartz, S.I., Schevach, E.M., Rosenthal, A.S., and Green, I.: Analogous functions of macrophages and Langerhans cells in the initiation of the immune response. J. Invest. Dermatol., 71:59–64, 1978.
22. Rowden, G., Lewis, H.G., and Sullivan, A.K.: Ia antigen expression on human epidermal Langerhans cells. Nature, 268:247, 1977.
23. Rowden, G., and Lewis, M.G.: Langerhans cells: involvement in pathogenesis of mycosis fungoides. Brit. J. of Derm., 95:665–672, 1976.
24. Van Leeuwen, A.W.F.M., Meijer, C.J.L.M., van Vloten, W.A., Scheffer, E., and de Man, J.C.H.: Further evidence for the T cell nature of the atypical mononuclear cells in mycosis fungoides. Virch. Archiv B Cell Path, 21:179–187, 1976.
25. Tan, R.S., Butterworth, C.M., McLaughlin, H., Malka, S., and Samman, P.: Mycosis Fungoides – a disease of antigen persistence. Brit. J. of Derm., 91:607–615, 1974.
26. Van der Loo, E.M., van Muijen, G.N.P., van Vloten, W.A., Beens, W., Scheffer, E., and Meijer, C.J.L.M.: C type virus like particles specifically localized in Langerhans cells of skin and lymph nodes of patients with Mycosis Fungoides and Sézary's syndrome. Virch. Archiv B Cell Path., 31:193–203, 1979.
27. Brownlee, T.R., and Murad, T.M.: Ultrastructure of Mycosis Fungoides. Cancer, 26:686–698, 1970.

28. Fisher, E.R., Horvat, B.L., and Wechsler, H.L.: Ultrastructural features of mycosis fungoides. Am. J. Clin. Pathol., 58:99–110, 1972.
29. Lutzner, M.A., Hobbs, J.W., and Horvath, P.: Ultrastructure of abnormal cells in Sézary's syndrome, mycosis fungoides and parapsoriasis en plaque. Arch. Derm., 103:375–386, 1971.
30. Brouet, J.C., Flandrin, G., and Seligmann, M.: Indications of the thymus derived nature of the proliferating cells in six patients with Sézary's syndrome. N. Engl. J. Med., 289:341–344, 1973.
31. Edelson, R.L., Kirkpatrick, C.H., Shevach, E.H., Schein, P.S., Smith, R.W., Green, I., and Lutzner, M.A.: Preferential cutaneous infiltration by neoplastic thymus derived lymphocytes. Morphologic and functional studies. Ann. Int. Med., 80:685–692, 1974.
32. Van Leeuwen, A.W.F.M., Meijer, C.J.L.M., and de Man, J.C.H.: T cell membrane characteristics of "mycosis cells" in the skin and lymph node. J. Invest. Derm., 65:367–369, 1975.
33. Broder, S., Edelson, R.L., Lutzner, M.A., Nelson, D.L., McDermott, R.P., Daim, M.E., Golman, C.K., Meade, B.D., and Waldman, T.A.: The Sézary syndrome: A malignant proliferation of helper T cells. J. Clin. Invest., 58: 1297–1306, 1976.
34. Worman, C.P., Burns, G.F., and Barker, C.R.: Evidence for the presence of a receptor for IgM on the pathological cells of Sézary's syndrome. Clin. Exp. Immunol., 31:391–396, 1978.
35. Flaxman, B.A., Zelazny, G., and Scott, E.J. van: Non specificity of characteristic cells in mycosis fungoides. Arch. Derm., 104:141–147, 1971.
36. Yeckley, J.A., Weston, W.L., Thorne, E.G., and Krueger, G.G.: Production of Sézary-like cells from normal human lymphocytes. Arch. derm., 111:29–33, 1975.
37. Samman, P.D.: The natural history of parapsoriasis en plaque (chronic superficial dermatitis) and prereticulotic poikoloderma. Brit. J. Derm., 87:405–411, 1972.
38. Van Vloten, W.A., van Duyn, P., and van Schaberg, A.: Cytodiagnostic use of Feulgen DNA measurement in cell imprints from the skin of patients with mycosis fungoides. Brit. J. Derm., 91:365–371, 1974.
39. Meijer, C.J.L.M., van der Loo, E.M., van Vloten, W.A., van der Velde, E.A., Scheffer, E., and Cornelisse, C.J.: Early diagnosis of mycosis fungoides and Sézary's syndrome by morphometric analysis of lymphoid cells in the skin. Cancer, 46:158–165, 1980.
40. Litovitch, T.L., and Lutzner, M.A.: Quantitative measurements of blood lymphocytes from patients with chronic lymphocytic leukemia and the Sézary Syndrome. J. Natl. Cancer Inst., 53:75–77, 1974.
41. Habbema, J.D.F., and Hermans, J.: Selection of Variables in Discriminant Analysis by F. Statistic and Error Rate. Technometrics, 19:487–493, 1977.
42. Rappaport, H., and Thomas, L.B.: Mycosis Fungoides. The pathology of extracutaneous involvement. Cancer, 34:1198–1229, 1974.
43. Scheffer, E., Meijer, C.J.L.M., and Vloten, W.A. van: Dermatopathic lymphadenopathy and lymph node involvement in mycosis fungoides. Cancer, 45:137–148, 1980.
44. Edelson, R.L.: Cutaneous T cell lymphoma: Mycosis Fungoides, Seźary Syndrome and other variants. J. Am. Acad. Dermatol., 2:89–106, 1980.

27. CUTANEOUS T CELL LYMPHOMAS: CLINICAL ASPECTS

W.A. VAN VLOTEN AND L. HAMMINGA

INTRODUCTIION

Cutaneous lymphomas offer the great advantage that the earliest manifestations of the disease in the skin can be easily studied, and as long as the disease remains confined to the skin, a dermatological approach to the treatment with specific regimes confined to the skin is appropriate. This stresses the importance of early diagnosis and staging of the disease.

Three cutaneous T cell lymphomas can be distinguished: mycosis fungoides, Sézary's syndrome, and the disease of Woringer-Kolopp.

Woringer-Kolopp's disease

Woringer-Kolopp's disease or pagetoid reticulosis is a very rare lymphoma of the skin characterized by the presence of a monomorphic tumor growth in the epidermis. Cytomorphological characteristics of the tumor cells show striking similarities to the atypical lymphoid cells in mycosis fungoides and Sézary's syndrome (1, 2). Woringer-Kolopp's disease is considered an epidermotropic variant of mycosis fungoides.

Sézary's syndrome

Sézary's syndrome, first described in 1938, is a rare disease characterized by an infiltrated erythroderma, pruritus, alopecia, hyperkeratosis of palms and soles, onychodystrophy, lymphadenopathy, and atypical lymphocytes in the peripheral blood (3, 4). The atypical lymphocytes (Sézary cell), which are characterized by a high nucleus-to-cytoplasma ratio, deep nuclear indentations, and condensed chromatin along the nuclear membrane, are present in the blood, skin, lymph nodes, and bone marrow (5).

Immunological and functional studies of these cells indicate them to be T-lymphocytes (6), probably helper T-cells (7).

Cytogenetic studies showed abnormal karyotypes with aneuploidy and marker chromosomes, but none of them consistently (8, 9). Different therapeutic modalities have been used, such as chlorambucil, leucopheresis,

J.G. van den Tweel et al. (eds.), Malignant Lymphoproliferative Diseases, 355–368
All rights reserved.
Copyright © 1980 by Martinus Nijhoff Publishers bv, The Hague/Boston/London.

and antilymphocyte globulin (10). According to the literature and our own experience, the best results can be obtained with chlorambucil 4 mg daily and prednisone 20 mg daily. Additional therapy with topical application of nitrogen mustard may be helpful (5, 10).

Mycosis fungoides

Mycosis fungoides is a T-cell lymphoma which begins in the skin. It has a great variability as to clinical pattern and histopathological alterations, and can therefore give many diagnostic difficulties. Mycosis fungoides is an uncommon disease and an estimate of 2 new cases per million population per year seems reasonable (11). In The Netherlands, with a total population of 14 million (12), 20 new cases were reported in 1978. In most large series males preponderate with a ratio of 3:2 (13). No definite association with genetic, occupational, environmental, geographic, or racial factors has been reported.

A long period (average 7 years) of unspecific skin lesions precedes the development of specific lesions allowing clinical and histological diagnosis, which is usually made in between the age of 50 and 70 years.

During the course of the disease, lymph nodes and visceral organs may become involved in the disease process, which has a fatal outcome occurring about 3–4 years after biopsy diagnosis. The main clinical points to be discussed are diagnosis, staging and therapy.

DIAGNOSIS

For many years three typical clinical stages in the development of skin lesions, called the Alibert-Bazin stages, have been recognized, i.e.:

1) the premycotic or eczematous stage,
2) the plaque or infiltrative stage, and
3) the tumor stage.

The first signs of mycosis fungoides may consist of erythematous, slight scaling and slightly infiltrated patches varying in color from red to violet. These patches can be diffuse or clearly demarcated, round, oval, annular, or horseshoe-shaped, and be distributed over the trunk and extremities in variable numbers (Figure 1a). In the first stage the lesions have a transient character; they appear and disappear. The premycotic lesions can begin as eczema and may be confused with seborrhoic dermatitis and in some cases with psoriasis, or with the benign form of parapsoriasis en plaques. The benign form of parapsoriasis en plaques, also called chronic superficial

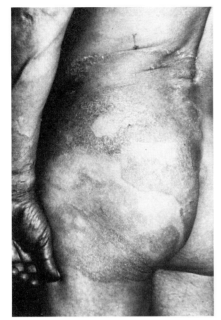
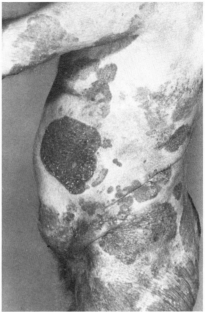
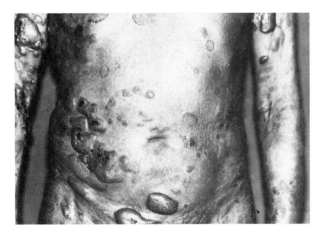

Figure 1. The three stages of mycosis fungoides.
(a) Premycotic stage.
(b) Plaque stage
(c) Tumor stage

dermatitis, has been distinguished from the prereticulotic form which can develop into mycosis fungoides (14).

In the plaque stage more persistent infiltrated lesions develop. They are round or oval and have a brick-red, smooth, slightly scaling surface and a typical cushionlike appearance and consistency. The plaques increase in size and several may coalesce, forming arciform and annular lesions (Figure 1b).

In the tumor stage, tumors may arise in plaques, in premycotic lesions, or in apparently normal skin. They are broad-based and hemispherical and can vary in size from one centimeter to ten centimeters. Small tumors coalesce, forming large lobulated tumor masses which may ulcerate in the center (Figure 1c).

It is the large raised ulcerated tumor which deserves the name fungating tumor. It is rarely seen today, since patients are referred in an early stage. The patient's general health is remarkably good until the terminal period.

Sings of poor prognosis include lymphadenopathy, blood lymphopenia with a decrease of circulating T cells and an increase of null cells, a depressed cellular reactivity, and internal dissemination (15, 16, 17).

HISTOPATHOLOGY

Histologically, mycosis fungoides is characterized by the presence in the skin of a bandlike polymorphous infiltrate in the upper dermis consisting of lymphocytes, histiocytes with an admixture of eosinophils, and plasma cells. In this infiltrate large cerebriform mononuclear cells, called mycosis cells, can be recognized. These cells invade the epidermis either diffusely or form Pautrier abscesses (18). Electron-microscopical investigation and the use of ultrathin sections may be helpful for the diagnosis of mycosis fungoides (19, 20). In early stages histological differentiation from parapsoriasis en plaques and chronic eczema may be difficult. It has been shown by several authors that these cerebriform mononuclear cells in mycosis fungoides have T-cell membrane characteristics (21, 22, 23, 24). The morphological aspects of the mycosis cells are dealt with in chapter 26 by Meijer et al. in this volume.

DNA CYTOPHOTOMETRY

Tumor cells in many different malignant processes show an increased nuclear DNA content and an abnormal chromosome complement. Since some of the cells in mycosis fungoides have an abnormal DNA content, this criterion is used to differentiate beginning mycosis fungoides from benign skin disorders (25).

We performed DNA cytophotometry on cell imprints made from skin biopsies. After fixation and hydrolysis, the preparations were stained with

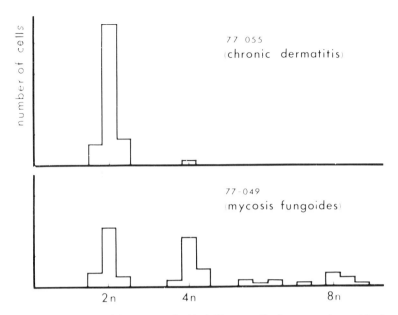

Figure 2. Feulgen-DNA histograms of skin-infiltrate cells from a patient with chronic dermatitis (top) and a patient with mycosis fungoides (bottom). The measured cells were taken at random. 2n = diploid DNA value.

the pararosanilin Schiff reagent, rinsed in sulphite solution, dehydrated, and mounted in Caedax. Cytophotometry was performed with the Zeiss scanning microscope (SMP), using the Arrayscan computer program (26). The total absorbance per cell nucleus gives the total amount of chromophore in the field measured, which is a measure of the DNA content of the cell nucleus. A histogram visualizes the distribution of the DNA values of the measured cells (Figure 2). Nonmalignant skin diseases have invariably shown a unimodal DNA distribution with a peak in the diploid region; some tetraploid cells can be found.

Initially, measurements were done at random, which resulted in a criterion of 5% tetraploid cells for a normal histogram. At present, cells are measured selectively, i.e., atypical-looking and hyperchromatic cells, and only aneuploid and polyploid cells are considered abnormal.

In mycosis fungoides, DNA histograms showed a markedly aneuploid and polyploid distribution of DNA values. DNA cytophotometry was performed in 175 patients suspected clinically and/or histopathologically of having a malignant cutaneous lymphoma (Table 1). Normal DNA histograms were found in 106, and during the follow-up period 96 of these were found to have a benign skin disease. Ten patients with a normal DNA histogram developed a cutaneous lymphoma. This discrepancy may be due to cell sampling.

Table 1. Results of DNA cytophotometry of skin infiltrate cells in 175 patients suspected of having malignant cutaneous lymphoma.

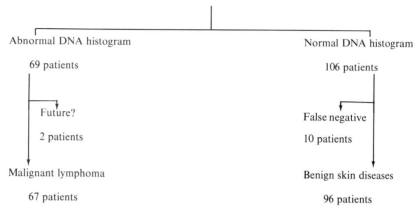

Sixty-nine of the 175 patients showed an abnormal DNA histogram with aneuploid and hypertetraploid DNA values. Of these, 67 developed a malignant lymphoma of the skin, as established clinically and histologically, during the follow-up period of 6 years. Recently, computer-assisted morphometry of the nuclei of lymphoid cells in the skin was carried out (27). The results, which are given in chapter 26 by Meijer et al., show good correlation with the results of the DNA measurements. The use of DNA cytophotometry and morphometry can be of additional and objective help in the diagnosis of early mycosis fungoides.

STAGING

When the diagnosis is made, a staging procedure is carried out to obtain information on the extent of the disease. For staging, we use a modified classification according to Fuks (15) in which the skin condition is related to the dissemination of the disease (Table 2).

Staging investigations include among others, blood morphology, and chemistry, urine analysis, chest radiography, liver and spleen scintigraphy, excision of enlarged lymph nodes, lymphangiography, bone marrow examination, and testing with DNCB and recall antigens for the evaluation of cellular reactivity.

LYMPH NODE PATHOLOGY

Histological differentiation between dermatopatic lymphadenopathy and early mycosis fungoides involvement of the lymph node is difficult, especially

Table 2. Staging classification of mycosis fungoides (modified after Fuks (17)).

	Premycotic *a*	*Plaques* *b*	*Tumor* *c*
I. Mycosis fungoides of the skin			
II. Mycosis fungoides of the skin with dermato- pathic lymphadenopathy			
III. Mycosis fungoides of the skin with lymph- node involvement			
IV. Mycosis fungoides of the skin with visceral involvement			

when the number of clearly recognizable mycosis cells is small (28). Recently, we described histopathological criteria for lymph-node involvement in mycosis fungoides (29), and these are summarized in chapter 29 by Scheffer and Meijer. Additional criteria were obtained from DNA measurements. DNA cytophotometry of lymph-node imprints was carried out in 25 patients with mycosis fungoides (30). Of 10 patients with histologically demonstrated dermatopathic lymphadenopathy, 8 showed a normal DNA histogram and 2 an abnormal DNA histogram. Nine of these ten patients had a sustained remission.

Twelve out of 15 patients with histologically established mycosis fungoides involvement of the lymph-nodes showed an abnormal DNA histogram with hypertetraploid DNA values; the other 3 had a normal DNA

Table 3. DNA cytophotometry of 25 lymph nodes in mycosis fungoides.

Histology	*DNA histogram*		Follow-up
	Normal	*Abnormal*	
DL	8	2	9 R 1 PR
MF	3	12	3 R 5 PR 7 died

DL = dermatopathic lymphadenopathy.
MF = lymph node with mycosis fungoides involvement.
R = sustained remission.
PR = partial remission.

histogram. Seven of these 15 patients died and 5 achieved only partial remission after therapy (Table 3).

In this group of 25 patients there is good correlation between the results
of DNA cytophotometry and lymph-node histology.

LYMPHOGRAPHY AND LIVER AND SPLEEN SCINTIGRAPHY

Lymphography has been reported in literature to be useful in the staging
of mycosis fungoides (31, 32). In our department, lymphagiographic results
have been evaluated with respect to lymph-node histology and follow-up
in 36 patients with mycosis fungoides in different stages of the disease (33).

Nonsuspect lymphograms were obtained in 12 patients of whom 3 had
definite mycosis fungoides involvement of the lymph-node, as demonstrated histologically.

Abnormal or suspect lymphangiograms were obtained in 24 patients, 13
of whom showed mycosis fungoides involvement of the lymph-nodes histologically (Table 4).

Liver and spleen scintigraphy never showed abnormalities in these 36
patients. The conclusion drawn from the results is that lymphography is not
a useful clinical tool in the staging of mycosis fungoides. It should be kept
in mind, however, that lymphography is not without risk of serious side
effects.

CHROMOSOME ANALYSIS

In mycosis fungoides abnormal circulating lymphoid cells are very rarely
seen in routine blood smears except during the terminal period, when a
leucaemic phase sometimes develops. However, ultrastructural analysis
showed the presence of a small number of cerebriform mononuclear cells

Table 4. Lymphography in 36 patients with mycosis fungoides.

| | Lymphangiogram | |
	Nonsuspect	Abnormal or suspect
Nonsuspect		
No palpable lymph nodes	6	6
Dermatopathic lymphadenopathy	6	2
Dermatopathic lymphadenopathy with mycosis fungoides invol- vement	4	12

in the peripheral blood of patients in earlier stages of mycosis fungoides (34). Abnormal karyotypes have been shown in cells from the skin and lymph-nodes (35).

We performed G-banded chromosome analysis on peripheral blood lymphocytes after phytohaemagglutinin stimulation in 16 patients with mycosis fungoides in different stages of the disease. A number of chromosome abnormalities were observed in 7 of these patients in the later stage of the disease.

Four patients showed similar marker chromosomes in multiple copies, some of them without a clearly visible centromere. Double minute chromosomes were found in 2 patients. Correlation was found between the presence of chromosomal abnormalities in the circulating blood lymphocytes and the course of the disease (36).

THERAPY

Many therapeutic modalities have been used in the past such as local radiotherapy, topical cortico-steroids, ultraviolet light, and various cytostatic agents. In the last few years, there has been a tendency to use much more aggressive therapy in the early stages in order to obtain a complete cure. Since the disease begins in the skin, these more aggressive therapies are limited to the skin.

In stages I and II (i.e., mycosis fungoides of the skin without lymph-node involvement) the patients are treated with: (a) total skin electron-irradiation, (b) topical nitrogen mustard, or (c) 8-methoxypsoralen followed by long-wave ultraviolet irradiation (PUVA).

TOTAL SKIN ELECTRON-IRRADIATION

With 4 MeV electron irradiation, superficial layers of the skin can be treated to a depth of about 1.2 cm; at greater depth there is a rapid fall-off in the dose delivered. Therefore, electron-beam therapy has become a welcome addition in the treatment of premycotic and plaque stage mycosis fungoides (15, 37). In Leiden 4 MeV electron-beam irradiation has been given to 28 patients during the last 4 years. Twice a week for 10 weeks the patient is irradiated with the six-field technique. A total of 3,500 rad is given. Results are very promising (Figure 3a, b); however, several patients have shown recurrences of small mycosis fungoides lesions. These patients were subsequently treated with topical nitrogen mustard, which proved to be an adequate form of treatment. Side effects of total skin electron-irradiation are a dry scaling of the skin, temporary nail loss and alopecia, and oedematous hands and feet (38).

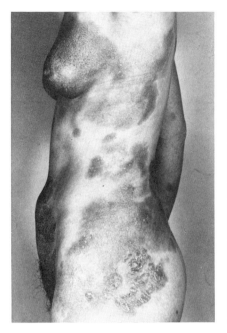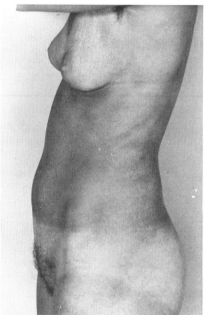

Figure 3. (a) Plaque stage of mycosis fungoides before treatment. (b) The same patient 4 years after total skin electron-irradiation.

TOPICAL NITROGEN MUSTARD

Whole-body topical appliation of a dilute aqueous solution of mechlorethamine hydrochloride (nitrogen mustard) has been shown to be effective in the early stages of mycosis fungoides (39). This therapy can also be used for a long time as maintenance treatment, and the frequency of application be adjusted according to the response and irritation encountered (40).

For this form of treatment, 10 mg mechlorethamine HCl powder is dissolved in 40 ml of water just before application. The patients are instructed to apply the freshly prepared solution daily over the entire body. Care must be taken to avoid the eyes. Some of the patients treated with topical nitrogen mustard may develop a delayed hypersensitivity reaction which, however, appears to have a beneficial effect on the course of mycosis fungoides.

PHOTOCHEMOTHERAPY (PUVA)

Recently, patients with mycosis fungoides in an early stage have been treated successfully with 8-methoxy-psoralen orally followed by irradiation of the skin with long-wave ultraviolet light (UVA) (41, 42). After an initial course of irradiations a maintenance scheme can be given with success, especially in the premycotic stage.

In stages III and IV (i.e., mycosis fungoides of the skin with lymph node and/or visceral involvement) the patients are treated with cytostatic drugs. Many different monocytostatic drugs have been used for mycosis fungoides, but the duration of response has been short and no prolongation of survival has been demonstrated. Mention is made of: *alkylating agents* such as mechlorethamine (13, 43), chlorambucil (44), and cyclophosphamide (13, 45); *antimetabolites* such as methotrexate (46, 44) and azaribine (47); *cytostatic antibiotics* such as actinomycin (44), bleomycin (48, 49) and adriamycin (50).

More recently, attention has been paid to the use of polycytostatic regimes to obtain a synergistic effect. Several combinations of cytostatics are being used at the moment in different countries, but reports of large trials are not yet available.

In The Netherlands two polycytostatic regimes are in use, one comprising COP (Cyclophosphamide, Oncovin, Prednisone), and the other MOPP (Mechlorethamine, Oncovin, Procarbazine, and Prednisone). Recently, we have treated patients with extensive plaque and tumor-stage mycosis fungoides and lymph-node involvement (stages III and IV) with total skin electron-irradiation followed by an intermittent COP regime. This combination seems very promising.

COOPERATIVE STUDY GROUPS ON MYCOSIS FUNGOIDES

Cutaneous lymphomas are rare and the clinician is often confronted with many problems in the management of patients with these diseases. For this reason, several multidisciplinary and multicenter study groups have been established during the last few years to evaluate diagnosis and therapy; and preliminary results have recently been reported. These groups are the Mycosis Fungoides Cooperative Study Group in the United States (51), which is sponsored by the National Cancer Institute; the Scandinavian Mycosis Fungoides Study Group (52, 53, 54); the Dutch Mycosis Fungoides Study Group (12), the Scottish Dermatological Society's Mycosis Fungoides Register (55); and the French Study Group on Mycosis Fungoides (56).

ACKNOWLEDGEMENTS

Part of this work was supported by the Konigin Wilhelmina Fonds D 76–35. We wish to thank Dr. M. van der Ploeg of the Department of Histochemistry and Cytochemistry of the University of Leiden for Cytophotometric facilities and his stimulating discussions and advice, and Miss Els A. Pet for technical assistance.

Note: During the preparation of the proofs, the Proceedings of the Workshop on Cutaneous T Cell lymphoma appeared in Cancer Treatment Report, 63:561–736, 1979.

REFERENCE

1. Braun Falco, O., Marghescu, S., and Wolff, H.H.: Pagetoïde Retikulose Morbus Woringer-Kolopp. Hautarzt, 24:11–21, 1973.
2. DeGreef, H., Holvoet, C., van Vloten, W.A., Desmet, V., and de Wolf-Peters, C.: Woringer-Kolopp disease. Cancer, 38:2154–2165, 1976.
3. Sézary, A., and Bouvrain, J.: Erythrodermie avec présence de cellules monstreuses dans le derme et le sang circulant. Bull. de la Société francaise de dermatologie et de syphiligraphie, 45:254–260, 1938.
4. Winkelmann, R.K., and Linman, L.W.,: Erythroderma with atypical lymphocytes (Sézary syndrome). Amer. J. Med., 55:192–198, 1973.
5. Hamminga, L., Hartgrink-Groeneveld, C.A., and van Vloten, W.A.,: Sézary's syndrome: a clinical evaluation of eight patients. Brit. J. Derm., 100:291–296, 1979.
6. Brouet, J.C., Flandrin, G., and Seligmann, M.: Indication of the thymusderived nature of the proliferating cells in six patients with Sézary's syndrome. New Eng. Med., 289:341–344, 1973.
7. Broder, S., Edelson, R.L., Lutzner, M.A., Nelson, D.L., McDermott, R.P., Durm, M.E., Golman, C.K., Meade, B.D., and Waldman, T.A.: The Sézary syndrome. A malignant proliferation of helper T cells. J. Clin. Invest., 58:1297–1307, 1976.
8. Bosman, F.T., and van Vloten, W.A.: Sézary's syndrome: a cytogenetic cytophotometric and autoradiographic study. J. Pathol., 118:49–57, 1976.
9. Lutzner, M.A., Emerit, J., Durepaire, R., Flandrin, G., Grupper, Ch., and Prunieras, M.: Cytogenetic, cytophotometric and ultrastructural study of large cerebriform cells of the Sézary syndrome and description of a small cell variant. J. Nat. Cancer Inst., 50:1145–1162, 1973.
10. Winkelman, R.K., Perry, H.O., Muller, S.A., Schroeter, A.L., Jordon, R.E., and Rogers, R.S.: Treatment of Sézary's syndrome. Mayo Clinic proceedings, 49:590–592, 1974.
11. Brehmer-Andersson, E.: Mycosis fungoides and its relation to Sézary's syndrome, lymphomatoid papulosis and primary cutaneous Hodgkin's disease. Acta dermatovenereologica, 56: supplement 75, 1976.
12. Hamminga, L., and van Vloten, W.A.:Report of the Dutch Mycosis fungoides study group. Brit. J. Derm., 102:477–478, 1980.
13. Epstein, E.H., Levin, D.L., Croft, J.D., and Lutzner, M.A.: Mycosis fungoides. Medicine, 15:61–72, 1972.
14. Samman, P.D.: The natural history of parapsoriasis en plaques (chronic superficial dermatitis) and prereticulotic poikiloderma. Brit J. Derm., 87:405–411, 1972.
15. Fuks, Z.Y., Bagshaw, M.A., and Farber, E.M.: Prognostic signs and the management of the mycosis fungoides. Cancer, 32:1358–1395, 1973.
16. Van der Harst-Oostveen, C.J.G.R., and van Vloten, W.A.: Delayed-type hypersensitivity in patients with mycosis fungoides. Dermatologica, 157:129–135, 1978.
17. Nordqvist, B.C., and Kinney, J.P.: T and B cells and cell-mediated immunity in mycosis fungoides. Cancer, 37:714–718, 1978.
18. Lever, W.F., and Schaumberg-Lever, G.: Histopathology of skin diseases 5th ed. J.B. Lippingcott. Cy. Philadelphia, Toronto, 1975.
19. Braun Falco, O., Schmoeckel, C., and Wolff, H.H.: The ultrastructure of

mycosis fungoides of Sézary syndrome and of Woringer-Kolopp's disease (pagetoid reticulosis). Bull. du Cancer, 64:191–208, 1977.

20. Lutzner, M.A., Hobbs, J.W., and Horvath, P.: Ultrastructure of abnormal cells. Arch. Derm. Suppl. (Chicago), 103:375–386, 1971.

21. Burg, G., and Braun Falco, O.: Morphological and functional differentiation and classification of cutaneous lymphomas. Bull. du Cancer, 64:225–240, 1977.

22. Edelson, R.L.: Membrane properties of the abnormal cells of cutaneous T cell Lymphomas. Ann. Intern. Med., 83:548–552, 1975.

23. Van Leeuwen, A.W.F.M., Meyer, C.J.L.M., van Vloten, W.A., Scheffer, E., and de Man, J.C.H.: Further evidence for the T cell nature of the atypical mononuclear cells in mycosis fungoides. Virchows Arch. B Cell Path., 21:174–187, 1976.

24. Lutzner, M.A., Edelson, R., Schein, P., Green, I., Kirkpatrick, C., and Ahmed A.: Cutaneous T cell lymphomas: The Sézary's syndrome, mycosis fungoides and related disorders. N.I.H. Conference. Ann. Intern. Med., 83:534–552, 1975.

25. Van Vloten, W.A., van Duijn, P., and Schaberg, A.: Cytodiagnostic use of Feulgen–DNA measurements in cell imprints from the skin of patients with mycosis fungoides. Brit J. Derm., 91:365–371, 1974.

26. Van der Ploeg, M., van den Broek, K., Smeulders, A.W.M., Vossepoel, A., and van Duijn, P.: Hidacsys. Computer programm for interactive scanning cytophotometry. Histochemistry, 54:273–288, 1977.

27. Meijer, C.J.L.M., van der Loo, E.M., van Vloten, W.A., van der Velde, E.A., Scheffer, E., and Cornelisse, C.J.: Early diagnosis of mycosis fungoides and Sézary's syndrome by morphometric analysis of lymphoid cells in the skin. Cancer, in press.

28. Rappaport, H., and Thomas, L.B.: Mycosis fungoides: the pathology of extra-cutaneous involvement. Cancer, 34:1198–1220, 1974.

29. Scheffer, E., Meyer, C.J.L.M., and van Vloten, W.A.: Dermatopathic lympha-denopathy and lymphnode involvement in mycosis fungoides. Cancer, 45:137–148, 1980.

30. Van Vloten, W.A., Scheffer, E., and Meyer C.J.L.M.: DNA cytophotometry of lymphnode imprints from patients with mycosis fungoides. J. Invest. Derm. 73:275–277, 1979.

31. Escovits, E.S., Soulen, R.L., van Scott, E.J., Kalmanson, J.D., and Barry, W.E.: Mycosis fungoides; a lymphographic assesment. Radiology, 112:23–27, 1974.

32. Fuks, Z.Y., Castellino, R.A., Carmel, J.A., Farber, E.M., and Bagshaw, M.A.: Lymphography in mycosis fungoides. Cancer, 34:106–112, 1974.

33. Hamminga, L., Mulder, J.D., Evans, C., Scheffer, E., Meyer, C.J.L.M., and van Vloten, W.A.: Staging lymphography with respect to lymphnode histology, treatment, follow-up in patients with mycosis fungoides. Cancer, in press.

34. Meyer, C.J.L.M., van Leeuwen, A.W.F.M., van der Loo, E.M., van de Putte, L.B.A., and van Vloten, W.A.: Cerebriform (Sézary like) mononuclear cells in healthy individuals: morphologically distinct population of T cells. Virchows Archiv. B Cell Path., 25:95–104, 1977.

35. Erkman Balis, B., and Rappaport, H.: Cytogenetic studies in mycosis fungoides. Cancer, 34:626–633, 1974.

36. Van Vloten, W.A., Pet, E.A., and Geraedts, J.P.M.: Chromosome studies in mycosis fungoides. Submitted for publication.

37. Hoppe, R.L., Fuks, Z., and Bagshaw, M.A.: The rationale for curative radio-

therapy in mycosis fungoides. J. Radiation Oncology, Biol. Phys., 2:843–851, 1977.

38. Van Vloten, W.A., Vermey, J., and de Vroome, H.: Total skin electron irradiation in mycosis fungoides. Dermatologica, 155:28–35, 1977.
39. Van Scott, E.J., Kalmanson, J.D.: Complete remissions of mycosis fungoides lymphoma induced by topical nitrogen mustard (HN$_2$). Cancer, 32:18–30, 1973.
40. Vonderheid, E.C., van Scott, E.J., Johnson, W.C., Grekin, D.A., and Asbell, S.O.: Topical chemotherapy and immunotherapy of mycosis fungoides. Arch. Dermatol., 113:454–462, 1977.
41. Gilchrest, B.A., Parrish, J.A., Tannebaum, L., Haynes, H.A., and Fitzpatrick, T.B.: Oral methoxsalen photochemotherapy of mycosis fungoides. Cancer, 38:683–689, 1976.
42. Roenigk, H.M.: Photochemotherapy for mycosis fungoides. Arch. Dermatol, 113:1047–1051, 1977.
43. Van Scott, E.J., Grekin, D.A., Kalmanson, J.D., Vonderheid, E.C., and Barry, W.E.: Frequent low doses of intravenous mechlorethamine for late stage mycosis fungoides lymphoma. Cancer, 36:1613–1618, 1975.
44. Wright, J.C., Lyons, M.M., and Walker, D.G.: Observations on the use of cancer chemotherapeutic agents in patients with mycosis fungoides. Cancer, 17:1045–1062, 1964.
45. Van Scott, E.J., Auerbach, J., and Clendenning, W.F.: Treatment of mycosis fungoides with cyclophosphamide. Arch. Derm., 85:107–109, 1962.
46. McDonald, C.J., and Bertino, J.R.: Treatment of mycosis fungoides lymphoma: effectivenes of infusions of methotrexate followed by oral citrovorum factor. Cancer treatment Reports, 62:1009–1014, 1978.
47. McDonald, C.J., and Calabresi, P.: Azaribine for mycosis fungoides. Arch. Dermatol, 103:158–167, 1971.
48. De Bast, C., Moriame, N., and Wanet, J.: Bleomycine in mycosis fungoides and reticulum cell lymphoma. Arch. Derm., 404:508–512, 1971.
49. Van Vloten, W.A., and Polano, M.K.: Bleomycine therapy in mycosis fungoides. Dermatologica, 150:50–57, 1975.
50. Levi, J.A., Wiggs, C.H., and Wiernik, P.H.: Adriamycin therapy in advanced mycosis fungoides. Cancer, 39:1967–1970, 1977.
51. Editorial: Mycosis fungoides cooperative study. Arch. Derm., 111:457–459, 1975K
52. Groth, O., Molin, L., Thomsen, K., Grunnet, E., Helbe, L., Holst, R., Michaëlsson, G., Nilsson, E., Roupe, G., Schmidt, H., and Skogh, M.: Tumour stage of mycosis fungoides treated with bleomycin and methotrexate; Report from the Scandinavian Mycosis Fungoides Study Group. Acta. Dermatovener., 59:59–64, 1979.
53. Molin, L., Thomsen, K., and Volden, G.: Mycosis fungoides plaque stage treated with topical nitrogen mustard with and without attempts at tolerance induction: Report from the Scandinavian mycosis fungoides study group. Acta Dermatoven, 59:64–68, 1979.
54. Thomsen, K.: Scandinavian mycosis fungoides study group. Bull. du Cancer, 64:287–290, 1977.
55. MacKie, R.: Evaluation and staging in the Scottisch Dermatological Society mycosis fungoides register. Bull. du Cancer, 64:279–286, 1977.
56. Communoqué: Etude de groupe du mycosis fungoïde. Ann. Dermatol Venereol. (Paris), 106:191–192, 1979.

28. SYSTEMIC MANIFESTATIONS OF MYCOSIS FUNGOIDES

H. RAPPAPORT

For many years the precise position of mycosis fungoides (MF) in the spectrum of malignant lymphomas was not known. Unlike other malignant lymphomas, mycosis fungoides always originates in the skin and many be preceded by a possibly preneoplastic "premycotic" stage in which clearcut histologic features of malignancy are either lacking or equivocal. In the advanced lesions, the cells show great variability, particularly in size, which has led to the erroneous conclusion that the cellular proliferation is histiomonocytic in nature. The data in the literature as to the incidence of extracutaneous involvement vary greatly both in living patients and in autopsy series. Lymph node enlargement is a common occurrence. It may be due dermatopathic lymphadenopathy or actual involvement of the lymph nodes by MF, or both. From a review of published reports, one could never be absolutely sure as to how many of the cases included in a reported series were malignant lymphoma cutis rather than MF. Finally, students of the disease were divided between those who indicated that when MF does progress beyond the skin, the extracutaneous lesions are either reticulum cell sarcoma, lymphosarcoma, or Hodgkin's disease, and others who felt that MF is a well defined and pathologically recognizable entity throughout its entire course (1, 8).

There was also uncertainty whether the cells of the so-called Sézary syndrome, now considered as the "erythrodermic" form of MF (4), were or were not identical with the circulating tumor cells that were observed in the classical or Alibert form of MF. Recent observations now have clearly established that MF and Sézary syndrome are malignant lymphoproliferative diseases of the T-lymphocyte type (2, 3, 5) and that the great variation in the appearance of the proliferating cells in tissue sections in advanced MF represents increasing cellular atypia as we find it in other neoplastic disorders. Thus, a change in cellular morphology that occurs in the course of a patient's illness should not be considered as a change into a different type of malignant lymphoma (10).

Extracutaneous lesions are a manifestation of metastatic spread of the disease from the skin. In the lymph node, they are at first subtle and may be difficult to recognize by routine histological methods. Both electron

J.G. van den Tweel et al. (eds.), Malignant Lymphoproliferative Diseases, 369–372
All rights reserved.
Copyright © 1980 by Martinus Nijhoff Publishers bv, The Hague/Boston/London.

microscopy (9, 12) and karyotype analysis (6) have been more sensitive methods in demonstrating nodal involvement than routine tissue sections. It has also been established that the incidence of extracutaneous involvement is high. In our series of 45 patients, extracutaneous involvement was demonstrable at postmortem examination in 32 (10). Our postmortem studies seem to indicate that lymph-node involvement was always associated with visceral involvement (10) and strongly suggests that whatever barrier to the spread of the disease exists, it is present between the skin and the lymph nodes and not between the lymph nodes and the viscera. In contrast, we found visceral involvement in four out of 16 patients without histologically demonstrable lymph node involvement at autopsy. This could be a sampling problem and would tend to indicate that a negative lymph node biopsy does not necessarily prove that the patient does not have visceral involvement.

Thus it seems that a positive lymph node biopsy is the best indicator of extracutaneous involvement and probably of visceral spread. Whether a staging laparotomy in the presence of a negative lymph-node biopsy offers additional information and guidance for therapy has not, as yet, been clearly established (7, 15).

In our cases, the incidence of visceral involvement is higher than in most other reported series. It is of interest that all patients in whom the autopsy did not reveal evidence of extracutaneous involvement died of the infectious complications and had a shorter survival than those who had visceral MF, one-third of whom actually died as a result of involvement of vital organs (10, 11). It is possible that the patients in whom life can be prolonged by successful control of infectious complication are more likely to develop visceral MF than those who succumb early from infection, that is, before the disease runs its complete course.

The microscopic features of visceral MF are highly characteristic and usually readily distinguishable from those of other malignant lymphomas (10). Such characteristic features include (a) involvement of the paracortical zone of the lymph node and of the periarterial (T-zones) of the spleen (14); (b) the only slight cellular atypia during the early phases of the disease which makes the recognition of the cells of MF difficult; (c) the demonstration of cells with highly convoluted (cerebriform) nuclei which are at times large and hyperchromatic; (d) the tendency to infiltrate the organs diffusely without destroying pre-existing parenchyma; (e) the finding in some areas of individual tumor cells rather than of cohesive cell masses; (f) the unusually high incidence of pulmonary involvement which was higher than that of the spleen, liver, and bone marrow; and (g) an affinity of the tumor cells for epithelium which was evident not only in the skin and oral mucous membranes but also in some viscera. The involvement of the lungs and the myocardium, particularly the conduction system (11) was sufficiently severe in some cases to be a primary cause of death.

In summary, our pathologic observations indicate that MF is a malignant lymphoma invariably arising in the skin and in the classical or Alibert form, preceded by a so-called "premycotic" phase in which clear-cut morphologic evidence of neoplasia may be lacking. The disease spreads from the skin by the lymphatic or hematogenous route to lymph nodes and viscera, but the nodal and visceral lesion are morphologically recognizable as MF and should not be confused with other malignant lymphomas. In some instances the lesions of MF may be composed of tumor cells which are so atypical that the picture may resemble a so-called pleomorphic reticulum cell sarcoma. In rare instances, Sternberg-Reed cells have been reported (10, 13) but the clinical picture and the pathological evolution of the disease in no way resemble Hodgkin's disease. Early lymph-node involvement may be difficult to diagnose histologically, and supportive studies, including electron microscopy and karyotype analysis may be useful. Involvement of lymph nodes is a strong indicator of visceral involvement and there is, at the present time, no clear evidence that surgical staging by laparotomy contributes appreciably to the assessment of the extent of the disease and the choice of therapy.

REFERENCES

1. Bluefarb, S.M.: Is mycosis fungoides an entity? Arch. Derm. Syph., 71:293, 1955.
2. Broome, J.D., Zucker-Franklin, D., Weiner, M.S., Branco, C., and Nussenzweig, V.: Leukemic cells with membrane properties of thymus-derived (T) lymphocytes in a case of Sézary's syndrome. Morphologic and immunologic studies. Clin. Immunol. Immunopath., 1:319–329, 1973.
3. Brouet, J.C., Flandrin, G., and Seligmann, M.: Indications of the thymus-derived nature of the proliferating cells in six patients with Sézary syndrome. N. Engl. J. Med., 289:341–344, 1973.
4. Clendenning, W.E., Brecher, G., and Van Scott, E.J.: Mycosis fungoides. Relationship to malignant cutaneous reticulosis and the Sézary syndrome. Arch. Derm. Syph., 89:785–790, 1964.
5. Edelson, R.L., Kirkpatrick, C.H., Shevach, E.M., Schein, P.S., Smith, R.W., Green, I., and Lutzner, M.A.: Preferential cutaneous infiltration by neoplastic thymus-derived lymphocytes. Morphologic and functional studies. Ann. Intern. Med., 80:685–692, 1974.
6. Erkman-Balis, B., and Rappaport, H.: Cytogenetic studies in mycosis fungoides Cancer, 34:626–633, 1974.
7. Griem, M.L., Moran, E.M., Ferguson, D.J., Mettler, F.A., and Griem, S.F.: Staging procedures in mycosis fungoides. Br. J. Cancer (2), 31:362–367, 1975.
8. Lapiére, S.: The realm and frontiers of mycosis fungoides. J. Invest. Derm., 42:101–103, 1964.
9. Lutzner, M.A.: Cellular identities in the malignant lymphomas. In: Dermato-

logy in general practice, pp. 573–577, Fitzpatrick, T.B., Arndt, K.A., Clark, W.H., Jr., Eisen, A.Z., Van Scott, E.J., and Vaughn, J.H., (eds.), McGraw Hill, New York, 1971.

10. Rappaport, H., and Thomas, L.B.: Mycosis fungoides: The pathology of extracutaneous involvement. Cancer, 34:1198, 1974.

11. Roberts, W.C., Glancy, D.L., and DeVita, V.T.: Heart in malignant lymphoma (Hodgkin's disease, lymphosarcoma, reticulum cell sarcoma and mycosis fungoides). A study of 196 autopsy cases. Am. J. Cardiol., 22:85–107, 1968.

12. Rosas-Uribe, A., Variakojis, D., Molnar, Z., and Rappaport, H.: Mycosis fungoides. An ultrastructural study. Cancer, 34:634–645, 1974.

13. Strum, S.B., Park, J.K., and Rappaport, H.: Observations of cells resembling Sternberg-Reed cells in conditions other than Hodgkin's disease. Cancer, 26:176–190, 1970.

14. Thomas, L.B., and Rappaport, H.: Mycosis fungoides and its relationship to other malignant lymphomas. In: The reticuloendothelial system: IAP monograph No. 16, pp. 243–261, Rebuck, J.W., Berard, C.W., and Abell, M.R., (eds.), Williams and Wilkins, 1975.

15. Variakojis, D., Rosas-Uribe, A., and Rappaport, H.: Mycosis fungoides. Pathologic findings in staging laparotomies. Cancer, 33:1589–1600, 1974.

29. EARLY INVOLVEMENT OF LYMPH NODES IN MYCOSIS FUNGOIDES

E. SCHEFFER AND C.J.L.M. MEIJER

INTRODUCTION

The recognition of lymph node involvement in mycosis fungoides (MF) is important because it is associated with a poor prognosis and determines the choice of therapy (1–6).

Histological diagnosis of partial or total replacement of the lymph-node architecture by atypical lymphoreticular tissue will not be too difficult for the pathologist in most cases, whereas early involvement—i.e., without disturbance of the lymph node architecture—may be quite difficult to establish. Peripheral lymph nodes from MF patients, when excised as part of a staging procedure, usually show the histological features of dermatopathic lymphadenopathy (DL) without effacement of the lymph-node architecture by MF infiltration. Since DL may develop in patients with a form of chronic dermatosis unrelated to MF, it seems important to have criteria for the recognition of early MF involvement of dermatopathic lymph nodes from MF patients.

Skin lesions in MF have a hallmark: the mycosis cell (6, 7). An identical cell type in Sézary's syndrome (SS) is the Sézary cell. This cell type was originally defined electron-microscopically (8), but is quite well recognizable light-microscopically in histological sections of good quality. Its outstanding characteristic is its strongly indented, cerebriform nucleus. This cell type has therefore been termed the cerebriform mononuclear cell (CMC). Several investigators have stressed the nonspecificity of CMC for MF or SS, because such cells, though notably smaller than the typical mycosis or Sézary cells, have been observed in various dermatoses unrelated to MF (8–11) as well as in synovia from patients with rheumatoid arthritis (12) and in the blood of healthy individuals (13). CMC variants characterized by large and often hyperchromatic cerebriform nuclei have been described as light-microscopically diagnostic for MF and SS (4, 5, 7, 14).

CMC not only have T-cell membrane characteristics (15–23) but also show T-cell behavior, since they home in the paracortical areas of lymph nodes (24). It is therefore hardly surprising that they occur mainly in the paracortical areas (8) and are to be expected in increased numbers in the

J.G. van den Tweel et al. (eds.), Malignant Lymphoproliferative Diseases, 373–385
All rights reserved.

enlarged paracortical areas of dermatopathic lymph nodes. CMC have indeed been described in dermatopathic lymph nodes from patients with diseases unrelated to MF (25, 26). Several authors have stated that the presence of mycosis cells in clusters or sheets is obligatory for the diagnosis of MF involvement of lymph nodes (3, 4, 5, 27). Therefore, to recognize early involvement of dermatopathic lymph nodes, it is necessary to scrutinize these lymph nodes for the presence of CMC with large nuclei: such larger cells might then be considered mycosis cells.

Characteristically, in DL the paracortical areas are moderately to greatly enlarged due to the accumulation of histiocytic cells with abundant cytoplasm and lymphocytes. At lower magnification, these areas have a rather pale appearance. Many of the histiocytic cells have been identified as interdigitating reticulum cells and Langerhans cells electron-microscopically (25), the latter containing Langerhans-cell or Birbeck granules. Some histiocytic cells contain melanin and presumably contain lipid, because they have a foamy cytoplasm. Scattered among these cells there are many lymphocytes, some of which have deeply indented, cerebriform nuclei; such CMC occur mainly within the paracortical areas.

HISTOLOGICAL INVESTIGATION OF LYMPH NODES FROM MF PATIENTS

To diagnose early MF involvement, it was felt necessary to discriminate between lymph nodes with and without CMC larger than those found in dermatopathic lymph nodes from patients with diseases unrelated to MF. For this reason, a partially retrospective histological study of 30 inguinal lymph nodes from 24 MF patients was performed (26). Most of these lymph nodes had been excised as part of the clinical staging procedure, and others had been obtained at autopsy. The diagnosis MF was based on clinical and histological criteria. The skin lesions had been present from 1 to 10 years. Ten dermatopathic lymph nodes, either originating from patients with unrelated diseases or excised on suspicion of malignancy, were used as controls. All lymph node sections were carefully scrutinized for the presence of CMC, the smallest and the largest of which were selectively chosen for measurement. CMC nuclei were measured with a calibrated ocular and the largest nuclear diameter was recorded. In view of the limited accuracy of this method, the values were recorded in 0.5-micron classes. To avoid differences due to any histotechnical variations, the range of small lymphocyte nuclear diameters was also determined in the same way and proved to be remarkably constant in different sections.

HISTOLOGICAL CATEGORIES

The histological alterations in these lymph nodes were classified into 4 histological categories: DL with CMC not larger than those in the controls (Category I), DL with CMC larger than those in the controls (Category II), and partial replacement (Category III) and total replacement (Category IV) of lymph-node architecture by atypical lymphoreticular tissue (Table 1). These histological categories have been extensively described elsewhere (26). Category I is identical with DL in patients without MF or a related disease (Figure 1). In Category II, besides the presence of larger CMC, there generally tend to be many more CMC, not only within but also outside the paracortical areas. Furthermore, there generally tend to be more eosinophils and large lymphoid cells than in Category I (Figure 2). These seem to be minor criteria, however (Table 2). In Category III there is partial replacement of the lymph-node architecture by atypical lymphoreticular tissue. In some of our cases a few Sternberg-Reed cell-like cells were found (Figure 3). Pre-existent parts of lymph-node tissue generally show a Category II histological picture. Category IV represents diffuse lymph-node involvement with effacement of the lymph-node structure (Figure 4).

CORRELATION OF THE HISTOLOGICAL FINDINGS WITH THE RESULTS OF DNA CYTOPHOTOMETRY AND THE CLINICAL COURSE

The histological findings were correlated with the results of cytophotometrical measurements of the DNA content of the cell nuclei in imprints of the same lymph nodes and with the clinical course (28–30). Follow-up periods ranged from 1 to 6 years (Table 3).

The lymph nodes from 8 patients were assigned to Category I; in general, these patients responded well to therapy and had normal DNA values. One patient, however, showed only a partial response.

Table 1. Histological alterations in inguinal lymph nodes from patients with mycosis fungoides.

Category I: DL* – l.n.d.c.** of CMC*** *not larger* than in controls
Category II: DL – l.n.d.c. of CMC *larger* than in controls
Category III: Focal replacement of lymph node architecture
Category IV: Total replacement of lymph node architecture by atypical lymphoreticular tissue

---

  *DL = dermatopathic lymphadenopathy.
 **l.n.d.c. = largest nuclear diameter class.
***CMC = cerebriform mononuclear cells.

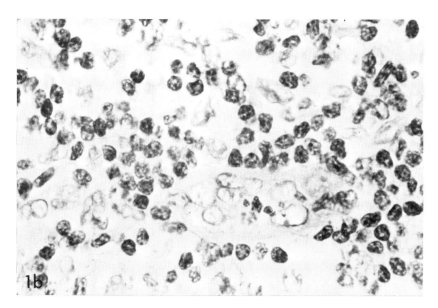

Figure 1. (a) Part of lymph node from patients with MF, showing dermatopathic lymph-adenopathy (DL). Parts of two secondary follicles and part of a greatly enlarged paracortical area (PCA) are shown (Category I). × 54.4.
(b) Part of PCA of same lymph node (detail of Figure 1a), showing an epitheloid venule lined by endothelial cells and surrounded by histiocytes, small lymphocytes, and cerebriform mononuclear cells (CMC). The largest diameter of the CMC nuclei does not exceed that of CMC in control dermatopathic lymph nodes (Category I). × 544.

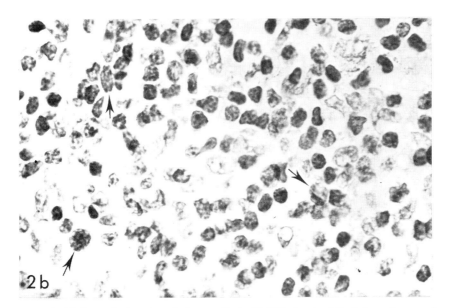

Figure 2. (a) Part of a lymph node from patient with MF, showing DL. A few primary and secondary follicles and an enlarged PCA are shown (Category II). × 54.4.

(b) Part of PCA of same lymph node (detail of Figure 2a), showing an epitheloid venule lined by endothelial cells and surrounded by histiocytes, small lymphocytes and CMC (Category II). There are CMC with largest nuclear diameter exceeding that of CMC in Category I and in control dermatopathic lymph nodes (arrows). × 544.

Table 2. Criteria for the diagnosis of early MF involvement in lymph nodes showing dermatopathic lymphadenopathy.

Main criterion: Presence of CMC* with a largest nuclear diameter class larger than that of CMC in controls (7.1–7.5 μm).

Minor criteria:
1) Numerous CMC in and outside paracortical areas.
2) Moderate number of large lymphoid cells in paracortical areas.
3) Moderate to large numbers of eosinophils in paracortical areas.

---

*CMC = cerebriform mononuclear cells.

The lymph nodes from 12 patients were classified as Category II; 6 of these patients died within $3\frac{1}{2}$ years. The other 6 generally responded less well to therapy than the patients in Category I; only partial remissions could be obtained in most cases. The DNA content of cells in imprints was abnormal in 6 out of 11 cases; in 5 cases the values were normal but 2 of these 5 patients died. In one case DNA cytophotometry was not performed.

The poor clinical course of patients whose lymph nodes were assigned to Categories III and IV is in accordance with the literature. One patient is still alive but the follow-up period is relatively short (1 year). CMC in these categories generally tend to be somewhat larger; the DNA values were abnormal in all of these cases.

DISCUSSION

Recently, Lennert (31) described criteria for distinguishing DL associated with MF from DL associated with other, nonneoplastic diseases of the skin, on the basis of a re-evaluation of 8 dermatopathic lymph nodes from patients diagnosed clinically as having MF, histologically as cases of DL. For the early diagnosis of MF in lymph nodes, Lennert gives—in short—the following criteria. Large numbers of Lutzner cells (CMC) are present in the outer cortex, and particularly in the marginal sinus, subsinusoidal regions of the cortex, and paracortical areas. The Lutzner cells are prominent due to their polymorphism. Numerous mitotic figures (in Lutzner cells) within the paracortical areas are suggestive of MF. Occasionally, infiltration of atypical cells is seen in the lymph node capsule. Germinal centers in the lymph node are often small or have completely vanished. Plasmocytosis of the medulla is usually slight, if present at all, and eosinophils are also few in number.

The results of the present study only agree partially with Lennert's criteria, namely, in that the number of CMC and their polymorphism (variability of the largest nuclear diameters) as well as the number of CMC occurring outside the paracortical areas tends to be higher in Category II lymph nodes. Mitotic figures may be found in paracortical areas of dermatopathic lymph

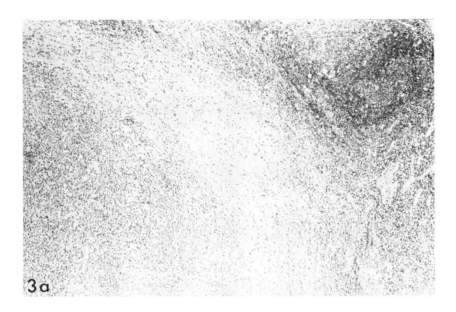

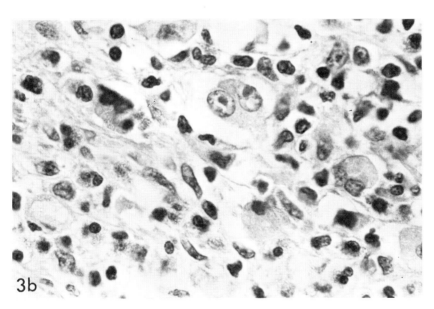

Figure 3. (a) Part of focus of atypical lymphoreticular tissue in lymph node from patient with MF. Part of the pre-existent lymph node tissue is visible, with a secondary follicle in the right upper corner (Category III). × 54.4.

(b) Detail of Figure 3a. An atypical binucleated cell, reminiscent of a Sternberg-Reed cell, several eosinophilic granulocytes, atypical lymphoid and histiocytic cells, and a few CMC are present. × 544.

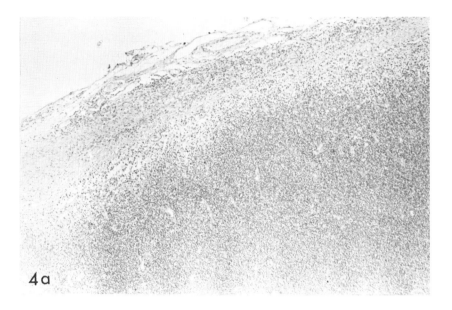

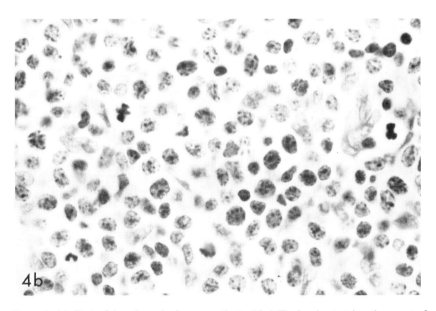

Figure 4. (a) Part of lymph node from a patient with MF, showing total replacement of lymph node architecture by diffuse proliferation of atypical lymphoreticular tissue (Category IV). × 54.4.

(b) Detail of Figure 4a, showing diffuse proliferation of atypical large lymphoid cells. A few CMC can be seen (Category IV). × 544.

Table 3. Relationship between histological picture of lymph node, largest nuclear diameter, and DNA content of cerebriform mononuclear cells and response to therapy of patients with MF. Follow-up periods range from 1 to 6 years.

	Histological picture	Largest nuclear diameter of largest CMC (μm)	Diagnosis	DNA content of CMC nuclei	Response to therapy	Died within 3½ years
Controls (n = 10)	DL	6.1–7.5	DL			
I. MF (n = 8)	DL	6.1–7.5	DL	8/8 N	7/8 R, 1/8 PR	
II. MF (n = 12)	DL	7.6–11.5	DL + early MF partial involvement	6/11 A, 5/11 N	4/12 R, 8/12 PR	6/12
III. MF (n = 3)	partial***	9.6–12.5* 7.1–11.0**	partial involvement	2/2 A	1/3 R, 2/3 PR	2/3
IV. MF (n = 1)	diffuse***	10.6–12.0	diffuse MF involvement	1/1 A	1/1 PR	1/1

DL = dermatopathic lymphadenopathy   A = abnormal   R = remission

   N = normal   PR = partial remission

MF = mycosis fungoides

* In MF foci.

** In remaining areas.

*** Replacement of lymph node architecture by atypical lymphoreticular tissue.

nodes unassociated with MF as well as in those of Category I lymph nodes. Some of our Category II lymph nodes showed an increased number of mitotic figures in the paracortical areas; this finding may, however, represent pro-liferation of histiocytic cells (interdigitating reticulum cells, Langerhans cells) as well as of CMC or other lymphoid cells. An increased mitotic rate might herald impeding progression to a frank lymphomatous stage (Catego-ries III and IV). Support for the assumption that the latter categories may indeed develop from Category II, is provided by the finding that in 4 patients the lymph nodes, either excised some time after the first excision or obtained at autopsy, fell into Categories III or IV, whereas the first lymph nodes to be excised had been classified as Category II. In the present study the state of the germinal centers and the number of plasma cells in the medulla were not helpful criteria for early MF involvement; the number of eosinophilic granulocytes tended to be higher in the Category II ("early involvement") lymph nodes than in those of Category I. The presence of CMC larger than those in the control dermatopathic lymph nodes appeared to be the main criterion for early MF involvement in the present study.

The development of early MF involvement of dermatopathic lymph nodes has been suggested to resemble the development of diagnostic MF lesions in the skin from the unspecific praemycotic stage (26). The Langer-hans cell, as recently pointed out by Rowden and Lewis (32), may be in-volved in the pathogenesis of the MF skin lesion, since it seems to represent the antigen-trapping cell in the epidermis; Tan et al. (33) have suggested that MF might result from antigen persistence causing specific reactive lympho-cytes to home in the skin. The early, nonspecific dermatosis seen in the development of MF might thus result from chronic exposure to antigen. The Langerhans cells seem not only to act as antigen-trapping cells in the epidermis but also to be capable of transporting the antigens on their surface, via the lymphatics, from the skin to the regional lymph nodes to initiate the cellular immune response (34, 35, 36) and, eventually, to reside in the paracortical areas and form a new site for homing of specific lym-phocytes. Since the Langerhans cells are closely related to the interdigitat-ing reticulum cells in the paracortical areas both morphologically and func-tionally, these cell types may even be identical.

Homing of CMC has been observed in paracortical areas of lymph nodes from MF patients (24, 26). Thus, involvement of lymph nodes in MF could be a phenomenon analogous to the development of the MF skin lesion. Eventually, as a result of persistent Langerhans cell-mediated antigen, a disturbance of immune response regulation could give rise to development of a malignant cell clone or clones. Besides entering the paracortical areas from the epitheloid venules, CMC might reach these areas by way of the draining lymphatics from the skin and the marginal sinus and other sinuses of the lymph node. Langerhans-cell-induced "transformation" of CMC could conceivably occur "en route" in the lymph vessels as well as in the skin and in the paracortical areas.

Atypical cells which seem to be "transition forms" between CMC and the atypical large lymphoid cells (immunoblasts) can be observed in Categories III and IV. This of course does not constitute proof that such cells originate from the CMC. However, in recent publications a few examples have been presented of anaplastic lymphomas no longer having the morphological characteristics of Sézary or mycosis cells but still displaying helper T-cell function in vitro (37) and histochemical T-cell markers (38), respectively.

Proliferation of histiocytic cells in paracortical areas in Category II and in the MF foci in Category III lymph nodes may also occur, because mitotic figures may be observed among such cells in these areas. According to Lennert, interdigitating reticulum cells found among the lymphoid cells, may be part of the neoplasm and not merely remnants of DL (31).

This may be one reason why, among various cases lymphomatous lymph nodes in the end stage of MF show marked variability.

REFERENCES

1. Epstein, E.H., Levin, D.L., Croft, J.D., Jr., and Lutzner, M.A.: Mycosis fungoides: survival, prognostic features, response to therapy and autopsy findings. Medicine, 51:61, 1972.
2. Fuks, Z.Y., Bagshaw, M.A., and Farber, E.M.: Prognostic signs and the management of mycosis fungoides. Cancer, 32:1385, 1973.
3. Variakojis, D., Rosas-Uribe, A., and Rappaport, H.: Mycosis fungoides – Pathologic findings in staging laparotomies. Cancer, 33:1589, 1974.
4. Rappaport, H., and Thomas, L.B.: Mycosis fungoides. The pathology of extra-cutaneous involvement. Cancer, 34:1198, 1974.
5. Thomas, L.B., and Rappaport, H.: Mycosis fungoides and its relationship to other malignant lymphomas. In: The reticuloendothelial system, chapter 12, International Academy of Pathology Monograph. Williams and Wilkins, Baltimore, 1975.
6. Van Vloten, W.A.: Cutaneous T cell lymphoma: Clinical aspects. This volume, chapter 27.
7. Lever, W.F., and Schaumburg-Lever, G.: Histopathology of skin diseases. J.B. Lippingcott, Philadelphia–Toronto, 5th. edition, 1975.
8. Lutzner, M.A., Hobbs, J.W., and Horvath, P.: Ultrastructure of abnormal cells in Sézary syndrome, mycosis fungoides, and parapsoriasis en plaque. A.M.A. Archives of Dermatology, 103:375, 1971.
9. Flaxman, B.A., Zelazny, G., and Van Scott, E.J.: Nonspecificity of characteristic cells in mycosis fungoides. A.M.A. Archives of Dermatology, 104:141, 1971.
10. Duncan, S.C., and Winkelmann, R.K.: Circulating Sézary cells in hospitalized dermatology patients. British Journal of Dermatology, 99:171, 1978.

11. Gisser, S.D., and Young, I.: Mycosis fungoides-like cells. Their presence in a case of pityriasic dermatitis with a comment on their significance as an indicator of primary T cell dyscrasia. The American Journal of Surgical Pathology, 1:97, 1978.
12. Van Leeuwen, A.W.F.M., Meijer, C.J.L.M., De Vries, E., Van de Putte, L. B.A., and De Man, J.C.H.: Atypical mononuclear (mycosis type or Sézary type) cells with T cell membrane characteristics in rheumatoid synovial fluids. Proceedings of the Koninklijke Nederlandsche Akademie van Wetenschappen, series C, Biological and medical sciences, 69:267, 1976.
13. Meijer, C.J.L.M., Van Leeuwen, A.W.F.M., Van der Loo, E.M., Van de Putte, L.B.A., and Van Vloten, W.A.: Cerebriform (Sézary-like) mononuclear cells in healthy individuals: a morphologically distinct population of T cells. Relationship with mycosis fungoides and Sézary syndrome. Virchows Archiv B, Cellular Pathology, 25:95, 1977.
14. Brehmer-Andersson, E.: Mycosis fungoides and its relations to Sézary's syndrome, lymphomatoid papulosis, and primary cutaneous Hodgkin's disease. A clinical, histopathologic and cytologic study of fourteen cases and a critical review of the literature. Acta Dermato-venereologica 56, suppl. 75, 1976.
15. Crossen, P.E., Mellor, J.E.L., Finlay, A.G., Ravick, M.R.E., Vincent, P.C., and Gurz, F.W.: The Sézary syndrome. Cytogenetic studies and identification of the Sézary cell as an abnormal lymphocyte. American Journal of Medicine 50:24, 1971.
16. Broome, J.D., Zucker-Franklin, D., Weiner, M.C., Bianco, C., and Nussenzweig, V.: Leukemic cells with membrane properties of thymus derived (T) lymphocytes in a case of Sézary's syndrome: morphologic and immunologic studies. Clinical Immunology and Immunopathology, 1:319, 1973.
17. Brouet, J.C., Flandrin, G., and Seligmann, M.: Indications of the thymus derived nature of the proliferating cells in six patients with Sézary's syndrome. The New England Journal of Medicine, 289:341, 1973.
18. Edelson, R.L., Kirkpatrick, C.H., Shevach, E.M., Schein, P.S., Smith, R.W., Green, I., and Lutzner, M.A.: Preferential cutaneous infiltration by neoplastic thymus-derived lymphocytes in morphologic and functional studies. Annals of Internal Medicine, 80:685, 1974.
19. Robinowitz, B.N., Noguchi, S., and Roenigk, H.H.: Tumor cell characterization in mycosis fungoides. Cancer, 37:1747, 1976.
20. Van Leeuwen, A.W.F.M., Meijer, C.J.L.M., and De Man, J.C.H.: T cell membrane characteristics of "mycosis cells" in the skin and lymph node. The Journal of Investigative Dermatology, 65:367, 1975.
21. Broder, S., Edelson, R.L., Lutzner, M.A., Nelson, D.L., McDermott, R.P., Durm, M.E., Golman, C.K., Meade, B.D., and Waldmann, T.A.: The Sézary syndrome. A malignant proliferation of helper T cells. Journal of Clinical Investigation, 58:1297, 1976.
22. Edelson, R.L.: Recent advances in the cutaneous T cell lymphomas. Bulletin du Cancer, 64:209, 1977.
23. Burg, G., Rodt, H., Grosse-Wilde, H., and Braun-Falco, O.: Surface markers and mitogen response of cells harvested from cutaneous infiltrates in mycosis fungoides and Sézary's syndrome. The Journal of Investigative Dermatology, 70:257, 1978.
24. Van Leeuwen, A.W.F.M., Meijer, C.J.L.M., Van Vloten, W.A., Scheffer, E., and De Man, J.C.H.: Further evidence for the T cell nature of the atypical

mononuclear cells in mycosis fungoides. Virchows Archiv B, Cellular Pathology, 21:179, 1976.

25. Rausch, E., Kaiserling, E., and Goos, M.: Langerhans cells and interdigitating reticulum cells in the thymus-dependent region in human dermatopathic lymphadenitis. Virchows Archiv B, Cellular Pathology, 25:327, 1977.

26. Scheffer, E., Meijer, C.J.L.M., and Van Vloten, W.A.: Dermatopathic lymphadenopathy and lymph node involvement in mycosis fungoides. Cancer, 45, 137, 1980.

27. Rosas-Uribe, A., Variakojis, D., Molnar, Z., and Rappaport, H.: Mycosis fungoides: an ultrastructural study. Cancer, 34:634, 1974.

28. Van Vloten, W.A., Van Duijn, P., and Schaberg, A.: Cytodiagnostic use of Feulgen-DNA measurements in cell imprints from the skin of patients with mycosis fungoides. British Journal of Dermatology, 91:365, 1974.

29. Van Vloten, W.A., Schaberg, A., and Van der Ploeg, M.: Cytophotometric studies on mycosis fungoides and other cutaneous reticuloses. Bulletin du Cancer, 64:249, 1977.

30. Van Vloten, W.A., Scheffer, E., and Meijer, C.J.L.M.: DNA-cytophotometry of lymph node imprints from patients with mycosis fungoides. The Journal of Investigative Dermatology, 73, 275, 1979.

31. Lennert, K., in collaboration with N. Mohri, H. Stein, E. Kaiserling, and H.K. Müller-Hermelink: Malignant lymphomas other than Hodgkin's disease. Springer-Verlag, Berlin–Heidelberg–New York, 1978, p. 175.

32. Rowden, G., and Lewis, M.G.: Langerhans cells: involvement in the pathogenesis of mycosis fungoides. British Journal of Dermatology, 91:665, 1976.

33. Tan, R.S.H., Butterworth, C.M., McLaughlin, H., Malka, S., and Samman, P.D.: Mycosis fungoides – a disease of antigen persistence. British Journal of Dermatology, 91:607, 1974.

34. Shelley, W.B. and Juhlin, L.: Langerhans cells form a reticuloepithelial trap for external contact antigens. Nature, 261:46, 1976.

35. Silberberg-Sinakin, I., Thorbecke, G.J., Baer, R.L., Rosenthal, A.S., and Berezowski, V.: Antigen-bearing Langerhans cells in skin, dermal lymphatics and in lymph node. Cell Immunology, 25:137, 1976.

36. Stingl, G., Katz, S.I., Shevach, E.M., Rosenthal, A.S., and Green, I.: Analogous functions of macrophages and Langerhans cells in the initiation of the immune response. The Journal of Investigative Dermatology, 71:59, 1978.

37. Lawrence, E.C., Broder, S., Jaffe, E.S., Braylan, R.C., Dobbins, W.O., Young, R.C., and Waldmann, T.A.: Evolution of a lymphoma with helper T cell characteristics in Sézary syndrome. Blood, 52:481, 1978.

38. Schwarze, E.W., and Ude, P.: Immunoblastic sarcoma with leukemic blood picture in the terminal stage of mycosis fungoides. Virchows Archiv A, Pathological Anatomy and Histology, 369:165, 1975.

HODGKIN'S DISEASE

30. NATURAL HISTORY OF HODGKIN'S DISEASE IN RELATION TO NON-HODGKIN'S LYMPHOMA

H. KIM

INTRODUCTION

In malignant lymphomas, the histologic classification has been and still remains one of the most important prognostic indicators and the guide to clinicans for the proper management of their patients. This is true, in spite of the rapid advances in our knowledge of immunology and immunological characterization of human lymphoid tissue and its neoplasia (3, 27).

Following the first report in 1832 by Thomas Hodgkin (14) of his clinico-pathologic observations on seven patients, varied terminology applied to both Hodgkin's disease (15, 23, 25) and non-Hodgkin's lymphomas (2, 7, 8, 10, 21, 24, 26) has been confusing and classifications have been many and controversial. The histologic classification of Hodgkin's disease proposed by Lukes et al. (23), and modified at the Rye Conference (25) (Table 1) has been successfully applied to clinico-pathologic studies in many countries, leading to its universal acceptance.

In contrast to Hodgkin's disease, the histopathologic classification originally proposed by Rappaport (34) has been the subject of considerable controversy although it is still the most widely used after having demonstrated its applicability and usefulness, both clinically (4, 12, 13, 16, 37) and

Table 1. Hodgkin's disease.

Jackson and Parker	Lukes et al. (23)	Rye classification (25)
Paragranuloma ——	Lymphocytic and/or histiocytic —— a) Nodular b) Diffuse	Lymphocytic predominance
Granuloma	Nodular sclerosis —————— Mixed ———————— Diffuse fibrosis	Nodular sclerosis Mixed cellularity Lymphocytic depletion
Sarcoma ————————	Reticular	

J.G. van den Tweel et al. (eds.), Malignant Lymphoproliferative Diseases, 389–397

Table 2. Hodgkin's disease: Distribution according to histologic types.*

Lymphocyte predominance	63	(3%)
Nodular sclerosis	1307	(59%)
Mixed cellularity	602	(27%)
Lymphocyte depletion	169	(8%)
Unclassifiable	68	(3%)
Total	2209	(100%)

*Based on data of Repository Center for Lymphoma Clinical Studies, City of Hope National Medical Center, Duarte, California.

morphologically (19). According to the scheme, the lymphomas are subdivided according to architectural pattern as well as cytology and presumed degree of differentiation of the predominant cell (34). With the better understanding of our immune system and studies utilizing immunologic techniques, however, it has become apparent that this classification has scientific flaws as to both histogenetic and immunologic aspects. Recognizing this deficiency, many workers of different countries proposed different classifications for non-Hodgkin's lymphomas (2, 7, 8, 10, 21, 24, 26). Unfortunately only few clinicopathologic studies utilizing these different terminologies and classifications are available (29, 30, 39), and their validity, reproducibility, and applicability have not yet been entirely demonstrated.

HODGKIN'S DISEASE

Table 1 shows the realtionship between the classification of Lukes and Butler (23) which led to the Rye modification (25) and the original Jackson and Parker classification (15) that they replaced. Unlike the classification of non-Hodgkin's lymphomas which are based on functional and morphologic features of neoplastic cells, the Hodgkin's disease is classified according to the cellular background and the relative abundance of Hodgkin's cells including Reed-Sternberg cells. Table 2 represents unpublished data of the Repository Center for Lymphoma Clinical Studies showing the distribution of 2,209 Hodgkin's disease cases according to the Rye histologic classification. Lymphocyte predominance type carries the most favorable prognosis. It is characterized by lymphocyte-rich cellular milieu and sparsely scattered Sternberg-Reed cells. So-called L and H cells are also characteristic of this type. The discovery of nodular sclerosing type was the most significant contribution of Lukes and Butler's classification (23). Previously it was buried under the "granuloma" category of the Jackson and Parker classification. This subgroup shows clusters of lacunar cells circumscibed by varying amounts of birefringent collagen (23). This is the most frequent histologic type of Hodgkin's disease, comprising 59% in the United States. It shows a predilection for the mediastinum and female sex (9). The prognosis for this type is favorable. The mixed cellularity Hodgkin's disease shows more abundant Hodgkin's cells and Sternberg-Reed cells usually in a polymorphous cellular environment composed of lymphocytes, plasma cells, and eosinophils in varying proportions. Prognosis is generally not as favorable as the two previous groups. The least favorable prognostically is the lymphocyte depletion. This type is characterized by the paucity of lymphocytes in the background and shows numerous Hodgkin's cells ("reticular") (23) or, in some instances, diffuse fibrosis with a relatively small number of Hodgkin's cells ("diffuse fibrosis") (23). According to the study of Bearman et al. (1) confirmining the results of others (31), this is the most aggressive form of Hodgkin's disease, but it does not necessarily have a rapidly fatal clinical course despite the advanced stage of disease at presentation. However, the improvement of the overall survival (79% at five years and 62% at ten years) (18) in recent years has reduced the prognostic significance of the histopathologic classification of Hodgkin's disease.

Surgical staging procedures

High accuracy of the lymphographic studies (5) and diagnostic laparotomy for the staging of Hodgkin's disease (11, 17) have significantly contributed to our understanding of both Hodgkin's disease and non-Hodgkin's lymphomas. Both procedures are now routinely used for the staging of Hodgkin's disease and in selected cases for non-Hodgkin's lymphomas as well.

From the data accumulated by the routine use of highly accurate lymphangiogram studies and staging laparotomies, the following information has become available (40): (a) if left supraclavicular lymph node is involved, the frequency of subdiaphragmatic nodal involvement is 40%; (b) if right supraclavicular lymph node is involved, the frequency of subdiaphragmatic nodal involvement is only 8%; (c) in the presence of retroperitoneal disease, left cervical involvement can be anticipated; (d) if Hodgkin's disease is apparently confined to subdiaphragmatic sites, a "blind" left scalene fat pad biopsy should be performed; (e) it is unusual to have lower abdominal involvement without upper nodal or splenic involvement; (f) in patients who present with isolated mediastinal involvement, biopsy of a palpable right supraclavicular lymph node or a blind right scalene biopsy may alleviate the need for mediastinoscopy or thoracotomy. We also learned that laparotomy will prove to be of most help if: (a) patient has stage 1A with low cervical nodes or stage 2A or 3A disease for which radiotherapy alone is planned; (b) suspicious lymphangiogram and radio-therapy alone is planned; (c) splenomegaly is present; (d) fertile women requiring oophoropexy (38). On the other hand, laparotomy is not necessary if patients has: (a) stage 1A disease with high cervical nodes and negative lymphangiogram; (b) stage 1A or 2A with mediastinal disease only; (c) stage 1B, 2B, 3B or 3A disease for which chemotherapy is planned, and (d) high risk patient (38).

NON-HODGKIN'S LYMPHOMAS

Table 3 shows distribution of non-Hodgkin's lymphomas according to Rappaport classification. This is based on 3,779 cases accumulated at The Repository Center for Lymphoma Clinical Studies, City of Hope National Medical Center, Duarte, California. Non-Hodgkin's lymphomas are composed of widely different histologic categories with equally divergent clinical manifestations (27). The comprehensive and detailed review of natural history for each histologic category of non-Hodgkin's lymphomas, therefore, is beyond the scope of this presentation. In the United States, diffuse "histiocytic" lymphoma and poorly differentiated lymphocytic lymphoma with varying degrees of nodularity represent two most common histologic types (Table 3). They account for 27% and 25% respectively of all non-Hodgkin's lymphomas.

Nodular lymphoma, poorly differentiated lymphocytic type corresponds

Table 3 Non-Hodgkin's lymphomas: Distribution according to Rappaport Classification.*

	N	D	N & D	UNCL	Totals	
Well-differentiated lymphocytic	5	222	3	3	262	7.0%
Intermediate-differentiated lymphocytic	3	9	6	15	33	0.9%
Poorly-differentiated lymphocytic	835	397	196	72	1500	39.6%
Lymphoblastic	0	63	0	14	77	2.0%
Mixed-cell type	235	126	92	30	483	12.8%
Histiocytic	55	957	103	180	1295	34.3%
Burkitt's	0	7	1	4	12	0.3%
Undifferentiated non-Burkitt's	0	35	0	27	62	1.6%
Unclassified	2	18	0	35	55	1.5%
Totals	1135	1834	401	409	3779	100.0%

*Based on data of Repository Center for Lymphoma Clinical Studies, City of Hope National Medical Center, Duarte, California; N – Nodular; D – Diffuse. N & D – Nodular and Diffuse; UNCL – Pattern not specified.

to small cleaved follicular center cell lymphoma of Lukes and Collins (24, 26) and centroblastic/centrocytic lymphoma of Kiel classification (21). This represents the most common type of non-Hodgkin's lymphomas of adults. It rarely occurs before the age of thirty. In spite of the widespread nature with bone marrow involvement in up to 85% of the patients from its inception (28, 35), it is generally a slowly progressive disease (16, 33) without cure and remissions are always followed by relapses. For this reason, aggressive combination chemotherapy is usually not indicated. In a recent study of selected patients with stage 3 and 4 non-Hodgkin's lymphomas of favorable histologic types including nodular lymphoma, poorly differentiated lymphocytic type, no significant actuarial survival difference was noted between those who were treated according to protocol and those who did not receive therapy (32).

Diffuse "histiocytic" type is morphologically, functionally and clinically heterogeneous (3, 24, 26, 27, 30). Utilizing Lukes and Collins classification, it represents, at least, the five following categories: (a) large cleaved, (b) large noncleaved, (c) B-immunoblastic, (d) T-immunoblastic, (e) true histiocytic (24, 26, 30). In our experience, 78% of Rappaport's diffuse "histiocytic" lymphoma represent large noncleaved follicular center cell lymphoma (Table 4) (30). We are not certain, however, what proportion of this histologic category represents either immunoblastic or centroblastic according to Kiel classification. Our data (30) and those of others (39) indicate that the large cleaved subcategory does indeed have a better prognosis compared with the remainder of the large cell lymphoma (Table 4). The large noncleaved follicular center cell lymphoma represents the second most common type of non-Hodgkin's lymphoma in the United States. It occurs at all ages and typically has an aggressive clinical course with rapidly fatal outcome (30). Median survival is usually less than one year although bone

Table 4. Diffuse lymphomas.

	Rappaport		Lukes and Collins		
Cell type	No. of cases	Median Survival (months)	Cell type	No. of cases	Median Survival (months)
"Histiocytic"	54	8	Large cleaved	5	22 P = 0.08
			Large noncleaved	42	7
			B-Immunoblastic	6	6
			True histiocytic	1	5

From Nathwani et al. (30).

marrow involvement occurs in less than 10% of the patients at the onset (16, 35).

Surgical staging procedures

As in Hodgkin's disease, we learned, from lymphographic studies (5) and diagnostic laparotomies (6, 22, 36, 41), that non-Hodgkin's lymphoma also spreads in a predictable manner to anatomically contiguous sites (13, 18). Table 5 shows the relationship of histology to site in Hodgkin's disease (9) and non-Hodgkin's lymphomas (19) based on Stanford experience. The mesenteric lymph nodes, which are very seldon involved in Hodgkin's disease, are involved in a high proportion of non-Hodgkin's lymphomas (12, 13, 19, 22). Since these nodes are not effectively covered with the in-verted-Y field, a modification of technique became necessary to assure the adequate irradition, while providing effective protection to the kidneys (18). In addition, non-Hodgkin's lymphomas involve bone marrow, Waldeyer's ring and liver more often than in Hodgkin's disease. The following infor-mation was obtained from these lymphographic studies and diagnostic laparotomies (13): (a) spread of non-Hodgkin's lymphomas in a predictable manner by a contiguous involvement in 57% to 100% depending on the initial site of the disease; (b) subdiaphragmatic involvement in nodular lymphoma is 100% if the patient has bilateral supraclavicular disease and is more than 75% if the patient has unilateral supraclavicular disease; (c) subdiaphragmatic involvement in diffuse lymphoma is present in 81% of the patients if bilateral supraclavicular disease is present, while 42% is involved when left supraclavicular disease is noted; (d) hepatic involvement

Table 5. Relationship of histology to site in Hodgkin's disease and non-Hodgkin's lymphomas (Stanford University Series).*

Site	Hodgkin's disease (9) cases, %	Non-Hodgkin's lymphomas (19) cases, %
Abdomen	46	61
Spleen	42	34
Access. spleen	27	33
Splenic hilar nodes	56	54
Paraaortic nodes	30	40
Mesenteric nodes	6	56
Liver	4	16
Gastrointestinal tract	0	6
Bone marrow	4	22
Mediastinum	58	17
Waldeyer's ring	< 1	4

* Based on preoperative clinical evaluation and surgical staging procedures.

is always associated with simultaneous involvement of the spleen; and (e) 20% of the patients with positive laparotomies, multiple histologies were noted in different sites leading to major changes in therapy in half (10%). These multiple histologies are comprised not only of different histologic types of non-Hodgkin's lymphoma (19, 22) but also may be composed of Hodgkin's disease and non-Hodgkin's lymphoma (12, 19).

REFERENCES

1. Bearman, R.M., Pangalis, G.A., and Rappaport, H.: Hodgkin's disease, lymphocyte depletion type. A clinicopathologic study of 39 patients. Cancer, 41:293–302, 1978.
2. Bennett, M.H., Farrer-Brown, G., and Henry, K.: Classification of non-Hodgkin's lymphomas. Lancet, 2:405–406, 1974.
3. Berard, C.W., Jaffe, E.S., Braylan, R.C., Mann, R.S., and Nanba, K.: Immunologic aspects and pathology of malignant lymphomas. Cancer, 42:911–921, 1978.
4. Bloomfield, C.D., Goldman, A., Dick, F., Brunning, R.D., and Kennedy, B.J.: Multivariate analysis of prognostic factors in the non-Hodgkin's malignant lymphomas. Cancer, 33:870–879, 1974.
5. Castellino, R.A., Billingham, M., and Dorfman, R.F.: Lymphographic accurancy in Hodgkin's disease and malignant lymphoma with a note on the "reactive" lymph node as a cause of most false positive lymphograms. Invest. Radiol., 9:155–165, 1974.
6. Chabner, B.A., Johnson, R.E., Young, R.C., Canellos, G.P., Hubbard, S.P., Johnson, S.K., and DeVita, V.T.: Sequential nonsurgical and surgical staging of non-Hodgkin's lymphoma. Ann. Intern. Med., 85:149–154, 1976.
7. Dorfman R.F.. Classification of non-Hodgkin's lymphoma. Lancet 1:1295, 1974.
8. Dorfman, R.F.: Classification of non-Hodgkin's lymphoma. Lancet, 2:961, 1974.
9. Dorfman, R.F.: Relationship of histology to site in Hodgkin's disease. Cancer Res., 31:1786–1793, 1971.
10. Gerard-Marchant, R., Hamlin, I., and Lennert, K.: Classification of non-Hodgkin's lymphomas. Lancet, 2:406–408, 1974.
11. Glatstein, E., Guernsey, J.M., Rosenberg, S.A., and Kaplan, H.S.: The value of laparotomy and splenectomy in the staging of Hodgkin's disease. Cancer, 24:709–718, 1969.
12. Goffinet, D.R., Castellino, R.A., Kim, H., Dorfman, R.F., Fuks, Z., Rosenberg, S.A., Nelson, T., and Kaplan, H.S.: Staging laparotomies in unselected previously untreated patients with non-Hodgkin's disease. Cancer, 32:672–681, 1973.
13. Goffinet, D.R., Warnke, R., Dunnick, N.R., Castellino, R., Glatstein, E., Nelsen, T.S., Dorfman, R.F., Rosenberg, S.A., and Kaplan, H.S.: Clinical and surgical (laparotomy) evaluation of patients with non-Hodgkin's lymphomas. Cancer Treat. Rep., 61:981–992, 1977.
14. Hodgkin, T.: On some morbid appearance of the absorbent glands and spleen. Med. Chir. Trans., 17:68–114, 1832.

15. Jackson, H., Jr., and Parker, F.: Hodgkin's disease. II. Pathology. N. Engl. J. Med., 231:35–44, 1944.
16. Jones, S.E., Fuks, Z., Bull, M., Kadin, M.E., Dorfman, R.F., Kaplan, H.S., Rosenberg, S.A., and Kim, H.: Non-Hodgkin's lymphomas. IV. Clinicopathologic correlation in 405 cases. Cancer, 31:806–823, 1973.
17. Kadin, M.E., Glatstein, E., and Dorfman, R.F.: Clinicopathologic studies of 117 untreated patients subjected to laparotomy for the staging of Hodgkin's disease. Cancer, 27:1277–1294, 1971.
18. Kaplan, H.S.: Hodgkin's kisease and other human malignant lymphomas: Advances and prospects–G.H.A. Clowes Memorial Lecture. Cancer Res., 36:3863–3878, 1976.
19. Kim, H. and Dorfman, R.F.: Morphological studies of 84 untreated patients subjected to laparotomy for the staging of non-Hodgkin's lymphomas. Cancer, 33:657–674, 1974.
20. Kim, H., Hendrickson, M.R., and Dorfman, R.F.: Composite lymphoma. Cancer, 40:959–976, 1977.
21. Lennert, K., Mohri, N., and Stein, H.: The histopathology of malignant lymphoma. Br. J. Haematol., suppl., 31:193–203, 1975.
22. Lotz, M.J., Chabner, B., DeVita, V.T., Johnson, R.E., and Berard, C.W.: Pathological staging of 100 consecutive untreated patients with non-Hodgkin's lymphomas. Extrameduallary sites of disease. Cancer, 37:266–270, 1976.
23. Lukes, R.J., Butler, J.J., and Hicks, E.B.: Natural history of Hodgkins disease as related to its pathologic picture. Cancer, 19:317–344, 1966.
24. Lukes, R.J., and Collins, R.D.: Immunological characterization of human malignant lymphomas. Cancer, 34:1488–1503, 1974.
25. Lukes, R.J., Craver, L.F., Hall, T.C., Rappaport, H., and Ruben, P.: Report of the Nomenclature Committee. Cancer Res., 26:1131, 1966.
26. Lukes, R.J., Parker, J.W., Taylor, C.R., Tindle, B.H., Cramer, A.D., and Lincoln, T.L.: Immunologic approach to non-Hodgkin lymphomas and related leukemias. Analysis of results of multiparameter studies of 425 cases. Semin. Hematol., 15:322–351, 1978.
27. Mann, R.B., Jaffe, E.S., and Berard, C.W.: Malignant lymphomas—A conceptual understanding of morphologic diversity. A review. Am. J. Pathol., 94:105–192, 1979.
28. McKenna, R.W., Bloomfield, C.D., and Brunning, R.D.: Nodular lymphoma: Bone marrow and blood manifestations. Cancer, 36:428–440, 1975.
29. Meugé, C., Hoerni, B., De Mascarel, A., Durand, M., Richaud, P., Hourni-Simon, G., Chauvergne, J., and Lagarde, C.: Non-Hodgkin malignant lymphomas. Clinicopathologic correlations with the Kiel classifications. Retrospective analysis of a series of 274 cases. Europ. J. Cancer, 14:587–592, 1978.
30. Nathwani, B.N., Kim, H., Rappaport, H., Solomon, J., and Fox, M.: Non-Hodgkin's lymphomas. A clinicopathologic study comparing two classifications. Cancer, 41:303–325, 1978.
31. Neiman, R.S., Rosen, P.J., Lukes, R.J., Lymphocyte depletion Hodgkin's disease: A clinicopathological entity. New Engl. J. Med., 288:751–755, 1973.
32. Portlock, C.S., and Rosenberg, S.A.: No initial therapy for Stage III and IV non-Hodgkin's lymphomas of favorable histologic types. Ann. Intern. Med., 90:10–13, 1979.
33. Quazi, R., Aisenberg, A.C., and Long, J.C.: The natural history of nodular lymphoma. Cancer, 37:1923–1927, 1976.

34. Rappaport, H.: In Atlas of tumor pathology, Section 3, Fascicle 8, Washington, P.C., 1966.
35. Rosenberg, S.A.: Bone marrow involvement in the non-Hodgkin's lymphomata. Br. J. Cancer (Suppl. II), 31:261–264, 1975.
36. Rosenberg, S.A., Dorfman, R.F., and Kaplan, H.S.: The value of sequential bone marrow biopsy and laprotomy and splenectomy in a series of 127 consecutive untreated patients with non-Hodgkin's lymphomata. Br. J. Cancer, suppl. II, 31:221–227, 1975.
37. Rosenberg, S.A., Dorfman, R.F., and Kaplan, H.S.: A summary of the results of a review of 405 patients with non-Hodgkin's lymphoma at Stanford University. Br. J. Cancer, suppl. II, 31:168–173, 1975.
38. Shohet, S.B., Newcom, S.R.: Hodgkin's disease, Western J. Med., 127:487–496, 1977.
39. Strauchen, J.A., Young, R.C., De Vita, V.T. Jr., Anderson, T., Fantone, J.C., and Berard, C.W.: Clinical relevance of the histopathological subclassification of diffuse "histiocytic" lymphoma. N. Engl. J. Med., 299:1382–1387, 1978.
40. Sweet, D.L., Kinnealey, A., and Ultmann, J.E.: Hodgkin's disease: Problems of staging. Cancer, 42:957–970, 1978.
41. Veronesi, U., Musumeci, E., Pizzetti, F., Gennari, L., and Bonadonna, G.: The value of staging laparotomy in non-Hodgkin's lymphomas (with emphasis on the histiocytic type). Cancer, 33:446–459, 1974.

31. IMMUNOPATHOLOGY OF HODGKIN'S DISEASE

C.R. TAYLOR

Hodgkin's disease acquired its eponymous title at the suggestion of Samuel Wilks who described (in 1865 (78)) several of the cases initially reported by one of his predecessors at Guy's Hospital, Thomas Hodgkin. The importance of Hodgkin's original paper was not so much his autopsy description of seven cases of enlargement of the lymph gland and spleen, for as Hodgkin himself said, "Others must have observed this finding at autopsy;" but rather his interpretation of the significance of this observation: "This appears to be a primary affectation of the lymph gland" (29). Wilks clearly distinguished this disease process from lardaceous disease (or amyloid) on the one hand, and from tuberculosis on the other, and was further impressed by the unique nature of the process: "This process of Hodgkin is distinct from tuberculosis and from cancer" (78).

With the growing sophistication of light microscopy and the development of routine sectioning and staining procedures, the diagnosis of Hodgkin's disease came to be based primarily upon histologic criteria. Many of the criteria that current generations of pathologists have learned to rely upon were described during the early days of light microscopy from 1870 onwards. For example, the bizarre polyploid giant cells of Hodgkin's disease were identified by Langhans, Greenfield and others some 30 years prior to the more detailed descriptions of Sternberg and Reed (1898 (64) and 1902 (56) respectively). In addition, the striking pattern of nodular sclerosis in Hodgkin's disease was clearly described by Andrewes in 1902 (4), though its prognostic significance was not fully appreciated until the work of Hanson (1964 (28)) and Lukes and Butler (1966 (45)).

Of the seven cases originally described by Thomas Hodgkin on the basis of gross autopsy findings only four were judged by Fox (1926 (18)) to be true examples of this entity, the remainder representing either syphilis, tuberculosis, or conditions of uncertain nature.

That our diagnostic accuracy is a little higher today than it was in Hodgkin's time is attributable to more precise definition of the histologic criteria used at light microscopy, rather than to any enhanced understanding of the pathogenesis or nature of the disease process. The recognition of the various subgroups of Hodgkin's disease, of differing prognostic import, was of particular value in that it served to sharpen the morphologic criteria that

J.G. van den Tweel et al. (eds.), Malignant Lymphoproliferative Diseases, 399–416
All rights reserved.
Copyright © 1980 by Martinus Nijhoff Publishers bv, The Hague/Boston/London.

had existed for many years (see above). In addition, the general acceptance of the Jackson and Parker (1947 (33)), and later the Lukes and Butler (1966 (45)), subclassifications of Hodgkin's disease, serve to polarize the nomenclature in use, putting an effective stop to the proliferation of new terminology for Hodgkin's disease and related processes, that in the past had caused so much confusion (Wallhauser, 1933 (76)).

The adoption of the Lukes/Butler classification of subtypes of Hodgkin's disease, following the acceptance of the Rappaport classification of lymphomas (Rappaport et al., 1956 (55)), had other far reaching implications, particularly leading to the current view that a clear distinction exists between Hodgkin's disease and the so-called non-Hodgkin lymphomas. This view is now firmly entrenched but has not always been beyond debate, as witnessed by the opposing views revealed in later pages.

IMMUNOPATHOLOGY OF HODGKIN'S DISEASE

Having sketched, somewhat briefly, the background for the plot that follows, it is necessary to turn to the main theme of this paper, namely the immunopathology of Hodgkin's disease. Immunopathology in its broadest sense bears upon Hodgkin's disease chiefly in two respects. These, for convenience, will be considered separately, though they may in truth be partly interdependent. First, abnormalities of effector immune function clearly are present in Hodgkin's disease. They exist in some variety and have been described by many authors using diverse methods of examining immune function. These abnormalities will be recounted briefly. Second, abnormalities of immune function have been implicated as part of the pathogenesis of Hodgkin's disease. These theories are closely interwoven with current ideas concerning the nature and cellular derivation of the malignant cell of Hodgkin's disease, and with theories concerning the very nature of the disease process.

ABNORMALITIES OF IMMUNE FUNCTION IN HODGKIN'S DISEASE—CLINICAL AND LABORATORY ASPECTS

The immunological findings in Hodgkin's disease are complex and controversial. Based upon clinical studies of delayed hypersensitivity responses and upon analyses of B- and T-cell number and function, there is a general consensus of support for the occurrence of some degree of immune paresis of the cell-mediated type. Beyond this there is considerable disagreement.

IMMUNODEFICIENCY AND T-CELL FUNCTION

In Hodgkin's disease clinically evident immunodeficeincy is primarily of cell-mediated type. Immunoglobulin levels are normal or raised in active Hodgkin's disease as evidenced by the studies of Wagener et al. (75), who described increased levels of IgG and IgA in males and females alike, with further elevations of IgM restricted to females. Elevations of IgD and IgE have also been described ((12, 72), respectively), the latter most particularly in nodular sclerosing Hodgkin's disease. Although hypogammaglobulinaemia is rarely observed in Hodgkin's disease, the work of Weitzman and associates (77), demonstrating reduced titres of antibody to *H. influenzae*, suggests that more subtle defects exist and may contribute to the increased susceptibility of Hodgkin's disease patients to certain bacterial infections. Increased vulnerability to specific viral infections, as exemplified by Herpes zoster infection, appears to be related primarily to deficiency of cell-mediated immune function. The observations of reduced in vitro lymphocyte responses to Varicella/zoster antigen would seem to support this contention (59). Interestingly, this last effect was at least partly attributable to therapy, for it was much less obvious in newly diagnosed untreated patients.

Hancock and colleagues (26, 27) studied several different immune parameters in 60 patients with Hodgkin's disease and 42 patients with non-Hodgkin lymphoma. Skin tests (Candida, mumps, Trichophytin, streptokinase and old tuberculin), lymphocyte transformation studies (PHA), leukocyte migration assays (PPD and Candida), neutrophil function test (NBT, neutrophil bacterial killing), serum immunoglobulin determinations, and B- and T-cell analyses were performed. Deficits were detected most commonly in advanced Hodgkin's disease when every patient showed abnormalities of at least one of these tests. To what extent these abnormalities were attributable to treatment was unclear. Using a slightly different approach, Case and colleagues (11) performed skin tests for recall antigens and B- and T-cell assays on long-term (five year +) survivors of Hodgkin's disease. They found no difference in in vivo testing from the control group; the only abnormality detected was that lymphocytes from Hodgkin's disease patients responded less well to PHA in vitro.

Long et al. (41) reported decreased PHA responses and loss of MLC reactions (in vitro) by peripheral blood lymphocytes from 32 patients with untreated Hodgkin's disease. In contrast, Navone and Stramignoni (49) found the in vitro PHA response to be "nearly as high as in controls". Srichaikul et al. (68) were able to demonstrate decreased responses in stage III and stage IV disease only. Again there was the question as to what extent the observed deficiencies were attributable to therapy, or to extensive lymphoid involvement with destruction by advanced disease, or to some primary deficit intrinsic to the Hodgkin process.

The work of DeGast and Halie (14) addressed this question. Following a study of DNCB sensitization and PHA transformation in 61 untreated patients with Hodgkin's disease, the authors found that DNCB sensitization was progressively reduced in all stages from I to IV, but that the PHA response was not reduced in untreated stage I, even when limiting doses were used. Clearly, not all groups share this experience. Furthermore, attempts to correlate observed immune deficits with prognosis have generally proved unrewarding. For example, McCredie and colleagues (46) studied the PHA response and lymphocyte numbers in Hodgkin's disease, and only lymphopoenia at initial presentation showed any correlation with prognosis.

Björkholm and colleagues in the first of a series of papers (9) reported evidence of decreased MLC responses in 10 of 39 patients with Hodgkin's disease Further studies of histopathology, stage, sensitization with PPD, mumps and Candida antigen, together with examination of peripheral blood lymphocytes for mitogen response and surface markers produced one of the most comprehensive studies of "immunodeficiency in Hodgkin's disease and its relation to prognosis" (title of thesis by M. Björkholm, 1978, published in part in *Scandinavian Journal of Haematology*, Supplement 33). Björkholm and colleagues found decreased E-rosette scores and depressed mitogen responses but could not establish any clear correlation between these two parameters. Spontaneous lymphocyte transformation was, however, increased in Hodgkin's disease compared to controls and correlated with aggressive disease and systemic symptoms (30). Defective mitogen responses persisted up to 10 years following treatment (8) and a family study revealed some abnormalities in the healthy twins of Hodgkin's disease patients. After further detailed study of these observations, the authors concluded that the findings strongly suggested the presence of an exogenous factor (probably a virus) causing the depressed responses in relatives.

B- AND T-CELL NUMBERS

Findings differ according to whether studies are performed upon peripheral blood lymphocytes, or upon lymphocytes from involved or noninvolved lymph nodes or spleen.

Peripheral blood lymphocytes

In general the E-rosettes (T) scores have been reported as normal or reduced while SIg (presumptive B-cell) scores have been reported as normal or elevated. In almost all of these studies, results have been expressed as raw percentages without reference to the absolute lymphocyte count which is abnormal in many of these patients. When absolute T- and B-cell are computed, abnormalities are more often found, as exemplified by the report of Bensa et al. (6) that absolute numbers of B cells were increased in 30% of cases, while T-cell absolute numbers were diminished in 65%. Bensa and colleagues interpreted the increase in SIg-bearing cells as representing a true increase in B cells. Others have attributed the presence of increased numbers of SIg-bearing cells to other mechanisms, particularly the presence of an antibody absorbed to circulating T lymphocytes. For example, Grifoni and colleagues (25) described reduced numbers of IgM-bearing cells but a marked increase in IgG-bearing cells, attributable to adsorption of an anti-T-cell cytotoxic antibody of IgG class. Gajl-Peczalska and colleagues (20) also studied the absolute numbers of T and B cells and recorded normal values in 70% of peripheral blood specimens and in 60% of involved lymph nodes.

Just as the increased number of SIg-bearing cells may not truly reflect the B-cell population, so also the depression of E-rosette scores may give a false idea of the number of T cells present. For example, Björkholm and colleagues (8, 9) ascribed the low E-rosette scores observed in Hodgkin's disease to the presence of serum blocking factors, possibly ferritin or lipoprotein molecules, rather than due to an absolute reduction in T cells. This view is shared by Bodbrove and Fuks and coworkers, who were able to show that E-rosette scores were generally less than the "true" T cell scores, as determined by the use of an anti-T-cell serum, and that (19) this reduction of E-rosette score was attributable to the presence of a serum blocking factor. This factor appeared to be removed by overnight incubation of the peripheral blood lymphocytes and was claimed to be specific for Hodgkin's disease in reference to a control population of cancer patients and patients with non-Hodgkin lymphoma. Subsequently, Jaffe and Merryman (35) have partially confirmed these findings, but have pointed out that the same phenomenon of serum inhibition of PHA responses and restoration following incubation procedures has been observed in other diseases. Jaffe and colleagues thus concluded that "it seems premature to suggest this phenomenon as a basis for a diagnostic test (for Hodgkin's disease)." Interestingly, Amlot and Unger (2) had earlier reported the presence of an inhibitory factor in Hodgkin's disease serum of 11 of 54 patients with Hodgkin's disease. Of relevance in this context is the study of Moroz and colleagues (48) who described the presence of absorbed ferritin on the surface of lymphocytes in Hodgkin's disease. They speculated that the effect of levamisole in increasing E-rosette formation in Hodgkin's disease might be attributable to apoferritin release from the lymphocyte surface. This phenomenon was not considered to be unique to Hodgkin's disease.

Tissue lymphocytes

Assays of T- and B-cell numbers in peripheral blood in Hodgkin's disease do not correspond to assays of splenic lymphocytes undertaken in the same patients, whether the spleen is microscopically involved by Hodgkin's disease or free of involvement. For example, Hunter and colleagues (31) found increased numbers of T cells in spleeens with histological involvement by Hodgkin's disease (11 patients compared with six controls). Peripheral blood and noninvolved spleens showed T-cell levels within the normal range. Santoro and associates (60, 61) reported similar observations and speculated that this might be indicative of a local immunologic reaction against the Reed-Sternberg cell. However, the findings of Payne and colleagues (52), in a study of 24 cases of untreated Hodgkin's disease, contrast with the above findings, for these authors found elevated E-rosette scores both in involved nodes and in uninvolved spleen, but normal values in involved spleens. Again the number of SIg-positive lymphocytes present in some cases was found to be increased, and the authors speculated that this might be due to the presence of immunoglobulin-coated T lymphocytes (see above). Bentwich and collaborators (7) having also observed the recovery of rosette formation following overnight incubation in serum-free culture medium, speculated that the blocking factor might be antibody. This view clearly related to the observations of Grifoni, Tognella and colleagues (25, 73, 74) of the presence of a cytotoxic anti-T-cell antibody in Hodgkin's disease patients.

HODGKIN-ASSOCIATED ANTIGEN

Order and colleagues initially described two separate antigens, designated the F and S antigens, in tissue extracts of Hodgkin's disease (see Order (50)). The F antigen, studied by immunofluorescence, was observed to localize in areas of Hodgkin involvement in the spleen. These observations had been confirmed at least in part by Denton (15). Subsequently it became apparent that the Hodgkin's disease F antigen was closely related to ferritin. It has long been recognized that elevated serum ferritin levels may be found in malignant disease including Hodgkin's disease. According to figures cited by Jacobs and associates (34) serum ferritin levels were elevated in 44% of 108 patients with Hodgkin's disease, with a particularly high incidence in late stage nodular sclerosis. Jacobs and colleagues studied an additional 125 untreated patients and found "increasing concentrations of serum ferritin at each advancing stage of the disease, and high concentrations with systemic symptoms". There was no relationship to histologic type, but in view of the observations of Moroz and colleagues cited above, it is possible that these increased ferritin levels might play a part in the abnormalities of T-cell function observed in Hodgkin's disease.

Long and colleagues (41) have described a separate antigen that is apparently specific for Hodgkin's disease, but at present this antigen is detected in tissue culture cells and not in vivo. Carcassone and colleagues (10) detected yet another Hodgkin-related antigen using an immunofluorescence method and an antibody derived from rabbits immunized with Hodgkin tissue. These authors suggested that several separate antigens might occur in relation to Hodgkin's disease and that some of these might be of oncofetal type.

IMMUNOLOGIC PHENOMENA IN HODGKIN'S DISEASE

The cause of the systemic symptoms occurring in Hodgkin's disease has always been a mystery. Amlot and colleagues (1) and Kavai (39) investigated the possibility that circulating immune complexes might account for the production of systemic symptoms. Immune complexes were found in most cases of Hodgkin's disease, but no definite correlation was estbalished with the presence or absence of night sweats or fever. Long and colleagues (42, 43, 44) reported further studies of their tissue culture antigen and described evidence of formation of immune complexes of this antigen with autologous antibody in 29 of 90 patients with Hodgkin's disease. They speculated that these circulating complexes might explain some of the "paraimmune" phenomena reported in Hodgkin's disease, including the nephrotic syndrome.

Finally, a variety of lymphokines or chemotactic factors have been described in Hodgkin's disease, and it has been postulated that the presence of such factors may correlate with some of the histologic and immunologic findings. For example, Golding et al. (23) described the production of leukocyte inhibitor factor in Hodgkin's disease and noted a correlation with the decreased PHA response, possibly accounting for the observed immunodeficiency in Hodgkin's disease.

ABNORMALITIES OF IMMUNE FUNCTION IN THE PATHOGENESIS OF HODGKIN'S DISEASE

The pathogenesis, and by implication nature, of Hodgkin's disease has long been a focus of controversy and a stimulus to research. Hodgkin himself described the process as a "hypertrophy" of the lymphoid tissues, while Wilks in 1865 in rediscovering the disease seemed to favor a truly neoplastic state: "it must take its place in the rank of malignant diseases, or amongst those affections which are characterized by the development of new growths in the system" (78).

Thus the stage was set and the debate commenced. The old maxim that "tuberculosis follows Hodgkin's disease like a shadow" was given credence by the observation of Sternberg (in 1898 (64)) that eight of his 13 cases of Hodgkin's disease clearly had tuberculosis. Dorothy Reed (1902 (56)), though she shares credit for the description of the pathognomonic cell of Hodgkin's disease, disagreed with Sternberg that Hodgkin's disease was a peculiar form of tuberculosis and felt that it was in fact an independent entity, though often associated with tuberculosis. Reed felt that the histologic features were in keeping with an inflamatory process that clearly differed from any of the known sarcomas in histologic pattern and mode of behavior. An intensive, but thus far unsuccessful, search for an infectious etiologic agent followed, and concentrated in turn upon the tubercle bacillus including avian variants, diptheroid bacteria, brucella, various fungi, and finally a range of viruses. These areas of investigation parallel the time course for the discovery of these various organisms and the development of means of identifying them.

With the developing concepts of autoimmune disease in the decade around 1950, a further etiologic mechanism was suggested. In fact, the implication of immune mechanisms in the pathogenesis of Hodgkin's disease was perhaps anticipated by the observations of Rosenthal (58) who discussed the significance of tissue lymphocytes in the prognosis of lympho-granulomatosis (Hodgkin's disease).

Kaplan and Smithers (in 1959 (38)) were the first to propose formally the notion that Hodgkin's disease might represent a situation analogous to graft-versus-host disease, then recently demonstrated in experimental animals. Clinical similarities were apparent at that time. The origin of the "foreign grafted cells" remained a mystery, but one solution was proposed by Green and colleagues (1960 (24)), postulating the passage of maternal cells across to the foetus in utero. Subsequently, with the lack of any experimental basis, the theory of Kaplan and Smithers lay fallow for many years. However, the subsequent observation of the development of lymphoma in mice with chronic graft-versus-host disease (GVH—chronic allogeneic disease) led to a renewal of interest in some variation of this GVH hypothesis. The lymphomas developing in chronic allogeneic disease (5) resemble morphologically the pleomorphic reticulum cell sarcoma or the so-called Hodgkin-like lesion of the mouse. Detailed study of a number of these lymphomas has revealed a wide spectrum of morphological appearances in different strains and within individual mice (67). In some cases the tumors corresponded morphologically to immunoblastic sarcoma in man (otherwise classified as reticulum cell sarcoma or malignant lymphoma histiocytic), while in other cases the pleomorphic irregular mixture of cells comprising

the tumor produced resemblance to Hodgkin's disease, although the exact-
ing morphologic criteria demanded for the diagnosis of Hodgkin's disease
in man were not fulfilled in the murine model (67). A workable variant of this
GVH hypothesis has recently been presented by Gleichmann and colleagues
based on the occurrence of a graft-versus-host-like reaction between normal lymphocytes and antigenically altered lymphocytes that the host re-
gards as foreign cells (21).

ORIGIN AND NATURE OF THE NEOPLASTIC CELL

Central to the problem of the pathogenesis underlying Hodgkin's disease
is the continuing uncertainty of the nature of the neoplastic cells. Currently
the weight of scientific opinion would seem to favor a macrophage/histiocy-
tic derivation for the Reed-Sternberg cell (Table 1). In fact, we are quite
certain of the derivation of the Reed-Sternberg cell; it appears to develop
from the mononuclear variant, dubbed the Hodgkin cell by Moeschlin
(47), through a series of sequential morphologic changes recognized by
Sternberg and illustrated by Favre and Croizat (17), and more recently by
Anagnoustou et al. (3) in theoretical sequence. The multinucleate Reed-
Sternberg cell shows little evidence of proliferation (little DNA synthesis)

Table 1. Origin of the Hodgkin/Reed-Sternberg cell: Some recent studies.

Long et al. (42, 43, 44)	—	(culture studies) favored histiocyte
Stuart et al. (65)	—	(Marker studies) R-S cell negative with anti-monocyte antibody
Schmitt et al. (62)	—	(Marker studies) R-S cell nonmarking
Curran and Jones (13)	—	(Silver staining) R-S cell-dendritic histiocyte
Yam and Li (80)	—	(Cytochemical studies) R-S cell—lymphoid
Glick et al. (22)	—	(EM study) R-S cell—lymphoid
Papadimitriou et al. (51)	—	(Immunoperoxidase study) R-S cell possible related to some form of 'stem' cell
Kadin et al. (36)	—	(Short term culture marker studies) R-S cell—macrophage
Landaas et al. (40)	—	(Immunoperoxidase studies) R-S cell, probably not lymphoid
Poppema et al. (54)	—	(Immunoperoxidase study) R-S cell—not lymphoid
de Sousa et al. (16)	—	(Ecotaxis and ferritin) R-S cell–probably not lymphoid
Taylor (66, 69, 70, 71)*	—	(Immunoperoxidase studies) lymphoid in at least some cases; uncertain in others

*Taylor (69, 70, 71) gives a detailed bibliography of other postulated origins of the Reed-
Sternberg cell.

and may serve only as a convenient marker of the disease process, while the proliferating cell showing active DNA synthesis is the mononuclear cell. It is the origin of this latter cell that is in question.

The tissue culture studies of Kaplan and Gartner (37) and Long et al. (42, 43, 44) favor a histiocytic origin, although the behavioral characteristics of the cell lines derived by these two groups differ quite markedly. Pretlow and associates (79) have also cultured Reed-Sternberg cells sucessfully, but prefer to reserve judgment as to their cellular lineage.

An alternative view, for which I personally feel some sympathy, is that of a lymphocytic origin for the Hodgkin cell, and hence the Reed-Sternberg cell and the Hodgkin's disease process. This view is founded upon an hypothesis that permits a logical explanation of a number of the pathologic findings in Hodgkin's disease. It is supported by evidence that is not sufficiently clearcut to allow a definite conclusion. Mononuclear Hodgkin cells resemble immunoblasts morphologically and ultrastructurally (22). In addition, Reed-Sternberg-like cells can be observed in immunoblastic proliferations and in certain of the non-Hodgkin lymphomas of undoubted lymphocytic origin (68). In many cases, characteristic Reed-Sternberg cells can be shown to contain cytoplasmic immunoglobulin. They also bear some surface immunoglobulin (that may be adsorbed), but otherwise show no surface markers specific for either lymphocytes or monocytes. The cytoplasmic immunoglobulin is monoclonal only in a minority of cases (68) and monoclonality would be expected in any neoplasm derived from B lymphocytes or more precisely B immunoblasts. In most instances the characteristic Reed-Sternberg cells can be shown to react with both anti-κ and anti-λ sera, suggesting the presence of polyclonal immunoglobulin within individual cells, an observation favoring an exogenous origin of the cytoplasmic immunoglobulin by phagocytosis or by passive absorption. The observations of Papadimitriou et al (51) and Poppema and colleagues (54) of other serum proteins (namely α_1-chymotrypsin and α_1-antitrypsin) seem to support the idea of passive absorption as the mechanism. However, in the paper by Papadimitriou and colleagues, the intracellular immunoglobulin was observed to be restricted to a single heavy chain subclass in many cases, a finding that is difficult to explain except by in situ synthesis. Thus the observation of cytoplasmic immunoglobulin adds fuel to the controversy and cannot be taken as proof of a lymphocytic origin because of the confusing multiple staining pattern observed within individual cells in the majority of cases.

As noted above, polyploid cells resembling Reed-Sternberg cells are not uncommonly found in certain of the non-Hodgkin lymphomas, particularly in immunoblastic sarcoma of B-cell type. In a number of these cases it has been possible to show a monoclonal pattern of immunoglobulin in the neoplastic immunoblasts that comprise the majority of the tumor cell population, while the large bizarre cells that resemble Reed-Sternberg cells and clearly form part of the tumor on morphologic grounds show a multiple staining pattern like that seen in Reed-Sternberg cells. Recent studies of Isaacson and Wright (32) using a panel of antisera against lymphocyte markers (immunoglobulin components and J chain) and monocyte/ macrophages (lysozyme, α_1-antitrypsin) also fail to offer conclusive evidence of a lymphocytic origin for these bizarre giant cells.

A LYMPHOCYTIC ORIGIN—IMPLICATIONS (Table 2)

If Hodgkin's disease does ultimately prove to be lymphocytic in origin, this has far-reaching implications for our understanding of the process. The Reed-Sternberg cell and mononuclear Hodgkin cell, if derived from the immunoblast, must conform to the logistics of lymphocyte transformation illustrated in Figure 1 with immunoblasts representing the proliferating phase of the life cycle of the small lymphocyte. Not all of the cells of a neoplastic clone would be expected to be in the same phase of the cell cycle, and not all would have uniform morphologic appearances or behavioral characteristics, in strict analogy to B-cell lymphomas discussed elsewhere ("Interrelations of B Cell Lymphomas" and "Changing Concepts in Lymphoma Classification"—Taylor, this volume). Thus a variable proportion of the apparently normal small lymphocytes seen in Hodgkin's disease might in fact form part of the neoplastic clone, and the rate of proliferation of the clone would be reflected by the proportion of cells in the proliferative phase of the cycle, i.e. resembling immunoblasts or mononuclear Hodgkin cells. The differing prognostic importance of the histologic subtypes (lymphocyte predominant, mixed cellularity and lymphocyte depleted) might be explained in this way in analogy to the non-Hodgkin lymphomas (Figure 2). In an extension of the analogy both Hodgkin's disease and the non-

Table 2. Pathogenesis and nature of Hodgkin's disease.

A lymphocytic origin might explain:

Mixed histologic picture? (Figures 1 and 2)

Nodular (follicular) pattern?

Progression of LP → MC → LD? (Figure 2)

Relation of number of lymphocytes to prognosis? (Figure 2)

Difficulty of separating some HD from non-Hodgkin lymphoma?

Composite lymphoma and transmutations?

Resemblance to known lymphocytic neoplasms, rather than histiocytic?

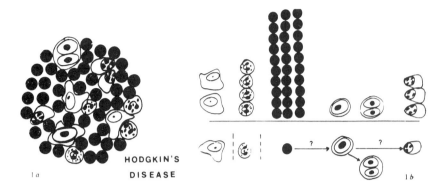

Figure 1. Histology of Hodgkin's disease related to lymphocyte transformation.
(a). Diagramatic representation of histological appearances of Hodgkin's disease. By current concepts only two of these cells (the Hodgkin cell or immunoblast and the Reed-Sternberg cell) are neoplastic; the remainder supposedly being reactive.
(b) Cellular components of Hodgkin's disease from diagram (a), composed according to cytological type, from left to right—histiocytes, eosinophils, small lymphocytes, immunoblast or mononuclear Hodgkin cell, Reed-Sternberg cell and plasma cells. It is postulated that the neoplastic Hodgkin and Reed-Sternberg cells are derived from neoplastic small lymphocytes by a parody of the normal process of lymphocyte transformation, possibly with a metabolic block in the cell cycle leading to polyploid giant cell forms. Thus a proportion of the normal appearing small lymphocytes might form part of the neoplasm, as might also any plasma cells derived from this neoplastic small lymphocyte population. The various proportions of these forms of the neoplastic cell would then determine the histologic subtype of Hodgkin's disease (see text and Figure 2).

Hodgkin lymphomas include variants that are distinguished chiefly by extensive sclerosis.

The not uncommon association of Hodgkin's disease and non-Hodgkin lymphomas (including formation of composite lymphomas) might also be explained along these lines, resurrecting an old belief once given strong support by reputable pathologists (Table 3). Finally, we may ask, if the follicles (nodules) of certain of the non-Hodgkin lymphomas are interpreted as indicative of the B-cell nature of these tumors (follicular lymphomas, follicular center cell lymphomas, centroblastic/centrocytic lymphomas, etc.), why is it that the nodules (follicles?) of certain forms of Hodgkin's disease (LP nodular, nodular sclerosis) are interpreted any differently?

Table 2 summarizes some of the logical deductions that follow the assumption of a lymphocytic origin for Hodgkin's disease. One other hypothesis should perhaps be considered, namely, that not all cases of Hodgkin's disease are alike. Different cases might have a different cellular origin (another old idea). The basic finding that defines a process as being Hodgkin's disease is the occurrence of the "characteristic" binucleate cells (Reed-Sternberg cells) in a mixed cell background. There may in fact be nothing "specific" about these binucleate cells. Henry Harris long ago (see page 630, Florey's *General Pathology*, Loyd-Lukes, 1970) showed that

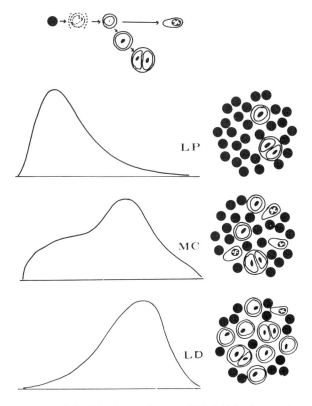

Figure 2. Progression of the Histologic subtypes of Hodgkin's disease: A possible analogy with progression of the non-Hodgkin lymphomas. (See Figure 1 in "Interrelations of B Cell Lymphomas"—Taylor, this volume).

The Reed-Sternberg/Hodgkin cell is depicted as taking origin during the lymphocyte transformation process. The neoplastic clone may consist of lymphocytes in addition to abnormal immunoblasts (Hodgkin cells). The latter represent the proliferating component; the more numerous they are the worse the prognosis. Thus a change in the proportion of lymphocytes to Hodgkin cells may be interpreted as a shift of the predominant cell cycle phase within the neoplastic population, in strict analogy with the proposed scheme interrelating the B-cell lymphomas (see Figure 2 in "Interrelations of B-Cell Lymphomas": interestingly the non-Hodgkin lymphomas could also be classified simply as lymphocyte predominant (LP), mixed cellularity (MC) and lymphocyte depleted (LD), much as in Hodgkin's disease, with similar prognostic implications. Sclerosing varieties of both disease processes also exist in parallel (nodular sclerosis, sclerosing non-Hodgkin lymphomas).

bizarre giant cells develop in culture conditions if one interferes artifically with late S phase or with mitosis. Development of a similar defect in a neoplastic cell population could conceivably produce binucleate or multinucleate cells of similar appearance (Reed-Sternberg cells) though their cellular lineage might be diverse (e.g. lymphoid cells in some, monocytoid cells in others, etc).

It must be stressed that the onus of proof is still upon us. Clearly there is more to Hodgkin's disease than meets even the most critical eye.

Table 3. Interrelations of lymphomas*

Oliver (1913)—"It is the predominate cell type which allows one to classify the tumour as lymphosarcoma, endothelioma [reticulum cell sarcoma] or Hodgkin's disease.... All constitute a series of neoplastic processes of the lymphatic glands, which differ not so much qualitatively as quantitatively."

Pullinger (1931)—"A group of diseaes of the reticulum exists in which proliferation is possible into one or several of the possible cell progeny."

Warthin (1931)—"Hodgkin's disease is a neoplasm and related genetically to the lympho-blastomas, of which both the aleukaemic and leukaemic forms are identical pathologically. Transition forms exist between all of these groups."

Ginsburg (1934)—extensively reviewed the opinions of Banti (1903), Gibbons (1906), Coley (1908), Mueller (1921), and McCartney (1928), in reaching his own conclusions that "they [Hodgkin's disease and lymphosarcoma] are merely variations of the same disease."

Herbut et al. (1945)—"These combinations can only be explained by considering the three diseases [Hodgkin's disease, lymphosarcoma, and reticulum cell sarcoma] as not only closely related, but as having a common neoplastic origin."

Willis (1948)—"I join Warthin, Ginsburg, Herbut et al., and others, who regard all tumours of lymphoid tissue as related variants of one disease.... The names used for the principal variants have descriptive and clinical value but do not denote distinct pathological entities."

Custer and Bernhard (1948)—"They are all mesenchymal tumors which vary only in degree and type of differentiation ... a striking fluidity in histologic pattern with transitions and combinations."

Gall (1962)—"To my distress I found that the patterns differed in the same patient in approximately one third of cases. It is true that the variations were often a matter of degree [i.e. Hodgkin's paragranuloma to Hodgkin's sarcoma, differentiated to undifferentiated lymphosarcoma, follicular to diffuse lymphosarcoma]; in rare instances, however, the lesions of Hodgkin's disease and of lymphocytic lymphoma were both detectable in the same individual."

---

* The originators of these unitarian views were considered by Robb-Smith to follow the "fluid lymphoma school." (52). References in Taylor (70, 71).

REFERENCES

1. Amlot, P.L., Slaney, J.M., and Williams, B.D.: Circulating immune complexes and symptoms in Hodgkin's disease. Lancet, 1:449–451, 1976.
2. Amlot, P.L. and Unger, A.: Binding of phytohaemagglutinin to serum substances and inhibition of lymphocyte transformation in Hodgkin's disease. Clin. Exp. Immunol., 26:520–527, 1976.
3. Anagnostou, D., Parker, J.W., Taylor, C.R., Tindle, B.H., and Lukes, R.J.: Lacunar cells of nodular sclerosing Hodgkin's disease. An ultrastructural and immunohistologic study. Cancer, 39:1032–1043, 1977.
4. Andrewes, F.W.: Discussion on lymphadenoma and its relation to tuberculosis. Trans. Path. Soc. London, 53:305–314, 1902.
5. Armstrong, M.Y.K., Gleichmann, E., Gleichmann, H., Beldotti, L., Andre-Schwartz, J., and Schwartz, R.S.: Chronic allogeneic disease. II. The development of lymphomas. J. Exp. Med., 132:417–439, 1970.

6. Bensa, J.C., Micouin, C., Schaerer, R., Sotto, J.J., and Hollard, D.: Quantitative study of T and B lymphocytes in Hodgkin's disease. Biomedicine 26:137–144, 1977.
7. Bentwich, Z., Cohen, R., and Brautbar, C.: Proceedings: T and B blocking factors in Hodgkin's disease. Isr. J. Med. Sci., 11:1382, 1975.
8. Björkholm, M., Holm, G., Mellstedt, H.: Immunologic profile of patients with cured Hodgkin's disease. Scand. J. Haematol., 18:361–368, 1977.
9. Björkholm, M., Holm, G., Mellstedt, H., and Pettersson, D.: Immunological capacity of lymphocytes from untreated patients with Hodgkin's disease evaluated in mixed lymphocyte culture. Clin. Exp. Immunol., 22:373–377, 1976.
10. Carcassone, Y., Favre, R., and Meyer, G.: Evidence for surface antigents on Hodgkin's disease cells. Cr. Acad. Sci., 280:1505–1507, 1975.
11. Case, D.C., Jr., Hanson, J.A., Corrales, E., Young, C.W., Dupont, B., Pinsky, C.M., and Good, R.A.: Depressed in vitro lymphocyte responses to PHA in patients with Hodgkin disease in continuous long remissions. Blood, 49:771–778, 1977.
12. Corte, G., Ferrarini, M., Tonda, P., and Bargellesi, A.: Increased serum IgD concentrations in patients with Hodgkin's disease. Clin. Exp. Immunol., 28:359–362, 1977.
13. Curran, R.C., and Jones, E.L.: Letter: Dendritic cells and B lymphocytes in Hodgkin's disease. Lancet, 2:349, 1977.
14. De Gast, G.C., and Halie, M.R.: Relation of cell-mediated immunity to staging, histology and prognosis in untreated patients with Hodgkin's disease. Neth. J. Med., 19:196–200, 1976.
15. Denton, P.M.: Immune responsiveness in Hodgkin's disease. Br. J. Cancer 28, suppl., 1:119–127, 1973.
16. de Sousa, M., Yang, M., Lopes-Corrales, E. Tan, C., Hansen, J.A., Dupont, B., and Good, R.A.: Ecotaxis: the principle and its application to the study of Hodgkin's disease. Clin. Exp. Immunol., 27:143–151, 1977.
17. Favre, M., and Croizat, P.: Caracteres generaux du granulome malin, tires de son etude anatomoclinique. Ann. Anat. Pathol., 8:838–900, 1931.
18. Fox, H.: Remarks on microscopical preparations made from some of the original tissue described by Thomas Hodgkin, 1832. Ann. Med. History, 8:370–374, 1926.
19. Fuks, Z., Strober, S., and Kaplan, H.S.: Interaction between serum factors and T lymphocytes in Hodgkin's disease. N. Engl. J. Med., 295:1273–1278, 1976.
20. Gajl-Peczalska, K.J., Bloomfield, C.D., Sosin, H., and Kersey, J.H.: B and T lymphocytes in Hodgkin's disease. Analysis at diagnosis and following therapy. Clin. Exp. Immunol. 23:47–55, 1976.
21. Gleichmann, E., Peters, K., Lattmann, E., and Gleichmann, H.: Immunologic induction of reticulum cell sarcoma: donor-type lymphomas in the graft-versus-host model. Eur. J. Immunol., 5:406–412, 1976.
22. Glick, A.D., Leech, J.H., Flexner, J.M., and Collins, R.D.: Ultrastructural study of Reed-Sternberg cells. Comparison with transformed lymphocytes and histiocytes. Am. J. Pathol. 85:195–208, 1976.
23. Golding, B., Golding, H., Lomnitzer, R., Jacobson, R., Koornhof, H.J., and Rabson, A.R.: Production of leukocyte inhibitory factor (LIF) in Hodgkin's disease. Spontaneous production of an inhibitor of normal lymphocyte transformation. Clin. Immunol. Immunopathol., 7:114–122, 1977.
24. Green, I., Inkelas, M., and Allen, L.B.: Hodgkin's disease: a maternal-to-foetal lymphocyte chimaera? Lancet, 1:30–32, 1960.

25. Grifone, V.: Human lymphoid cell studies and new problems in the treatment of lymphoproliferative diseases. In: Atti dei Convegni Lincei 20, p. 163, Accademia Nazionale dei Lincei, Roma, 1976.

26. Hancock, B.W., Bruce, L., Sugden, P., Ward, A.M., and Richmond, J.: Immune status in untreated patients with lymphoreticular malignancy—a multifactorial study. Clin. Oncol., 3:57–63, 1977a.

27. Hancock, B.W., Sugden, P., and Ward, A.M. Letter: Intensive investigation in management of Hodgkin's disease. Br. Med. J., 1:381, 1977b.

28. Hanson, T.A.S.: Histological classification and survival in Hodgkin's disease. A study of 251 cases with special reference to nodular sclerosing Hodgkin's disease. Cancer, 17:1595–1603, 1964.

29. Hodgkin, T.: On some morbid appearance of the absorbent glands and spleen. Trans. Med. Chir. Soc. London, 17:68–114, 1832.

30. Holm, G., Mellstedt, H., Björkholm, M., Johansson, B., Killander, D., Sundblad, R., and Söderberg, G.: Lymphocyte abnormalities in untreated patients with Hodgkin's disease. Cancer, 37:751–762, 1976.

31. Hunter, C.P., Pinkus, G., Woodward, L., Moloney, W.C., and Churchill, W.H.: Increased T lymphocytes and IgMEA-receptor lymphocytes in Hodgkin's disease spleens. Cell. Immunol., 31:193–198, 1977.

32. Isaacson, P., and Wright, D.H.: Anomalous staining patterns in immunohistologic studies of malignant lymphoma. J. Histochem. Cytochem, in press.

33. Jackson, H., and Parker, F.: Hodgkin's Disease and Allied Disorders. New York: Oxford University Press, Inc., 1947.

34. Jacobs, A., Slater, A., Whittaker, J.A., Canellos, G., and Wernik, P.H.: Serum ferritin concentration in untreated Hodgkin's disease. Br. J. Cancer, 34:162–166, 1976.

35. Jaffe, I.A., and Merryman, P.: Letter: Serum factors and T lymphocytes in Hodgkin's disease: correction. N. Engl. J. Med., 296:630, 1977.

36. Kadin, M.E., Stiles, D.P., Levy, R., and Warnke, R.: Exogenous immunoglobulin and the macrophage origin of Reed-Sternberg cells in Hodgkin's disease. N. Engl. J. Med., 299:1208–1214, 1978.

37. Kaplan, H.S., and Gartner, S.: "Sternberg-Reed" giant cells of Hodgkin's disease: cultivation in vitro, heterotransplantation, and characterization as neoplastic macrophages. Int. J. Cancer, 19:511–525, 1977.

38. Kaplan, H.S., and Smithers, D.W.: Auto-immunity in man and homologous disease in mice in relation to the malignant lymphomas. Lancet, 2:1–4, 1959.

39. Kavai, M., Berenyi, E., Palkovi, E., and Szegedi, G.: Letter: Immune complexes in Hodgkin's disease. Lancet, 1:1249, 1976.

40. Landaas, T.Ø., Godal, T., and Halvorsen, T.B.: Characterization of immunoglobulins in Hodgkin cells. Int. J. Cancer, 20:717–722, 1977.

41. Long, J.C., Aisenberg, A.C., and Samecnik, P.C.: An antigen in Hodgkin's disease tissue cultures: Fluorescent antibody studies. Proc. Natl. Acad. Sci., 71:2285–2289, 1974.

42. Long, J.C., Aisenberg, A.C., and Zamecnik, P.C.: Chromatographic and etectrophoretic analysis of an antigen in Hodgkin's disease tissue cultures. J. Natl. Cancer Inst., 58:223–227, 1977.

43. Long, J.C., Hall, C.L., Brown, C.A., Stamatos, C., Weitzman, S.A., and Carey, K.: Binding of soluble immune complexes in serum of patients with Hodgkin's disease to tissue cultures derived from the tumor. N. Engl. J. Med., 297:295–299, 1977.

44. Long, J.C., Zamecnik, P.C., Aisenberg, A.C., and Atkins, L.: Tissue culture studies in Hodgkin's disease: morphologic, cytogenetic, cell surface, and enzymatic properties of cultures derived from splenic tumors. J. Exp. Med. 145: 1484–1500, 1977.
45. Lukes, R.J., and Butler, J.J.: The pathology and nomenclature of Hodgkin's disease. Cancer Res., 26:1063–1081, 1966.
46. McCredie, J.A., Inch, W., and Sutherland, R.: Effect of splenectomy and radiotherapy on peripheral blood lymphocytes and prognosis in Hodgkin's disease. In: Neoplasm immunity: Mechanisms, pp. 145–147, Crispen, R.G., (ed.), ITR, Chicago, 1976.
47. Moeschlin, S., Schwarz, E., and Wang, H.: Die Hodgkinzellen als Tumorzellen. Schweiz. Med. Wochenschr., 80:1103–1104, 1950.
48. Moroz, C., Lahat, N., Biniaminov, M., and Ramot, B.: Ferritin on the surface of lymphocytes in Hodgkin's disease patients. A possible blocking substance removed by levamisole. Clin. Exp. Immunol., 29:30–35, 1977.
49. Navone, R., and Stramignoni, A.: PHA response of blood and lymph node lymphocytes in vitro in malignant lymphomas. Acta Haematol., 51:76–83, 1974.
50. Order, S.E.: Antigenic analysis of the lymphomata. Br. J. Cancer 31, Suppl., 2:128–139, 1975.
51. Papadimitriou, C.S., Stein, H., and Lennert, K.: The complexity of immuno-histochemical staining pattern of Hodgkin and Sternberg-Reed cells—demonstration of immunoglobulin, albumin, α_1-antichymotrypsin and lysozym. Int. J. Cancer, 21:531–541, 1978.
52. Payne, S.V., Jones, D.B., Haegert, D.G., Smith, J.L., and Wright, D.H.: T and B lymphocytes and Reed-Sternberg cells in Hodgkin's disease lymph nodes and nodes and spleens. Clin. Exp. Immunol., 24:280–286, 1976.
53. Peckham, M.J., and Cooper, E.H.: Proliferation characteristics of the various classes of cells in Hodgkin's disease. Cancer, 34:135–146, 1969.
54. Poppema, S., Elema, J.D., and Halie, M.R.: The significance of intracytoplasmic proteins in Reed-Sternberg cells. Cancer, 42:1793–1803, 1978.
55. Rappaport, H., Winter, W.J., and Hicks, E.B.: Follicular lymphoma: A re-evaluation of its position in the scheme of malignant lymphoma, based on a survey of 253 cases. Cancer, 9:792–821, 1956.
56. Reed, D.M.: On the pathological changes in Hodgkin's disease, with especial reference to its relation to tuberculosis. Johns Hopkins Hosp. Rep., 10:133–196, 1902.
57. Robb-Smith, A.H.T.: The interrelationship of lymphoreticular hyperplasia and neoplasia. In: The Effects of Environment on Cells and Tissues. Proceedings of the IX World Congress of Anatomic and Clinical Pathology. Amsterdam: Excerpta Medica, 1975, pp. 65–171.
58. Rosenthal, S.R.: Significance of tissue lymphocytes in the prognosis of lymphogranulomatosis. Arch. Path., 21:628–646, 1936.
59. Ruckdeschel, J.C., Schimpff, S.C., Smyth, A.C., and Mardiney, M.R., Jr.: Herpes zoster and impaired cell-associated immunity to the varicellazoster virus in patients with Hodgkin's disease. Am. J. Med., 62:77–85, 1977.
60. Santoro, A., Belpomme, D., and Mathé, G.: T and B spleen lymphocytes in Hodgkin's disease. Haematologica, 62:11–12, 1977.
61. Santoro, A., Caillou, B., and Belpomme, D.: T and B lymphocytes and monocytes in the spleen in Hodgkin's disease: the increase in T lymphocytes in involved spleens. Eur. J. Cancer, 13:355–359, 1977.

62. Schmitt, D., Alario, A., Perrot, H., and Thivolet, J.: Letter: Origin of Reed-Sternberg cell. Lancet, 2:137, 1977.
63. Srichaikul, T., Siriasawakul, T., Wibulyachainunt, S., Khantanaphar, S., Matangkasombut, P., Sirisinha, S., and Charupatana, C.: Immunologic studies in malignant lymphoma. Am. J. Clin. Pathol., 62:335–341, 1974.
64. Sternberg, C.: Ueber eine eigenartige unter dem Bilde der Pseudoleukämie verlaufende Tuberkulose des lymphatischen Apparates. Z. f. Heilk. 19:21–90, 1898.
65. Stuart, A.E., Williams, A.R.W., and Habeshaw, J.A.: Rosetting and other reactions of the Reed-Sternberg cell. J. Pathol., 122:81–90, 1977.
66. Taylor, C.R.: The nature of Reed-Sternberg cells and other malignant cells. Lancet, 2:802–807, 1974.
67. Taylor, C.R.: Immunohistological observations upon the development of reticulum cell sarcoma in the mouse. J. Pathol., 118:201–219, 1976.
68. Taylor, C.R.: Immunocytochemical methods in the study of lymphoma and related conditions. J. Histochem. Cytochem., 26:495–512, 1978.
69. Taylor, C.R.: Upon the nature of Hodgkin's disease and the Reed-Sternberg cell. Recent Results Cancer Res., 64:214–231, 1978.
70. Taylor, C.R.: A history of the Reed-Sternberg cell. Biomedicine, 28:196–203, 1978.
71. Taylor, C.R.: Hodgkin's disease and the lymphomas, vol. 3, Annual Research Review 1978, Eden Press, Montreal, Canada, and Churchill Longman Livingstone, Edinburgh/London, 1979.
72. Thomas, M.R., Steinberg, P., Votaw, M.L., and Bayne, N.K.: IgE levels in Hodgkin's disease. Ann. Allergy, 37:416–419, 1976.
73. Tognella, S., Mantovani, G., Del Giacco, G.S., Manconi, P.E., Cengiarotti, L., Floris, C., and Grifoni, V.: Effects of Hodgkin cytotoxic serum on blast transformation of normal and Hodgkin human peripheral blood lymphocytes. Tumori, 61:53–62, 1975a.
74. Tognella, S., Mantovani, G., Cengiarotti, L., DelGiacco, G.S., Manconi, P.E., and Grifoni, V.: Effects of Hodgkin cytotoxic serum on electrophoretic mobility of normal and Hodgkin peripheral blood lymphocytes. Tumori, 61:45–52, 1975b.
75. Wagener, D.J., Van Munster, P.J.J., and Haanen, C.: The immunoglobulins in Hodgkin's disease. Eur.. Cancer, 12:683–688, 1976.
76. Wallhauser, A.: Hodgkin's disease. Arch. Path., 16:522–562; 672–712, 1933.
77. Weitzman, S.A., Aisenberg, A.C., Siber, G.R., and Smith, D.H.: Impaired humoral immunity in treated Hodgkin's disease. N. Engl.. Med., 297:245–248, 1977.
78. Wilks, Sir. S.: Cases of enlargement of the lymphatic glands and spleen (or, Hodgkin's disease), with remarks. Guy's Hosp. Rep. 11:56–67, 1865.
79. Willson, .K.V., Zaremba, .L., Pretlow, T.J.: Functional characterisation of cells separated from suspensions of Hodgkin disease tumor cells in an isokinetic gradient. Blood, 50:783–797, 1977.
80. Yam, L.T., Li, C.Y.: Histogenesis of splenic lesions in Hodgkin's disease. Am. J. Clin. Pathol., 66:976–985, 1976.

32. THE RESULTS OF THE TREATMENT OF HODGKIN'S DISEASE: AN OVERVIEW OF CURRENT APPROACHES AND FUTURE DIRECTIONS*

S.A. ROSENBERG

INTRODUCTION

The results of the treatment of Hodgkin's disease have improved dramatically since 1960. Though long survivals and cures were being reported for some patients prior to that time, it is only in recent years that cure can be achieved for any stage of the disease and for the majority of all patients with Hodgkin's disease. The reasons for this success are many and will be discussed in this review. New problems and challenges are being identified in the management of patients with Hodgkin's disease as attention is being directed toward reducing the morbidity and complications of treatment programs without sacrificing the excellent curative results which are now possible

Overview of survival statistics

It is difficult to provide a generally accepted estimate of the probablity of cure for all patients with Hodgkin's disease. The problem is complicated because different medical centers have different patient populations with different prognoses. This is due in part to geographic variation and socio-economic characteristics, as well as to patient selection and referral patterns.

The situation is further complicated because treatment methods are changing relatively rapidly, usually before the true curative potential of former methods has been demonstrated. Palliative treatment has also improved considerably in the past decade so that even patients who are not cured are experiencing improved survival duration, not infrequently, of ten years or more.

Presently, the overall cure rate for all patients, with all stages of disease, treated initially at experienced major medical centers throughout the world,

* The studies reported herein were carried out in collaboration with Henry S. Kaplan, M.D., and supported, in part, by Grant CA-05838, from the National Cancer Institute, National Institutes of Health, Bethesda, Maryland, and by a gift from the Bristol-Myers Company.

J.G. van den Tweel et al. (eds.), Malignant Lymphoproliferative Diseases, 417–429

is estimated at 50 percent. At several research centers where the most modern methods are being developed, the cure rate is approaching 75 percent.

Survival rates are higher than cure rates at five years after diagnosis, but approach the cure rate at ten years. Late treatment complications which may result in death are occurring at five to ten years. Deaths from unrelated

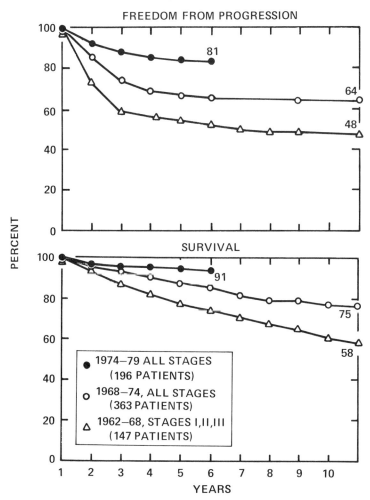

Figure 1. Results of treatment of 706 patients with Hodgkin's disease on protocol studies at Stanford during three periods, 1962–68, 1968–74, and 1974–79.

causes are being recorded more often as patients are being cured of Hodgkin's disease and entering the later decades of life. These factors pose
statistical problems in analyzing long-term results of the treatment of
Hodgkin's disease.

At Stanford University Medical Center, the survival and cure rates have
progressively improved for previously untreated patients entered on treatment protocols since 1962. Figure 1 shows the results of treatment of 706
patients during three periods of 1962–68, 1968–74, and 1974–79. The first
period included patients with clinical Stages I, II, and III disease, prior to the
use of routine laparotomy. The later two periods include patients with all
stages of disease, between 15 and 65 years of age. Deaths from all causes are
included in these survival analyses.

The current role of histopathologic subtype

The Rye modification of the Lukes-Butler system is an accepted useful
classification of Hodgkin's disease (1). There is no doubt that the four main
subtypes have different natural histories and prognoses. However, improved treatment results are reducing the differences in prognoses of the
groups (2).

The Stanford series of protocol patients has relatively few patients with
the lymphocyte predominance (LP) and lymphocyte depletion (LD) subtypes. Between 70 and 75 percent have had the nodular sclerosis (NS) type
and about 20 percent have mixed cellularity (MC). Figure 2 shows the minimal differences which now exist among the four subtypes in freedom from
relapse (FFR) and survival rates. Figure 3 demonstrates that there is no
difference in FFR, or "cure", rates between patients with NS and MC subtypes, though NS patients live somewhat longer once their disease has
relapsed. This is primarily due to survival differences in patients with
pathologic Stages IIIB and IV disease.

Though these recent observations are provocative, it should not be concluded that histologic subtype is of little or no importance. There are relatively few patients in the LP and LD categories. This is partially due to age
selection of this Stanford series and to the type of Hodgkin's disease which
is seen at our Medical Center. It is also due to the comparable success of
combination chemotherapy programs for all histologic subtypes (3).

It must also be emphasized that recent treatment programs are quite
aggressive. In order to achieve the high survival and cure rates, a significant number of patients are being managed with more treatment than necessary. As future treatment programs are devised to attempt to reduce the
morbidity, toxicity, and cost of these difficult regimens, the natural history
insight provided by the histologic subtypes will again become more important.

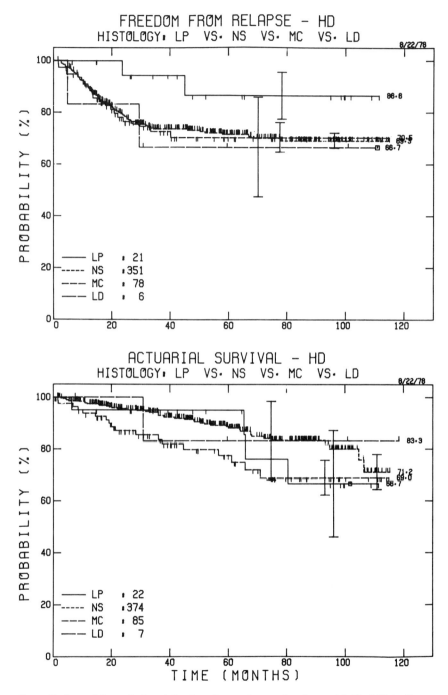

Figure 2. Actuarial survival and freedom from relapse of patients with Hodgkin's disease on protocol studies at Stanford since 1968, according to histologic type.

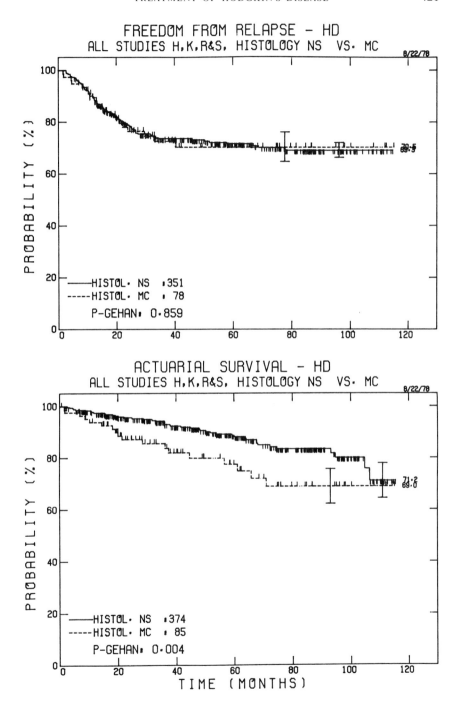

Figure 3. Actuarial survival and freedom from relapse of patients with Hodgkin's disease on protocol studies at Stanford since 1968, with nodular sclerosis and mixed cellularity types.

The current role of the staging classification for Hodgkin's disease

The staging system most widely used for patients with Hodgkin's disease is the Ann Arbor classification proposed in 1971 (4). This has been a useful system, emphasizing the important difference between clinical stage (CS) and pathologic stage (PS), the latter usually indicating that laparotomy and splenectomy have been employed.

As with histologic subtypes, the anatomical stage subgroups are losing their prognostic significance. Figure 4 shows the freedom from relapse, or "cure" rates, and survival rates of the four Ann Arbor stages as treated at Stanford since 1968. There are no important differences between the total groups of PS I and II patients, and even the PS IV group is showing markedly improved results. Symptomatic patients, as a total group, continue to have a poorer prognosis than asymptomatic patients. This is primarily due to the prognostic importance of systemic symptoms in patients with PS III and IV disease, rather than in PS I and II disease, at least in the Stanford series.

It must be emphasized, however, that management programs very much depend on the anatomic stage of the disease, even if the prognostic differences among the four major stages are being reduced.

The challenge to the Ann Arbor system is coming as prognostic groups are being sought to select more or less aggressive treatment programs. Specifically, there is need to identify subgroups which may require combined modality regimens of irradiation and chemotherapy in order to achieve high cure rates. It has been proposed by various groups and studies that patients with limited extranodal disease (5), the E-lesion of the Ann Arbor system; those with large mediastinal masses (6); or those with more widespread abdominal disease in the PS IIIA group (7, 8) are the patients not adequately identified by the Ann Arbor system to receive combined modality therapy.

None of these proposed prognostic subgroups has been confirmed in the Stanford series as requiring combined modality programs (9, 10). However, it may well be that these disease settings identify patients with risks of disease recurrence, if attention to meticulous detail of radiotherapy management is not carried out.

The Ann Arbor classification is helpful because it is widely accepted and easily applied, though there is some difficulty with the definition of the E lesion. However, experienced clinicians realize that patients with Hodgkin's disease present a continuum in terms of extent and severity, from the most favorable to the most serious. Systemic symptoms are sometimes minimal and may be difficult to recognize. In other patients, they are extreme and may be out of proportion to the apparent extent of disease. With each of the Stages II, III, and IV, there are extents and sites of disease which have different prognostic significances.

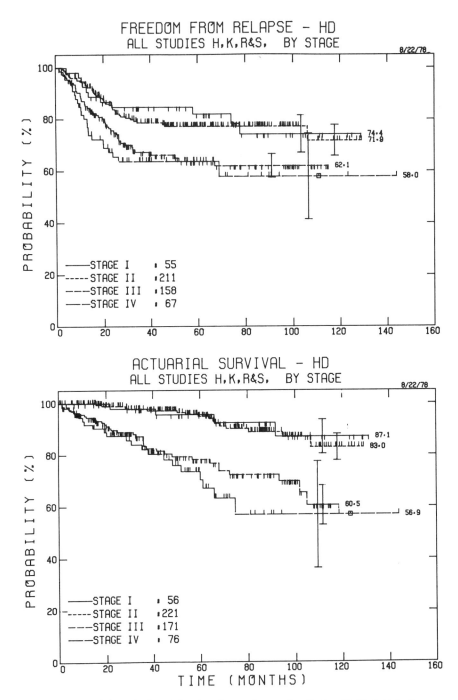

Figure 4. Actuarial survival and freedom from relapse of patients with Hodgkin's disease on protocol studies at Stanford since 1968, according to Ann Arbor Stage.

Current status of diagnostic studies

There has been some question about the routine requirement of the two major diagnostic methods which have contributed so significantly to the better understanding and management of patients with Hodgkin's disease. These are bipedal lymphography and diagnostic laparotomy with splenectomy.

The lymphogram is extremely important for evaluation of the iliac and retroperitoneal lymph nodes. Laparotomy is most important for identification of Hodgkin's disease of the spleen; to a lesser extent to identify involvement of lymph nodes outside of those seen well on lymphography; and, in occasional patients, to demonstrate Hodgkin's disease of the liver. The two procedures complement each other. One does not replace the other.

The lymphogram should be performed prior to laparotomy, if it is planned, so that the surgeon can be directed to the most suspicious, or abnormal, lymph nodes for biopsy. The lymphogram has the important added value for continued and long-term surveillance of the opacified lymph nodes, to determine the return to normal from abnormal after irradiation or chemotherapy. It also should be used to recognize extension or recurrence of of Hodgkin's disease after initial treatment programs. There is no satisfactory substitute for the bipedal lymphogram in the management of a patient with Hodgkin's disease.

The current role of exploratory laparotomy and splenectomy is more controversial. The surgical procedure carries with it a small but definite acute morbidity and a small risk of complications or death from late overwhelming bacterial sepsis. There seems to be little doubt that the benefits of the surgical procedure have outweighed the risks during the past decade.

However, as certain disease settings are being recognized in which the information gained from laparotomy would not change therapy programs, the more acceptable it is to avoid the surgical procedure for selected patients. The critical question, which is different in various major treatment centers is—"will the information gained from laparatomy change the treatment program?" If the answer is "no", then the procedure has only very limited benefit. At Stanford, the answer is still "yes". Patients with PS IIB disease are treated differently from those with PS IIIB and patients with PS I and IIA are treated differently from those with PS IIIA. Those with PS IIIA or B are treated differently from those with PS IVA or B. Therefore, diagnostic laparotomy and splenectomy are still performed routinely for Hodgkin's disease at Stanford unless Stage IV disease has been identified.

Radiotherapy of Hodgkin's disease

It must be emphasized that irradiation techniques continue to evolve and improve, resulting in higher cure rates and less morbidity.

Complications of radiation pneumonitis are only rarely serious, and symptomatic radiation carditis has virtually been eliminated by the proper use of subcarinal and apical cardiac blocks. Radiation myelitis should not occur as a complication of the treatment of Hodgkin's disease.

Radiotheraptists have developed techniques for treating the entire lung or hemithorax with low doses. The entire liver and upper abdomen can also be treated safely, and treatment results have probably improved because of these techniques.

The experienced radiotherapist prepares shaped fields for the individual patient, utilizes treatment simulators, and concentrates on treating areas often responsible for marginal recurrences. Gradually shrinking fields are utilized for large mediastinal or retroperitoneal nodal masses to minimize radiation morbidity.

As a result, radiation therapy remains the treatment of choice for patients with PS IA and IIA, PS IB and IIB, and PS IIIA Hodgkin's disease. Between 60 and 90 percent of patients with these stages of disease can be cured without the addition of chemotherapy in the primary treatment program (11). If the patient fails to be cured by irradiation alone, combination chemotherapy will result in subsequent cure after relapse in approximately half of the patients. This carries an overall curative potential of between 80 and 95 percent for all patients in these stages, including those with the E lesion.

Patients with PS IIIB or IV disease, however, are not adequately treated with irradiation alone and require combination chemotherapy from the onset (11).

Chemotherapy of Hodgkin's disease

The results of MOPP chemotherapy (nitrogen mustard, vincristine, procarbazine, and prednisone) of Hodgkin's disease have revolutionized the management of the disease. Numerous series have demonstrated the value of the combination chemotherapy (12). If properly utilized, approximately 80 percent of patients can achieve a complete remission of their disease with MOPP, and 40 percent can be cured of the disease with chemotherapy alone. In some series and certain disease settings, the chemotherapy results are even superior to these figures. DeVita's ten year experience reports a 52 percent overall cure rate, including 100 percent of a small group of 22 asymptomatic patients (3). Patients with bone marrow involvement appear to have the poorest prognosis for cure with MOPP chemotherapy (13).

The current questions in the chemotherapy management of Hodgkin's disease are:

1) Can combinations with less acute toxicity and less morbidity be shown to be as successful as MOPP?

2) Can the MOPP program be used for shorter periods of time, either in the therapeutic or adjuvant setting without compromising the results?

3) Which drug combination regimens are most successful in treating patients who have progressed during, or relapsed after, MOPP chemotherapy?

4) Can drug combination regimens be developed which are superior to the MOPP regimen, especially for the poorest prognostic subgroups?

This review will not attempt to discuss these questions since most of them cannot be answered due to lack of proper studies, though initial efforts are being made.

It must be emphasized, however, that the most serious long-term complications of MOPP chemotherapy are sterility in men (14, 15), and risks of late acute myelogenous leukemia (16); the latter is especially frequent and serious in patients receiving both irradiation and MOPP.

Combined modality therapy

In the past decade, the trend of investigators has been to test treatment programs which combine radiation therapy and combination chemotherapy for most stages of Hodgkin's disease. These studies, when properly carried out, have shown almost uniformly that the initial disease control results are improved. However, survival benefits have not been proved, or have been of borderline significance (11, 17). Evaluation of these treatment methods and trials have been complicated because of the long periods of time required to demonstrate survival benefits and because of improved ability of physicians to prolong survival and cure patients who have recurred after initial treatment.

Of very great concern has been the observation that hematologic malignancies are occurring in as many as 5 percent of patients who have received combined modality therapy. Acute myelogenous leukemia has been observed in many series and appears to be a much greater risk in patients who have received both forms of therapy. The risk increases with time, and it is not known what the peak risk will be, since the rate appears to still be rising at ten years after initial treatment (16). The acute leukemia is a type especially resistant to management, since it appears in a setting of hypoplasia or aplasia of the bone marrow, and complete remission inductions have been very difficult to achieve.

This same group of patients also appears to be at risk to develop a non-Hodgkin's lymphoma of poor prognosis (18). Histologically, it is an undifferentiated, or histiocytic, type in the Rappaport classification and is distinctly different from Hodgkin's disease. This malignancy also appears quite long after initial treatment, with the incidence rate still rising at ten years after therapy.

With these reservations in mind, the Stanford studies of combined modality therapy have been summarized in several recent reports (11, 19). Adjuvant MOPP, after total nodal irradiation, appears to have its greatest impact upon survival for patients with PS IIIA disease, and for the total group of asymptomatic patients. Adjuvant MOPP can adequately replace extended field radiation therapy to clinically uninvolved sites in an effort to control occult disease. A regimen of less acute toxicity, PAVe (procarbazine, alkeran, and vinblastine) is as effective an adjuvant as the MOP (P) program (prednisone withheld if mediastinal irradiation is used). Alternating chemotherapy and radiotherapy programs are resulting in imporved results for patients with PS IIIB disease (20).

Utilizing radiation therapy has not imporved results for patients with PS IV disease who have also been treated with MOPP (11). The group at Yale has reported good results by combining low dose irradiation with chemotherapy for patients with PS IV disease, but, unfortunately, the study was not a controlled trial and is difficult to evaluate (21).

Summary and future directions

The results of therapy for patients with Hodgkin's disease have dramtically improved. The factors responsible for this improvement are many, including improved histopathologic criteria and classifications, an accepted anatomic staging classification, improved diagnostic methods, advances in radiotherapy equipment and techniques, and greatly improved chemotherapy programs. A major reason for the improvement has been the collaboration of investigators in different disciplines, especially when new treatment methods have been subjected to carefully controlled clinical trials.

Despite these advances, however, many challenges remain. Patients are still dying of Hodgkin's disease either because the cure rate is not 100 percent for any disease setting or because improper treatment was utilized initially. The morbidity of the management programs is still excessive. Investigators must develop and properly evaluate treatment programs which can be safely utilized by more physicians and treatment centers, with reduced acute toxicity and reduced late treatment complications. The costs of treatment programs must be measured and compared in terms of life disruption, emotional stress, and physical damage. All must be minimized as much as possible, without compromising the excellent treatment results and cures which are now possible.

REFERENCES

1. Lukes, R.J.: Criteria for involvement of lymph node, bone marrow, spleen, and liver in Hodgkin's disease. Cancer Res., 31:1755–1967, 1971.
2. Torti, F.M., Dorfman, R.F., Rosenberg, S.A., et al.: The changing significance of histology in Hodgkin's disease. Proc. Am. Assoc. Cancer Res. – Am. Soc. Clin. Oncol., 20: (C545), 1979.
3. DeVita, V., Canellos, G., and Hubbard, S., et al.: Chemotherapy of Hodgkin's disease (HD) with MOPP: a 10 yr. progress report. Proc. Am. Assoc. Cancer Res. – Am. Soc. Clin. Oncol., 17:269 (C-131), 1976.
4. Carbone, P.P., Kaplan, H.S., and Musshoff, K., et al.: Report of the committee of Hodgkin's staging classification. Cancer Res., 31:1860–1861, 1971.
5. Levi, J.A., and Wiernik, P.H.: Limited extranodal Hodgkin's disease: unfavorable prognosis and therapeutic implications. Am. J. Med., 63:365–372, 1977.
6. Mauch, R., Goodman, R., and Hellman, S.: The significance of mediastinal involvement in early stage Hodgkin's disease. Cancer, 42:1039–1045, 1978.
7. Desser, R.K., Golomb, H.M., and Ultamann, J.E., et al.: Prognostic classification of Hodgkin's disease in pathologic stage III, based on anatomical considerations. Blood, 49:883–893, 1977.
8. Stein, R.S., Hilborn, R.M., and Flexner, et al.: Anatomic substages of stage III Hodgkin's disease: implications for staging, therapy, and experimental design. Cancer, 42:429–436, 1978.
9. Torti, F.M., Portlock, C.S., and Rosenberg, S.A., et al: Extranodal (E) lesions in Hodgkin's disease: prognosis and response to therapy. Proc. Am. Assoc. Cancer Res. – Am. Soc. Clin. Oncol., 19:367 (C-241), 1978.
10. Hoppe, R.T., Cox, R.S., and Rosenberg S.A., et al.: Prognostic factors in pathological stage IIIA Hodgkin's disease. Proc. Am. Assoc. Cancer Res. – Am. Soc. Clin. Oncol., 20: (C-576), 1979.
11. Rosenberg, S.A., Kaplan, H.S., and Glatstein, E.J., et al.: Combined modality therapy of Hodgkin's disease: a report on the Stanford Trials. Cancer, 42:991–1000, 1978.
12. DeVita, V.T. Jr., Lewis, B.J., and Rozencweig, M., et al.: The chemotherapy of Hodgkin's disease: past experiences and future directions. Cancer, 42:979–990, 1978.
13. Portlock, C.S., Robertson, A.C., and Turbow, M.M., et al.: MOPP chemotherapy for advanced Hodgkin's disease: prognostic factors in 242 patients. Clin. Res., 24:158A, 1976.
14. Sherins, R.J., and DeVita, V.T., Jr.: Effect of drug treatment for lymphoma on male reproductive capacity: studies of men in remission after therapy. Ann. Intern. Med., 79:216–220, 1973.
15. Chapman, R.M., Sutcliffe, S.B., and Rees, L.H., et al.: Cyclical combination chemotherapy and gonadal function: retrospective study in males. Lancet, 1:285–289, 1979.
16. Coleman, C.N., Williams, C.J., and Flint, A., et al.: Hematologic neoplasia in patients treated for Hodgkin's disease. N. Engl. J. Med., 297:1249–1252, 1977.
17. O'Connell, M.J., Wiernik, P.H., and Brace, K.C., et al.: A combined modality approach to the treatment of Hodgkin's disease: preliminary results of a prospectively randomized clinical trial. Cancer, 35:1055–1065, 1975.
18. Krikorian, J.G., Burke, J.S., and Rosenberg, S.A., et al.: Occurrence of non-

Hodgkin's lymphoma after therapy for Hodgkin's disease. N. Engl. J. Med., 300:452–458, 1979.

19. Rosenberg, S.A., and Kaplan, H.S.: The management of stages I, II, and III Hodgkin's disease with combined radiotherapy and chemotherapy. Cancer, 35:55–63, 1975.

20. Hoppe, R.T., Portlock, C.S., and Glatstein, E., et al.: Alternating chemotherapy and irradiation in the treatment of advanced Hodgkin's disease. Cancer, 43: 472–481, 1979.

21. Prosnitz, L.R., and Montalvo, R.L.: The therapy of Hodgkin's disease – 1978; a combined modality approach. Prog. Clin. Cancer, 7:97–112, 1978.

SECTION V
SPECIAL TOPICS

33. EPITHELIOID CELLULAR LYMPHOGRANULOMATOSIS (LYMPHOEPITHELIOID CELL LYMPHOMA): HISTOLOGIC AND CLINICAL OBSERVATIONS*

H. NOEL, D. HELBRON,* AND K. LENNERT

INTRODUCTION

In 1952, one of us (K.L.) (10) reported three cases of malignant lympho-granulomatosis (Hodgkin's disease) with a special morphology. Sternberg-Reed cells were very scarce in these cases, and the normal structure of the lymph node was replaced by small, locally or diffusely distributed clusters of epithelioid cells (Figure 1). The epithelioid-cell clusters were a constant finding in subsequent lymph-node biopsies and at autopsy. In 1968, Lennert and Mestdagh (14) published 30 cases characterized by massive infiltration by such groups of epithelioid cells, and distinguished this lesion from Hodgkin's disease with a high content of epithelioid cells and easily de-monstrable Sternberg-Reed cells. The latter group of cases did not show any important morphologic or clinical differences from classic Hodgkin's disease. In contrast, the former lesion, which was called epithelioid cellular lymphogranulomatosis (ECLg), appeared to be a special type of neoplasia. It occurred predominantly in the middle-aged and the elderly, showed no predilection for either sex, and displayed some notable clinical features, e.g. relatively frequent involvement of the tonsils, hepatosplenomegaly, and, occasionally, allergic reactions. The average survival time did not differ significantly from that of patients with Hodgkin's disease with mixed cel-lularity. However, typical Sternberg-Reed cells, were demonstrable in only a minority of the cases.

The latter finding, together with the observation of two cases showing transformation into "lymphosarcoma" instead of so-called Hodgkin's sarcoma and the occurrence of numerous epithelioid cell clusters in some cases of immunoglobulin-producing non-Hodgkin's lymphoma (13, 25) led Lennert later (13) to express some doubts as to whether all these lesions actually represented a variant of Hodgkin's disease. He therefore proposed the more neutral term lymphoepithelioid cell lymphoma (15). At about the same time, Dorfman (5, 6) and Lukes and Tindle (18) emphasized the dif-

*Supported by the Kind-Philipp-Stiftung.

J.G. van den Tweel et al. (eds.), Malignant Lymphoproliferative Diseases, 433–445.
All rights reserved.
Copyright © 1980 by Martinus Nijhoff Publishers bv, The Hague/Boston/London.

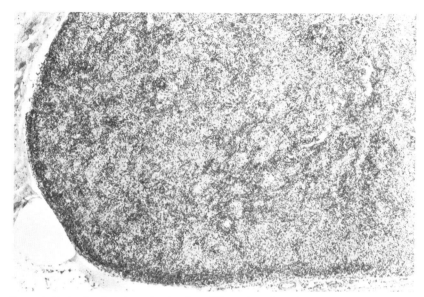

Figure 1. Part of a lymph node showing diffuse alteration of the normal structure, with numerous clusters of epithelioid cells. Hematoxylin and eosin. × 39.6

ficulties frequently encountered in the differential diagnosis between "immunoblastic lymphadenopathy" and what they called "Lennert's lymphoma", which they considered to be a separate entity. The latter became a subject of debate (24, 30). In 1976, Burke and Butler (2) described 15 cases, but could not determine the exact status of "Lennert's lymphoma" in relation to other malignant lymphomas or immunoblastic proliferations. Kim et al. (8) later regarded "Lennerts's lymphoma" as a variant of a non-Hodgkin's lymphoma and said that it resembled malignant lymphoma of the diffuse, mixed cell type. There have also been reports on isolated cases, some with evidence of an abundance of T lymphocytes (3, 4, 9, 19, 21, 26, 28).

In a recent study (20), we attempted to determine whether this disorder merits recognition as a separate clinicopathologic entity and, if so, to establish its position in the scheme of lymphoid neoplasia.

MATERIAL AND METHODS

A total of 136 cases were registered as "ECLg" in our department during the period between 1952 and 1976. Lymph-node biopsies from 114 of these cases were available for our study. The histologic picture was that of a mostly diffuse lymphoma with a polymorphic cytological picture and a large number of epithelioid cells occurring in disseminated clusters. There was no fibrosis or necrosis, and there were only occasionally multinucleate forms (Langhans giant cells). Epithelioid cells are large cells with pale, oval or round nuclei and a large amount of mainly eosinophilic cytoplasm. In the cases studied these cells did not show any definite signs of malignancy, but their nuclei were sometimes much larger than those of epithelioid cells present in reactive processes (e.g., sarcoidosis). The 114 cases with these features were diagnosed as ECLg, because they showed no evidence indicating any other classic type of lymphoma at the time of diagnosis.

The sections were stained with hematoxylin and eosin, Giemsa, periodic acid Schiff (PAS), and silver impregnation of reticulin (Gomori staining). Clinical data were obtained from questionnaires filled out at the time of biopsy or retrospectively from clinical reports kindly sent to us by the patients' physicians. Dates of death were established from public records up to 1 December 1976 and used to calculate survival rates by the life-table method.

RESULTS

Morphologic findings

On initial re-examination of the biopsy material it was already possible to distinguish two main groups of cases of ECLg. In the first group, the lymph-node architecture was usually completely effaced and pleomorphic lymphocytes predominated (Figure 2). This group included the biopsy specimens showing characteristic Sternberg-Reed cells. In the second group we found numerous plasma cells and plasma-cell precursors, but no Sternberg-Reed cells. The lymph-node architecture was indistinct, but not completely effaced. Several cases in this group exhibited some or all of the typical features of immunoblastic lymphadenopathy as defined by Lukes and Tindle (18). Besides these two main groups, there were some cases in which the diagnosis had to be changed and others in which it remained unclear (Table 1).

Hodgkin type

The first main group comprised 23 cases in which we found classic Sternberg-Reed cells, although there were extremely few. It was necessary to search for them with great care, and exhaustive search often revealed such cells in only one of the four sections examined per case. In three cases Sternberg-Reed cells were not seen in the first biopsy specimen but occured in the second or third. In eight cases we did not find Sternberg-Reed cells until autopsy. At autopsy, two cases showed uniform-appearing sarco-

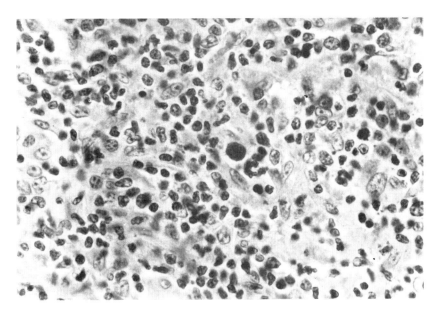

Figure 2. The same lymph node as in Figure 1. at a slightly higher magnification. Note the pleomorphic lymphocytes (T lymphocytes?) and one pyknotic Sternberg-Reed cell. Hematoxylin and eosin. × 396.

Table 1. Diagnosis after revision of 114 cases of "epithelioid cellular lymphogranulomatosis" (ECLG).

Diagnosis	n	%	Transition *Into sarcoma* (n)
Hodgkin type of ECLg (with Sternberg-Reed cells)	51	44.5	2
LgX type of ECLg (no Sternberg-Reed cells)	37	32.5	4
with parotid involvement	5		
Revised diagnosis	13	11.5	—
Hodgkin's disease with lymphocytic pre-dominance, nodular	1		
Hodgkin's disease with partial involve-ment	2		
Lymphoplasmacytoid immunocytoma	3		
Immunoblastic lymphoma	7		
Unclassifiable	13	11.5	
Total	114	100.	6

mas that had developed instead of lymphocytes and epithelioid cells. The sarcomas were composed of small, irregularly shaped "blast cells" and were thus distinguishable from the morphologic picture previously defined as Hodgkin's sarcoma. There were, however, still a few Sternberg-Reed cells.

The 11 cases in which the first biopsy specimen did not reveal any Sternberg-Reed cells, led us to re-examine the sections lacking such cells once again, now for other features that would permit assignment to the first main group. In sections with Gomori staining we found that the lymph-node structure was completely effaced in all areas showing ECLg infiltration. Cytologically, two types of cells appeared to be of diagnostic significance, viz.: large mononuclear basophilic cells and relatively small giant cells with multilobulated nuclei. The large mononuclear basophilic cells corresponded partially to the Hodgkin cells previously identified by Giemsa staining (11). Their cytoplasm was moderately abundant and grayish-blue. They had one large nucleus with a weakly stained nuclear membrane, weakly stained chromatin, and very large grayish-blue nucleoli. Besides these cells, there were similar but more basophilic cells with less abundant, deep-blue cytoplasm and deep-blue nucleoli and nuclear membrane. The mononuclear cells were definitely capable of mitosis, as indicated by the presence of large, sometimes typical mitotic figures. The cells with multilobated nuclei showed all the morphologic characteristics of Sternberg-Reed cells, but were smaller than typical Sternberg-Reed cells. It was often necessary to apply oil immersion in order to detect them (Figure 3). We consider that these small cells with multilobated nuclei may be interpreted as a type of Sternberg-Reed cell. The presence of such cells allowed us to classify a second subgroup of 28 cases as Hodgkin's disease and to assign them to the same group as the 23 definite cases of Hodgkin's disease described above, which otherwise showed the same morphology.

In this first main group the highly predominant lymphocytes were markedly pleomorphic. They had irregularly shaped nuclei with coarse chromatin and were relatively large (Figures 2 and 3). These cells were interspersed with medium-sized and large basophilic blast cells. A few plasma cells were also present. In addition, many cases showed a small or intermediate number of eosinophilic granulocytes, but only an occasional neutrophilic granulocyte. Occasionally, we found small foci of necrosis and small circumscribed areas of fibrosis. This first group was called the Hodgkin type of ECLg.

LgX type

The second main group comprised 37 cases. Instead of a predominance of lymphocytes, these cases showed numerous plasma cells and plasma-cell precursors, including immunoblasts. In contrast to the first group, there were neither Sternberg-Reed cells nor Hodgkin cells. Eosinophilic gran-

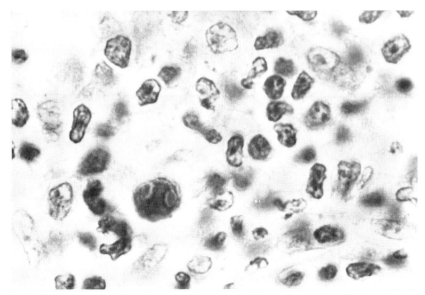

Figure 3. The same lymph node as in Figures 1 and 2 at a higher magnification, showing pleomorphic lymphocytes (T lymphocytes?) and one Sternberg-Reed cell of the small type with huge, inclusion-body-like nucleoli buried in folds of the nuclear membrane. Hematoxylin and eosin. × 9.900.

ulocytes were sometimes interspersed among the tumor cells. The most conspicuous feature was an increase in PAS-positive epithelioid venules, which were seen in all lymph-node regions, including the expanded capsule. Gomori staining often revelaed a relatively intact lymph-node structure. The capsule and connective tissue septa were usually well defined and often showed marked expansion and infiltration by lymphocytes, plasma cells, histiocytes, and epithelioid cells. The sinuses were sometimes intact, but sometimes no longer recognizable. The follicles and their germinal centers either had disappeared or showed regressive transformation and at times contained protein deposits. It is clear from these findings that the lesion is very similar to immunoblastic lymphadenopathy as defined by Lukes and Tindle (18) or angioimmunoblastic lymphadenopathy (7), which has been called lymphogranulomatosis X(LgX) by our research group (23). Therefore, we called this second main group the LgX type of ECLg.

The material of three cases in the second main group showed a more tumorlike appearance. The plasma cells and plasma-cell precursors formed relatively monotonous infiltrates. There were fewer epithelioid venules; instead, vessels with thin walls and flat endothelial cells predominated. In two of these cases, LgX had been diagnosed on the basis of previous biopsy findings. In four other cases, a true immunoblastic lymphoma developed out of LgX with the polymorphic picture described above. At autopsy, one other case showed the picture of lymphoplasmacytic immuno-cytoma.

The LgX type of ECLg also included a special variant that was associated with lymphoepithelial sialadenitis of the parotid gland, as seen in Sjögren's syndrome. The lymph-node lesions, however, differed somewhat histologi-cally from those in cases without involvement of the parotid gland, the former showing follicles with active germinal centers and fewer epithelioid venules.

The differences in the morphology of the lymph-node biopsies between the Hodgkin type and the LgX type are summarized in Table 2.

Revision of the diagnosis

In a third group comprising 13 cases, the diagnosis ECLg was found to be incorrect, and another type of malignant neoplasia was diagnosed after re-examination (Table 1). In one case the revised diagnosis was nodular para-granuloma (Hodgkin's disease with lymphocytic predominance, nodular type). Hodgkin's disease with partial lymph-node involvement was found in two cases. It is well known that groups of epithelioid cells are often

Table 2. Morphologic criteria for the diagnosis of epithelioid cellular lymphogranulomatosis in lymph-node biopsies.

	Hodgkin type	*LgX type*
Absolute		
Sternberg-Reed cells	+	—
Variants of Sternberg- Reed cells	+ ("dwarfs", "giant immunoblasts")	— Immunoblasts
Relative		
histology:		
Capsule	Fibrous or thinned, occasionally infiltrated and destroyed	Often infiltrated, with venules
Trabeculae	Usually absent	Often expanded by inflammation
Venules	Occasionally increased in number	Markedly or slightly in- creased in number
Fibrosis	Usually patchy, irregular	Often diffuse increase in reticulin fibers or around venules
cytology:		
Lymphocytes	Predominant	Moderate number
Plasma cells	Occasionally increased in number	Always increased in number, often markedly; frequently contains PAS$^+$ inclusions
Immunoblasts/ plasmablasts	Usually only a few	Often numerous
Eosinophils	+/−	+/−

demonstrable in both nodular paragranuloma and the early stages of Hodgkin's disease (12). Lymphoplasmacytoid immunocytoma was the revised diagnosis in three cases and immunoblastic lymphoma in seven cases. These two types of non-Hodgkin's lymphoma are not infrequently associated with a focal epithelioid cell reaction (13). Demonstration of monoclonality by the immunoperoxidase technique helped us to distinguish these cases from ECLg.

Unclassifiable cases

The last group contained 13 cases in which it was not possible to classify the lymph node lesions definitely according to the criteria applied for the first two groups. These cases will have to be investigated more thoroughly to determine their exact nature.

CLINICAL OBSERVATIONS

Age and sex distribution

Both types of ECLg occurred chiefly in late adult life, and rarely before the age of 40 years. The patients with the Hodgkin type ranged in age from 22 to 82 years, with a median of 60 years, and those with the LgXtype from 31 to 83 years, with a median of 59.5 years. The mean age of the patients with parotid involvement was 54 years (range– 41–70 years).

The Hodgkin type showed a slight predilection for women. In contrast, the LgX type without involvement of the parotid gland showed a distinct preference for men (1.9:1). Four of the five patients with involvement of the parotid gland were women.

Clinical presentation

In the Hodgkin group, localized (chiefly cervical) lymphadenopathy was nearly as common as generalized lymphadenopathy. The patients presented only occasionally with hepatomegaly, splenomegaly, or both. In the LgX group generalized lymphadenopathy had usually developed before diagnosis, sometimes within a period of only a few weeks. Hepatosplenomegaly was found in more than a third of the patients with the LgX type. About half of all patients with ECLg manifested fever. Pruritus was remarkably common among the patients with the LgX type. At the time of diagnosis, exanthema with itching was found only in patients with the LgX type (Table 3).

The LgX type with involvement of the parotid gland began with a tumor of the salivary gland that gradually increased in size. The contralateral salivary gland or regional lymph nodes became involved months or years later. Two of the female patients in this subgroup showed symptoms belonging to Sjögren's syndrome.

Table 3. Frequency of various signs and symptoms presented by patients with epithelioid cellular lymphogranulomatosis at the time of histological diagnosis.

	Hodgkin type (%)	LgX type (%)
Lymphadenopathy	100	100
generalized	56	77
localized	44	23
cervical	70	43
Involvement of tonsils	25	33
Hepatosplenomegaly	18	39
Fever	50	54
Pruritus	22	50
Exanthema	0	36

Laboratory findings

There were no significant differences between the blood pictures of the two main groups. Lymphocytopenia was frequent, whereas leukocytosis, eosinophilia, and monocytosis were only occasionally reported. The tuberculin test was usually negative in patients in both groups. Half of the patients with the LgX type showed a markedly elevated ESR (more than 50 mm in the first hour), whereas only a few patients with the Hodgkin type showed this elevation. Thirteen out of 22 patients with the LgX type had γ-globulin values higher than 1.7 g%, whereas most of the patients with the Hodgkin type had normal γ-globulin values.

Course and survival

In the Hodgkin group full remission could be obtained with radiotherapy (in stages Ia and IIa) or with combined chemotherapy (in Stages III and IV). Monochemotherapy proved to be inadequate or ineffective.

In the LgX group the period of remission obtained with cortisone was almost as long as that with monochemotherapy. Combined chemotherapy and cycles of radiation and cytostatic drugs led to complete remission, but death could not be prevented. The average period of remission was not longer than that obtained with cortisone or monochemotherapy alone.

There was no significant difference between the Hodgkin and LgX types with respect to the life expectancy after biopsy (Figure 4). The median survival time was 10.5 months for both groups. The five patients with involvement of the parotid gland, however, survived for years. Two of them died—one of an unrelated cause after 2 years, and the other, who had had Sjögren's syndrome for 3 years, after manifestation of generalized lymphoma 22 months after biopsy.

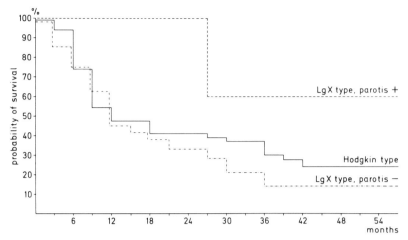

Figure 4. Actuarial survival of patients with the Hodgkin type (n = 47) and the lympho-granulomatosis X(lgX) type of epithelioid cellular lymphogranulomatosis with (+; n = 5) and without (−; n = 29) involvement of the parotid gland.

DISCUSSION

This retrospective study in 114 cases of epithelioid cellular lymphogranulo-matosis showed the presence of Sternberg-Reed cells in 51 cases (44.5%) although they were very scarce and difficult to find. We are therefore in-clined to consider such cases to represent a special variant of Hodgkin's disease. However, since the specificity of Sternberg-Reed cells for Hodgkin's disease is still a matter of discussion (27, 29), it is not possible to draw a final conclusion from this finding alone. We agree with several other in-vestigators, who have pointed to the importance of the pleomorphism of the lymphocytes predominating in the ECLg lesions (2, 5, 8). It is helpful to distinguish these cells from the cells with a mature appearance seen in "Hodgkin's disease with lymphocytic predominance, lymphocytic-histiocy-tic type, diffuse" (17). We attempted to demonstrate immunoglobulin in lymphocytes of ECLg and found that they were negative. They also dif-fered morphologically from centrocytes and other types of cells known to belong to the B-lymphocyte series. On the other hand, we have not been able to obtain fresh material to confirm the observations made by others (3, 9, 21, 28) in isolated cases where T-cell receptors were demonstrated. Some of these authors speculated that ECLg might be a T-cell lymphoma, although others (see e.g. (22)) have shown that T lymphocytes may constitute a majori-ty of the cells in some Hodgkin lesions.

If ECLg does indeed belong to the spectrum of Hodgkin's disease, it must be regarded as a special form whose main characteristic is a predilection for elderly individuals. This feature alone might account for the more advanced stage at presentation, the occasionally atypical manifestations, and the poorer prognosis of the disease in our series. These are common findings in Hodgkin's disease in elderly (16). A particularly high frequence of ECLg among patients with Hodgkin's disease involving Waldeyer's ring has also been reported by others (31).

The second main group comprising 37 cases (32.5%) of ECLg, fulfilled our criteria for lymphogranulomatosis X. The exact nature of LgX is still unclear. It includes the immunoblastic lymphadenopathy defined by Lukes and Tindle (18) and the angioimmunoblastic lymphadenopathy described by Frizzera et al. (7). In the present study we also made the surprising obser-vation that two cases of lymphoproliferative disease associated with Sjögren's syndrome (1) fell into the LgX type of ECLg, wheras three others showed the "lymphoepithelial lesions" with no manifestations of Sjögren's syndrome.

Although there are evident differences in the clinical presentation and apparently in the response to therapy between the two main groups of cases of ECLg, the prognosis is uniformly poor. This fact and the occurrence of some unclear cases in which we were unable to make a definite classification, increase the need for further investigation.

SUMMARY

Re-examination of sections from a series of 114 cases diagnosed as epithelioid cellular lymphogranulomatosis (ECLg) showed that 20% of the tumors represented Hodgkin's disease, since they contained characteristic Sternberg-Reed cells, although in very small numbers. A second group (24.5%) showed basically similar histologic and cytologic pictures but the tunor contained Sternberg-Reed cells of a small type only and also large basophilic mononuclear cells, some of which could be interpreted as Hodgkin cells. These cases too were interpreted as Hodgkin's disease. Thus, a total of 44.5% of the cases of ECLg were re-classified as the Hodgkin type. In all these cases there was a predominance of pleomorphic lymphocytes (T lymphocytes?). Such cases might represent a special type of Hodgkin's disease that occurs chiefly in elderly people. It is difficult to recognize the neoplasia as Hodgkin's disease, because sometimes Sternberg-Reed cells are not found in the first biopsy specimen, and when present there were invariably very few.

Besides the cases classified as Hodgkin's disease, there was a second main group related to so-called lymphogranulomatosis X (which partially corresponds to immunoblastic lym-phadenopathy). This group accounted for 32.5% of the cases of ECLg. Predominance of pleomorphic lymphocytes was not found in this group, which showed typical lymphocytes and numerous cells of the plasma-cell series. There were no Sternberg-Reed cells of any type. These cases showed certain special clinical features, but not enough to constitute a separate entity. In contrast to the first main group, the usual treatment for Hodgkin's disease did not lead to long-term remission.

In the third group of cases, the diagnosis had to be changed to Hodgkin's disease of another type, immunocytoma, or immunoblastic lymphoma. The fourth group comprised cases that were unclassifiable by the methods used in this study.

REFERENCES

1. Anderson, L.G., and Talal, N.: The spectrum of benign to malignant lympho-proliferation in Sjögren's syndrome. Clin. exp. Immunol., 9:199–221, 1971.
2. Burke, J.S., and Butler, J.J.: Malignant lymphoma with a high content of epithelioid histiocytes (Lennert's lymphoma). Amer. J. clin. Path., 66:1–9, 1976.
3. Delsol, G., Fabre, J., Familiades, J., and Ohayon, E.: Lennert's lymphoma (Letter to the Editor). Amer. J. clin. Path., 69:646, 1978.
4. Diebold, J., Reynes, M., Ricot, G., James, J.M., Zittoun, R., and Bilski Pas-quier, G.: Lymphome malin lympho-épithélioide (lymphome de Lennert). Nouv. Presse méd., 6:2145–2151, 1977.
5. Dorfman, R.F.:Letter to the Editor. Hum. Pathol. 6:264, 1975.
6. Dorfman, R.F., and Warnke, R.: Lymphadenopathy simulating the malignant lymphomas. Hum. Pathol., 5:519–550, 1974.
7. Frizzera, G., Moran, E.M., and Rappaport, H.: Angio-immunoblastic lym-phadenopathy with dysproteinemia. Lancet, I:1070–1073, 1974.
8. Kim, H., Jacobs, C., Warnke, R., and Dorfman, R.F.: Malignant lymphoma with a high content of epithelioid histiocytes: A distinct clinicopathologic entity and a form of so-called "Lennert's lymphoma". Cancer, 41:620–635, 1978.
9. Klein, M.A., Jaffe, R., and Neiman, R.S.: "Lennert's lymphoma" with trans-formation to malignant lymphoma, histiocytic type (immunoblastic sarcoma). Amer. J. clin. Path., 68:601–605, 1977.
10. Lennert, K.: Zur histologischen Diagnose der Lymphogranulomatose. Habil.-Schrift., Frankfurt A.M., 1952.
11. Lennert, K.: Histologische Studien zur Lymphogranulomatose. I. Die Cytologie der Lymphogranulomzellen. Frankfurt. Z. Path., 64:209–234, 1953a.
12. Lennert, K.: Studien zur Histologie der Lymphogranulomatose. II. Die diag-nostische Bedeutung der einzelnen Zellelemente. Frankfurt. Z. Path., 64:343–356, 1953b.
13. Lennert, K.: Pathologisch-histologische Klassifizierung der malignen Lym-phome. In: Leukamien und maligne Lymphome, pp. 181–194. Stacher, A., (cd.), Urban and Schwarzenberg, München-Berlin-Wien, 1973.
14. Lennert, K., and Mestdagh, J.: Lymphogranulomatose mit konstant hohem Epitheloidzellgehalt. Virchows Arch. A, 344:1–20, 1968.
15. Lennert, K., Mohri, N., Stein, H., and Kaiserling, E.: The histopathology of malignant lymphoma. Brit. J. Haemat., 31(Suppl.):193–203, 1975.
16. Lokich, J.J., Pinkus, G.S., and Moloney, W.C.: Hodgkin's disease in the elderly. Oncology, 29:484–500, 1974.
17. Lukes, R.J., and Butler, J.J.: The pathology and nomenclature of Hodgkin's disease. Cancer Res., 26:1063–1081, 1966.
18. Lukes, R.J., and Tindle, B.H.:"Immunoblastic lymphadenopathy" a hyperim-mune entity resembling Hodgkin's desease. New Engl. J. Med., 292:1–8, 1975.
19. MacGillivray, J.B., and Macintosh, W.G.: A case of Lennert's lymphoma. J. clin. Path., 31:560–566, 1978.
20. Noel, H., Helbron, D., and Lennert, K.: Die epitheloidzellige Lymphogranu-lomatose (sogenanntes "Lennert's lymphoma"). In: Lymphknotentumoren, pp. 40–45. Stacher, A., and Höcker, P., (eds.) Urban and Schwarzenberg, Mün-chen-Wien-Baltimore, 1979.
21. Palutke, M., Varadachari, C., Weise, R.W., Husain, M., and Tabaczka, P.:

Lennert's lymphoma, a T-cell neoplasm (Letter to the Editor). Amer. J. clin. Path., 69:643–646, 1978.

22. Payne, S.V., Jones, D.B., Haegert, D.G., Smith, J.L., and Wright, D.H.: T and B lymphocytes and Reed-Sternberg cells in Hodgkin's disease lymph nodes and spleens. Clin. exp. Immunol., 24:280, 1976.

23. Radaszkiewics, T., and Lennert, K.: Lymphogranulomatosis X. Klinisches Bild, Therapie and Prognose. Dtsch. med. Wschr., 100:1157–1163, 1975.

24. Robb-Smith, A.H.T.: Lennert Lymphoma (Letter to the Editor). Lancet, II:970, 1976.

25. Scheurlen, P.G., and Hellriegel, K.P.: "Epitheloidzellige Lymphogranulomatose" mit Gammopathie und Chromosomenaberratione Klin. Wschr., 49:597–604, 1971.

26. Staples, W.G., and Getaz, E.P.: "Lympho-epithelioid cellular lymphoma" (Lennert's lymphoma). A case report. S.Afr. med. J., 51:555–556, 1977.

27. Strum, S.B., Park, J.K., and Rappaport, H.: Observation of cells resembling Sternberg-Reed cells in conditions other than Hodgkin's disease. Cancer, 26:176–190, 1970.

28. Tindle, B.H., and Long, J.C.: Case Records of the Massachusetts General Hospital, Case 30. New Engl. J. Med., 297:206–211, 1977.

29. Tindle, B.H., Parker, J.W., and Lukes, R.J.: "Reed-Sternberg cells" in infectious mononucleosis? Amer. J. clin. Path., 58:607–617, 1972.

30. The Lennert Lymphoma. Editorial, Lancet II, p. 507, 1976.

31. Todd, G.B., and Michaels, L.: Hodgkin's disease involving Waldeyer's lymphoid ring. Cancer, 34:1769–1778.

34. THE PATHOLOGY OF CHILDHOOD LYMPHOMAS

H. KIM

INTRODUCTION

Malignant lymphomas and leukemias represent the most common malignancy in the pediatric age group with the reported annual incidence of 2300 new cases for leukemia and 700 new cases for malignant lymphomas (55). Of the latter, Hodgkin's disease accounts for 300 new cases and non-Hodgkin's lymphoma for the remainder (55). The prognostic significance and therapeutic implications of certain features in acute leukemia is well recognized. The features that have shown correlation with prognosis include: (a) lymphoblastic versus myeloblastic nature, (b) age at diagnosis, (c) race, (d) sex, (e) initial white blood cell count, (f) central nervous system involvement, (g) mass lesions, especially of the mediastinum, and (h) surface marker characteristics (9). These multiple prognostic indicators have been elaborated by many studies and there is little controversy or disagreement as to their prognostic relevance and therapeutic implications. There has also been a remarkable improvement in the prolongation of life expectancy in children with acute leukemias. On the other hand, there have been difficulties in assessing the value of treatment in children with non-Hodgkin's lymphoma. One major source of confusion has been the lack of satisfactory classification. Rappaport's classification (40), based on growth pattern and cytology of proliferating cells, has been applied successfully to numerous clinicopathologic studies throughout the world, especially in adult patients with non-Hodgkin's lymphomas (18). Unfortunately, this scheme did not show such a good correlation in the childhood lymphomas. This is, in part, due to the well-known fact that in childhood (a) nodular lymphomas are very rare (52) and (b) well-differentiated lymphocytic lymphomas and poorly-differentiated lymphocytic (small cleaved, follicular center cell type of Lukes and Collins (28) and centroblastic/centrocytic of the Kiel classification (25)) never or rarely occur (13, 31). In addition, malignant lymphoma, lymphoblastic (3, 35) now an established clinicopathologic entity, has been erroneously included among other diffuse non-Hodgkin's lymphomas (15). Based on these observations, Dorfman proposed a classification scheme for childhood lymphomas (13) (Table 1). Difficulties, however, still exist in distinguishing, on morphologic grounds, these dif-

J.G. van den Tweel et al. (eds.). Malignant Lymphoproliferative Diseases, 447–457

Table 1. Childhood lymphomas (13).

Lymphoblastic
  convoluted
  nonconvoluted
Large lymphoid
Histiocytic
Burkitt's lymphoma
Undifferentiated

ferent types of childhood non-Hodgkin's lymphomas. In this presentation, clinicopathologic and immunologic aspects of childhood non-Hodgkin's lymphomas will be briefly reviewed based on our own experience as well as those of others.

Classification

With the advance in knowledge of our immune system, varied terminology and classification has been proposed for non-Hodgkin's lymphomas (13, 25, 28). Of these, the classifications proposed by Lukes and Collins (28) and the Kiel classification (25) modified from Lennert are conceptually different from the traditional Rappaport classification (40). While there are many studies on childhood non-Hodgkin's lymphomas (6, 23, 24, 32, 33, 53, 54) there are no detailed clinicopathologic studies utilizing these newly proposed classifications. In spite of this, however, there is a good general concensus as to the nature and origin of malignant lymphoma, lymphoblastic (3, 35), and Burkitt's tumor (1, 2, 27, 56, 57). On the other hand, lack of knowledge prevails as to the nature of (a) so-called undifferentiated, non-Burkitt's type, (b) true histiocytic lymphoma, and, to a lesser extent, (c) large lymphoid tumors which morphologically correspond to large noncleaved follicular center cell lymphoma and B-immunoblastic sarcoma of Lukes and Collins (28). As to the surface characteristics of these lymphoma cells, the childhood non-Hodgkin's lymphomas can be subdivided into B cell, T cell, histiocytic, and "null" cell types (8, 9, 38, 39, 51) Table 2 shows generally accepted criteria for each of these categories.

Malignant lymphoma, lymphoblastic

Malignant lymphoma, lymphoblastic (35) is a distinct clinicopathologic entity. Its clinical and hematologic features include: (a) high male/female ratio (3, 9, 11, 17, 25, 35, 39, 41), (b) high incidence in children, adolescence, and young adults (3, 9, 11, 17, 25, 35, 39, 41, 49), (c) absence of cytopenia at clinical onset (35), (d) usual absence of splenomegaly (35), (e) frequent presentation with mediastinal mass (3, 9, 11, 17, 25, 35, 39, 49), (f) early

Table 2. Childhood non-Hodgkin's lymphoma functional classification.

B-cell lymphoma:
  Surface immunoglobin
T-cell lymphoma:
  Rosettes with unsensitized sheep erythrocytes
"Null" cell lymphoma:
  No monoclonal surface immunoglobulin, or sheep erythrocyte receptors
Histiocytic lymphoma:
  Phagocytosis, rosettes with erythrocytes—IgG antibody complexes, cytoplasmic esterase,
    no surface immunoglobulin

involvement of bone marrow and peripheral blood during the course of the disease (3, 9, 11, 17, 25, 35, 41, 49), and (g) frequent involvement of central nervous system and gonads (17, 35). Histologically, the lymphoblastic lymphoma has a distinctive appearance. The tumor is characterized by a diffuse proliferation of immature lymphoid cells which are indistinguishable from lymphoblasts of acute lymphoblastic leukemia and show a high mitotic index. Typically, they are distributed in the paracortical area of the lymph nodes with occasional sparing of lymphoid follicles. Nucleoli are often not clearly visible and, if present, they are usually single (Table 3). The tumor cells vary in size from 10 to 16 μm but the majority of the tumor cells measure about 12 to 14 μm (35). The cytoplasm is scanty and often not discernible in routine H & E sections. Immunologic studies have shown that the majority of lymphoblastic lymphoma are T-lymphocytic in origin (9, 14, 20, 21, 45) and a minority of "null" cell type. Tumor cells contain terminal deoxynucleotidyl transferase (TdT) enzyme (12, 22) which is normally found in thymocytes and their bone marrow precursors but not in mature peripheral T-lymphocytes (30). High TdT activity may be found in blastic transformation of chronic granulocytic leukemia (30, 43, 44, 47), in acute myeloblastic leukemia (46), and in human bone marrow lymphocytes (4, 10). A positive reaction for acid phosphatase has also been found to be quite characteristic for this lymphoma (25, 48). In our experience, 82% developed a full-blown leukemic picture during the course of the disease and 43% of them developed central nervous system and gonadal involvement (35). For this reason, it has been proposed that this lymphoma should be treated from its inception with chemotherapy according to protocols used in the treatment of acute lymphoblastic leukemias (35, 39, 49). Subsequent to our study of lymphoblastic lymphoma, it has been reported that not all of the malignant lymphomas with convoluted nuclei have T-cell markers (5, 17, 22) and that T-cell markers were demonstrable in some of the lymphoblastic lymphomas without convoluted nuclei (17, 22). This confirms our opinion that nuclear convolutions are not an absolute morphologic criteria for the identification of the neoplastic cells of lymphoblastic lymphoma as T-cells. The nuclear convolution does not appear to be an important morphologic

Table 3. Differential diagnosis.

	Lymphoblastic	Burkitt's Tumor	Undifferentiated, Non-Burkitt's
Starry sky	Rarely present	Always present	Variable
Nucleus	Variable	Uniform	Pleomorphic
Nucleolus	Single and indistinct when present	Multiple, distinct	Multiple, distinct
Cytoplasm	Usually imperceptible	Amphophilic to basophilic, moderate amount	Amphophilic to basophilic, variable
Pyroninophilia	Variable	Strong	Usually strong
Cytoplasmic Fat	Absent	Present	Variable

marker in ALL as well (37). Malignant lymphoma, lymphoblastic has also been reported in adults (42).

Burkitt's lymphoma corresponding to malignant lymphoma, lymphoblastic

Burkitt's lymphoma is another distinct clinicopathologic entity (1, 2, 27, 56, 57). Histologically, it is characterized by a diffuse proliferation of neoplastic lymphoid cells of uniform size and shape. It is considered to be a B-cell lymphoma of probable follicular center cell origin (29). Morphologically, no difference is noted between the African cases and the nonendemic form. Its rapid growth is reflected in histologic sections by many mitoses, and starry-sky pattern. Typically, the cytoplasm contains fat demonstrable by oily red 0 stain. This cytoplasmic fat and markedly dilated mitochondria explain the cytoplasmic vacuoles noted in the imprint preparations. Intense pyroninophilia is due to the large amount of polysomes in the cytoplasm. Kinetic studies in vivo and in vitro have identified Burkitt's lymphoma as the fastest growing neoplasm in man (57). Rapid interference with the vital structures and metabolism may result from this rapid cell proliferation and turnover. It also accounts, in part, for the sensitivity of Burkitt's lymphoma to alkylating and cell cycle specific agents (57). Cytogenetic studies of both African and North American Burkitt's lymphoma have shown translocation from 8q to 14q, not related directly to Epstein-Barr virus (19). Neoplastic cells also contain the Epstein-Barr virus genome in up to 97% of patients studied. This association has not been so strongly demonstrated in nonendemic cases of Burkitt's lymphoma although genome-positive cases have been identified. Clinically, there seem to be differences between endemic form and nonendemic

Burkitt's tumor (56, 57). In endemic areas it affects children with mean age of 7 years. Males are affected slightly more often than females. Characteristic sites of involvement include jaw in 50% of all patients, ovaries in 80% of females always bilaterally, and testis in 4–10% of males. Only one-third of testicular involvement is bilateral. Liver, spleen, mediastinum, and peripheral lymph nodes are usually spared. Involvement of abdominal viscera such as kidney is common as well as invasion of meninges and central nervous system. Massive bilateral involvement of the breasts is a dramatic manifestation of Burkitt's tumor in young women during pregnancy and lactation. In nonendemic cases the mean age is 11 years with male to female ratio of 2:1. In contrast to African cases, gastrointestinal tract is the most common site of involvement. The bone marrow and peripheral lymph nodes are involved more often than in endemic form (26).

Undifferentiated, non-Burkitt's type

Unlike malignant lymphoma, undifferentiated, Burkitt's type, there is considerable variation in size and shape of both cytoplasm and nuclei. Nucleoli are multiple and distinct as in Burkitt's tumor, but they are more often large and single and eosinophilic (Table 3).

The immunologic surface marker characteristics, clinical manifestations, and the natural history of this type of lymphoma are not well defined at this time.

"Histiocytic" lymphoma (Rappaport)

It is now well recognized that so-called "histiocytic" lymphoma of Rappaport (40) is immunologically and morphologically heterogeneous. According to the Lukes and Collins classification (28), this may be large cleaved, large noncleaved, B-immunoblastic, T-immunoblastic, or true histiocytic. According to the Kiel classification (25), it would be either centroblastic or immunoblastic. In our experience with mostly adult patients with non-Hodgkin's lymphomas, the majority of "histiocytic" lymphoma proved to be large noncleaved follicular center cell lymphoma. Table 4 shows distribution of 69 childhood non-Hodgkin's lymphomas treated at St. Jude Children's Research Hospital according to both Rappaport and Lukes and Collins classifications. Of the 69, 16 cases were classified as either B-immunoblastic or large noncleaved. Their combined incidence is almost the same as that of Burkitt's tumor. This is, however, not reflected in Lukes' own series of childhood lymphomas and leukemias shown in Table 5. According to this series of 84, 65 represented acute lymphoblastic leukemia of childhood, 13 convoluted lymphocytic lymphoma which is similar, if not identical, to malignant lymphoma,

Table 4. Childhood non-Hodgkin's lymphoma (St. Jude Children's Research Hospital) (34).

Rappaport		*Lukes and Collins*	
Lymphoblastic.		Lymphocytic,	
convoluted	20	convoluted	22
nonconvoluted	4	B-Immunoblastic	8
Undifferentiated	27	Large noncleaved	8
Histiocytic	11	Small noncleaved	19
Unclassifiable	7	Undefined	4
	—	Histiocytic (? True)	1
		Unclassifiable	7
Totals	69		69

lymphoblastic and 6 small transformed follicular center cell lymphoma which is an equivalent to Burkitt's tumor. It is not clear why, in this series, there are no cases of B-immunoblastic or large noncleaved follicular center cell lymphoma. In Dorfman's classification for childhood lymphomas (13), both B-immunoblastic and large noncleaved follicular center cell lymphomas would be classified as large lymphoid type. Regardless of the terminology, we do not know enough about this category of lymphoma in children and should be subject for a prospective study.

True histiocytic lymphoma

Only a small portion of lymphomas are proven to be true histiocytic in nature by immunologic and functional studies (28, 36). While equally rare, malignant histiocytosis is considered to be a true histiocytic malignancy (16). It is generally, however, not considered in the discussion of malignant lymphomas because of the usually systemic nature of the disease from its clinical onset (7, 50). This rapidly progressive systemic disease is character-

Table 5. Lukes and Collins (28a) childhood lymphomas and leukemias.

	No. of cases studied
U cell (undefined)	65*
(Includes 14 cases with < 20% rosettes)	
T cell	
Convoluted lymphocyte	13
B cell	
Small transformed (noncleaved) FCC diffuse	6
Total	84

Table 6. Childhood lymphomas and leukemias.

	T (14 Patients)	B (9 Patients)	Null (56 Patients)
Surface markers	T rosettes (100%) HTLA (100%) complement receptors often	Monoclonal IgM (100%)	HTLA positive in some cases; E, SmIg; complement negative
Age and sex	3–20 years Males (60%)	6–20 years Males and females	Peak incidence earlier than other groups (6 years)
Masses	Mediastinal (50%)	Abdominal (90%)	Seldom (2%)
Bone marrow involvement	Frequent (72%)	Often	Almost always (98%)
Morphology	Different from SmIg positive; similar to T positive	Characteristic "Burkitt" cell	Different from SmIg positive; similar to T rosette positive
Terminology	Lymphoblastic convoluted lymphocytic	Burkitt's tumor, nonendemic	Acute lymphoblastic leukemia

Modified from Kersey et al. in: Immunological diagnosis of leukemias and lymphomas, Vol. 20., p. 28, Thierfelder, G., Rodt, H., and Thiel, E. (eds), Springer-Verlag, Berlin, Heidelberg, New York, 1976.

ized by abrupt onset, fever, progressive pancytopenia, hepatosplenomegaly, and mild lymphadenopathy with or without jaundice. It is usually rapidly fatal with a median survival of 6 months (50). Characteristic lymph node biopsy shows distortion of the normal architecture but at least partial maintenance of a sinusoidal pattern. Neoplastic histiocytes show striking predilection for sinuses with gradual infiltration to the adjacent paracortical areas of lymph node. Cytologically, the neoplastic histiocytes are different from the cells of the other malignant lymphomas. They are much larger, and they have more pleomorphic nuclei with more abundant cytoplasm which is usually eosinophilic in character. One can demonstrate non-specific esterase in the cytoplasm and imprint preparation will usually demonstrate the phagocytic activity of these neoplastic cells. It would not be surprising to see the neoplastic cells in true histiocytic malignancy to preferentially proliferate in sites physiologically occupied by normal histiocytes such as the subcapsular and medullary sinuses of lymph nodes and the sinusoids of the spleen and liver. Malignant histiocytosis may indeed turn out to be a true histiocytic lymphoma.

SUMMARY

Childhood lymphomas can be morphologically divided into lymphoblastic lymphoma, Burkitt's tumor, undifferentiated lymphoma, non-Burkitt's type, true histiocytic lymphoma, and large lymphoid or "histiocytic" lymphoma (large noncleaved and B-immunoblastic of Lukes and Collins). Surface marker characteristics, age and sex distribution, and other pertinent features are summarized in Table 6 for lymphoblastic lymphoma, Burkitt's tumor, and ALL. We know little, at this time, about true histiocytic lymphoma apart from malignant histiocytosis, large noncleaved follicular center cell lymphoma or B-immunoblastic lymphoma in children. A prospective clinicopathologic as well as immunologic studies are required to identify the nature of these categories in children. The same is true for undifferentiated lymphoma, non-Burkitt's type in the Rappaport classification.

REFERENCES

1. Arseneau, J.C., Canellos, G.P., Banks, P.M., Berard, C.W., Gralnick, H.R., and DeVita, V.T.: American Burkitt's lymphoma: A clinicopathologic study of 30 cases. I. Clinical factors relating to prolonged survival. Am. J. Med., 58:314–321, 1975.
2. Banks, P.M., Arseneau, J.C., Gralnick, H.R., Canellos, G.P., DeVita, V.T., and Berard, C.W.: American Burkitt's lymphoma: A clinicopathologic study of 30 cases. II. Pathologic correlations. Am. J. Med., 58:322–329, 1975.
3. Barcos, M.P., and Lukes, R.J.: Malignant lymphoma of convoluted lymphocytes: A new entity of possible T-cell type. In: Conflicts in childhood cancer. An evaluation of current management, vol. 4, pp. 147–178, Sinks, L.F., and Godden, J.O., (eds.), Alan R. Liss, New York, 1975.
4. Barr, R.D., Sarin, P.S. and Perry, S.M.: Terminal transferase in human bone marrow lymphocytes. Lancet, 1:508, 1976.
5. Bloomfield, C.D., Frizzera, G., Gajl-Peczalska, K.J., Brunning, R.D., and Kersey, J.: Malignant lymphoma, lymphoblastic (MLLB) in the adult (abstract) Proc. Am. Soc. Clin. Oncol., 19:378, 1978.
6. Brecher, M.L., Sinks, L.F., Thomas, R.R.M., and Freeman, A.I.: Non-Hodgkin's lymphoma in children. Cancer, 41:1997–2001, 1978.
7. Byrne, G.E., Rappaport, H.: Malignant histiocytosis. In: Malignant diseases of the hematopoietic system. Gann monograph on cancer research no. 15, pp. 145–162, Akazaki, (ed.), Tokyo University Press, 1973.
8. Coccia, P.F.: Characterization of the blast cell in childhood non-Hodgkin's lymphoproliferative malignancies. Semin. Oncol., 4:287–296, 1977.
9. Coccia, P.F., Kersey, J.H., Gajl-Peczalska, K.J., Krivit, W., and Nesbit, M.E.: Prognostic significance of surface marker analysis in childhood non-Hodgkin's lymphoproliferative malignances. Am. J. Hematol., 1:405–417, 1976.
10. Coleman, M.S., Hutton, J.J., DeSimone, P., and Bollum, F.: Terminal deoxyribonucleotidyl transferase in human leukemia. Proc. Natl. Acad. Sci. USA, 71:4404, 1974.
11. Cooke, J.V.: Mediastinal tumor in acute leukemia. A clinical and roentgenoligic study. Am. J. Dis. Child., 44:1153–1177, 1932.
12. Donlon, J.A., Jaffe, E.S., and Braylan, R.C.: Terminal deoxynucleotidyl transferase activity in malignant lymphomas. N. Engl. J. Med., 297:461–464, 1977.
13. Dorfman, R.F.: Pathology of the non-Hodgkin's lymphomas: New classifications. Cancer Treat. Rep., 61:945–951, 1977.
14. Gajl-Pcezalska, K.J., Bloomfield, C.D., Coccia, P.F., Sosin, H., Brunning, R.D., and Kersey, J.H.: B and T cell lymphomas. Analysis of blood and lymph nodes in 87 patients. Am. J. Med., 59:657–685, 1975.
15. Glatstein, E., Kim, H. Donaldson, S.S., Dorfman, R.F., Gribble, T.J., Wilbur,

J.R., Rosenburg, S.A. and Kaplan, H.S.: Non-Hodgkin's lymphomas. VI. Results of treatment in childhood. Cancer, 34:204–211, 1974.

16. Jaffe, E.S., Shevach, E.M., Sussman, E.H., Frank, M., Green I., Berard, C.W.: Membrane receptor sites for the identification of lymphoreticular cells in benign and malignant conditions. Brit. J. Cancer 31 (suppl. 2): 107–120, 1975.

17. Jaffe, E.S., Braylan, R.C., Frank, M.M., Green, I., and Berard, C.W.: Heterogeneity of immunologic markers and surface morphology in childhood lymphoblastic lymphoma. Blood, 48:213–222, 1976.

18. Jones, S.E., Fuks, Z., Bull, M., Kadin, M.D., Dorfman, R.F., Kaplan, H.S., Rosenberg, S.A., and Kim, H.: Non-Hodgkin's lymphomas. IV. Clinicopathologic correlation in 405 cases. Cancer, 31:806–823, 1973.

19. Kaiser-McCaw, B., Epstein, A.L., Kaplan, H.S., and Hecht, F.: Chromosome 14 translocation in African and North American Burkitt's lymphoma. Int. J. Cancer, 19:482–486, 1977.

20. Kaplan, J., Mastrangelo, R., and Peterson, W.D., Jr.: Childhood lymphoblastic lymphoma, a cancer of thymus-derived lymphocytes. Cancer Res., 34:521–525, 1974.

21. Kersey, J., Nesbit, M., Hallgren, H., Sabad, A., Yunis, E., and Gajl-Peczalska, K.: Evidence for origin of certain childhood acute lymphoblastic leukemias and lymphomas in thymus-derived lymphocytes. Cancer, 36:1348–1352, 1975.

22. Koziner, B., Filippa, D.A., Mertelsmann, R., Gupta, S., Clarkson, B., Good, R.A., and Siegal, F.P.: Characterization of malignant lymphomas in leukemic phase by multiple differentiation markers of mononuclear cells. Correlation with clinical features and conventional morphology. Am. J. Med., 63:556–567, 1977.

23. Landberg, T., Garwicz, S. and Akerman, M.: A clinico-pathological study of non-Hodgkin's lymphomata in childhood. Br. J. Cancer (Suppl. II), 31:332–336, 1975.

24. Lemerle, M., Gerard-Marchant, R., Sancho, H. and Schweisguth, O.: Natural history of non-Hodgkin's malignant lymphoma in children. A retrospective study of 190 cases. Br. J. Cancer (suppl. II), 31:324–331, 1975.

25. Lennert, K., Mohri, N., Stein, H., and Kaiserling, E.: The histopathology of malignant lymphomas. Brit. J. Haemat., 31 (suppl.):193–203, 1975.

26. Levine, P.H. and Cho, B.R.: Burkitt's lymphoma: Clinical features of North American Cases. Cancer Res., 34:1219–1221,1974.

27. Levine,P.H.,Cho,B.R., Connelly, R.R., Berard, C.W., O'Connor, G.T., Dorfman, R.F., Easton, J.M., and DeVita, V.T.: The American Burkitt Lymphoma Registry: A progress report. Ann. Intern. Med., 83:31–36, 1975.

28. Lukes, R.J., and Collins, R.D.: Immunologic characterization of human malignant lymphomas. Cancer, 34:1488–1503, 1974.

28a. Lukes, R.J., and Collins, R.D.: Lukes-Collins classification and its significance. Cancer Treat. Rep., 61:971–979, 1977.

29. Mann, R.B., Jaffe, E.S., Braylan, R.C., Nanba, K., Frank, M.M., Ziegler, J.L., Berard, C.W.: Non-endemic Burkitt's lymphome. A B cell tumor related to germinal centers. New England J. Med., 295:685–691, 1976.

30. McCaffrey, R.P., Harrison, T.A., Parkman, R., and Baltimore, D.: Terminal deoxynucleotidyl transferase activity in human leukemic cells and in normal human thymocytes. N. Eng. J. Med., 292:775, 1975.

31. Murphy, S.B.: Current concepts in cancer. Childhood non-Hodgkin's lymphoma. N. Eng. J. Med., 299:1446–1448, 1978.

32. Murphy, S.B.: Management of childhood non-Hodgkin's lymphoma. Cancer Treat. Rep., 61:1161–1173, 1977.

33. Murphy, S.B.: Prognostic features and obstacles to cure of childhood non-Hodgkin's lymphoma. Semin. Oncol., 4:265–271, 1977.
34. Murphy, S.B., and Hustu, H.O.: Personal communication.
35. Nathwani, B.N., Kim, H., and Rappaport, H.: Malignant lymphoma, lymphoblastic. Cancer, 38:964–983, 1976.
36. Nathwani, B.N., Kim, H., Rappaport, H., Solomon, J., and Fox, M.: Non-Hodgkin's lymphomas. A clinicopathologic study comparing two classifications, Cancer 41, 303–325, 1978.
37. Pangalis, G.A., Nathwani, B.N., Rappaport, H., and Rosen, R.B.: Acute lymphoblastic leukemia: Correlation of nuclear morphology with clinical presentation, response to therapy, and survival. Cancer, 43:551–557, 1979.
38. Pinkel, D., Hustu, H.O., Aur, R.J.A., Smith, K., Borella, L.D., and Simone, J.: Radiotherapy in leukemia and lymphoma of children. Cancer, 39:817–824, 1977.
39. Pinkel, D., Johnson, W. and Aur, R.J.A.: Non-Hodgkin's lymphoma in children. Br. J. Cancer (Suppl. II), 31:298–323, 1975.
40. Rappaport, H.: In: Atlas of Tumor Pathology, section 3, fasc. 8, Washington, D.C., 1966.
41. Ravindranath, Y., Kaplan, J., and Zeulzer, M.D.: Significance of mediastinal mass in acute lymphoblastic leukemia. Pediatrics, 55:889–893, 1975.
42. Rosen, P.J., Feinstein, D.I., Pattenhale, P.K., Tindle, B.H., Williams, A.H., Cain, M.J., Bonorris, J. B., Parker, J.W., and Lukes, R.J.: Convoluted lymphocytic lymphoma in adults. A clinicopathologic entity. Ann. of Intern. Med., 89:319–324, 1978.
43. Sarin, P.S., Anderson, P.N., and Gallo, R.C.: Terminal deoxynucleotidyl transferase activities in human blood leukocytes and lymphoblast cell lines: High levels in lymphoblastic cell lines and blast cells of some patients with chronic myelogenous leukemia in acute phase. Blood, 47:11, 1976.
44. Sarin, P.S., and Gallo, R.C.: Terminal deoxynucleotidyl transferase in chronic myelogenous leukemia. J. Biol. Cehm., 249:8051, 1974.
45. Smith, J.L., Barker, C.R., Clein, G.P., and Collins, R.D.: Characterization of malignant mediastinal lymphoid neoplasm (Sternberg sarcoma) as thymic in origin. Lancet, 1:74–77, 1973.
46. Srivastava, B.I.S., Kan, S.A., Minowada, J., Gomez, A., and Rakowski, I .: Terminal deoxynucleotidyl transferase activity in blastic phase of chronic mylogenous leukemia. Cancer Res., 27:3612–3618, 1977.
47. Srivastava, S., Khan, S.A., and Henderson, E.S.: High terminal deoxynucleotidyl transferase activity in acute myelogenous leukemia. Cancer Res., 36: 3847, 1976.
48. Stein, H., Petersen, N., Gaedicke, G., Lennert, K., and Landbeck, G.: Lymphoblastic lymphoma of convoluted or acite phosphatase type—A tumor of T precursor cells. Int. J. Cancer, 17:292–295, 1976.
49. Sullivan, M.P.: Treatment of lymphoma. Cancer, 35:991–995, 1975.
50. Warnke, R.A., Kim, H., Dorfman R.F.: Malignant Histiocytosis (Histiocytic meduallary reticulosis). I. Clinicopathologic study of 29 cases. Cancer, 35: 215–230, 1975.
51. Williams, A.H., Taylor, C.R., DPhil, B., Higgins, G.R., Quinn, J.J., Schneider, B.K., Swanson, V., Parker, J.W., Pattengale, P.K., Chandor, S.B., Powars, D., Lincoln, T.L., Tindle, B.H., and Lukes, R.J.: Childhood lymphoma-leukemia. I. Correlation of morphology and immunological studies. Cancer, 42:171–181, 1978.

52. Winberg, C.D., Nathawani, B.N., and Rappaport, H.: Nodular (follicular) lymphomas in children and young adults: A clinicopathologic study of 64 patients. Lab. Invest., 40:56, 1979.
53. Wollner, N., Burchenal, J.H., Lieberman, P.H., Exelby, P., D'Angio, G., and Murphy, M.L.: Non-Hodgkin's lymphoma in children. A comparative study of two modalities of therapy. Cancer, 37:123–134, 1976.
54. Wollner, N., Lieberman, P., Exelby, P., D'Angio, G. Burchenal, J., Fang, S., and Murphy, M.L.: Non-Hodgkin's lymphoma in children: Results of treatment with $LSA_2\text{-}L_2$ protocol. Br. J. Cancer (suppl. II), 31:337–342, 1975.
55. Wollner, N.: Non-Hodgkin's lymphoma in children. Ped. clinics North Am., 23:371–378, 1976.
56. Wright, D.H.: Burkitt's lymphoma and infectious mononucleosis. In: Comprehensive immunology. series 4: The immunopathology of lymphoreticular neoplasms, pp. 391–424, Towmey, J.J., and Good, R.A., (eds.), Plenum Medical, New York and London, 1978.
57. Ziegler, J.L.: Burkitt's lymphoma. Med. Clinics North Am., 61:1073–1082, 1977.

35. EXTRANODAL LYMPHOMAS

H. KIM

INTRODUCTION

Though malignant lymphomas are usually considered to be neoplasms of lymph nodes and other lymphoid tissue such as spleen, bone marrow, thymus, and Waldeyer's ring, substantial portions of malignant lymphoma arise from other sites such as gastro-intestinal tract, skin, lung, salivary glands, orbit and gonad, etc. If we exclude lymphomas which arise from lymph node and other lymphoid tissue, malignant lesions primary in extranodal site comprise 17.5% of the non-Hodgkin's lymphomas reported in the United States. Distribution of extranodal lymphomas according to their site of origin is listed in Table 1. The relative frequency of extranodal lymphomas may be higher in different countries; Israel 36%, Finland 28%, East Germany 47% and Italy 48%. Most of extranodal lymphomas are non-Hodgkin's lymphomas and Hodgkin's disease is extremely rare. In spite of the relative prominance of extranodal lymphomas, information on the subject is rather sparse in literature and even when they are available, it is usually difficult to analyze the data. This is due to difficulty in assembling an adequate series of a single site, lack of uniform criteria for inclusion, and utilization of different terminology and mode of therapy.

Information on the distribution according to histologic types of extranodal lymphomas is difficult to obtain. Many reports are based on retrospective analysis and still use terms such as reticulum cell sarcoma. For the purpose of this presentation, Rappaport's terminology will be utilized for non-Hodgkin's lymphomas in conjuction with, if information is available, Lukes and Collins classification. Since the time and space is limited, primary lymphomas of only selected sites will be considered in this presentation. However, pertinent articles are listed in the reference section for other sites not discussed at this presentation.

J.G. van den Tweel et al. (eds.), Malignant Lymphoproliferative Diseases, 459–467
All rights reserved.
Copyright © 1980 by Martinus Nijhoff Publishers bv, The Hague/Boston/London.

Table 1. Distribution of extranodal lymphomas in the United States.*

	End results Group of Cancer Registries 1950–1964		Third National Survey 1969–1971		Surveillance, Epidemiology and end results 1973–1975	
Stomach	346	27.3%	253	28.3%	227	27.8%
Small bowel	110	8.7%	119	13.3%	118	14.4%
Skin excluding MF	110	8.7%			Data not collected	
Connective tissue	90	7.1%	68	7.6%	69	8.4%
Colon and rectum	82	6.5%	73	8.2%	60	7.3%
Salivary gland	69	5.4%	42	4.7%	49	6%
Bone	69	5.4%	51	5.7%	39	4.8%
Lung	53	4.2%	39	4.4%	41	5%
Thyroid	36	2.8%	34	3.8%	26	3.2%
Breast	33	2.6%	13	1.5%	21	2.6%
Orbit	32	2.5%	19	2.1%	24	2.9%
Testis	23	2.8%	30	3.4%	20	2.4%
All other sites	215	17%	153	17%	123	15.1%
All cases	1268	100.0%	894	100.%	817	100.%

* Excluding nasopharanx, pharynx, tonsils, and retroperitoneum.

STOMACH

Malignant lymphoma accounts for about 5% of all gastric malignancies. The stomach is the most common site of extranodal lymphoma (Tables 1 and 2). Most common clinical complaints of presentation are ulcer symptoms. The gastric lymphoma occurs in adults and the median age varies from 45 years to over 60 years in different series. Males are more often affected with male to female ratio of 1–3.5 to 1. They are usually single and present most commonly in regions of antrum, pylorus and lesser curvature. They vary in size from 0.3cm to 30cm in diameter (average diameter: 9 to 11 cm). Histologically about $\frac{3}{4}$ of the cases are "histiocytic" and the remainder are lymphocy-

Table 2. Lymphomas of the gastrointestinal tract: distribution according to location.

Stomach	48	(41%)
Small bowel	37	(31.6%)
Ileocecal	13	(11.1%)
Appendix	2	(1.7%)
Large bowel	11	(9.4%)
Multiple G.I. sites	6	(5.1%)
Total	117	(100%)

Lewin et al.: Cancer 42:693–707, 1978.

tic with rare cases of Hodgkin's disease. They are mostly diffuse and nodular lymphomas are not common. Prognosis varies from 35 to 59% for a five-year survival and 20 to 37% for ten-year survival. It depends upon (a) histology and stage of disease, (b) size and depth of infiltrate, and (c) status of the regional lymph node spread. However, the size of the lesion, depths of infiltrate, and lateral extent of lesion and clinical or gross findings do not help us in differentiating benign reactive lymphoid lesions from malignant lymphomas. Correct interpretation depends upon identification of cellular composition and cytology of the infiltrate. In neoplastic infiltrates, the cellular population is uniform in contrast to most reactive lesions which are composed of polymorphous mixture of various cells including small and large lymphocytes, eosinophils, and plasma cells. As a general rule, well-differentiated lymphocytic proliferation are usually reactive in the stomach. The feature which is often of help in distinguishing lymphomas from reactive infiltrates is the relationship of an associated ulcer with the infiltrate. In lymphomas, a bulk of the lesion forms the basis of an ulcer whereas, in reactive lesions, ulcer bed is composed of granulation tissue and much of the infiltrates are to each side of the ulcer. Table 3 shows differential features of gastric lymphomas and gastric lymphoid hyperplasia.

INTESTINAL TRACT

Primary lymphomas of the intestinal tract account for 15 to 22% which is second only to the stomach in frequency of all extranodal non-Hodgkin's lymphomas. Distribution of lymphomas according to each segment of the intestinal tract is shown in Table 2. In the small intestine, malignant lymphomas represent 20% of all malignancies, while it represents less than 0.5% of all

Table 3. Gastric lymphoid tumors: differential features.

	Lymphoma	*Hyperplasia*
Cell population	Uniform	Polymorphic
Cell maturation	Immature or malignant	Mature
Germinal centers	Absent	Often present
Necrosis	Present or absent	Absent
Pattern	Uniform, Monotonous	Nodular, Discontinous
Margins	Uniform	Irregular
Fibrosis	Little	Moderate to marked
Ulcer	Tumor base	Usually fibrotic
Localization	Superficial or deep	Usually confined to wall
Lymph nodes	Reactive or tumor	Reactive

Platz, C.E.: In Proceedings of "Tutorial on Neoplastic Hematopathology", presented in cooperation with the City of Hope National Medical Center and the University of Chicago Center for Continuing Education, Henry Rappaport, M.D., Director, Febr., 1980.

Table 4. Gastrointestinal lymphomas: clinical features.

		Intestine		
	Stomach	*Small*	*Large*	*Ileocecal*
Number of patients	28	24	8	13
Age Average	60	45	58	37
Range	31–82	3–77	52–77	7–70
Sex				
M:F	1.1:1	3.2:1	0.6:1	3.3:1
Presenting symptoms and signs (%)				
Abdominal pain	75	75	50	100
Anorexia	32	16	12	23
Nausea and vomiting	39	50	25	38
Diarrhea	0	0	50	38
Constipation	10	8	0	7
Weight loss	18	50	12	31
GI bleeding	32	37	62	29
Abdominal mass	14	29	25	29

Modified from Lewin et al.: 42:693–707, 1978.

primary malignancies in the colon and rectum. If we consider all patients with malignant lymphomas, approximately 10% show evidence of gastro-intestinal tract involvement at the time of their clinical presentation. Clinical features of gastro-intestinal lymphomas are listed in Table 4. As in primary gastric lymphomas, the lymphomas of the intestinal tract usually present with a single lesion. Multiple lesions occur in 10 to 20% of cases. Five year survival for lymphomas of the intestinal tract including those of the stomach varies from 30 to 45%. In the series of Lewin et al., the survival was not significantly affected by the involvement of the regional lymph node. Dissemination beyond the regional lymph node, however, is of great prognostic significance with no patients having such a dissemination living for more than two years. In the series of Lewin et al., the best results were seen in the group of patients who received radiotherapy in addition to surgery.

SKIN

Excluding mycosis fungoides or Sézary syndrome, malignant lymphomas primary of the skin accounts for 8.7% of all extranodal lymphomas (Table 1). Unlike in mycosis fungoides or Sézary syndrome, a majority of patients present with a solitary nodule of the head and neck. The histology varies in different series. In the series of Long et al., lymphocytic type of either nodular

Table 5. Histopathologic findings in malignant lymphoma of the skin.

1) Location of infiltrate: dermal	16/25
subcutaneous	9/25
2) Sparing of Grenz zone:	16/25
3) Epidermis: — no change	17/25
— ulceration, spongiosis, atrophy, etc.	8/25
— Darier-Pautrier abscesses	0/25
4) Adnexa and other skin structures: usually involved	
5) Perivascular or transmural infiltration of dermal blood vessels	

Long et al.: Cancer 38:1282–1296, 1976.

or diffuse comprised 76% while "histiocytic" comprised only 12%. According to the same series, lymphomas of the skin eventually disseminate with involvement of the lymph node and viscera six months to five years after the onset in the majority of the patients. The median survival was 3.7 years and disseminated lymphoma was the cause of deaths in 64%. Table 5 shows the summary of histopathologic findings in malignant lymphomas of the skin.

LUNG

The primary lymphoma of the lung is extremely rare. Usually patients are asymptomatic and pulmonary masses are detected on routine X-rays of the chest. Radiographically these may vary from small coin lesions to large masses involving the entire lung. Pleural effusion or lymphadenopathy may be associated. The tumors usually abut on the pleural surface. Table 6 details the differential features of pulmonary lymphoma and pseudolymphoma.

Table 6. Pulmonary-lymphoid tumors: differential diagnosis.

Pseudolymphoma	*Lymphoma*
Mixed cell infiltrate	Uniform infiltrate
Infiltrate mature	Infiltrate mature or immature
Germinal centers	No germinal centers
Septal growth pattern	Usually solid pattern
Peripheral septal	Periphery encapsulated
Usually solitary lesion	Solitary or multiple nodules
Bronchi involved but intact	Destruction of bronchial cartilage
Pleura not involved discontinuously	Seeding of pleura
Hilar nodes not involved	Hilar nodes negative or involved

Platz, C.E.: In Proceedings of "Tutorial on Neoplastic Hematopathology", presented in cooperation with the City of Hope National Medical Center and the University of Chicago Center for Continuing Education, Henry Rappaport, M.D., Director, Feb., 1980.

GONADS

Lymphomas account for about 5% of testicular tumors and it is the most common form of malignant disease of testis in men over 60 years of age. There are no distinguishing clinical features and frequently an erroneous diagnosis of germ cell tumor is made. Over 50% of all bilateral testicular tumors are malignant lympomas. According to Paladugu et al., the most common histology in testis is "histiocytic" and, in ovary, poorly-differentiated lymphocytic. All testicular and the majority of ovarian lymphomas are diffuse and most are non-Hodgkin's lymphomas. A striking feature in their series was the high frequency of vascular invasion (41%) in testicular lymphomas which was reflected in a high incidence (86%) of noncontiguous lung involvement at autopsy, suggesting hematogenous spread. Although the patient may present with clinical Stage I disease, the survival may still be short. The gonadal lymphomas usually disseminate early after detection of gonadal masses.

BIBLIOGRAPHY

General

Cutler, S.J., and Young, J.L., (eds.): Third national cancer survey: Incidence data. N.C.I. monograph No. 41.

Freeman, C., Berg, J.W., and Cutler, S.J.: Occurrence and prognosis of extranodal lymphomas. Cancer, 29:253–260, 1972.

Goffinet, D.R., Warnke, R., Dunnick, N.R., Castellino, R., Glatstein, E., Nelsen, T.S., Dorfman, R.F., Rosenberg, S.A., and Kaplan, H.S.: Clinical and surgical (laparotomy) evaluation of patients with non-Hodgkin's lymphomas. Cancer Treat. Rep., 61:981–992, 1977.

Hande, K.R., Reimer, R.R., and Fisher, R.I.: Comparison of nodal primary versus extranodal primary histiocytic lymphoma. Cancer Treat. Rep., 61:999–1000, 1977.

Levi, J.A. and Wiernik, P.H.: Limited extranodal Hodgkin's disease: Unfavorable prognosis and therapeutic implications. Am. J. Med., 63:365–372, 1977.

Matas, A.J., Hertel, B.F., Rosai, J., Simmons, R.L., and Najarian, J.S.: Post-transplant malignant lymphoma: Distinctive morphologic features related to its pathogenesis. Am. J. Med., 61:716–720, 1976.

Rudders, R.A., Ross, M.E., and DeLellis, R.A.: Primary extranodal lymphoma: Response to treatment and factors influencing prognosis. Cancer, 42:406–416, 1978.

Saltzstein, S.L.: Extranodal malignant lymphomas and pseudolymphomas. Pathol. Annu. pp. 159–184, 1969.

Torti, F.M., Portlock, C.S., Rosenberg, S.A., and Kaplan, H.S.: Extranodal (E) lesions in Hodgkin's disease (HD) prognosis and response to therapy (meeting abstract). Proc. Am. Assoc. Cancer Res., 19:367, 1978.

Unpublished data: Surveillance, epidemiology and end results (SEER) program, Biometry Branch, NCI.

Gastrointestinal tract

Chiles, J.T., and Platz, C.E.: The radiographic manifestations of pseudolym-phoma of the stomach. Radiology, 116:551–556, 1975.

Hande, K.R., Fisher, R.I., DeVita, V.T., Chabner, B.A., and Young, R.C.: Diffuse histiocytic lymphoma involving the gastrointestinal tract. Cancer, 1984–1989, 1978.

Henry, K. and Farrer-Brown, G. Primary lymphomas of the gastrointestinal tract. I. Plasma cell tumours. Histopathol., 1:53–76, 1977.

Hoerr, S.O., McCormack, L.J., and Hertzer, N.R.: Prognosis in gastric lymphoma. Arch. Surg., 107:155–158, 1973.

Jacobs, D.S.: Primary gastric malignant lymphoma and pseudolymphoma. Am. J. Clin. Pathol., 40:379–394, 1963.

Joseph, J.I. and Lattes, R.: Gastric lymphosarcoma. Am. J. Clin. Pathol., 45:653–669, 1966.

Kahn, L.B., Selzer, G., and Kaschula, R.O.C.: Primary gastrointestinal lymphoma. A clinicopathologic study of fifty-seven cases. Am. J. Dig. Dis., 17:219–232, 1972.

Lewin, K.J., Kahn, L.B., and Novis, B.H.: Primary intestinal lymphoma of "West-ern" and "Mediterranean" type, Alpha chain disease and massive plasma cell infiltration. A comparative study of 37 cases. Cancer, 31:2511–2528, 1976.

Lewin, K.J., Ranchod, M., and Dorfman, R.F.: Lymphomas of the gastrointestinal tract. A study of 117 cases presenting with gastrointestinal disease. Cancer, 42:693–707, 1978.

Lim, F.E., Hartman, A.S., Tan, E.G., Cady, B., and Meissner, W.A.: Factors in the prognosis of gastric lymphoma. Cancer, 39:1715–1720, 1977.

Nassar, V.H., Salem, P.A., Shahid, M.J., Alami, S.Y., Balikian, J.B., Salem, A.A., and Nasrallah, S.M.: "Mediterranean abdominal lymphoma" or immunopro-liferative small intestinal disease. Part II: Pathological aspects. Cancer, 41:1340–1354, 1978.

Ranchod, M., Lewin, K.J., and Dorfman, R.F.: Lymphoid hyperplasia of the gas-trointestinal tract: A study of 26 cases and review of the literature. Am. J. Surg. Pathol., 2:383–400, 1978.

Rappaport, H., Ramot, B., Hulu, N., and Park, J.K.: The pathology of so-called Mediterranean abdominal lymphoma with malabsorption. Cancer, 29:1502–1511, 1972.

Wright, C.J.: Pseudolymphoma of the stomach. Hum. Pathol., 4:305–318, 1973.

Skin

Caro, W.A. and Helwig, E.B.: Cutaneous lymphoid hyperplasia. Cancer, 24:487–502, 1969.

Clark, W.H., Mihm, M.C., Reed, R.J., and Ainsworth, A.M.: The lymphocytic in-filtrates of the skin. Hum. Pathol. 5:25–43, 1974.

Connors, R.C., and Ackerman, A.B.: Histologic pseudomalignancies of the skin. Arch. Dermatol. 112:1767–1780, 1976.

Edelson, R.L.: Recent advances in the cutaneous T cell lymphomas. Bull. Cancer, 64:209–224, 1977.

Long, J.C., Mihm, M.C., and Quazi, R.: Malignant lymphoma of the skin: A clinicopathologic study of lymphoma other than mycosis fungoides diagnosed by skin biopsy. Cancer, 38:1282–1296, 1976.

Lutzner, M., Edelson, R., Schein, P., Green, I., Kirkpatrick, C., and Ahmed, A.:
  Cutaneous T-cell lymphomas: The Sézary Syndrome, mycosis fungoides, and
  related disorders. Ann. Int. Med., 83:534–552, 1975.
Valentino, L.A., and Helwig, E.B.: Lymphomatoid papulosis. Arch. Pathol., 96:
  409–416, 1973.
Wolk, B.H.: Primary malignant lymphoma cutis. CMA J., 117:750–753, 1977.

Salivary gland

Hyman, G.A., and Wolfe, M.: Malignant lymphomas of the salivary glands. Review
  of the literature and report of 33 new cases, including four cases associated
  with the lymphoepithelial lesion. Am. J. Clin. Pathol., 65:421–438, 1975.
Talal, N., Sokoloff, L., and Barth, W.F.: Extrasalivary lymphoid abnormalities in
  Sjögren's Syndrome (reticulum cell sarcoma, "Pseudolyphoma", macroglobulinemia). Am. J. Med., 43:50–65, 1967.

Bone

Boston, H.C., Dahlin, D.C., Ivins, J.C. and Cupps, R.E.: Malignant lymphoma
  (so-called reticulum cell sarcoma) of Bone. Cancer, 34:1131–1137, 1974.
Reimer, R.R., Chabner, R.A., Young, R.C., Reddick, R., and Johson, R.E.: Lym-
  phoma presenting in bone: Results of histopathology, staging, and therapy.
  Ann. Int. Med., 87:50–55, 1977.
Shoji, H., and Miller, T.: Primary reticulum cell sarcoma of bone. Significance of
  clinical features upon the prognosis. Cancer, 28:1234–1244, 1971.
Stein, R.S., Ultmann, J.E., Byrne, G.E., Moran, E.M., Golomb, H.M., and Oetzel,
  N.: Bone marrow involvement in non-Hodgkin's lymphoma: Implications for
  staging and therapy. Cancer, 37:629–636, 1976.

Lung

Jenkins, B.A., and Salm, R.: Primary lymphosarcoma of the lung. Br. J. Dis. Chest,
  65:225–237, 1971.
Saltzstein, S.L.: Pulmonary malignant lymphomas and pseudolymphomas: Classification, therapy, and prognosis. Cancer, 16:928–955, 1963.

Thyroid

Burke, J.S., Butler, J.J., and Fuller, L.M.: Malignant lymphomas of the thyroid:
  A clinical pathologic study of 35 patients including ultrastructural observations. Cancer, 39:1587–1602, 1977.
Heimann, R., Vannineuse, A., DeSloover, C., and Dor, P.: Malignant lymphomas
  and undifferentiated small cell carcinoma of the thyroid: A clinicopathologic
  review in the light of the Kiel classification for malignant lymphomas. Histopathol., 2:201–213, 1978.

Breast

Mambo, N.C., Burke, J.S., and Butler, J.J.: Primary malignant lymphomas of the
  breast. Cancer, 39:2033–2040, 1977.

Wiseman, C. and Liao, K.T.: Primary lymphoma of the breast. Cancer, 29:1705–1712, 1972.

Orbit

Blodi, F.C., and Gass, J.D.: Inflammatory pseudotumor of the orbit. Brit. J. Ophthal, 52:79–93, 1968.

Garner, A.: Pathology of "pseudotumors" of the orbit: A review. J. Clin. Pathol., 26:639–648, 1973.

Kelly, A., Rosas-Uribe, A., and Kraus, S.T.: Orbital lymphomas and pseudo-lymphomas. A clinicopathologic study of eleven cases. Am. J. Clin. Pathol., 68:377–396, 1977.

Schwarze, E. -W., Radaszkiewicz, T., Pülhorn, G., Goos, M., and Lennert, K.: Maligne und benigne Lymphome des Auges, der Lid- und Orbitalregion. Virchows Arch. A. Path. Histol. 370:85–86, 1976.

Testis

Gowing, N.F.: Malignant lymphoma of the testis. In: Pathology of the testis, pp. 334-355, R.C.B., Pugh, (ed.), Blackwell Scientific Publications, London, 1976.

Paladugu, R.R., Bearman, R.M., and Rappaport, H.: Malignant lymphoma with primary manifestation in the gonad: A clinicopathologic study of 38 patients. Cancer, 45:561–571, 1980.

Raute, M., and Wurster, K.: Das maligne Lymphom des Hodens: Unter besonderer Berücksichtigung des Reticulosarkoms. Virchows Arch. A. Path. Anat. Histol. 363:239–272, 1974.

Robb, W.A.: Lymphoma of the testis. J.R. Coll. Surg. Edinb., 23:28, 1978.

Sussman, E.B., Hajdu, S.I., Lieberman, P.H. and Whitmore, W.F.: Malignant lymphoma of the testis: A clinicopathologic study of 37 cases. J. Urol., 118: 1004–1007, 1977.

Talerman, A.: Primary malignant lymphoma of the testis. J. Urol. 118:783–786, 1977.

Central nervous system

Henry, J.M., Heffner, Jr., R.R., Dillard, S.H., Earle, K.M., and Davies, R.L.: Primary malignant lymphomas of the central nervous system. Cancer, 34: 1293–1302, 1974.

Schneck, S.A., and Penn, I.: De-novo brain tumours in renal-transplant Recipients. Lancet pp. 983–986, May 15, 1971.

Taylor, C.R., DPhil, B., Russell, R., Lukes, R.J., and Davis, R.L.: An immunohistological study of immunoglobulin content of primary central nervous system lymphomas. Cancer, 41:2197–2205, 1978.

36. HAIRY-CELL LEUKEMIA

J. JANSEN, H.R.E. SCHUIT, C.J.L.M. MEIJER AND W. HIJMANS

INTRODUCTION

Hairy-cell leukemia (HCL; leukemic reticuloendotheliosis) is a rare form of chronic leukemia. The clinico-pathological entity HCL, which accounts for about 2% of all leukemias, was established in 1958 by Bouroncle and coworkers (1). Splenomegaly, without prominent lymphadenopathy, and pancyopenia were described as the typical manifestations. In the peripheral blood, mononuclear cells with hairlike projections of the cell membrane were present. The course of the disease was slowly progressive and some patients had already survived for many years.

Much attention has been paid to this disease, particularly in the last decade. Retrospective studies of large numbers of patients have shown that the clinical picture at diagnosis may differ considerably from the typical presentation with massive splenomegaly and pancytopenia. Cases without splenomegaly or with very high leukocyte counts have been reported. A rapidly progressive course has been observed in some patients, with death occurring within a few months after the onset of symptoms (2–6).

CLINICAL ASPECTS

The history of the patients is rather unspecific, with complaints of general weakness and fatigue. Infectious episodes, especially of pneumonia, are frequent. Between 25 and 40% of the patients are discovered at routine check-up, which shows splenomegaly, cytopenia, or abnormal cells in the peripheral blood. The clinical features at diagnosis are given in Table 1, the laboratory data in Table 2. Additional laboratory findings are severe monocytopenia (in at least 90% of cases) and moderate leuko-erythroblastosis. The neutrophil alkaline-phosphatase index is increased in most patients. Gamma-globulin levels are normal or elevated, and only sporadically decreased. M proteins are extremely rare.

The malignant cells of HCL have round, bilobular, or even clefted nuclei with a spongy appearance, and "hairy" cytoplasmic projections resulting in a indistinct cell border. In these cells Yam et al. (7) demonstrated the presence

J.C. van den Tweel et al. (eds.). Malignant Lymphoproliferative Diseases, 469–479
All rights reserved.
Copyright © 1980 by Martinus Nijhoff Publishers bv, The Hague/Boston/London.

Table 1. Clinical features at diagnosis in 3 retrospective studies.

	Sebahoun et al. (5) (n = 131)	Golomb et al. (3) (n = 71)	Jansen et al. (4) (n = 135)
Age: median (range)	52 (—)	— (22–79)	52 (19–78)
M:F	4	3.7	4.6
Splenomegaly (%)	71	83	90
Hepatomegaly (%)	33	19	29
Lymphadenopathy (%)	17	38	28
Haem. diathesis (%)	30	34	28

of acid phosphatase activity that was resistant to tartaric acid. This cytochemical reaction, due to isoenzyme 5 of acid phosphatase, occurs in 90% of the cases of HCL; although it is not pathognomonic for HCL, it is very helpful in establishing the correct diagnosis. Electron microscopically, the hairy cell shows long cytoplasmic villi, few cytoplasmic lysosomes, and an oval, frequently indented, nucleus. In the hairy cells of 50% of the patients hollow cylindrical structures representing ribosome-lamella complexes can be observed (8). These complexes are typical of HCL, but they are not pathognonomic. Identical structures have been reported in other lymphoproliferative disorders and in monoblastic leukemia (2).

The clinical features and the peripheral-blood film most often point to the diagnosis; nevertheless, histological examination of spleen and/or bone-marrow tissue is mandatory for an unequivocal diagnosis. Bone-marrow biopsy is the best diagnostic procedure; the biopsy specimen always shows diffuse infiltration, but sometimes only partial infiltration is present. The bone marrow is less tightly packed than in malignant lymphoma or in CLL. Increased amounts of reticulin fibers are usually observed and are responsible for the dry tap that is obtained in 30–50% of the patients when bone-

Table 2. Laboratory data at diagnosis in 3 retrospective studies.

	Sebahoun et al. (5) (n = 131)	Golomb et al. (3) (n = 71)	Jansen et al. (4) (n = 135)
	%	%	%
anemia (Hb < 12 g/dl)	78	82	83
leukocytes (< 5,000/mm³)	80	64	68
(> 10,000/mm³)	8	18	16
neutrophils (< 1,000/mm³)	63	—	75
(< 500/mm³)	33	—	35
hairy cells (< 500/mm³)	70	—	—
(< 100/mm³)	—	—	11
platelets (< 100,000/mm³)	73	56	83

marrow aspiration is attempted. The spleen is diffusely involved and, microscopically, the splenic architecture is replaced by a loose infiltrate that fills the red-pulp cords, whereas the white pulp is decreased or absent. Most of the spleens show "pseudo-sinuses", vascular lesions lined by hairy cells and filled with erythrocytes (6, 9).

Actuarial survival curves show that median survival in HCL is about 4–5 years from the onset of symptoms (Figure 1). A few patients have a rapidly progressive course and die within a year after the onset of symptoms. About one-third of the patients survive for more than 10 years, sometimes without any specific therapy. There are only few parameters that correlate with life-expectancy. Females probably do better than males. The hemoglobin level, neutrophil count, and degree of splenomegaly have been reported to be of prognostic value in some, but not all, retrospective studies (3–5).

The effect of therapy is difficult to assess in as rare a disease as HCL. Splenectomy is very probably beneficial, but no controlled studies have been performed. Splenectomy and nonsplenectomy groups were not comparable in most series. In a retrospective analysis of comparable groups of 24 sple-nectomized and 51 nonsplenectomized patients (collected partly from Leiden University Hospital material and partly from the literature), we did not find a significantly better survival for the splenectomy group after 2 years (4). A large-scale retrospective study based on the analysis of data from many institutions is now in progress to find out which patients in particular benefit from splenectomy. Other therapeutic measures are not of documen-

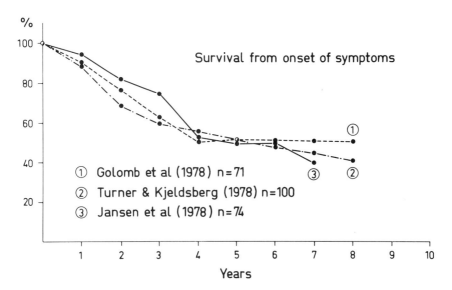

Figure 1. Actuarial survival curves for HCL.

ted value. Corticosteroids have been employed with varying success. Low-dose cytotoxic therapy (e.g., cyclophosphamide 50–100 mg/day p.o.) has been advocated by Catovsky (2), and a few patients have benefitted from high-dose cytotoxic therapy. Perhaps the general opinion that all cytotoxic therapy should be withheld in HCL, will have to be revised in the near future.

As could be expected in patients with cytopenia, infection and—to a smaller degree—bleeding are the leading causes of death. Pneumonia and sepsis in particular occur frequently. Neutropenia, monocytopenia, impaired chemotaxis, B-lymphocytopenia, and decreased T-cell function may all contribute to the susceptibility to infections.

ORIGIN OF THE HAIRY CELL

The origin of the hairy cell, the malignant cell of HCL, is the subject of much debate. The earliest studies of the 1970s already divided the investigators into two groups. Some authors detected on the cells surface-bound immunoglobulins (sIg) that were often monoclonal with respect to light chains; and the hairy cells were therefore considered to be B-lymphocytic cells (10, 11). Others observed phagocytosis by hairy cells and considered the cells to be monocytic in origin (12). The sIg was interpreted by these workers as bound, either via the Fc receptor present on most hairy cells or in some other way. Some workers have concluded that hairy cells are hybrid cells (half lymphocyte/half monocyte) (13) or derive from an as yet unknown type of cell (14).

In recent years, new arguments for a monocytic or a lymphocytic origin of hairy cells have been put forward almost continuously. Arguments for a monocytic origin are shown in Table 3, those for a lymphocytic origin in Table 4.

Our group studied hairy cells with multiple techniques in an attempt to classify HCL. The techniques used can be subdivided into 4 groups: immunofluorescence studies, rosette studies, phagocytosis studies, and cytochemical/histochemical studies.

Table 3. Evidence supporting a monocytic origin of hairy cells.

Phagocytosis of latex particles, bacteria, etc.
Bactericidal activity
Avid FcIgG receptors
Cytochemistry (nonspecific esterase; acid phosphatase)
Endogenous peroxidase activity in electron microscopy
Adherence to glass
Peripheral monocytopenia

Table 4. Evidence supporting a lymphocytic origin of hairy cells.

Intrinsic monoclonal surface Ig
Intracytoplasmic Ig
Ig production in vivo and in vitro
Lymphocyte-specific antigens
Rosettes with mouse erythrocytes
Peripheral B-lymphocytopenia

Immunofluorescence

As already mentioned, there is much disagreement about the intrinsic nature of the sIg found on hairy cells; do these cells synthesize their sIg or take it up from the serum? Freshly collected hairy cells of some patients show flourescence with all kinds of labeled antiserum, i.e., with all anti-heavy-chain and both anti-light-chain antisera. It has been claimed that this polyclonal pattern is due to binding of the Fc part of the antisera by the Fc receptor of the hairy cells. Therefore, the use of F(ab')2 fragments of antisera has been advocated (11). In our view, however, the polyclonal pattern is due to the uptake of serum immunoglobulins by hairy cells, possibly by trapping between the villous projections of the cell membrane. The finding that fluorescence was not obtained with any labeled antiserum in a patient whose cells were known to have very avid—or dense—Fc receptors, argues against the role of Fc receptor binding as the cause of polyclonal fluorescence patterns. Mild fixation with diluted formaldehyde (0.04%; 10 min) always changed the polyclonal patterns (κ and λ) into monoclonal (κ or λ) patterns, probably by removing the bound Ig. This technique gave the same results as incubation in serum-free medium for one or more hours. The hairy cells of some patients showed a monoclonal pattern with respect to light chains even without fixation or incubation.

In all probability the monoclonal picture indicates true intrinsic sIg. It is not easy to explain how hairy cells could pick up Ig of only one light-chain type unless a M-protein is present. Many groups have tried to study the intrinsic nature of sIg by stripping the sIg from the cells with trypsin; at least some of these groups were able to document the reappearance of sIg (15).

Many investigators have reported δ, $\mu\delta$, or γ on the surface of hairy cells (11, 14, 16). Multiple heavy-chain determinants have seldom been detected. However, Catovsky (2), Burns et al. (15), and our group (17) found multiple heavy-chain determinants in a large percentage of the cases. Catovsky and Burns et al. found $\gamma\mu\delta$ very often; we observed many combinations: $\alpha\delta$, $\alpha\mu\delta$, $\gamma\mu\delta$, $\gamma\delta$ and $\alpha\gamma$ (Table 5). Some cases of HCL showed no intrinsic sIg (2, 17). Intracytoplasmic immunoglobulins were present in only 4/21 cases studied by our group (3 × μ, 1 × γ) (17); others have reported larger num-

Table 5. Heavy-chain patterns in 3 series of patients with HCL.

	Catovsky (2)	Burns et al. (15)	Jansen et al. (17)
μ	1		
$\mu\ \delta$	3	1	1
$\gamma\ \mu\ \delta$	4	5	1
$\gamma\ \delta$			1
γ	1	7	6
δ	2		
$\alpha\ \delta$	1		4
$\alpha\ \mu\ \delta$			2
$\alpha\ \gamma\ \mu\ \delta$		2	
$\alpha\ \gamma$			3
negative	1		2
	n = 13	n = 15	n = 20

bers (15). In some instances hairy cells have been reported to produce immunoglobulins in vitro (15). We have demonstrated this capacity of the cells in at least one patient. Thus, many findings point to the capacity of hairy cells to produce immunoglobulins in vitro and in vivo.

Rosette studies

The study of surface receptors on hairy cells cannot contribute much to the discussion about the origin of the cell. Both B lymphocytes and monocytes probably carry receptors for the Fc part of IgG (FcIgG) and for the third factor of complement (C_3). Receptors for the Fc part of IgM (FcIgM) and for mouse erythrocytes (Em) have been described on lymphocytes only. Most patients with HCL undoubtedly have malignant cells with receptors for the Fc part of IgG, as demonstrated with EAIgG rosettes or with labeled antigen-antibody complexes. With both techniques we found a wide range of densities of FcIgG receptors. The hairy cells of some patients evoked hardly any rosettes of erythrocytes coated with IgG, whereas the cells of other patients formed EAIgG rosettes almost without exception. The results obtained by Burns et al. (15), all of whose cases of HCL gave rise to a very high percentage of EAIgG rosetting cells, can probably be attributed to larger number of IgG molecules on the indicator cells. At least some cases without any EAIgG rosettes reported in the literature are ascribable to a rather unsensitive indicator system (human erythrocytes with anti-Rh (D) IgG).

Probably, the hairy cells of most patients also evoke EAIgM rosettes, thus indicating the presence of a receptor for the Fc part of IgM (18). We found such a receptor on varying numbers of hairy cells, which again suggests a spectrum of densities of this receptor. Our cases without detectable FcIgM receptors might have been positive if a more sensitive indicator system had been used.

In our and others' experience hairy cells never evoked EAIgMC rosettes, which suggests that the cells lack a receptor for C_3. Nevertheless, some authors have reported the presence of C_3 receptors. The explanation that EAIgM rosettes may have been responsible for "false-positive" EAIgMC rosettes seems unlikely, because EAIgM controls were often negative, and in our hands EAIgMC rosettes were always negative, even when many EAIgM rosettes were formed. Thus, some cases of HCL may have receptors for C_3, but the majority do not. Hairy cells often evoke rosettes of mouse erythrocytes (Em) (2). We found some positive cases, but we have not studied this subject in great detail.

There are only a few reports of cases in which hairy cells evoked spontaneous rosette formation with sheep erythrocytes (19). Four cases have been observed that seem to represent cases of T-cell HCL. The cells of these patients formed E rosettes, did not carry sIg, and did not evoke EAIgG or EAIgMC rosettes. Cawley et al. (20) studied a patient whose cells showed both T- and B-cell features (E rosettes, anti-T-cell antiserum, sIg, and FcIgG and FcIgM receptors). We have studied two patients with a similar type of HCL (21). However, in these patients only the hairy cells of the peripheral blood showed T- and B-cell characteristics (E rosettes, anti-T-cell antiserum, sIg, intracytoplasmic Ig in one case, FcIgG receptors). The hairy cells of the spleens showed only B-cell features. The bone marrow of the only patient studied in this respect contained two populations: one with T- and B-cell features and the other with only B-cell features. After splenectomy hairy cells with only B-cell features appeared in the peripheral blood, which indicates that this population had been selectively sequestrated by the spleen.

Phagocytosis

Very convincing pictures have been published of hairy cells containing particles (bacteria, latex, zymosan, cell debris, platelets, or even erythrocytes) completely surrounded by cytoplasm, thus suggesting that these particles had been phagocytosed. Since the only evidence of phagocytosis by hairy cells derives from light and electron microscopy, these pictures could be due to "pseudo-phagocytosis", i.e., overprojection in light microscopy or tangential sectioning in electron microscopy. We therefore used bacteriological, biochemical, and microscopical techniques in an attempt to determine whether hairy cells are true phagocytes (22).

Lysostaphin, a staphylolytic enzyme, kills only extracellular staphylococci. In our control studies on normal and leukemic monocytes, the enzyme did not kill intracellular (truly phagocytosed) bacteria. After phagocytosis of *Staphylococcus aureus*, incubation of hairy cells with lysostaphin reduced the number of bacteria by 95%, which indicates that almost all of the bacteria were extracellular. Microscopical controls also indicated that the hairy cells did not contain bacteria after lysostaphin treatment. The few monocytes that were present still contained bacteria.

Lanthanum nitrate stains the outer membrane of cells in transmission electron microscopy. When this heavy metal was added during the fixation procedure for electron microscopy of monocytes that had phagocytosed latex particles, the membranes of the phagosomes were not stained because these membranes no longer belonged to the outer cell membrane at the time of staining. However, under the same conditions, the membranes of the "phagosomes" of hairy cells were coated with lanthanum, which indicates that these "phagosomes" still belonged to the outer cell membrane; in other words, the latex particles lay in deep invaginations of the outer cell membrane. Elemental X-ray micro-analysis proved that the coating of the "phagosomes" of hairy cells indeed consisted of lanthanum; the phagosomes of monocytes showed only background activity of lanthanum comparable with the amount over the nucleus.

Hairy cells did not show increased oxygen consumption on exposure to bacteria in the presence of serum, whereas leukemic and normal monocytes showed such an increase without exception. All these findings argue against a "professional phagocyte" status of hairy cells. There is no hard evidence that hairy cells truly phagocytose particles. These cells trap particles between the long villous protrusions of the cell membrane, but probably do not internalize the particles.

Cytochemistry

The cytochemical patterns of B lymphocytes, monocytes, and hairy cells are listed in Table 6. Acid phosphatase resistance to tartaric acid is caused by isoenzyme 5; activity of this isoenzyme can be observed in CLL, lymphosarcoma-cell leukemia, and prolymphocytic leukemia although far lower levels than in HCL. Nonspecific esterase, with α-naphthyl butyrate as a substrate, is negative in B lymphocytes. The typical pattern observed in HCL, characterized by some scattered fine granules, can also be observed in the malignant cells of patients with plasma-cell leukemia and prolymphocytic leukemia. Peroxidase activity is never observed in hairy cells at the light-microscopical level. Reyes et al. (23) detected endogenous peroxidaselike activity in hairy cells at the ultrastructural level. The pattern was similar to that seen in resident macrophages, with activity in the nuclear envelope and in the rough endoplasmic reticulum. It should be kept in mind, however, that many other cells besides professional phagocytes show peroxidaselike activity at the ultrastructural level.

In summary the results of our studies indicate that hairy cells are essentially nonphagocytic cells. These hairy cells have receptors and cytochemi-

Table 6. Cytochemical patterns of hairy cells, monocytes, and B-lymphoctyes.

	Hairy cells	Monocytes	B-lymphocytes
Peroxidase	0	$\pm$ — +	0
Nonspecific esterase	0 — $\pm^a$	+ — + + + [b]	0 — $\pm$
Acid phosphatase			
— tartrate	+ — + + +	+ — + + +	0 — $\pm^c$
+ tartrate	$\pm$ — + +	0	0
Lyszoyme	0	+ — + +	0

[a] granular staining; [b] diffuse (cytoplasmic staining); [c] only after stimulation

cal patterns compatible with B-lymphocytic cells, carry intrinsic monoclonal surface Ig, and sometimes even show intracytoplasmic Ig or produce Ig in vitro or in vivo. In our view, it seems clear at present that hairy cells must be B-lymphocytic cells. Other findings — for instance the presence of lympho-cyte-specific antigens, and the long-term intravascular circulation — all fit into the concept that HCL is a B-lymphocyte disorder.

An interesting point is to try to localize the maturation "arrest" of HCL and to fit this leukemia into the scheme of lymphoproliferative disorders. Burns et al. (15) have postulated that the hairy cell is a kind of memory-B-cell, and Lennert (24) placed hairy cells near the centrocytes, B2 lympho-cytes, and ("reticular") plasma cells. Hairy cells have been shown to carry surface Ig often exhibiting multiple heavy-chain determinants. This would locate the cell at a stage somewhat later in B-cell ontogeny than the cells of CLL, probably, in the "switch" from small μ-bearing lymphocyte to more mature Ig containing lymphocyte. This is in accordance with recent findings by Vessière-Louveaux et al. (to be published (25)), who found that the fre-quency of the combination $\alpha\mu\delta$ is second to that of $\mu\delta$. Furthermore, the combined results in Table 5 show that 60% of the patients had γ on the sur-face of their cells, which also suggests a rather late stage of B-cell differentia-tion. Thus, the cases of HCL with intracytoplasmic Ig would be the most mature, the cases without intracytoplasmic Ig and with $\mu/\mu\delta$ on the cell surface the most immature. The rather wide spectrum of maturation of the cells in individual cases of HCL, might be related with the variable density of membrane receptors (FcIgG, FcIgM, and C_3) and the variable cytochemical pattern (acid phosphatase, nonspecific esterase).

REFERENCES

1. Bouroncle, B.A., Wiseman, B.K., and Doan, C.A.: Leukemic reticuloendothe-liosis. Blood, 13:609–630, 1958.
2. Catovsky, D.: Hairy-cell leukaemia and prolymphocytic leukaemia. Clin. Haemat., 6:245–268, 1977.

3. Golomb, H.M., Catovsky, D., and Golde, D.W.: Hairy-cell leukemia. A clinical review based on 71 cases. Ann. Intern. Medic., 89:677–683, 1978.

4. Jansen, J., Hermans, J., Remme, J., den Ottolander, G.J., and Lopes Cardozo, P.: Hairy-cell leukaemia. Clinical features and effect of splenectomy. Scand. J. Haemat., 21:60–71, 1978.

5. Sebahoun, G., Bouffette, P., and Flandrin, G.: Hairy-cell leukemia. Leukem. Res., 2:187–195, 1978.

6. Turner, A., and Kjeldsberg, C.R.: Hairy-cell leukemia: A review. Medicine (Baltimore), 57:477–499, 1978.

7. Yam, L.T., Li, C.Y., and Finkel, H.E.: Leukemic reticuloendotheliosis. The role of tartrate-resistant acid phosphatase in diagnosis and splenectomy in treatment. Archiv. Intern. Medic., 130:248–256, 1972.

8. Katayama, I., Li, C.Y., and Yam, L.T.: Ultrastructural characteristics of the hairy cells of leukemic reticuloendotheliosis. Amer. J. Pathol., 67:361–370, 1972.

9. Nanba, K., Soban, E.J., Bowling, M.C., and Berard, C.W.: Splenic pseudosinuses and hepatic angiomatous lesions. Distinctive features of hairy-cell leukemia. Amer. J. Clin. Pathol., 67:415–426, 1977.

10. Haak, H.L., de Man, J.C.H., Hijmans, W., Knapp, W., and Speck, B.: Further evidence for the lymphocytic nature of leukaemic reticuloendotheliosis (hairy-cell leukaemia). Brit. J. Haemat., 27:31–38, 1974.

11. Fu, S.M., Winchester, R.J., Rai, K.R., and Kunkel, H.G.: Hairy-cell leukemia: proliferation of a cell with phagocytic and B-lymphocyte properties. Scand. J. Immunol., 3:847–851, 1974.

12. King, G.W., Hurtubise, P.E., Sagone, A.L., LoBuglio, A.F., and Metz, E.N.: Leukemic reticuloendotheliosis. A study of the origin of the malignant cell. Amer. J. Medic., 59:411–416, 1975.

13. Seligmann, M.: B-cell and T-cell markers in lymphoid proliferation. N. Eng. J. Medic., 290:1483–1484, 1974.

14. Braylan, R.C., Jaffe, E.S., Triche, T.J., Nanba, K., Fowlkes, B.J., Metzger, H., Frank, M.M., Dolan, M.S., Yee, C.L., Green, I., and Berard, C.W.: Structural and functional properties of the "hairy-cells" of leukemic reticuloendotheliosis. Cancer, 41:210–227, 1978.

15. Burns, G.F., Cawley, J.C., Worman, C.P., Karpas, A., Barker, C.R., Goldstone, A.H., and Hayhoe, F.G.J.: Multiple heavy-chain isotypes on the surface of the cells of hairy-cell leukemia. Blood, 52:1132–1147, 1978.

16. Golomb, H.M., Vardiman, J., Sweet, D.L., Simon, D., and Variakojis, D.: Hairy-cell leukaemia: evidence for the existence of a spectrum of functional characteristics. Brit. J. Haemat., 38:161–170, 1978.

17. Jansen, J., Schuit, H.R.E., van Zwet Th.L., Meijer, C.J.L.M., and Hijmans, W.: Hairy-cell leukaemia: A B-lymphocytic disorder. Brit. J. Haematol., 42:21–34, 1979.

18. Burns, G.F., Cawley, J.C., Barker, C.R., Goldstone, A.H., and Hayhoe, F.G.J.: New evidence relating to the nature and origin of the hairy cells of leukemic reticuloendotheliosis. Brit. J. Haemat., 36:71–84, 1977.

19. Saxon, A., Stevens, R.H., and Golde, D.W.: T-lymphocyte variant of hairy-cell leukemia. Ann. Intern. Medic., 88:323–326, 1978.

20. Cawley, J.C., Burns, G.F., Nash, T.A., Higgy, K.E., Child, J.A., and Roberts B.E.: Hairy-cell leukemia with T-cell features. Blood, 51:61–69, 1978.

21. Jansen, J., Schuit, H.R.E., Schreuder, G.M.Th., Muller, H.P., and Meijer

C.J.L.M.: Distinct subtype within the spectrum of hairy-cell leukemia. Blood, 54:459–467, 1979.

22. Jansen, J., Meijer, C.J.L.M., van der Valk P., de Bruijn, W.C., Leijh, P.C.J., den Ottolander, G.J., and van Furth, R.: Phagocytic potential of hairy cells. Scand. J. Haematol., 23:69–79, 1979.

23. Reyes, F., Gourdin, M.F., Farcet, J.P., Dreyfus, B., and Breton-Gorius, J.: Synthesis of a peroxidase activity by cells of hairy-cell leukemia: a study by ultrastructural cytochemistry. Blood, 52:537–549, 1978.

24. Lennert, K.: Malignant lymphomas other than Hodgkin's disease. Springer Verlag; Berlin-Heidelberg-New York, 1978.

25. Vessière-Louveaux, M.Y.R., Hijmans, W., and Schuit, H.R.E.: Multiple heavy-chain determinants on the membrane of the small lymphocytes in blood (to be published).

37. THE PROGNOSTIC RELEVANCE OF LEUKEMIC CELL TYPING IN ACUTE LYMPHOBLASTIC LEUKEMIA

R. WILLEMZE

INTRODUCTION

For a number of patients with acute lymphoblastic leukemia (ALL), mainly children, current treatment regimens may be adequate, but a large proportion still dies from the disease within a few years.

Clinicians have long suspected that ALL represents a heterogenous group of diseases differing as to certain clinical and hematological findings, cytological and cytochemical characteristics of the malignant cells, and prognosis. The discovery of a sign or symptom with prognostic value at the time of diagnosis would allow the selection of a group of bad-risk patients for therapy with alternative treatment schedules. In this context, a variety of prognostic signs and symptoms have been described during the last ten years. However, heterogeneity persisted within each group of patients.

This paper deals with several aspects of the clinical staging, the cytological and cytochemical characteristics of the blast cells, and the immunological typing of these cells in relation to each other and to the prognosis of patients with ALL.

CLASSIFICATIONS OF ALL (Table 1)

Clinical criteria

Traditionally, the clinical staging of the disease has been used for classification.

Age has been found to be an important determinant of survival time (Figure 1). The overall median survival time of children up to 14 or 15 years of age treated on the basis of the ALL protocols of the Dutch Childhood Leukaemia Study Group (S.N.W.L.K.), is 4 to 5 years (1) compared with 2 years for 75 adolescent and adult patients with ALL treated at the Nijmegen (Prof. C. Haanen) and Leiden University Hospitals during recent years (2, 3). Within the children's group, patients under 2 years and over 9 years of age appear to have an adverse prognosis, and within the adult group,

J.G. van den Tweel et al. (eds.), Malignant Lymphoproliferative Diseases, 481–487.
All rights reserved.
Copyright © 1980 by Martinus Nijhoff Publishers bv, The Hague/Boston/London.

Table 1. Various approaches to the classification of acute lymphatic leukemia.

According to clinical criteria:
   age
   leukocyte and blast cell or thrombocyte counts enlargement of spleen, liver,
   or lymph nodes extramedullary involvement
According to cytological criteria:
   cytochemical criteria (P.A.S., acid phosphatase, esterase, etc.)
   cell size, nucleoli
According to immunological criteria:
   B, T, and non-B, non-T cell types.

patients over 40 years at the time of diagnosis a significantly worse one
(4, 5).

A variety of clinical signs including enlargement of lymph nodes, liver,
and spleen, the presence of a mediastinal mass, involvement of testes and/or
meninges, low initial leukocyte and thrombocyte counts, have been found to

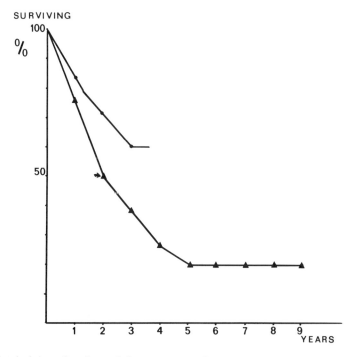

Figure 1. Survival time after diagnosis for two groups of ALL patients.
●—● survival curve of 215 children treated according to ALL protocol II of the Dutch
Childhood Leukaemia Study Group (1973–1977);
■—■ survival curve of 75 adolescent and adult patients treated at the Nijmegen and
Leiden University Hospitals (1970–1977).

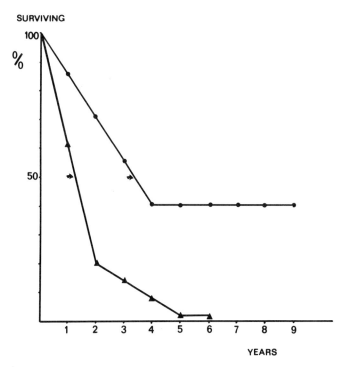

Figure 2. Survival time after diagnosis for adult patients with ALL treated at the Nijmegen and Leiden University Hospitals.
●—● survival curve of patients with initial leukocyte counts lower than $20 \times 10^9/1$;
■—■ survival curve of patients with initial leukocyte counts higher than $20 \times 10^9/1$.

be important for the prediction of the duration of the first remission and survival times.

Much attention has been given to the initial leukocyte count and the presence of a mediastinal mass. A mediastinal mass at the time of dignosis has been reported in 10–15% of the children with ALL, and appears to be associated with a short duration of remissions and median survival times of approximately one year (6). The initial leukocyte count or blast-cell count is important in that patients with initial cell levels of between 20 and $100 \times 10^9/1$ in the blood have a worse prognosis than patients with lower malignant cells. But both groups do substantially better than the group with cell numbers over $100 \times 10^9/1$, although there is no difference in the percentage of patients in the 3 groups who achieve a complete remission (6).

In adult patients the initial leukocyte count also appears to be predictive for the length of the first remission and the survival time (Figure 2). Although the prognostic value of hepato-splenomegaly has been reported for children as well as adults, we found no relationship in our series of adult patients (5, 7).

Cytological criteria

Cytomorphological characteristics of the blast cells at the time of diagnosis have been reported to be important for the patient's prognosis. The degree of positivity of the periodic-acid Schiff (PAS) reaction of the bone marrow lymphoblasts has been found to have predictive value in that strong positivity was associated with an increased duration of remission and survival time. In recent studies, however, PAS positivity did not appear to correlate very well with prognosis (8).

Several authors have tried to distinguish distinct cytological subclasses of ALL. Mathé et al. (9) distinguished 5 cell types in ALL, i.e. the microlymphoblastic, prolymphocytic, macrolymphoblastic, prolymphoblastic, and immunoblastic types, in order of increasingly unfavorable prognosis, and independent of other well-known factors such as age and tumor-load. Bennett et al. (10) could identify only three of these subclasses of lymphoblasts, and Flandrin et al. (11) also distinguished three classes of malignant cells in ALL. All authors claim that their classifications correlate well with prognosis in large groups of patients (11).

Use of the size of the lymphoblasts as a prognostic criterion has led to conflicting results. Pantazopoulos and Sinks (12) found a good prognosis for patients with less than 10% large cells, but Murphy et al. (13) were unable to confirm these findings. Necheles et al. (14), who used a computer-assisted automated microscope, concluded that a combination of the percentage of large lymphoblasts and the percentage of cells with no visible cytoplasm, may have prognostic relevance. Lee et al. (15) analyzed several features and found that the lower the percentage of large cells and the lower the number of nucleoli per cell, the longer the duration of remission and survival time. They reported these features to be independent of age and leukocyte count at diagnosis.

As shown recently, the percentage of cells with nuclear convolutions is not a prognostically important feature (16). The French-American-British Cooperative Group proposed that ALL be divided into 3 subgroups, L_1, L_2, and L_3, on the basis of cytological features. No prognostic value has been reported so far, however.

The disadvantage of all of these cytological classifications of blast cells in ALL is that most of the methods have not proved to be reproducible for other investigators.

Immunological criteria

Recently, considerable attention has been focussed on the surface characteristics of the leukemic cells, and a distinction has been made between ALL with T-cell, B-cell, or non-T-, non-B-cell characteristics (6, 18). The non-T-, non-B-cell group has been subdivided into two types, the majority reacting with a specific anti-ALL serum (called common ALL) in children, the remainder, called the null cell subtype, being nonreactive with this serum.

Roughly 2–5% of these types of ALL, including Burkitt's type, are detected by B-cell antisera, and approximately 20% have T-cell characteristics, the others lacking B- or T-cell markers. It is apparent that this latter group is even more heterogenous, since it presumably includes pre-B and pre-T cells. The percentages may vary, depending on the tests used, but they probably also hold for the adult patients with ALL (Table 2) (19). Blast cells satisfying B-cell criteria comprise Burkitt's type acute leukemia and the leukemias with cytological features suggestive of poorly differentiated lymphocytic lymphoma.

In children the duration of the first remission and the survival time in T-cell type ALL are significantly shorter than in non-T-cell ALL (4, 6, 18). In adults, however, conflicting data have been reported on the length of the first remission and survival time (Table 3) (18, 19).

No differences have been found between the percentages of patients achieving complete remission in the T-cell and non-T-cell groups.

CORRELATIONS BETWEEN CLINICAL, CYTOLOGICAL, AND IMMUNOLOGICAL CRITERIA

Correlations have been reported between clinical presentation, cytological characteristics, and immunological factors. The ALL with T-cell characteristics appears to be associated with tumoral presentation of the disease more often than the non-B-, non-T-cell type is (6, 18). A mediastinal mass is seen in children in 50–80% of the T-cell group as against approximately 5% of the non-B-, non-T-cell type of ALL. It has been suggested that this latter group represents the pre-T-cell variant.

Table 2. Results of blast-cell typing of adult ALL patients (n = 15) treated at the Leiden University Hospital (1976–1978)*

B-cell type	1
T-cell type	5
Non-B, non-T-cell type	9

*Studies performed by G.M.Th. Schreuder (Dept. of Immunohematology (Prof. J.J. van Rood)). B-cells defined by the presence of surface immunoglobulins and anti-Ia sera; T-cells defined by E-rosette method and anti-T cell serum (Merieux).

Table 3. Clinical characteristics of the adult ALL patients treated at the Leiden University Hospital (1976–1978), according to blast-cell typing.

	T-cell type	*Non-T, non-B cell type*
No. of patients	5	9
Age (median)	20 years	21 years
Initial leukocyte count (median)	$110 \times 10^9/1$	$9 \times 10^9/1$
Mediastinal involvement	4 of 5	0 of 9
Complete remission	all	all
Duration of remission	7 to 17 months	3 to 33 months
Survival time	18 to 28 months	6 to 35 months

A high initial leukocyte count is found in the majority of the cases of T-cell type ALL. However, in children with initial leukocyte counts higher than $100 \times 10^9/1$, the T-cell and non-B-, non-T-cell variants are equally distributed, whereas there are three times more cases of non-B-, non-T-cell than of T-cell ALL among patients with initial leukocyte counts lying higher than $20 \times 10^9/1$ (6).

Belpomme, Mathé and Davies reported a relationship between their cytological classification of ALL and the immunological surface characteristics of these cells (20). The acid phosphatase stain is positive in the majority of the T-cell blasts and negative in almost all other ALL variants (21).

The reason for the lack of predictive value of some of the parameters in adults may be the (overall) worse treatment results in adults rather than the existence of a different type of ALL, although there is evidence that the non-T-cell type of ALL in adults represents a more heterogenous group than the corresponding type in children.

In conclusion it may be said that although many problems remain to be resolved in the field of cell-membrane markers, it is apparent that this work is the first serious attempt to distinguish separate groups of ALL on the basis of a patholophysiologic feature. The question of whether the membrane phenotype of the leukemic cells represents an important prognostic factor, independent of the well-known and more easily obtainable clinical risk factors, is still unsettled. The initial attempts to intensify the treatment of bad-risk ALL children (22) did not improve the duration or remission and the survival time, and it seems probable that different, rather than more intensive, therapy schedules are needed for the successful treatment of these patients.

REFERENCES

1. Van der Does-van den Berg, A. (Stichting Nederlandse Werkgroep Leukemie bij kinderen (SNWLK)): Resultaten van behandeling van acute lymfatische leukemie bij kinderen in Nederland (1965–1976). In: Het medisch jaar 1978, p. 181–194, Scheltema en Holkema, Utrecht, Bohn, 1978.

2. Willemze, R., Hillen, H., Hartgrink-Groeneveld, C.A. et al.: Treatment of acute lymphoblastic leukemia in adolescents and adults. Blood, 46:823–834, 1975.
3. Willemze, R., Hillen, H., and den Ottolander, G.J. et al.: Acute lymphatische leukaemie bij adolescenten en volwassenen. Ned. Tijdschr. Geneesk., in press.
4. Frei, E., and Sallan, S.E.: Acute lymphoblastic leukemia: treatment. Cancer, 42:828–838, 1978.
5. Ruggero, D., Baccarani, M., and Gobbi, M. et al.: Adult acute lymphoblastic leukaemia. Study of 32 patients and analysis of prognostic factors. Scand. J. Haematol. 22:154–164, 1979.
6. Chessells, J.M., Hardisty, R.M., and Rapson, N.T. et al.: Acute lymphoblastic leukaemia in children: classification and prognosis. Lancet II: 1307–1309, 1977.
7. Nijmegen and Leiden series of adult A.L.L. patients.
8. Shaw, M.T.: Lack of prognostic value of the periodic Acid Schiff Reaction and blast cell size in childhood acute lymphocytic leukemia. Amer. J. Hematol., 2:237–243, 1977.
9. Mathè, G., Pouillart, P., and Sterescu, M. et al.: Subdivision of classical varieties of acute leukemia. Correlation with prognosis and cure expentancy. Eur. J. Clin. Biol. Res., 16:554–560, 1971.
10. Bennett, J.M., Klemperer, M.R., and Segel, G.B.: Survival prediction based on morphology of lymphoblasts. Rec. Res. Cancer Res., 43:23–27, 1973.
11. Flandrin, G ., Bernard, J.: Cytological classification of acute leukemias. A survey of 1400 cases. Blood Cells, 1:7–15, 1975.
12. Pantazopoulos, N., and Sinks, L.F.: Morphological criteria for prognostication of acute lymphoblastic leukemia. Brit. J. Haematol., 27:25–30, 1974.
13. Murphy, S.B., Borella, L., and Sen. L. et al.: Lack of correlation of lymphoblast cell size with presence of T-cell markers or with outcome of chilhood acute lymphoblastic leukaemia. Brit. J. Haematol., 31:95–101, 1975.
14. Necheles, T.F., Brenner, J.F., and Fristensky, R. et al.: The computer-assisted morphological classification of acute leukemia. I. Preliminary results. Biomedicine (Exp.), 25:241–244, 1976.
15. Lee, S.L., Kopel, S., and Glidewell, O.: Cytomorphological determinants of prognosis in acute lymphoblastic leukemia in children. Sem. Oncol., 3:209–217, 1976.
16. Pangalis, G.A., Nathwani, B.N., and Rappaport, H. et al.: Acute lymphoblastic leukemia: the significance of nuclear convolutions. Cancer, 43:551–557, 1979.
17. Bennett, J.M., Catovsky, D., and Daniel, M.T. et al.: Proposals of the classification of the acute leukaemias. Brit. J. Haematol., 33:451–458, 1976.
18. Brouet, J.C., and Seligmann, M.: The immunological classification of acute lymphoblastic leukemias. Cancer, 42:817–827, 1978.
19. Bitran, J.D.: Prognostic value of immunologic markers in adults with acute lymphoblastic leukemia. New Engl. J. Med., 299:1317, 1978.
20. Belpomme, D., Mathé G., Davies, A.J.S.: Clinical significance and prognostic value of the T-B immunological classification of human primary acute lymphoid leukemias. Lancet, I:557–558, 1977.
21. Catovsky, D., Cherchi, M., and Greaves, M.F. et al.: Acid-phosphatase reaction in acute lymphoblastic leukaemia. Lancet, I:749–751, 1978.
22. Aur, R., Simone, J., and Hustu, O. et al.: Multiple combination therapy for childhood acute lymphocytic leukemia (A.L.L.). Blood, 52(S1):238, 1978.

38. THE SIGNIFICANCE OF FINE-NEEDLE ASPIRATION CYTOLOGY FOR THE DIAGNOSIS AND TREATMENT OF MALIGNANT LYMPHOMAS

P. LOPES CARDOZO

INTRODUCTION

Fine-needle aspiration biopsy of a palpable nodule thought to be a lymph node, is a minor procedure. On request, the cytologist can give a preliminary answer well within an hour if he makes use of an instant Giemsa stain (less than 5 minutes).

Because of the ease of the procedure and the reliability of the results in experienced hands the lymph-node aspiration biopsy has become a "first-visit method" in some clinics. It is also the most subtle tool for the demonstration of recurrence.

Obviously, it is not always certain that the target is actually a lymph node. The cytologist may encounter salivary gland lesions, cysts, material from the thyroid, Warthin's (Albrechts-Artz's) tumor, Schmincke-Regaud's tumor, etc. Furthermore a benign lymph node may be found instead of a lymphoma, and surgical biopsy may not be rendered necessary. It is not within the scope of this subject to enter into the differential diagnosis of benign processes, such as bacterial infections, viral infections, toxoplasma, tuberculosis, or simple hyperplasia. A fairly good (lymph-node) cytologist can distinguish such nodes from lymphomas. It is, however, recommended that in such cases the aspirated material remaining in the syringe be handed over to the bacteriologist, the parasitologist, the serologist, and/or the virologist, for confirmation.

In cases of metastatic nonlymphomatous malignancy, surgical biopsy may be rendered superfluous by the cytological investigation. For lymphoma the situation is different. In leukemic cases, where blood and bone-marrow films and the clinical picture are sufficient to establish the diagnosis, histology is usually not requested by the hematologist. Otherwise, surgical biopsy and histological examination are required for confirmation of the cytologist's diagnosis in each new patient. This is reasonable, because the lesion does not regress spontaneously and other nonsurgical methods can only produce indirect support for the cytologist's grave diagnosis of Hodgkin's disease and non-Hodgkin's lymphoma.

J.G. van den Tweel et al. (eds.), Malignant Lymphoproliferative Diseases, 489–502.
All rights reserved.
Copyright © 1980 by Martinus Nijhoff Publishers bv, The Hague/Boston/London.

Nevertheless, modern histology in lymphoma is based mainly on cytological features. Because the cytologist is in a better position to evaluate the cells as such, our axiom is, broadly speaking, not only that the cytologist's diagnosis should be supported by a histological diagnosis, but also that the reverse should be stipulated (provided one has a good lymph-node cytologist).

TECHNIQUE

The needle

The needles should be extremely fine, with a 0.6–0.7 mm outer diameter (23–22 gauge) and a short and thin bevel. The length of the needle is chosen in accordance with the depth required. Usually, 5 cm or even shorter will do for a palpable target. Sometimes a longer needle, e.g. 15 cm, is needed for transabdominal or intrapelvic punctures under fluoroscopic monitoring in lymph nodes visualized by lymphadenography.

The syringe (Figure 1)

Although a cytological diagnosis can sometimes be reached from a poor smear made at a puncture performed with an ordinary syringe, it is a basic rule

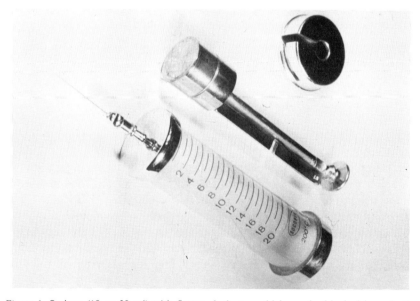

Figure 1. Syringe (10 or 20 ml) with flattened plunger which can be blocked in aspiration position.

always to use equipment providing automatic suction during the puncture. This can be achieved in two ways: many cytologists use the Franzén or Stormby technique (in which case a puncture should usually be done three times in one session), but we recommend the use of a 10ml or a 20ml Record® syringe with a flattened and blockable plunger. (The blocking lamella can be made and the plunger flattened by hand in any hospital with a technical service; this makes the syringes inexpensive and easily available.)

Procedure

The thumb and index finger of the left hand are used for fixation (Figure 2). If the target is highly movable, the middle finger is placed behind the lump for additional support. The right hand guides the needle, which is held like a pencil. The needle must be stabbed through the skin; the quicker this is done, the less pain is felt. The skin and subcutis are usually not anesthetized; otherwise 2% lidocaine® is used.

We prefer to maintain the suction during withdrawal of the needle to prevent any spillage of material in the needle tract.

Directly after the puncture, the spot is firmly pressed with a piece of cotton wool by either an assistant or the patient for about 5 minutes. Meanwhile, the cytologist or the cytotechnologist prepares the smears in the same

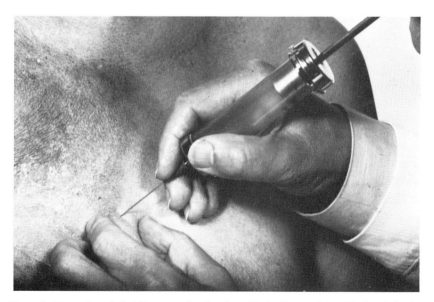

Figure 2. The syringe is held between the thumb and index finger of the right hand, the tips of the index and middle fingers guiding the needle. The wrist, hand, and finger are kept relaxed and flexible, as for writing.

way as for bone-marrow smears or by spreading the cells by repeated force-ful blowing over the slide with the syringe.

With the above-described technique the change of metastatic spread along the needle tract can be neglected (von Schreeb et al. (10)).

The cytologist of course must be very familiar with the cytology of the target organ, i.e., the lymph node, and the hematocytological picture, and have some knowledge of the clinical indications and implications.

The stain

The best stain for all kinds of fine-needle aspiration cytology is the (May-Grünwald) Giemsa (MGG) stain (or some other Romanowsky stain). The wealth of cytoplasmic detail given by this stain, as well as the simplicity of the method, its quickness, air-drying (allowing e.g. the use of cytochemical stains), low costs, flexibility, etc., are major advantages.

MAIN CYTOLOGICAL PATTERNS AND FEATURES OF SMEARS IN (1,023) LYMPHOMA CASES (HODGKIN'S AND NON-HODGKINS'S LYMPHOMA)

MATERIAL

Our material comprises 1,023 cases of primary malignant lymphoma.

A.   Of these, about a half (523) are cases of Hodgkin's disease, which has always been a favorite subject of European cytologists. Cytologists are in a particularly good position to establish this diagnosis at the earliest possible stage, because both the Hodgkin's and Reed-Sternberg giant cells are very characteristic and easy to find in the MGG-stained smears. Moreover, it is not difficult to distinguish three of the types i.e., lymphocyte predominance (LP), mixed-cellularity (MC), and the lymphocyte depletion (LD). More skill is needed to diagnose the Lukes' nodular sclerosis (NS) type, but the ex-perienced needle-aspiration cytologist often recognizes the greater resis-tance during the performance of the puncture, and will find the lacunar cells (Figure 3).

In our department the results of cytology and histology do not differ significantly. Especially in the early cases, cytology is very effective. In our experience the number of discrepancies between the cytological and his-tological diagnosis is very low.

B.   The *main* cytological patterns in non-Hodgkin's lymphoma (NHL) (generally divided into two malignancy groups, one low-grade (I–IV) and the other high-grade (V–VIII):

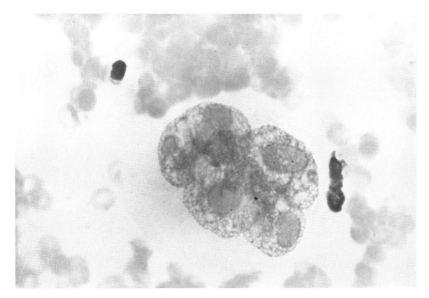

Figure 3. Cytological picture of lymph node in Hodgkin's disease (NS type). A Reed-Sternberg giant cell (lacunar cell) with reticular chromatin and giant blue nucleoli. The cytoplasm is abundant and transparent, containing only a few vacuoles.

LOW-GRADE MALIGNANT NON-HODGKIN'S LYMPHOMA

I. *Lymphocytic types*

1) Chronic lymphocytic leukemia (CLL) (both the B-cell and the T-cell (1–2%) types). Suspicion of the T-cell type of chronic lymphocytic leukemia may be raised by the presence of cells with more clefts (although the surface is not as complex and deeply indented as in Sézary's cells) and from a unipolarly positive acid phosphatase stain (situated in the Golgi apparatus). Sometimes there is azurophilic granulation suggesting a T-cell origin.
2) Prolymphocytic leukemia, which is both a cytological and a clinical entity, characterized by massive splenomegaly, small lymph nodes and a high lymphocytic blood count, as described by Galton and Dacie (2) and accepted by European hematologists.
3) Special cell types of "lymphocytic lymphoma" are:
(a) Hairy cell leukemia
(b) Mucosis fungoides and Sézary's lymphoma.

N.B. The convoluted-cell type of lymphoma does not belong to the low-grade malignant group. Because this is a highly malignant T-cell type, we have listed it under ALL (see below).

II. *Centrocytic lymphomas*

Here we have perhaps two subtypes:

1) The least dedifferentiated type, with coarse marbled chromatin and inconspicuous nucleoli (perhaps corresponding with some of Lukes' small cleaved cells). In smears, several cells show marked identation (Figure 4). 2) The "blastic" type of the centrocyte (from the hematologist's point of view), with densely granular or still more dedifferentiated, even a densely reticular chromatin and a single slightly pronounced central nucleolus. This second type of centrocyte has a polygonal, slightly anisokaryotic and slightly clefted (jagged, not concave) nucleus. These nuclear contours may give them a mosaic appearance. This type which was shown both in sections and in smears by Schwarze and Lennert at the Weimar Congress of the E.F.C.S. (7a), possibly corresponds with Lukes's large cleaved cells.

There is a gradual transition from this type to the true centroblastic cells. This accounts for a gray zone in which some pathologists already classify a

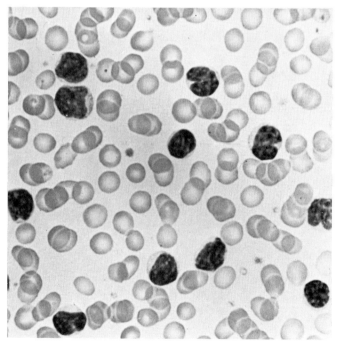

Figure 4. Centrocytoma with leukemic blood film, showing small cleaved cells with marbled chromatin.

lesion as centroblastic, whereas the cytologist still calls this a centrocytoma.

III. *Centrocytic/centroblastic lymphomas*

The bulk of the cases represent with a follicular pattern. In these CC/CB lymphomas one finds many true (large) centroblasts with a diameter of 12–14 μ, two or three marginal nucleoli, and a narrow rim of blue cytoplasm. They are mixed together with the centrocytes, which still dominate the field. The nuclear pattern is therefore somewhat anisokaryotic and even more so because some macrophages are often found as well.

IV. *Immunocytoma*

Immunocytoma is not a final diagnosis but a morphological categorial classification (Figures 5 and 6). Supportive data must be obtained biochemically, sometimes virologically, immunochemically (or even topographically

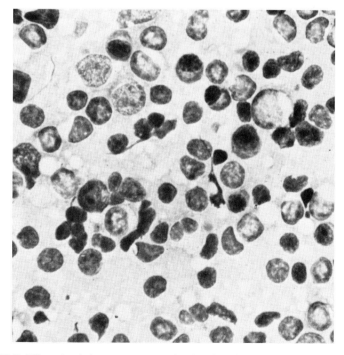

Figure 5. Well-differentiated immunocytoma, showing lymphocytes, prolymphocytes, an exceptional centroblast, plasma cells, and transitional cells between plasma cells and immunoblasts.

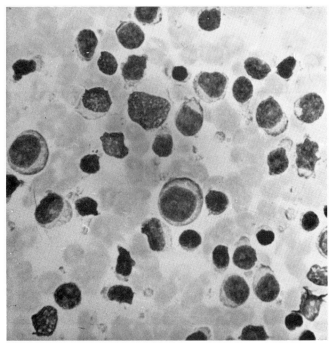

Figure 6. Polymorphous ("pleomorphic") immunocytoma. Besides the elements of the immunocytoma, one sees more primitive cells and the large true immunoblasts. In the terminal stage the immunoblasts may replace all other cell types, leading to a true immunoblastoma.

and geographically, as for Mediterranean lymphoma) to arrive at a precise diagnosis. In some cases we do not use the term immunocytoma and immediately jump to a final diagnosis, e.g., in obvious cases of myeloma or macroglobulinemia, diagnosed from material obtained by bone-marrow aspiration biopsy performed because of a clinically established paraproteinemia.

THE HIGH-GRADE MALIGNANT GROUP OF NHL

The highly malignant lymphomas, a category comprising about 30% of all NHL, comprise the "lymphoblastic", centroblastic, and immunoblastic lymphomas. These tumors always have a fine reticular chromatin structure and are rich in mitotic figures, although especially the prophases are not always recognized easily by the cytologically inexperienced morphologist. Sometimes one also finds numerous pairs of "twin cells", indicating a moderate anisokaryosis associated with fast growth.

V. Lymphoblastic lymphomas

The term *lymphoblast* is used in two cases:

For Burkitt's (type) tumor

Here we use not only a Giemsa and a PAS stain, but also an oil-red O stain. One also has to find macrophages in the smear among the small transformed and often (not always) vacuolized, nicely round "lymphoblasts" with a diameter of 8–10 μ (Figure 7). These blast cells can have either one central nucleolus or two peripheral nucleoli. Perhaps they could better be called small-type centroblasts; in Lukes' classification they represent small noncleaved follicular center cell lymphoma.

For acute lymphocytic leukemias (ALL)

The term lymphoblast, which is so generally accepted in hematology, now has little application in lymphoma pathology. There is a considerable overlap here, because broadly speaking the diagnosis ALL is made from the blood film and the bone-marrow and lymphnode histology is not requested.

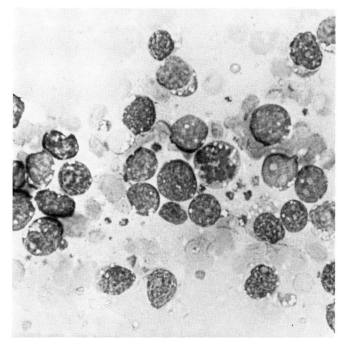

Figure 7. A true Burkitt's lymphoma from Africa. Small noncleaved nuclei, some with peripherally situated nucleoli (small type of centroblast). The cytoplasm often has vacuoles. Some of these vacuoles may contain neutral fat. Some macrophages are usually found.

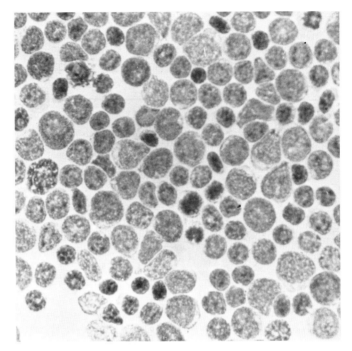

Figure 8. T-cell lymphoma of the convoluted type, showing mitotic figures, and many twin cells. The nuclei of the large cells have irregular outlines. Some of the cells have a "monocytoid" appearance.

In most cases of ALL the cell type is one of the accepted NH cell types: centroblasts, Burkitt's type "blasts", and immunoblasts. A special blastic cell type is Lukes' convoluted type (Figure 8).

VI. *Centroblastoma*

The term centroblast is perhaps a bit more restricted than Lukes' large noncleaved cell. Centroblasts are a well-defined blastic cell type (Figure 9). They are slightly enlarged cells, 12–14 μ in diameter. Centroblasts have a narrow monotonous strongly basophilic rim of cytoplasm which may contain some small vacuoles. The densely reticular chromatin is set in a round or ellipsoid but nearly round nuclear membrane to which two or three and sometimes four prominent but moderately enlarged nucleoli are attached. Cytochemically, the centroblast is a rather inert cell which occasionally shows some PAS-positivity.

If several of these cells are present, usually together with many cytologically related but less well-defined transformed lymphocytes, the diagnosis

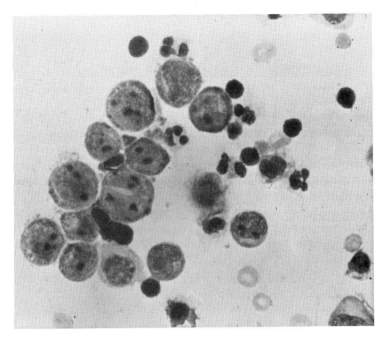

Figure 9. Large noncleaved cells (centroblasts) in a terminal stage of Mediterranean lymphoma.

is *centroblastoma*, which is equivalent to Lukes' tumor of the large non-leaved cell type.

VII. *Immunoblastoma*

The third malignant tumor in this group is derived from the immunoblast. When this is the dominant cell type, the tumor is called an immunoblastoma (immunoblastic sarcoma). These cells are often distinctly larger than the centroblasts. They may have one large central nucleolus or two to four usually paracentrally dispersed medium-sized nucleoli. Apart from the nucleolar pattern and the often larger cell size, the immunoblast usually has a clear para- or perinuclear zone, whereas the outer zone of the cytoplasm is generally strongly basophilic. Although the majority of the immunoblastomas have B-cell characteristics, a few are immunoblasts with T-cell features and still others are of the null-cell type.

VIII. *T-zone lymphoma*

Finally, we must mention the *T-zone lymphoma* (Lennert). Our cases included a mixture of a small cell type (8 μ) and a "blastic" type (14–16 μ). The small cells have either a marbled or a coarse and dense chromatin pattern.

The large blastic cell type has an often unilaterally indented or even a lobulated nuclear outline. This is quite different from the firm round outline of the centroblast.

In the highly dedifferentiated ("poorly differentiated") T-zone lymphoma we found many mitoses and a pronounced anisokaryosis. There were many twin cells in these cases. Twin cells are pairs of cells lying rather close together and having roughly the same size and shape. In the large blastic T cells the nucleoli were often situated centrally and not peripherally.

Although *histio(cytic) sarcoma* is not considered to belong to the malignant lymphomas, there is reason to mention it here. In the first place, cases of this kind, including Scott and Robb-Smith's histiocytic medullary reticulosis (8), are clinically treated as lymphomas. More important still are cases like those of Skoog and Feagler (9), in which the cell type started as true "lymphoblastic", but gradually transformed into a true histiocytic type with extensive phagocytosis.

Characterized by its cytological features, histio(cytic) sarcoma is of monocytic origin and thus is not a true NHL. This applies to its cytological MGG patterns, its phagocytic properties, and the electron-microscopical appearance. The α-naphthyl-acetate or -butyrate stain is often positive together with the acid phosphatase stain.

After MGG staining the cells are large with an ovoid or bean-shaped nucleus. Chromatin is densely (granulo) reticular. Generally, two to three usually medium-sized nucleoli are visible. Sometimes there are three or four nucleated ellipsoid giant cells with nuclei of the same size and hsape as those of the mononuclear tumor cells. When we find positive bone-marrow smears of leukemic blood film, we prefer to apply the refined bone marrow histology of Burkhardt (1), although the ordinary HE technique is also advocated by many histopathologists using the Yamshidi needle.

TERMINOLOGY PROBLEMS

It is difficult to compare our results with the histological findings in our material, because most pathologists in the Netherlands still use Rappaport's classification. For instance, we had many cases where our cytological diagnosis was (polymorphous) immunocytoma, whereas the histologist labeled the same lymphosarcoma and reticulosarcoma. Also we had histological reports reading reticulosarcoma in cases we diagnosed as histiosarcoma with leukemic blood film and bone marrow involvement. So too with Burkitt's type lymphoma, where the histologist noted lymphosarcoma. Other histological diagnoses which were difficult to compare were "reticulosis", followed or preceded by lymphosarcoma; and "leukemia" or "reticulosarcoma", which we termed acute lymphatic leukemia or acute myeloid leukemia.

However, a few points are beyond doubt. Once a (hemato) cytologist is familiar with lymph-node cytology and has the opportunity to use the Giemsa stain *routinely*, he is as safe as a histologist in making unequivocal diagnosis of malignancy. If one hesitates it is never a highly malignant case, and one will ask for a blood film and sometimes a bone-marrow smear. Also, when clinical doubt remains, one will repeat the aspiration after some weeks. If the problem is not solved within a month, one may ask for a surgical biopsy, but this means that the clinical observation and follow-up of the node are sacrified. If surgical biopsy is done routinely, many imprint smears must be made from the excised node before fixation. This is necessary because:

1) the cytology may reach a definite diagnosis;
2) the cytology can provide additional information; and
3) the cytology needs the material for comparison with future needle biopsies.

It is essential to distinguish some non-Hodgkin's lymphomas from other small-cell malignancies, particularly oat-cell and other small-cell anaplastic carcinomas. A unique feature of several oat-cell carcinomas is the wealth of minute nuclear off-springs. This very characteristic phenomenon is not seen in lymphomas. Moreover, in oat-cell carcinoma of the lung nucleoli are hardly visible or more often not visible at all, which is not the case in most lymphomas. Cytochemistry, particularly with use of, for instance, peroxiase staining or the Sudan black B, DOPA, and/or Schmorl stain may be helpful for the differential diagnosis in such cases.

DISCUSSION

The clinical use of lymph-node cytology, when performed with the Giemsa (Wright) stain and in the hands of a cytologist who is familiar with hematocytology, is an almost ideal method. Its usefulness in daily routine is already evident from the following eight points:

1) Cytology monitors diagnoses of would-be lymphomas, such as cysts, lipomas, atheromas, hernias, diseases of the salivary glands, etc.
2) Cytology recognizes reactive processes of the lymph-nodes and can provide material for microbiological, cytochemical, and other purposes.
3) In expert hands cytology is as reliable as histology for the recognition of metastatic malignancy.
4) Cytology recognizes the cell types of which a malignant lymphoma is composed. Since the Kiel and Lukes classifications of lymphomas are based on exactly these cell types (preferably stained with a Romanowsky stain, such as Giemsa), these are good classifications for cytologists to adopt, which would also promote comparability of results.

5) The cytologist can biopsy three and more sites at a time, thus contributing quickly and substantially to the staging of the tumor.
6) Cytology is the least invasive method to obtain conclusive evidence of recurrence of the tumor at an early stage.

REFERENCES

1. Burkhardt, R.: Bone marrow and bone tissue. Color atlas of clinical histopathology, Springer Verlag, Berlin, Heiderlberg, New York, 1971.
2. Galton, D.A.G., and Dacie, J.V.: Classification of the acute leukaemias. Blood cells 1, pp. 17–24, Springer-Verlag, Berlin, Heidelberg, New York, 1975.
3. Lennert, K.: Malignant lymphomas. Springer Verlag, Berlin, Heidelberg, New York, 1978.
4. Lopes Cardozo, P.: De cytologische diagnostiek van de ziekte van Kahler. Ned. Tijdschrift v. Geneesk., 103 :778–785, 1959.
5. Lopes Cardozo, P.: The cytological diagnosis of lymph node aspirations. Acta Ctyol., 8:194–205, 1974.
6. Lopes Cardozo, P.: An atlas of clinical cytology. Heinemann, London, Lippincott, Philadelphia, Chemie Verlag, Weinheim, 1976.
7. Mandema, E.: Over het multipel myeloom, het solitaire plasmacytoom en de macroglobulinaemia. Thesis, Groningen, 1956.
7a. Schwarze, E.-W., und Lennert, K.: Histologie und Zytologie der non-Hodgkin Lymphome. Vorlesung, 6th European Congress of Cytology, Weimar, 1976.
8. Scott, R.B., and Robb-Smith, A.H.T.: Histiocytic Medullary Reticulosis. Lancet, II:194–198, 1939.
9. Skoog, D.P., and Feagler, J.R.: T Cell Acute Leukaemia, terminating as malignant histiocytosis. Am. J. Med., 64:678–682, 1978.
10. Von Schreeb, T., Arner, D., Skovsted, G. and Wikstand, N.: Renal carcinoma. Is there a risk of spreading tumour cells in diagnostic puncture? Scand. J. Urol. Nephrol., 1:270–276, 1967.

INDEX

Abnormal immune proliferations 200
Acid α-naphythyl acetate esterase 141
Acid nonspecific esterase 16, 317
Acid nonspecific α-naphythyl acetate
  esterase 138
Acid phospatase 138, 143
  tartrate-resistant 138, 144
Acute lymphoblastic leukaemia 288,
  481, 499
  common antigen (CALLA) 13, 42
  cytological criteria 484
  immunological criteria 184
  subtypes
    non-B, non-T-cell type 144, 193
    null cell type 206, 320
    pre-B-cell type 320
    T-cell type 206, 320, 485
  survival time 482
Acute myeloid leukaemia 253
Aggregated IgG 93
Alkaline phospatase 138, 145
Alloantigens
  in helper cells 52, 77
  in suppressor cells 52, 77
Alpha l-antitrypsin 408
Alpha-chain disease 202, 251
Alpha l-chymotrypsin 408
Alpha-naphthyl acetate esterase 140
Amyloidosis (primary) 249, 261
Anaplastic lymphoid neoplasms 259
Angioimmunoblastic lymphadenopathy
  273
Anomalous staining (immunoperoxidase)
  122, 125
Antibody dependent cell cytotoxicity
  (see also Killer cells) 40, 92
Antigenic stimulation 18
Anti-idiotype antibodies 97, 287
Antisera
  anti Ia sera 485
  anti TH₁ sera 98
  in immunoperoxidase 115
  in fluorescence studies 136
Ataxia telangiectasia 81

B-cell (see also Pre-B-cells) 89, 119,
  181, 182, 282
  activation 79
  antigen-dependent differentiation 18
  antisera 485
  associated antigens, human 98
  determined stem cells 17
  differentiation 17, 31, 33
  immature types 17
  immunoblasts 9, 24
  lymphoblasts 38
  lymphocytes 13
  of the follicular center 91
  physiology 250
  regions 65, 200, 216
  subsets
    B1 17
    B2 18
  transformation 190
  virgin B-cells 33
Birbeck granules 343
Bone-marrow 3, 15
Burkitt's type lymphoma (Burkitt's
  tumor) 192, 215, 289, 450, 499
Bursa of Fabricius 3

Camera lucida studies 190
Cell-membrane markers 488
  of B-cells 14, 23, 39, 51, 316
  of T-cells 14
Cellular immunity 49
Centroblasts
  in germinal centers 9, 18
  in malignant lymphoma 216, 218, 497
Centrocytes
  fate of 19
  in germinal centers 9, 19
  in malignant lymphoma 213, 215, 216
Cerebriform mononuclear cell 119,
  308, 342, 344, 373
Chloroacetate esterase, naphthol-AS-D
  139, 145
Chronic lymphocytic leukemia 230,
  290

immunoperoxidase staining 125
of B-cell type 141, 231, 281, 288, 290
of T-cell type 141, 322
acid phosphatase staining 306
of helper T-cells 322
of suppressor T-cells 322
Cleaved cells, cytological aspects 496
Complement receptors 23, 39, 40, 89, 91
in B-cell differentiation 17, 18
on B-cells (B lymphocytes) 6, 89
on germinal center cells 91
on T-cells 320
Composite lymphomas 189, 288, 410
Convoluted cell lymphoma: see
Malignant lymphoma, convoluted cell type
Convoluted lymphocyte 191
Cutaneous T-cell lymphoma 341
C-type viruses 344
DNA cytophotometry 349
Cytocentrifuge preparations 102
Cytochemical methods 137
Cytoplasmic immunoglobulins 21, 86, 95, 115, 121, 408

Dendritic cells: see Reticulum cell, dendritic type
Dermatopathic lymphadenitis 64
Dermatopathic lymphadenopathy 373
Differentiation antigens 51, 86, 97, 103
Double secretors 254

Ecotaxis 64
Endothelial venules 8
Enzymatic stripping 95
Enzyme-labeled antibodies 112
Epi-illumination 133
Epithelioid-cell lymphogranulomatosis 433
Epithelioid venules 306
E-rosettes 87, 88, 121, 196
Extranodal lymphomas 459
distribution 460

F(ab)₂ fragment 95
Fc receptor 40, 60, 91, 92
Ferritin 126
Fetal liver 15
Fine-needle aspiration biopsy 491
Fixation techniques 116, 126
Fluid lymphoma school 177, 285, 291, 412
Follicular center 11, 188
reactive types 189
starry-sky pattern 19, 190
Follicular center cell 11, 281

lymphomas 119, 122, 191, 281, 282, 290
Bulky disease 225
large-cell subtype 226
large cleaved 165, 314
large non-cleaved 166, 314
small cleaved 164, 190
small non-cleaved, non-Burkitt 165, 192
survival 225
Follicular mantle lymphocytes 19
Follicular structures (B-area) 6
Formalin 116
Frozen sections 91

Germinal center 9
cell lymphomas (see also Follicular center cell lymphomas) 213
development 11
precursor cell 11
reaction 18
immunologic properties of the cells 20
Giemsa stain 491, 494
Graft-versus-host disease 406
Gut-associated lymphoid tissue 32

H-2 antigen 52
Hairy-cell leukemia 141, 144, 233, 469
Hashimoto's disease 203
Heavy-chain disease 232
of γ- and μ-chain types 246
Helper cell activity 92
Helper cells: see T-cell
Histiocytes 191
Histiocytic lymphoma
neoplasm of phagocytes 194, 452
Rappaport 451
Histiocytic medullary reticulosis 502
Histiocytic sarcoma 502
Hodgkin's disease 66, 125, 175, 194, 299, 399, 426, 494
associated antigen 404
cells 408, 409
classification
Ann Arbor 422
Jackson and Parker 390
Lukes and Butler 390
development of AML 426
diagnostic studies 424
etiology 405
histopathologic subtypes 419
and HLA 72
immunological studies 401–405
lymphography 424
pathogenesis 400, 405
Reed-Sternberg cells 399

staging classification 422
survival rates 418, 419
treatment 425–427
HLA 98
  in Hodgkin's disease 72
  in leukemias 74
  in non-Hodgkin lymphomas 73
Human T-lymphocyte antigen (HTLA)
  15
Hybridomas 99
Hydrolases 137
Hypogammaglobulinemia 192

Ia-antigens 98
  like antigens 13, 41
  of mice 98
Idiotype 97
Idiotypic immunoglobulin 287, 289
Ig-isotype diversity 39
Immunoblastic lymphadenopathy 203,
  273, 434
Immunoblastic sarcoma (lymphoma)
  119, 121, 128, 193, 213, 283, 296
  B-cell type 144, 195, 200, 281, 290,
  312, 408
  in immunoblastic lymphadenopathy
  203, 213
  T-cell type 203, 326
Immunoblastoma (cytological aspects)
  501
Immunoblasts 121, 181, 281, 318
Immunocytochemistry 153
Immunocytoma: see Malignant lym-
  phoma, lymphoplasmacytic
Immunofluorescence 111, 113, 229
  methods 133
Immunoglobulin 126
  expression 38
  molecules 135
Immunohistology 111
Immunomicrosphere 93
Immunoperoxidase 93, 111, 113, 122,
  287, 408
  anomalous staining 122, 125
  technique 113
Immunostimulation 57
Immunotolerance 57
Imprint smears 502
Inhibitory serum factors 88
Interfollicular tissue 191
Intrafollicular B-cell transforma-
  tion 190

J-chain 116, 409

Kiel-classification 178, 205, 293
Killer cells 40, 102

Lactoferrin 126
Lacunar cell (cytological aspects) 495
Langerhans cells 62, 65, 343, 374
Lanthanum nitrate 476
Lennert's lymphoma 433, 434
Leukemia-associated antigens 99
Leukemia, lymphoblastoid type 81
Leukemic reticuloendotheliosis 469
Low-grade malignant lymphoma 144,
  201
Lutzner cells 378
Lymph-node aspiration biopsy 491
Lymphoblast 189, 499
Lymphocyte circulation 181, 288
Lymphocyte homing 181, 290
Lymphocyte transformation 181, 188,
  284
Lymphocytic lymphoma: see Malig-
  nant lymphoma, lymphocytic 288
Lymphoepithelioid cell lymphoma 433
  age and sex distribution 440
  clinical presentation 440
  Hodgkin type 435
  LgX type 437
  survival 441
Lymphoid stem cells 32, 33
Lymphoid system, normal elements 3
Lymphoid tissue 64
Lymphoma classification, clinical
  relevance 204
Lymphomatoid papulosis 341
Lymphosarcoma (cytology) 412
Lysostaphin 475
Lysozyme 115, 121, 126, 127, 409

Macroglobulinaemia (see also
  Waldenström's disease) 249
Macrophages (see also Reticulum cells)
  57
Major histocompatibility complex 52
Malignant lymphoma
  Ann Arbor classification 297
  bone-marrow 297, 300
  centroblastic 213, 218, 222
  centroblastic, centrocytic 66, 213,
  216, 221
    incidence 218
  centrocytic 215, 222, 226, 496
    disease-free survival rates 226
  childhood 447
  classification 281
  computerized axial tomography 297
  convoluted cell type 198, 283, 289,
  310, 311
  cytological aspects 497
  diagnostic studies 296
  Dorfman classification 204

extranodal sites   225
favorable types   298
histiocytic, diffuse   296, 312
histologic diagnosis   127
historical aspects   176
isotope scans   297
Kiel classification   178, 205, 293
laparotomy   297
local irradiation   299
low- and high-grade   213
Lukes-Collins classification   178,
   296, 393
lymphoblastic   213, 300, 448
   Burkitt's type: see Burkitt's type
   lymphoma
   of the convoluted cell type   142
   of the mature thymocytic subtype
     321
   of the peripheral T-cell type   321
   of the prethymocytic subtype   321
   of the prothymocytic subtype   321
   and leukemias of the T-cell type
     319
lymphocytic
   of the T-cell type   322
   well differentiated   281
lymphogram   297
lymphoplasmacytic   119, 123, 144,
   192, 283, 497
   prognosis   247
   subtypes   245
   transformation   247
management   296, 298
nodular   221
nodular, mixed   298
radiation therapy   300
Rappaport classification   177, 204,
   296, 392
small lymphocytic lymphoma   125
surgery   299, 300
treatment   298, 300
ultrastructural characteristics   149
undifferentiated, non-Burkitt   451
unfavorable types   299
WHO classification   178, 205
whole body irradiation   299
Mediterranean lymphoma   498, 501
Memory cells   18
Mitogens   50
Monoclonal gammopathy, benign
   118, 249, 254
Monoclonal paraproteinemia   245, 246
Monoclonality
   in malignant lymphoma   95, 102, 287
   in multiple myeloma   118
Mononuclear phagocyte system   58
Monospecific antiglobulin sera   101
Mouse erythrocytes   97

Multiparameter studies   196
Multiple myeloma   118, 119, 232, 253,
   254, 281, 283, 287
   hyperviscosity syndrome   258
   renal failure   258
   terminating in acute leukemia   259
Mycosis cell   373
Mycosis fungoides   269, 307, 324, 341,
   373
   Birbeck granules   374
   DNA cytophotometry   375
   in lymph nodes   349
   interdigitating reticulum cells   374
Myelopoietic lineage   13

Naphthol-A.S.-D.-chloroacetate esterase:
   see Chloroacetate esterase
Neuraminidase   88
Nonspecific esterase   99, 138
   neutral   60, 61
5'-nucleotidase   60
Null cell   15, 92, 103, 173, 182, 193

Ontogeny
   of the human B-cells   31
   of the human lymphnodes   63
Oxidoreductases   137

PAP methods   112, 114
Paracortex: see Paracortical area
Paracortical area   6, 188, 290
Paraprotein idiotype   253
PAS reaction   137
Periarteriolar lymphocyte sheath   6
Peroxidase reaction   139
Phagocytosis   475
Phase contrast microscopy   135
Phenotypes   103
Plasmablast   24
Plasma cell   18, 24, 34, 245, 281
   reaction   18, 23
Plasmacytoid cells   245, 252
Plasmacytoid lymphocytic lymphoma:
   see Malignant lymphoma, lympho-
   plasmacytic
Plasmacytomas, immunosuppressive
   types   254
Pluripotent stem cell   13
Pokeweed mitogen   79
Polyacrylamide   97
Polyclonal immunoglobulin   252
Polymer beads   97
Polyribosomes   7
Postfollicular B-cell transformation
   190
Pre-B-cells   17, 32, 33, 64
Prelymphomatous states   202
Pre-T-cells   191

Prethymocytes 15, 316
Primary follicles 18
Primary immune response 18
Professional phagocyte 476
Prolymphocytic leukemia 144, 231
Prothymocytes 15, 317
Pseudo-phagocytosis 475
Pulmonary lymphoid tumors 463

Receptors
  for EB virus 43
  for mouse erythrocytes (E) 17
  for polyacrylic acid beads 13
  for sheep E (see also E-rosettes) 315
Recirculation of lymphocytes 8
Reed-Sternberg cell 404, 407
  cytology 494
  origin 409
Reticuloendothelial system 58
Reticulosarcoma 176
Reticulum cell 57, 58, 177
  dendritic type 8, 60, 190
  fibroblastic type 59
  histiocytic type 61, 216
  interdigitating type 8, 62, 343
    ATPase reaction 62
  in malignant lymphoma 66
  sarcoma 125, 412
Richter's syndrome 201
Rosette methods 86
Rosette test 78
Rough endoplasmic reticulum 7, 245

Sarcoidosis 65
Secretory Ig 24
Senescence and lymphoma development
  203
Sézary cell 373
Sézary syndrome 80, 142, 269, 307,
  324, 342, 373
Signet ring cell lymphoma 217
Sternberg-Reed cells (see also Reed-
  Sternberg cells) 66
Surface glycoprotein 43
Surface immunoglobulin 6, 17, 24,
  38, 86, 93, 115, 121, 196
Surface markers 77, 86, 115, 120, 123,
  182, 282
  studies 312

T/B-cell dichotomy 253
T-cell 119, 181, 182, 282
  ALL 311
  antisera 98, 475
  areas 62
  cell-membrane determinants 50
  CLL 306

cytotoxic 16, 55, 318
development 15
differentiation and characterization
  49
functional properties 50
γ cells 95
helper cells 16, 55, 79, 102, 318
immunoblastic lymphoma (sarcoma)
  213, 312
immunoblasts 9, 16
interaction 78
leukemic cell lines 81
lymphoblasts 38
lymphoblastic lymphoma: see M.L.
  lymphoblastic
lymphocytes 53
  acid phosphatase 99
  acid esterase, α-naphtyl 51
  azurophil granules 16, 317
  in FCC tumors 215
  maturation of 53
  subsets of 77
lymphomas 285
  small lymphocytic 305, 306
maturation and differentiation 315
mature lymphocytes 54
μ cells 78
neoplasm 315
  classification 315
physical properties 50
regions 65
subpopulations 54
suppressor cells 16, 55, 80, 92, 102,
  306, 318
suppressor-activator cell 82
suppressor-effector cell 82
suppressor-precursor cell 82
zone 188
  acid phosphatase 309
  lymphoma 66, 213, 309, 325, 501
Terminal deoxynucleotidyl transferase
  13, 51, 100
Thymocytes 16, 317
  acid phosphatase staining 15
  maturation of 15
Thymus 3, 54
  anlage 15
  epithelial cells 15
Tolerance induction 17
Twin cells 498

U cell (see Null cell)

Waldenström's disease (see also
  Macroglobulinaemia) 192, 232, 246,
  283
Woringer-Kolopp's disease 432

UN